# Shortell and Kaluzny's
# Health Care Management

## Organization Design
## and Behavior

### Sixth Edition

# Shortell and Kaluzny's Health Care Management Organization Design and Behavior

## Sixth Edition

**Lawton Robert Burns**

University of Pennsylvania

**Elizabeth H. Bradley**

Yale University

**Bryan Jeffrey Weiner**

University of North Carolina at Chapel Hill

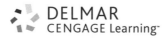
DELMAR
CENGAGE Learning™

Australia • Brazil • Japan • Korea • Mexico • Singapore • Spain • United Kingdom • United States

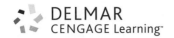

**Shortell and Kaluzny's Health Care Management: Organization Design and Behavior, Sixth Edition**
**Lawton Robert Burns, Elizabeth H. Bradley, and Bryan Jeffrey Weiner**

Vice President, Editorial: Career Education and Training Solutions: Dave Garza

Director of Learning Solutions: Matthew Kane

Senior Acquisitions Editor: Tari Broderick

Managing Editor: Marah Bellegarde

Product Manager: Natalie Pashoukos

Editorial Assistant: Nicole Manikas

Vice President, Marketing: Career Education and Training Solutions: Jennifer Baker

Marketing Director: Wendy Mapstone

Senior Marketing Manager: Michelle McTighe

Marketing Coordinator: Scott Chrysler

Production Director: Carolyn Miller

Production Manager: Andrew Crouth

Senior Content Project Manager: Kenneth McGrath

Senior Art Director: Jack Pendleton

Compositor: PreMediaGlobal

For product information and technology assistance, contact us at **Cengage Learning Customer & Sales Support, 1-800-354-9706**

For permission to use material from this text or product, submit all requests online at **www.cengage.com/permissions**. Further permissions questions can be e-mailed to **permissionrequest@cengage.com**

Library of Congress Control Number: 2010941718

ISBN-13: 978-1-4354-8818-2

ISBN-10: 1-4354-8818-0

**Delmar**
5 Maxwell Drive
Clifton Park, NY 12065-2919
USA

Cengage Learning is a leading provider of customized learning solutions with office locations around the globe, including Singapore, the United Kingdom, Australia, Mexico, Brazil, and Japan. Locate your local office at: **international.cengage.com/region**

Cengage Learning products are represented in Canada by Nelson Education, Ltd.

To learn more about Delmar, visit **www.cengage.com/delmar**

Purchase any of our products at your local college store or at our preferred online store **www.cengagebrain.com**

Printed in the United States of America
1 2 3 4 5 6 7 14 13 12 11 10

# CONTENTS

## PART ONE
### Introduction / 1

## PART TWO
### Micro Perspectives / 63

**PART THREE**
**Macro Perspectives / 281**

# CONTRIBUTORS

**Jeffrey A. Alexander, PhD**

Richard C. Jelinek Professor of Health Management
and Policy School of Public Health
University of Michigan
Ann Arbor, Michigan

**Jane Banaszak-Holl, PhD**

Associate Professor of Health Management and Policy,
School of Public Health
Associate Research Scientist, Institute of Gerontology
University of Michigan
Ann Arbor, Michigan

**Elizabeth H. Bradley, PhD, MBA**

Professor of Health Policy and Administration
Director, Health Management Program
Director, Yale Global Health Initiative
Yale School of Public Health
New Haven, Connecticut

**Lawton Robert Burns, PhD, MBA**

The James Joo-Jin Kim Professor, Professor of Health
Care Management, and Director of the Wharton
Center for Health Management and Economics
The Wharton School, University of Pennsylvania
Philadelphia, Pennsylvania

**Martin P. Charns, MBA, DBA**

Professor of Health Policy and Management School of
Public Health, Boston University
Director HSR&D Center for Organization, Leadership and
Management Research (COLMR)
VA Boston Healthcare System
Boston, Massachusetts

**Jon Chilingerian, PhD**

Associate Professor of Human Services Management
Director of the AHRQ Doctoral Training Program
Director of the Brandeis University-Tufts School of
Medicine MD-MBA Program
The Heller School for Social Policy and Management
Brandeis University
Waltham, Massachusetts

**Ann F. Chou, PhD**

Associate Professor of Health Administration and Policy
Department of Health Administration and Policy College
of Public Health
University of Oklahoma
Oklahoma City, Oklahoma

**Ann Leslie Claesson, PhD, PSP, FACHE**

Faculty
Capella University
Minneapolis, Minnesota

**Thomas D'Aunno, PhD**

Professor of Health Policy and Management
Mailman School of Public Health, Columbia University
New York, New York

**Mark L. Diana, MBA, MSIS, PhD**

Assistant Professor, Department of Health Systems
Management
Tulane University
New Orleans, Louisiana

**Amy C. Edmondson, PhD**

Novartis Professor of Leadership and Management
Harvard Business School
Boston, Massachusetts

**Bruce Fried, PhD**

Associate Professor and Director, Residential Masters
Programs
Department of Health Policy and Management
University of North Carolina at Chapel Hill
Chapel Hill, North Carolina

**Mattia J. Gilmartin RN, PhD**

Associate Professor
Hunter College, Hunter-Bellevue School of Nursing,
City University of New York
New York, New York

**Christian D. Helfrich, MPH, PhD**

Research Investigator
Northwest Health Services Research and Development
Center of Excellence
VA Puget Sound Health Care System
U.S. Department of Veterans Affairs
Seattle, Washington

**Timothy Hoff, PhD**

Associate Professor of Health Policy and Management
University at Albany School of Public Health
Rensselaer, New York

**Peter D. Jacobson, JD, MPH**

Professor of Health Law and Policy
Director, Center for Law, Ethics, and Health
University of Michigan School of Public Health
Ann Arbor, Michigan

**John R. Kimberly, PhD**

Henry Bower Professor of Entrepreneurial Studies
Professor of Management
Professor of Health Care Management
Professor of Sociology
Executive Director, Wharton/INSEAD Alliance
The Wharton School, University of Pennsylvania
Philadelphia, Pennsylvania

**Kristin Madison, JD, PhD**

Professor of Law
University of Pennsylvania Law School
Philadelphia, Pennsylvania

**Ann Scheck McAlearney, ScD**

Associate Professor, Health Services Management
and Policy
College of Public Health, Ohio State University
Columbus, Ohio

**Eilish McAuliffe, MSc, MBA**

Director of the Centre for Global Health
Director of Health Services Management
Senior Lecturer in Health Policy and Management
Trinity College
Dublin, Ireland

**Mario Moussa, PhD, MBA**

Adjunct Senior Fellow
Leonard Davis Institute of Health Economics
University of Pennsylvania
Philadelphia, Pennsylvania

**Ingrid M. Nembhard, PhD, MS**

Assistant Professor
Yale University School of Public Health
Yale University School of Management
New Haven, Connecticut

**Dr. Kevin W. Rockmann, PhD**

Associate Professor, School of Management
George Mason University
Fairfax, Virginia

**Lauren Taylor, MPH**

Research Associate
Yale School of Public Health
New Haven, Connecticut

**Sharon Topping, PhD**

Professor of Management
College of Business
University of Southern Mississippi
Hattiesburg, Mississippi

**Karen A. Wager, DBA**

Professor and Associate Dean for Student Affairs
Medical University of South Carolina
Charleston, South Carolina

**Stephen L. Walston, PhD, FACHE**

Professor of Health Administration and Policy
Department of Health Administration and Policy College
    of Public Health
University of Oklahoma
Oklahoma City, Oklahoma

**Bryan J. Weiner, PhD**

Professor, Department of Health Policy and Management
UNC Gillings School of Global Public Health
Chapel Hill, North Carolina

**Gary Young, JD, PhD**

Professor and Chairman, Department of Health Policy
    and Management
Boston University School of Public Health
Boston, Massachusetts
    *and*
Associate Director
Center for Organization, Leadership, and Management
    Research
Department of Veterans Affairs
Boston, Massachusetts

**Edward J. Zajac, PhD**

James F. Beré Professor of Organization Behavior
J. L. Kellogg Graduate School of Management
Northwestern University
Evanston, Illinois

# FOREWORD

For twenty five years and five editions we have attempted to provide an integrative perspective to the organization and management of health services; presenting the major management theories, concepts, and practices of the day. We have also provided practical illustrations and guidelines to assist managers and prospective managers in the provision of health services in a variety of settings.

As we go to press we have entered the era of health care reform, presenting new and perhaps not so new challenges and opportunities. Under the leadership of Rob Burns, Elizabeth Bradley and Bryan Weiner, the invited chapter authors have provided a thoughtful and in-depth analysis of the theories, concepts and approaches that managers and prospective managers need to address the critical issues in the provision of health services as well as meet the challenges and opportunities resulting from health care reform.

The passage of health care reform brings a great deal of uncertainty as it attempts to address the long standing problems of access, quality, cost containment and significant disparities under unprecedented economic conditions. Much has changed as reflected in the mandates regarding access to coverage, coverage itself, the role of public and private programs and health insurance exchanges as well as the role of comparative effective studies, payment reforms, accountable care organizations and patient-centered medical homes.

While these represent significant changes in the operation of the delivery system, the fundamental managerial challenges remain and will continue to require skillful attention if health care and the various delivery organizations are to realize their potential. Issues of maintaining a motivated workforce, assuring state of the art practice patterns, coordinating various disciplines and specialties to the benefit of patient care and accommodating an ever expanding technology within a market economy that would benefit the patient and the larger community have been and will continue to be the major responsibility of management.

This 6th edition provides readers with the relevant theories, concepts, tools, and applications to address operational issues that managers face on a daily basis. As described in the lead chapter the key challenge facing organizations and their managers is to deliver "value"—the ratio of quality to cost. While this has always been a concern, the reality of present day economics and the developing science has made this imperative.

The book is divided into three sections. The first section provides two insightful introductory chapters presenting the challenges of providing health services and some of the conceptual maps necessary to help guide managers in the decision making process and providing a framework for understanding the role and contributions of management and leadership within a variety of health care settings.

The next section focuses on the Micro Perspective— Managing the Internal Environment. This perspective addresses the classic issues of organization design, motivation, communications, power, organizational learning, performance/ quality improvement and managing groups and teams. Each chapter provides an "In Practice" scenario that sets the scene for the concepts and tools for effective management.

The last section, the Macro Perspective—Managing the External Environment, focuses on the organizational context and addresses the challenge of achieving competitive advantage, and managing alliances. Four new chapters will help prepare managers for the uncertainty of the years ahead. These include the challenges of managing an ever expanding information technology, consumerism, an increasingly complex regulatory environment and finally the recognition that we live in a globalized world.

Health services management has come of age and Burns, Bradley and Weiner and their colleagues have presented the theories, concepts and guidelines that future managers will need to succeed in the years ahead.

**Stephen M. Shortell, Ph.D**
> Blue Cross of California Distinguished
> Professor of Health Policy & Management
> Professor of Organizational Behavior,
> Haas School of Business and Dean, School
>   of Public Health
> University of California, Berkeley
> Berkeley, California

**Arnold D. Kaluzny, Ph.D**
> Professor Emeritus of Health and Policy &
>   Management,
> Gillings School of Global Public Health, and Senior
>   Research Fellow
> Cecil G. Sheps Center for Health Services Research,
> University of North Carolina at Chapel Hill,
> Chapel Hill, North Carolina

# PREFACE

## INTRODUCTION

This book is intended for those interested in a systemic understanding of organizational principles, practices, and insights pertinent to the management of health services organizations. The book is based on state-of-the-art organization theory and research with an emphasis on application. Although the primary audience is graduate students in health services administration, management, and policy programs, the book will also be of interest to undergraduate programs, extended degree programs, executive education programs, and practicing health sector executives interested in the latest developments in organizational and managerial thinking. It is also intended for students of business, public administration, medicine, nursing, pharmacy, social work, and other health professions who will assume managerial responsibilities in health sector organizations or who want to learn more about the organizations in which they will spend the major portion of their professional lives. Previous editions have been translated into Polish, Korean, Ukrainian, and Hungarian, and we look forward to the book's continued use by our international colleagues.

## TEXT APPROACH

The sixth edition broadens the view of health care sector beyond the traditional focus on hospitals and other provider organizations to include suppliers, buyers, regulators, public health and financing organizations. It offers a more comparative, global perspective on how the United States and other countries address issues of health and health care. Additionally, the book discusses managerial implications of

emerging issues in health care such as public reporting, pay for performance, information technology, retail medicine, ethics, and medical tourism. Finally, this sixth edition expands upon a major theme of the fifth edition: health care leaders must effectively design and manage health care organizations while simultaneously influencing and adapting to changes in environmental context. Managing the boundary between the internal organization and its external environment is therefore a central task of healthcare leadership.

## ORGANIZATION

The organization of the book reflects this expanded theme. Part 1 provides an overall perspective on the health care sector, discusses the distinctive challenges facing health care organizations, and examines the roles of leaders and managers in influencing organizational culture, performance, and change. Part 2 focuses on core leadership and managerial tasks within organizations. These include motivating people, guiding teams, designing structure, coordinating work, communicating effectively, exerting influence, resolving conflict, negotiating agreements, improving performance, and managing innovation and change. Part 3 describes the broader context in which health care organizations operate and discusses the managerial implications of several emerging trends and issues. These include the growth of strategic alliances in the health sector, the expansion and complexity of health law and regulation, the uses and challenges of health information technology, the rise of consumerism in health care, and the global interconnectedness of health systems.

The sixth edition includes a new introductory chapter (Chapter 1) and new chapters focusing on improving quality

(Chapter 9), strategic thinking (Chapter 10), health policy and regulation (Chapter 12), health information technology (Chapter 13), consumerism and ethics (Chapter 14), and global health and health care management (Chapter 15). It combines several chapters that appeared in the fifth edition in order to highlight connections among important managerial and organizational issues that can be easily missed when the issues are discussed in separate chapters. Two prominent examples are Chapter 3, which includes organization design, work design, and coordination; and Chapter 7, which includes power and politics, conflict management, and negotiation. Finally, several chapters that also appeared in the fifth edition have been thoroughly revised and updated, including the chapters of leadership and management (Chapter 2), communication (Chapter 6), and innovation and learning (Chapter 8).

# FEATURES

The sixth edition continues several popular features from the fifth edition. These include:

- An explicit list of topics provided at the beginning of each chapter
- Specific behaviorally-oriented Learning Objectives highlighted at the beginning of each chapter
- A list of Key Terms that readers should be able to define and apply as a result of reading each chapter
- An "In Practice" column describing a practical situation facing a health services organization.
- A section in several chapters called "Debate Time," which poses a controversial issue or presents divergent perspectives to stimulate the reader's thinking.
- Comprehensive Managerial Guidelines and Summary points at the conclusion of each chapter.
- Discussion Questions that help reinforce chapter concepts.

# NEW TO THIS EDITION

The sixth edition includes the seven new chapters described above as well as two new features. First, a brief case study appears in each chapter, with questions designed to stimulate discussion and encourage application of concepts and principles to practical managerial and organizational issues. Second, a glossary appears at the end of the book, which includes all of the key terms and their definitions.

# INSTRUCTOR RESOURCES

## Instructor Companion Site

The Instructor Companion site for this text offers many valuable support materials. To access the Instructor Companion site, go to http://login.cengage.com.

*If you have a Cengage SSO account:* Sign in with your e-mail address and password.

*If you do not have a Cengage SSO account:* Click Create My Account and follow the prompts.

The following support materials are included:

- **Electronic Instructor's Manual**—The Instructor's Manual that accompanies this book includes an overview of the In Practice and Debate Time material from the text; suggested solutions to the end-of-chapter discussion questions and case studies; teaching tips and exercises; complimentary reading lists; suggested solutions to the Vignette material in the study guide; and an overview of additional Debate Time material from the study guide.

- **PowerPoint presentations**—This book comes with Microsoft PowerPoint slides for each chapter. They're included as a teaching aid for classroom presentation, to make available to students on the network for chapter review, or to be printed for classroom distribution. Instructors, please feel free to add your own slides for additional topics you introduce to the class.

- **ExamView®**—ExamView®, the ultimate tool for objective-based testing needs, is a powerful test generator that enables instructors to create paper, LAN, or Web-based tests from test banks designed specifically for their Cengage Course Technology text. Instructors can utilize the ultra-efficient QuickTest Wizard to create tests in less than five minutes by taking advantage of Cengage Course Technology's questions banks, or customize their own exams from scratch.

- **Sample Course Syllabus**—The Sample Syllabus was developed to help instructors customize specific course titles.

## WebTutor on Blackboard and WebCT

- **WebTutor**—Designed to accompany specific Delmar, Cengage Learning textbooks, WebTUTOR™ is an eLearning software solution that turns everyone in your classroom or training center into a front-row learner. Blackboard and WebCT components are offered across all of our disciplines. Each WebTutor may include chapter learning objectives, online course preparation, study sheets, glossary flashcards, discussion topics, Web links, and an online forum to exchange notes and questions. In addition online chapter quizzes are provided in various formats including, matching exercises, completion, and multiple-choice questions with immediate feedback for correct and incorrect answers. Multiple-choice questions also include rationales for right and wrong choices. Whether you want to Web-enhance your class, or offer an entire course online, WebTUTOR™ allows you to focus on what you do best, teaching.

**WebTutor on Blackboard (ISBN 1-4354-8815-6)**

**WebTutor on WebCT (ISBN 1-4354-8816-4)**

# STUDENT RESOURCES

To access additional course materials, please visit the Student Companion site at www.cengagebrain.com. At the CengageBrain.com home page, search for the ISBN of your title (from the back cover of your book) using the search box at the top of the page. This will take you to the product page where these resources can be found.

The Student Companion site for this text provides the following support materials:

- **Electronic Study Guide**—The Study Guide includes Vignettes which present additional case study material followed by critical thinking questions; assignments for the students to complete either in class or on their own to help them practice the skills they will need on the job; and additional Debate Time scenarios.

# ABOUT THE AUTHORS

Lawton Robert Burns is the James Joo-Jin Kim Professor, and Professor of Health Care Management in the Health Care Management Department at the Wharton School, University of Pennsylvania. He is also Director of the Wharton Center for Health Management and Economics. His research focuses on hospital-physician relationships, strategic change, integrated health care, supply chain management, health care management, formal organizations, physician networks and physician practice management firms. Dr. Burns is the author of, and contributor to several books, as well as numerous articles, on Health Care Management. He is the recipient of numerous grants, awards and Fellowships and has held many academic positions throughout his career. Dr. Burns has also provided expert witness testimony for the federal government as well as for the private sector. He is a member of the Academy of Management, the American Hospital Association and the Association for Health Services Research. Lawton R. Burns has a Bachelor of Arts Degree in Sociology and Anthropology, a Master's Degree in Sociology and a Doctor of Philosophy Degree in Sociology.

Elizabeth H. Bradley, Ph.D. is a Professor of Epidemiology and Public Health at the Yale School of Public Health, where she directs the Health Management Program and Global Health Concentration. She is also the Director of the Yale Global Health Initiative. She has extensive academic and research experience in the public health arena and is the recipient of numerous honors and research grants. Her research focuses on health services, with an emphasis on management and quality improvement. Dr. Bradley is a member of the Gerontological Society of America, the Academy of Health, and the Association of University Programs in Health Administration. She is a faculty Associate of the American College of Healthcare Executives and a full member of the Yale Cancer Center Prevention/Control Program. She is also the author of over one hundred published papers and the author of, and contributor to, numerous books and articles in the health field. Elizabeth Howe Bradley has a Bachelor of Arts Degree in Economics, a master of Business Administration and a Doctor of Philosophy Degree in Health Policy and Health Economics.

Bryan J. Weiner is a Professor in the Department of Health Policy and Management, Gillings School of Global Public Health at the University of North Carolina at Chapel Hill. He is the author of, and the contributor to, numerous books and articles. He is a member of the Academy of Health, the Academy of Management, the American Public Health Association, and the Society for Behavioral Medicine. Dr. Weiner has a Bachelor of Arts Degree in Psychology, a Master of Arts Degree in Organizational Psychology, and a Doctor of Philosophy Degree in Organizational Psychology.

# ACKNOWLEDGMENTS

We believe that the major strength of this text is the diversity of the talented authors, who contributed multiple perspectives, experiences, skills, and expertise to each chapter. The new and substantially revised chapters reflect the breadth and depth of the authors' expertise, as well as their fresh perspectives. We wish to acknowledge with gratitude the immeasurable contribution that Stephen Shortell and Arnold Kaluzny have made in the fields of health care management research and education. As scholars, advisors, mentors, and colleagues, they have deeply influenced our work and our professional lives. Through the five editions of this book, over the past twenty five years, they have helped educate a generation of health services researchers, policy makers, managers, and health professionals. We hope that the sixth edition sustains the tradition of excellence that these gentlemen have established.

Finally, we wish to acknowledge Lauren Taylor and Rachelle Alpern for their excellent editorial assistance.

Lawton Robert Burns
University of Pennsylvania

Elizabeth H. Bradley
Yale University

Bryan Jeffrey Weiner
University of North Carolina at Chapel Hill

# PART ONE

# Introduction

# Chapter 1

# The Management Challenge of Delivering Value in Health Care: Global and U.S. Perspectives

**Lawton Robert Burns, Elizabeth H. Bradley, and Bryan J. Weiner**

## CHAPTER OUTLINE

- **The Challenge: Deliver Value**
- **Challenge of Rising Health Care Costs: Supply- and Demand-Side Drivers**
- **Other Challenges Exacerbating the Value Challenge**
- **Complexity of the U.S. Health Care System**
- **Why Changing the Health Care System Is So Difficult**
- **Systemic Views of U.S. Health Care**
- **Organization and Management Theory**
- **Summative Views of Organization Theory**
- **Organization Theory and Behavior: A Guide to This Text**

## LEARNING OBJECTIVES

**After completing this chapter, the reader should be able to:**

1.  Understand the challenge of delivering value in health care
2.  Identify the major forces affecting the delivery of health services
3.  Distinguish the similarities and differences in the forces shaping health services globally
4.  Understand why it is difficult to change the health care industry
5.  Develop a system view of health care delivery
6.  Understand the different types of firms operating in a health care system
7.  Identify, understand, and apply the major perspectives and theories on organizations to real problems facing health care organizations
8.  Develop mental agility in analyzing problems from multiple theoretical lenses

# KEY TERMS

| | |
|---|---|
| Ambidexterity | Iron Triangle |
| Bending the Cost Curve | Macro Perspective |
| Bounded Rationality | Micro Perspective |
| Bureaucracy | Open Systems Theory |
| Classical School of Administration | Population Ecology |
| Complex Adaptive System | Resource Dependence Theory |
| Contingency Theory | Scientific Management School |
| Decision-Making School | Social Network Approach |
| Evidence-Based Medicine | Strategic Management Perspective |
| External Environment | System Perspectives |
| Health Systems | Triple Aim |
| Hospital-Physician Relationships | Value |
| Human Relations School | Value Chain |
| Institutional Theory | |

## IN PRACTICE: The GAVI Alliance

The Global Alliance for Vaccines and Immunization (GAVI) was launched at the World Economic Forum on January 31, 2000. GAVI was a partnership of developing countries, organizations involved in international development and finance, the pharmaceutical industry, and philanthropic organizations. The Bill and Melinda Gates Foundation provided seed funding of $750 million for GAVI, followed by funding from several countries. GAVI was established to improve the distribution of new and underused vaccines to low-income countries and thereby reduce childhood mortality and morbidity, and increase the health status of these populations (Martin and Marshall, 2003; Milstien et al., 2008; GAVI Alliance, 2010).

A number of managerial challenges faced the GAVI Alliance in achieving its goals. First, the vision of the GAVI Alliance had to motivate local countries to participate in this vaccination program and gradually increase their own funding for it. Second, local countries needed to accept the responsibility to deliver the vaccine programs and the attendant results. Third, these countries had to help develop and manage local infrastructure to deliver the vaccines to rural populations—often referred to as the last hundred yards or miles of the supply chain. This meant the countries needed not only transportation and distribution networks but also a cadre of local health care workers with training in vaccine storage and administration. Fourth, the GAVI Alliance had to manage diverse stakeholders including the World Health Organization (WHO), the World Bank, UNICEF, large pharmaceutical firms that manufactured the vaccines, and the Gates Foundation. Fifth, the GAVI Alliance had to operate with a lean structure such that bureaucracy did not slow its progress. Sixth, the alliance had to develop leverage over pharmaceutical firms to purchase the needed drugs at a lower cost which local countries could afford. Last, the GAVI Alliance needed a clear governance structure with defined responsibilities for partners.

Between 2000 and 2009, GAVI directly supported the immunization of 256.7 million children for Hepatitis B, Haemophilus influenzae type B (Hib), and yellow fever. GAVI also speeded up population access to underused vaccines, strengthened health and immunization systems, and helped spawn innovative public-private partnerships (PPPs) in financing to expand vaccine coverage in 72 developing countries (GAVI Alliance, 2010). In January 2010, 10 years after the initiation of the GAVI Alliance, The Gates Foundation committed an additional $10 billion over the next 10 years.

---

**IN PRACTICE:  The GAVI Alliance  *(Continued)***

Despite its success, GAVI has not been without its problems. Although the alliance necessarily focused heavily on developing partnerships and initiating vaccine coverage, less attention was paid to implementation of plans and mobilization of resources for ongoing treatment (in-country follow-up). One reason may be that vaccine costs have risen both absolutely and as a percentage of the total health expenditures, and vaccinations may not be the top priority of developing-country governments (Milstien et al., 2008; Muraskin, 2004). Finally, the alliance partners need to grapple with the large supply chain "system costs" required to handle, transport, and store the drugs (Lydon et al., 2008) and the issue of securing long-term financial commitments from its partners.

---

# CHAPTER PURPOSE

A central challenge in delivering health care services in the new millennium is the challenge of delivering value. *Value* is created when additional features of quality or customer service desired by a customer can be provided at the same cost or price, or when a given set of features of quality or customer service can be delivered at a lower cost or price relative to other producers. Although investments in health care delivery can improve health status, which in turn can support economic growth and political stability (Burns, D'Aunno, and Kimberly, 2003; Esty et al., 1999; Sachs, 2001), still the value of health investments are not always transparent. For instance, despite evidence of the benefits of immunization coverage (Martin and Marshall, 2003; World Health Organization, 1996) and a steady increase globally during the 1970s and 1980s, immunization coverage declined sharply in the 1990s due to curtailed government funding in low-income countries. The GAVI Alliance entered in 2000 and, during its first 10 years, averted four million deaths and immunized a quarter of a billion children against deadly or disabling diseases (GAVI Alliance, 2010).

Why was this approach not already taken? To effect major changes in health care delivery and increase value, as the GAVI Alliance has, organizations require extraordinary approaches. Such approaches critically hinge on several management competencies. These include assembling (global) alliances, clarifying the governance structure of the alliance, developing the local health care infrastructure to deliver the needed services, balancing global and local commitments, and developing local ownership of health initiatives. Managerial skills (including but not limited to developing alliances, negotiating governance and roles, conflict management, managing change, forging strategic plans and leadership) are critical components of the manager's "tool kit" in any health care system.

# THE CHALLENGE: DELIVER VALUE

The key challenge facing health care firms is to deliver **value**, defined as the quotient of quality divided by cost. That is, firms are asked to deliver a higher level of quality at the same cost, the same level of quality at a lower cost, or higher quality at a lower cost. This challenge has been proposed to (a) providers, in the form of accountable care organizations (ACOs) and pay-for-performance, (b) suppliers, in the form of demonstrating the comparative clinical effectiveness of their products (versus alternate therapies), and (c) insurers and providers, in the form of value-based purchasing.

In order to create and deliver value, health care organizations must find a way to address three health policy goals of our health care system since the late 1920s: improve the quality of care, improve access to care, and reduce cost and cost acceleration—e.g., **bending the cost curve**, or the reducing of health spending relative to projected trends (Commonwealth Fund, 2007a).

Numerous health services researchers have questioned whether all three goals are simultaneously attainable (Chen, Jha, Guterman et al., 2010; Katz, 2010) or require a balancing act (Berwick et al., 2008). The achievement of these three goals is sometimes referred to as the **iron triangle** of health care (Kissick, 1994). Picture an equilateral triangle, with three equal angles of 60 degrees, and assume that each angle is one of these three policy goals. Any effort to address one policy angle widens that angle (e.g., access) at the expense of one or both of the other two angles (e.g., quality or cost). For example, the recent health insurance reform in the United States—the Patient Protection and Affordable Care Act—expands insurance coverage to 30 million citizens, but its savings will reportedly be more than offset by higher expenditures (and escalating costs) resulting from the expansion of coverage (CMS, 2010).

Provider organizations in the health care industry have nevertheless been periodically challenged to accomplish the quality and cost goals at the same time. In July 2009, providers from 10 U.S. markets convened in Washington to discuss how they deliver care to the Medicare population that is above average in quality and below average in cost, compared with national data contained in the Dartmouth Atlas (Institute for Healthcare Improvement, 2009). In past decades, providers have been asked to demonstrate a similar value (quality/cost) proposition using a series of management techniques, such as total quality management (e.g., reducing process variation and simultaneously raising the level of process performance), supply chain management (e.g., standardizing products to achieve consistency in use and lower unit cost), and clinical integration (standardizing care paths and protocols to reduce clinical practice variations and improve quality of care). In this past decade, the Institute of Medicine (2001) articulated six "aims for improvement" in a high-performing health care system: care should be safe, effective, patient-centered, timely, efficient, and equitable. The balancing of broad health policy goals is apparent on a global scale as well. The World Health Organization (WHO, 2000) uses three criteria to rank national **health systems**: health status (similar to quality), responsiveness to the expectations of the population (similar to access), and social and financial risk protection (similar to cost).

# CHALLENGE OF RISING HEALTH CARE COSTS: SUPPLY- AND DEMAND-SIDE DRIVERS

One reason why the health system is challenged to deliver value is that the denominator—health costs—has been rising steadily over time and proven difficult to restrain.

Health costs in the United States have been rising at roughly 3–4 percent annually (net of inflation) for the past six decades (Altman, 2010). Some have argued that public and private sector efforts work to temporarily rein in this rate of increase, only to see the cost escalation return (Altman and Levitt, 2002).

Why do costs rise inexorably? Many experts argue that the underlying driver of rising costs is technology and its broad application to new patients and patient indications (Aaron and Ginsburg, 2009; Commonwealth Fund, 2007b; Congressional Budget Office, 2008). Following Weisbrod (1991), technological improvements spur higher prices, higher demand, and higher costs—all of which call for greater insurance coverage for the new technology, which then drives further technological innovation. Technology contributes to rising costs in other ways. In contrast to other industries, health care technology is often a complement rather than a substitute for labor—e.g., requiring many technicians to utilize the new equipment. Moreover, providers often compete for patients based on the sophistication of the services and equipment they offer, leading to expensive excess capacity and duplication in a local market ("technology wars"). Insurance is another driver of rising costs, as broader coverage (e.g., for more people, or more benefits) increases demand and thus health spending, as well as the attendant problem of moral hazard (Arrow, 1963) whereby the insured utilize more health care than they would if they paid for services out of pocket (i.e., from their own resources without insurance).

There are several supply- and demand-side drivers of rising health costs. On the supply side, costs are driven by imperfect information markets whereby purchasers and consumers of health care are not able to discern quality differences perfectly among health care providers, make few repeat purchases, and enjoy less transparency of pricing, which allows great variation in the economic rents earned by providers of the same product or service. Such rents also result from provider market power. Costs are also driven in part by providers' practice of defensive medicine, providers' focus on acute rather than chronic care or prevention, and poor coordination of services among providers. Finally, costs are driven by geographic variations in the supply of hospital beds and specialist physicians, which may induce demand (Roemer, 1961).

## GEOGRAPHIC VARIATION IN HEALTH CARE SPENDING: A CLOSER LOOK

Health care expenditures in the United States have been rising for years, but per capita spending on health care varies widely across the country. In 2004, for example, Medicare expenditures per beneficiary ranged from roughly $4,000 in Utah to $6,700 in Massachusetts. Even greater differences appear in comparisons of smaller geographic units and individual medical providers. Some estimate that Medicare spending would decrease by 29 percent if spending in medium- and high-spending areas matched spending in low-spending areas (Wennberg, Fisher, and Skinner, 2002).

Why does health care spending vary so much across the country? The reasons are complex and difficult to tease apart. Differences in prices of health care services and severity of illness play an important role, but together these factors account for only half of the geographic variation in spending. Regional differences in the supply of specialist physicians and health care facilities are also thought to play a role. Regional differences in provider willingness to adopt new technologies or provide costly treatments that might or might not improve health care outcomes are also thought to increase costs.

Scholars and policy makers looking to slow the rate of growth in health care expenditures ("bend the cost curve") point to organized delivery systems that focus on coordinated care and prevention as a promising way to reduce the costs associated with the efficiencies, misaligned incentives, and poor quality attributed to the highly fragmented nature of the health care system that currently exists in the United States. In his efforts to promote health reform, for example, President Barack Obama praised the Mayo Clinic in Minnesota and the Cleveland Clinic in Ohio as examples of hospitals providing the highest-quality care at costs well below the national norm, and suggested that all providers in the country practice their type of medicine.

## DEBATE TIME: Defensive Medicine

Do physicians order unnecessary tests out of fear of being sued by patients? If so, how much does "defensive medicine" contribute to the escalating costs of medical care in the United States? These issues are hotly debated. On the one hand, physicians practicing in high-liability specialties like obstetrics report that they routinely order more tests than are medically necessary in order to reduce the risk that they will end up in court (Studdert et al, 2005). In a recent *Wall Street Journal* article, a physician noted, "Doctors get sued for failure to diagnose and not ordering tests... It's something that I do think about and in some cases it does influence my decision" (Searcey and Goldstein 2009). Pointing to escalating malpractice insurance premiums, some professional associations and lawmakers argue that significant cost savings could be achieved in the U.S. health care system through the passage and enactment of tort reform (e.g., limiting the size of malpractice liability awards). Others, however, argue that defensive medicine and malpractice liability do not contribute significantly to overall health care costs. According to a recent study, total spending on medical malpractice was $30 billion in 1997, a substantial amount to be sure, but less than 1 percent of total U.S. health care spending (Towers Perrin, 2008). Estimating the cost of defensive medicine is especially difficult because physicians order tests and procedures for many reasons that are difficult to disentangle. For example, fear of being sued can be mixed with the desire to provide the best care possible. Also, physicians can increase their incomes by ordering more tests and performing more procedures.

What do you think?

- How much defensive medicine occurs? How much do you think it contributes to health care spending? What, if anything, should be or could be done about it? What are the costs and benefits of the strategies you propose?

- Medical malpractice liability insurance is increasing at an alarming rate for some specialties and in some states. What, if anything, should or could be done about it? What are the costs and benefits of the strategies you propose?

On the demand side, costs are driven by the tax-free treatment of health care benefits (which contributes to richer health benefit packages and induces moral hazard), as well as public and private sector financing of health care through a third-party payment system of insurers and other fiscal intermediaries outside the patient-provider relationship. Favorable tax treatment and a third-party payer system combine to insulate the consumer/patient from the true cost of the health care services they demand. In addition, demand is driven by a country's national wealth, the expectations of its population, the highly technological nature of health care services, and the health behaviors of its population. These supply and demand drivers are listed in Table 1.1.

There are a handful of axioms governing the demand side of this vast system that may be peculiar to health care. The first is that technological innovations and their application are desired by providers, desired by patients, and drivers of rising health care costs ("the technological imperative") (Fuchs, 1986; Gelijns and Rosenberg, 1994). A second axiom is that technology drives specialization in the medical (and nursing) field, which further drives up health care costs. A third axiom is that every citizen deserves the finest health care now made available by these technological developments (often defined as the product or service offered by my firm) as long as someone else pays for it. Another axiom following from the technological imperative is that cost and price are the key issues germane to all parties. Indeed, the one issue that currently unites the entire value chain in health care is reimbursement; many analysts anticipate that it will be the patient/consumer that unites the chain in the future. Finally, technological innovation and its attendant costs spur the spread of insurance coverage for such innovation, which increases spending on innovation, which fuels yet more innovation (Weisbrod, 1991).

# OTHER CHALLENGES EXACERBATING THE VALUE CHALLENGE

Complicating the difficulty of providing value, health care systems face a number of other challenges. These include: increasing patient demand and expectations, increasing payer and societal demands for accountability, unexpected epidemiological shifts, calls for greater patient safety, increasing complexity, strains on federal and state government budgets, inadequate supply of primary care practitioners, reported shortages of specialists and other health personnel, erosion of the public's trust in physicians and hospitals, growing concerns over privacy of personal health information, lack

## TABLE 1.1  Supply- and Demand-Side Drivers of Health Costs

| Supply-Side Drivers | Demand-Side Drivers |
| --- | --- |
| Imperfect information regarding price and quality | Tax treatment of health care benefits |
| Provider market power | Third-party payment system |
| Non-price competition (e.g., technology wars) | Breadth and depth of insurance coverage |
| Technology and its diffusion | Moral hazard |
| Geographic variations | Rising national income |
| Poor coordination among providers | Poor healthy behaviors |
| Fee-for-service payment systems | Private sector financing of care, which supplements public spending, encourages greater coverage, and may promote cost-shifting |
| Excess capacity | |
| Acute care focus of delivery system | |
| Limited primary care | |
| Malpractice fears and pressures | |

of transparency in prices and information, conflicts of interest and incentives, lack of consumerism, lack of efficient and effective use of information technology, and provider resistance to change (Porter and Teisberg, 2006; Herzlinger, 2006; Dranove, 2008).

On top of these challenges one can lay a series of delicate balancing acts that health care firms (and society as a whole) must deal with beyond the value equation. These include: meeting rising demand and expectations with finite resources (both capital and labor), addressing chronic care needs with an acute care–based delivery system, fostering population-based models of care amidst a system based on physicians in small groups or solo practice, sharing information while respecting patient privacy, incorporating modern therapeutic and technological advances while restraining the rate of growth in cost, and promoting wellness behaviors in a system which finances acute care seeking.

# THE CHALLENGES ARE GLOBAL

The problems, issues, and challenges facing the health care industry are global, confronting health care systems in many countries (see Chapter 15). As an illustration, Table 1.2 identifies some of the common issues and problems facing the health care systems of India, China, and the United States. These countries have populations that are quickly aging—true especially of China, and increasingly so for both India and the United States. All three countries face a huge epidemiologic transition from acute care to chronic illness, with underdeveloped systems for dealing with chronic care (especially true in the East). Populations in all three countries have developed more sedentary lifestyles, with increasing incidence of diabetes, obesity, and hypertension. All three countries have populations with substantial national wealth that are now demanding more health care services and thereby increasing health care costs rapidly. Not surprisingly, all three countries also report that health care costs are a major source of personal and family bankruptcy. Finally, all three countries face the common issue of how to balance the demand for technological innovation by providers and patients with its high cost.

At the same time, there are several major divergences between these health care systems (see Table 1.3). The U.S. health care system compared with India or China spends a

**TABLE 1.2  Parallel Concerns in the United States, India, and China**

- Concern with iron triangle
- Concern with high hospital costs as cause of impoverishment/bankruptcy
- Concern with the high costs of technology
- Concern with geographic disparities in health status
- Concern with conflicts of interest and supplier-induced demand
- Concern with prices as driver of rising health care costs
- Concern with lifestyle issues and behaviors
- High number of specialists
- Hospital waste and inefficiency
- Lack of a primary care system
- Fee-for-service payment system
- Mixture of financing mechanisms: government, employer, individual
- Fragmentation in government ministries/bureaucracy
- Low consumer information
- Competing spending priorities (education, social services, health) at the local government level

much higher proportion of its gross domestic product on health care and provides a higher level of insurance coverage to its population. While health insurance programs are now spreading across India (increasingly private sector) and China (mostly public sector), they provide coverage for a limited range of services (e.g., focused until recently on hospital inpatient care). Hospital ownership patterns also diverge widely. China's hospital system is almost entirely public sector (although the country recently announced its intention to allow more entry by private hospitals), while India's formerly public sector hospital system has seen the emergence of a thriving private sector comprised of multi-hospital systems (e.g., Apollo, Fortis, Wockhardt, and MaxHealthcare). By contrast, much of the U.S. hospital market is voluntary and nonprofit in character. Such differences and commonalities suggest that management strategies to meet

## TABLE 1.3 Areas of Divergence: United States versus India and China

- Health care spending per capita
- Percentage of national health expenditures (NHE) accounted for by patient out-of-pocket spend
- Development of private health insurance
- Depth and breadth of insurance coverage
- Presence of centralized purchasers
- Percentage of NHE spent on drugs
- Tradition of private sector ownership of hospitals
- Development of the central government's role in health care
- Development of governance mechanisms to monitor providers

the value challenge must consider the local context, but may nevertheless share many similar elements. As Chapter 15 notes, these strategies may encompass prospective payment systems, enhanced provider reimbursement rates, patient marketing and recruitment, etc.

# COMPLEXITY OF THE U.S. HEALTH CARE SYSTEM

As of the writing of this book in early 2010, the United States still lacks a single national health insurance program (other than the Medicare program for the elderly) to pay for health care. Thus, one confronts a variety of mechanisms to finance health care by federal, state, and local governments, as well as employers, individuals, and philanthropic organizations. The U.S. system also has a fully developed **value chain** (i.e., interlinked activities among a set of firms whereby suppliers provide raw material inputs to manufacturers who process them and produce outputs for downstream markets) (Burns, 2002; Porter, 1985). For example, the United States has thousands of product manufacturers (pharmaceuticals, biotechnology, medical-surgical supplies, capital equipment, medical devices, and information technology), wholesalers and distributors, hospitals, physicians, nursing homes, pharmacies, home health agencies, insurers and insurance brokers, and employers offering health insurance coverage

to their employees. It also has hundreds of group-purchasing organizations and public health agencies; 50 State Medicaid programs; a vast federal **bureaucracy** (literally, government by bureaus or offices), which finances care, delivers health care services, regulates providers, approves new innovation, funds basic and applied research, and provides public health; and lots of niche firms offering pharmacy benefit management and disease management services (see Figure 1.1). This is a huge industry with lots of stakeholders, divergent interests and perspectives, and entrenched positions.

Effective management of any one sector of this system requires not only an understanding of the competitive developments within that sector, but also an understanding of the other sectors, what is taking place within them, and how they interact with one another. Some of the health care managerial approaches and actions over the last decade reflect cross-sector understanding and efforts. Such efforts include but are not limited to managing under new pay-for-performance (P4P) systems developed by both public and private sector payers; working with outside vendors (e.g., hotel chains, consulting firms, General Electric) to improve customer service, patient flow, and revenue cycle management; working with information technology companies to develop and implement electronic medical records (EMR) systems (see Chapter 13); hospitals partnering with physicians to improve quality of care or develop new ambulatory care sites; and hospitals working with group purchasing organizations (GPOs) to lower supply costs.

# WHY CHANGING THE HEALTH CARE SYSTEM IS SO DIFFICULT

In addition to being complex, the health care system is slow to change. There are several reasons for this. First, the industry is heavily regulated at both the state and federal levels by myriad agencies and professional associations. The federal government is also the dominant payer, reimbursing health care via administered prices. Market forces have thus given way to more regulation and piecemeal legislative action (due to legislative gridlock) at the federal level (Altman and Rodwin, 1988; Field, 2007).

Second, consumerism is a newcomer to health care. Until recently, consumerism was stifled by the prevalence of third-party payment and first-dollar coverage, the old sociological view of the patient playing the "sick role" (Parsons, 1951), the

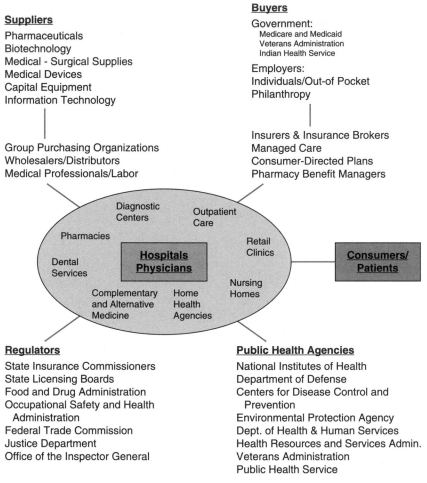

**Figure 1.1** System View of the U.S. Health Care Industry.
SOURCE: Delmar, Cengage Learning.

prevalence of customized transactions, infrequent (and few repeat) purchases, uncertainty over product quality, and the fact that roughly three-quarters of all monies spent were on products and services previously unseen by the patient. Today, consumerism can be found in a number of areas: consumer-directed health plans (CDHPs) and health savings accounts (HSAs), boutique/concierge medicine offered by physicians seeking to avoid managed care organizations (MCOs), complementary and alternative medicine (CAM), personal health records (PHRs), direct-to-consumer (DTC) advertising by pharmaceutical and medical device firms, health care financial services (smart cards), employer wellness programs, and consumer cost-sharing programs (see Chapter 14).

However, in most of these areas, consumer engagement is not widespread.

Third, health care delivery is heavily influenced by the medical profession, which controls (directly or indirectly) up to 85 percent of all spending (Sager and Socolar, 2005). While physicians do compete with one another, they nevertheless enjoy a monopoly or near monopoly over most important decisions governing resource allocation, including: prescribing an ethical pharmaceutical, performing a surgical procedure, scheduling a laboratory or imaging test, and admitting a patient to a hospital bed. Freidson (1970) long ago discussed the professional dominance of physicians. Physicians are

**IN PRACTICE:** Does Pay-for-Performance Work? The Case of the Premier Hospital Quality Incentive Demonstration

In 2003, the Centers for Medicare and Medicaid Services (CMS) and Premier Inc., a large national GPO, launched the Premier Hospital Quality Incentive Demonstration (PHQID) to determine if economic incentives are effective at improving the quality of inpatient care. Hospitals participating in the PHQID collected and submitted data on 33 quality measures for five clinical conditions: health failure, acute myocardial infarction, community-acquired pneumonia, coronary-artery bypass graft, and hip and knee replacement. For each clinical condition, hospitals performing in the top decile (i.e., 10 percent) received a 2 percent bonus in addition to their usual Medicare payment. Hospitals in the second decile received a 1 percent bonus. Hospitals that underperformed on quality indicators were liable for a 1–2 percent financial penalty in the third year. Between 2003 and 2007, CMS awarded more than $36.5 million to high-performing hospitals (Premier, 2009). Bonuses averaged $71,960 per year and ranged from $914 to $847,227 (Lindenauer et al., 2007).

Premier has trumpeted the success of the PHQID. According to its studies, participating hospitals raised their overall quality by an average of 17.2 percent over four years (Premier, 2009). Participating hospitals saved the lives of an estimated 4,700 heart attack patients and provided 500,000 additional evidence-based clinical services and recommendations (e.g., smoking cessation, pneumococcal vaccination, and discharge instructions) to more than 1.5 million patients treated in the five clinical areas covered by the demonstration. Finally, Premier reports that, by March 2008, participating hospitals outperformed nonparticipating hospitals by an average of 6.9 percentage points on 19 quality measures also used by Hospital Compare, the federal government's scorecard for hospital quality (Premier, 2009).

Academic research tells a somewhat different story. For example, Lindenauer et al. (2007) matched 207 PHQID hospitals to 406 hospitals that did not participate in the demonstration but publicly reported the same quality-performance data through Hospital Compare. They found that, over a two-year period from 2003 to 2005, the PHQID hospitals showed significantly greater improvement than hospitals that engaged in public reporting only. However, the overall difference was modest (about 3 percent) after statistically adjusting for other factors. Using somewhat different data sources, Ryan (2009) found no evidence that PHQID had a significant effect on risk-adjusted 30-day mortality or risk-adjusted 60-day cost for acute myocardial infarction, heart failure, pneumonia, or coronary artery bypass graft.

So, did the program work? The answer depends on several questions: (1) what is the relevant time frame, (2) which comparison group is most appropriate, (3) which quality indicators matter most, (4) what statistical procedures are most suitable, and (5) what additional factors need to be considered in the analysis? In 2007, CMS approved a two-year extension of the PHQID, modified the program's incentive payment structure, and committed $12 million per year in additional incentives.

largely autonomous, community-based entrepreneurs with (until recently) little employment relationship with hospitals in which many of these decisions are made. Due to professional training and the legal distinction between the hospital and its medical staff, hospitals have historically been challenged to alter the practice patterns and behaviors of their physicians.

Fourth, most of the nongovernmental sectors in health care have consolidated over the past two to three decades, thereby reducing competition, conferring market power and fostering higher prices. Consolidation has occurred in the following

sectors (time periods): pharmaceuticals (late 1980s to the present), pharmaceutical wholesalers (1980s–1990s), medical devices (1990s), hospitals (1990s), insurers (1990s), group purchasing organizations (1990s), and pharmacy benefit managers (1990s–2000s). These trends have fostered the emergence of several bilateral monopolies (e.g., big insurers negotiating with large hospital systems) in local markets.

Fifth, the delivery of hospital care (which accounts for roughly 30 percent of national health expenditures) is heavily dominated by nonprofit institutions, such as nonprofit community hospitals and municipal/state-owned facilities. Investor-owned facilities comprise only about 15–20 percent of the hospital sector—a percentage that has remained relatively flat for decades. Nonprofit hospital ownership and accountability to local boards and communities (rather than shareholders) may mitigate against pressures to alter their missions, strategies, and operating practices. Theory suggests that nonprofits exhibit relatively poor supply response to changes in demand, more limited entrepreneurship owing to constraints on the distribution of earnings, and choice of optimization of various outcomes (e.g., quantity of services provided, focus on physician convenience and returns) rather than profits (Hansmann, 1987). The empirical evidence here is generally equivocal outside of the nursing home industry.

Sixth, health care delivery is largely local. Physicians are licensed to practice in a given state and, like most hospitals, generally draw their patients from the local geographic area. Insurance companies are likewise licensed and regulated at the state level, and credential and contract with provider networks in local markets. Local markets have different configurations of power among key stakeholders (e.g., employers, insurers, hospitals, local government, etc.), which necessitate tailored strategies by manufacturers in order to sell their products. While there has been much talk about medical tourism, more domestic tourism (e.g., to regional centers of excellence) than foreign tourism (e.g., to Thailand or India) seems to take place (Deloitte, 2009). The largely local character of health care certainly complicates (and perhaps mitigates against) any concerted efforts to try to change the system from above.

Seventh, there is a widespread lack of valid data about quality and cost in health care. Until recently, most patient-provider transactions were captured and stored in paper-based systems (e.g., physician notes, patient charts, and medical records). This made it nearly impossible to analyze practice patterns to improve care quality and efficiency. To the extent that good patient care data existed, it rested in the hands of insurers who reimbursed providers for the care but did not share the granular information with them. This information asymmetry benefited insurers at the bargaining table with providers. In 2009, President Obama's stimulus package included funding for the diffusion of electronic medical records (EMRs) across physician offices to begin to address problems of data capture, although the issues of data validity and complexity of interpretation remain.

Eighth, and finally, efforts to change the health care system using business practices imported from the outside have repeatedly come up short (Arndt and Bigelow, 2000a; Burns and Pauly, 2002; Westphal, Gulati, and Shortell, 1997). One reason is that these practices have been adopted for normative reasons (e.g., to look efficient, to satisfy boards they are improving efficiency, and/or to imitate what other forward-looking organizations in the market are doing) as well as, or sometimes rather than, rational reasons (e.g., to remedy their operating problems). This would explain, for example, why hospitals have not invested more time and capital in the implementation of any given practice, or the coordination and integration among multiple practices, but rather pursued a series of discrete practice solutions over time (see Table 1.4) as they have come into vogue (flavor-of-the-month management) (Pfeffer and Sutton, 2006). Another reason is that such practices may not fully consider the institutional differences noted above and thus are not customized to health care settings.

Given the managerial problems that need to be confronted in health care, and given the complexity of the health care system and its peculiarities, what approaches seem fruitful for

## TABLE 1.4  Business Practices Adopted by Hospitals 1985–2010

- Corporate restructuring/holding companies
- Corporate diversification into new businesses
- Theory Z management
- Total quality management/continuous quality improvement (TQM/CQI)
- Horizontal integration (e.g., mergers & acquisitions)
- Vertical integration (physician acquisition, continuum of care, insurance)
- Strategic alliances with physicians and hospital networks
- Reengineering / work restructuring
- Product line management / service line management
- Customer focus / patient-centered care
- Focused factories
- Lean manufacturing and the Toyota Production System

addressing them? One approach is to apply system analysis to glean insights into the behavior of complex settings. Another approach is to apply organization and management theory. The next two sections sketch out some of these perspectives and how they might be usefully applied.

# SYSTEMIC VIEWS OF U.S. HEALTH CARE

Descriptions of the health care industry in the United States often begin with a discussion of whether it is a "system." Webster's dictionary defines a system as a complex unity formed of many often diverse parts subject to a common plan or serving a common purpose. Clearly, the U.S. health care industry does not meet this standard. As noted above, the multiple players have different goals (**triple aim**) and divergent interests ("patients need my product/service, you should pay for it," consolidation versus competition, integrated versus niche models).

Is a system view important? We think so, for many reasons. First, from a **macro perspective**, health outcomes are determined by an array of forces and factors that spans much more than a nation's health care infrastructure. There are multiple systems frameworks that describe these forces and factors (Shakarishvili, 2009). Hsiao (2003) and the World Health Organization (2000) have each developed a generic framework for the overall structure of any country's health care system. These frameworks describe several background forces (environment, nutrition, sanitation, professional training, and others) that affect the policy levers available to a system. These levers ("control knobs") include financing, payment, organization, regulation, and behavior. These control knobs are modeled to impact intermediate health system outcomes (efficiency, quality, and access) which in turn produce the ultimate health outcomes of health status, financial risk protection, and satisfaction (see Figure 1.2). Berwick et al.'s (2008) triple aims of any health system—improving the experience of care, improving the health of populations, and reducing per capita costs of care—resemble the intermediate outcomes described by Hsiao.

Second, as noted earlier, there are so many interdependent players that a systemic view helps to organize them and their interactions. Figure 1.1 provides such a framework for the U.S. context. Providers of health care services occupy the middle of the diagram for a specific reason: they are the main focus of everyone else. Buyers reimburse them for services rendered to

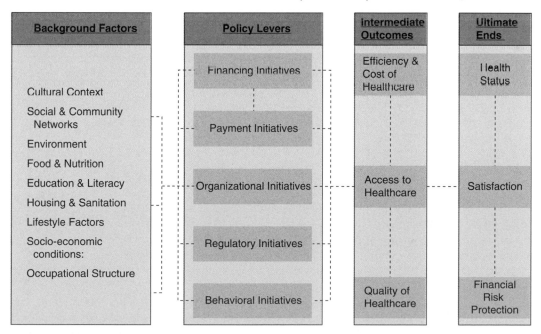

**Figure 1.2** The Health Care System.
SOURCE: Delmar, Cengage Learning.

their employees/beneficiaries; suppliers seek to sell them their products; regulators spend much of their time overseeing their quality/safety environment and their competitive conduct; and public health agencies seek to enhance population health by financing research and educational activities undertaken by providers as well as exercising oversight generally outside the direct provision of health care services. For the two parties in the upper-left and upper-right portions of the diagram (suppliers and buyers, respectively), two sets of intermediaries channel their services to providers.

This suggests a third reason for the importance of system views. The concept of a value chain (Porter, 1985)—i.e., a firm or industry's input, throughput, and output activities that are served by a host of support functions—suggests that value is created along this collection of activities and requires effective partnerships. Value can be created by making the appropriate make-versus-buy decisions on how much of the value chain to occupy. For example, should providers operate their own insurance vehicles or contract with payers in the local market? Much of health care today is undertaking an analysis of make-buy decisions with this system view in mind. Pharmaceutical firms are now considering whether or not they should shed their research and development arms, allow such functions to be performed by smaller and more nimble actors like biotechnology firms, and concentrate their efforts on the sales and marketing functions. Conversely, hospitals are now considering whether they should assume more of the functions of the group purchasing organizations they have historically contracted with and do their own in-house contracting. Historically, suppliers have deliberated whether or not they should serve as their own wholesalers/distributors, while employers/buyers have experimented with operating their own provider networks.

A system view is important for a fourth reason. Management theory teaches that successful innovation requires concomitant changes among the system's components (sectors) to achieve congruence or "fit" (Senge, 2006; Tushman and O'Reilly, 1997). Similar thinking has been applied to the U.S. health care system: payment reforms in the buyer sector must be accompanied by corresponding reforms in the provider delivery system. Thus, for proposed payment changes—pay-for-performance, gainsharing, or bundled payment—to work, provider organizations require new models of physician-hospital collaboration (Burns, Goldsmith, Muller, 2010). More broadly, efforts to reform one sector of the health care system must consider their impacts on the others to assess congruence with their interests and resources.

Fifth, as noted above, organizations within the health care industry have increasingly consolidated into systems over the past two decades with the stated objective of being more efficient, but may not operate as such. While mergers and acquisitions (M&A) have received a lot of attention (both by the merging firms and the media), post-merger integration activities have not. It is not clear that large multiunit systems can operate in a systemic fashion, extract scale economies from their operations, increase their productivity, add value, and address the multiple goals of access, quality, and acceptable cost. Systemic views of newly consolidated health care organizations and their potential (if any) to add value may thus be in society's interest. Indeed, between 2002 and 2004, the Federal Trade Commission (FTC) and Department of Justice (DOJ) conducted a series of workshops to assess the competitive and efficiency benefits of horizontal and vertical forms of consolidation (FTC/DOJ, 2004).

Thus, for example, despite the continuation of larger mergers (Pfizer and Wyeth, Merck and Schering Plough), research suggests that pharmaceutical M&A does not improve research productivity or profitability over the long term (Burns, Nicholson, and Evans, 2005). Instead, there are now suggestions that "big pharma" needs to "get small," perhaps by de-verticalizing their value chains, shedding their R&D activities, and focusing on a smaller set of activities. Similarly, the hospital systems that developed during the 1990s have devolved into more decentralized collections of autonomous operating units rather than centralized operations acting in concert (Burns and Muller, 2008). Indeed, the systems lens of federalism (the appropriate division of federal and state powers) suggests alternative ways for these hospital systems to organize themselves.

# ORGANIZATION AND MANAGEMENT THEORY

Schools of management thought have evolved over the past century to provide conceptual maps of how to deal with internal and external challenges. These conceptual maps include theories of how things work, what causes what, and how to act. The theories are not mutually exclusive and can serve as multi-dimensional or multilayered models to guide managerial action. Executives benefit from being familiar with, and adept at using, many of these conceptual maps. This is no easy task; it is akin to being ambidextrous, both left-brain and right-brain, and more a fox than a hedgehog (Berlin, 1953).

# Early Writings on Bureaucracy and Organization

Western management theory received its early impetus in the writings of Max Weber (1964), a German sociologist writing about the Prussian civil service in the late nineteenth century. Weber described the prominent features of this "bureaucracy" (literally, government by bureaus or offices) in terms of offices and officeholders, a vertical hierarchical ordering of these offices into organizational pyramids, a horizontal division of labor that separated offices and their functions, the use of explicit procedures to govern activities, the presence of records and files, and the selection of officeholders based on achievement rather than ascription. For Weber, bureaucracy was that form of administrative organization that operated under legal authority and was capable of the highest level of efficiency.

Research suggests that the bureaucratic model of organization is technically efficient and even superior to other forms under certain environmental, technological, and task conditions (Lawrence and Lorsch, 1967; Woodward, 1967). There is also considerable research on how to apply this model to the six common pathologies of the bureaucratic division of labor (Bacharach, Bamberger, and Conley, 1990):

- Role overlap (duplication): two roles perform the same task
- Role gap (accountability): neither role performs the needed task
- Role underuse (boredom): role not assigned enough tasks
- Role overload (burnout): role assigned too many tasks
- Role ambiguity (anxiety): role not clear what the tasks are
- Role conflict (stress): role's tasks are at cross-purposes

Bureaucracies are endemic to all organizations, including those in the health care industry. The degree of bureaucracy tends to be associated with both the firm's size and age. Thus, bureaucracy is less pronounced in small work groups and entrepreneurial startups (e.g., biotechnology firms) and more pronounced in hospitals and large consolidated firms (e.g., pharmaceuticals). Hospitals are peculiar bureaucracies in that they feature a "dual hierarchy"—a centralized system governing the nonmedical activities and a decentralized, collegial one governing the medical staff (Begun, Luke, and Pointer, 1990; Pool, 1991). Physician group practices, the majority of which are quite small, are peculiar in that they feature consensual governance rather than a bureaucracy. As many researchers have noted, physicians dislike and distrust authority (Burns and Wholey, 2000).

There is nothing inherently evil in bureaucracy, even though in modern parlance it has taken on a negative connotation of poor service, lack of responsiveness, and inscrutable, byzantine operation. At its essence, management and bureaucracy are all about "control." The word "manage" derives from the French word *manege*, used in dressage, meaning to put a horse through its paces (Braverman, 1974). The challenge for the modern manager is to utilize the clarifying elements of bureaucracy (e.g., to resolve the six pathologies above) while at the same time avoiding the classic bureaucratic pitfalls of too many hierarchical levels that separate executives at the top from frontline workers down below, or too many horizontal divisions or units that effectively create boundaries inside and outside the firm, which impede interaction and the flow of information, or too many rules and regulations, which stifle creative problem-solving. Chapters 3, 4, and 8 in this book consider these issues.

---

## IN PRACTICE: Efforts to Deal with Bureaucratic Dysfunctions

Considerable research has highlighted the dysfunctional consequences of bureaucracy including its inward focus (rather than focus on the client or the environment), its tendency to rigidity and inertia, and its stultifying effects on individual creativity and thus organizational change. Nothing has changed here; as late as the 1980s and 1990s, major firms such as General Electric (GE) used change programs like "Work-Out" to attack their bureaucracies (Ulrich, Kerr, and Ashkenas, 2002). After downsizing its workforce, GE found that the remaining managers and employees had more work and responsibilities to handle. To reduce the load, they gathered employee suggestions for how to get non-value-adding work out of GE's processes (hence, the title of the program). The company discovered that Work-Out was more than just trimming excess work, however. It was also an "exercise" work-out for employees to study and diagram their work processes, as well as a mechanism for conflict resolution as different departments worked out their differences in how processes overlapping their areas might be simplified.

# Frederick Taylor and Scientific Management

The **scientific management school** (Taylor, 1911) extended the Weberian model by explicitly emphasizing the "control" element of bureaucracy. Scientific management was an attempt to apply the methods of science to increasingly complex problems of controlling work in rapidly growing firms (Braverman, 1974). For example, Frederick Taylor employed time-motion studies to analyze a steelworker's task into its simplest components and then systematically improve the worker's performance of each component to maximize productivity and ensure conformity to the one best way of production. Such thinking became embedded in assembly-line technologies like auto making by industrialists like Henry Ford.

Scientific management had an enormous impact on management practice and theory for decades to come. Of particular importance to us are three assumptions. First, Taylor assumed that workers were guided by intuition and variable training, and thus were unable to perform their tasks in the best way. Instead, armed with scientific techniques (e.g., time-motion studies), management must control every aspect of the labor process and dictate precisely how it should be done. Workers were left with no discretion in their jobs, while managers were vested with all decision making regarding task design. This separation of decision making at the top from execution/implementation down below in the firm came to pervade all management and strategy thinking (Mintzberg, 1994). A second related assumption was that management needed to closely supervise workers to ensure adherence to standardized tasks and prevent any "soldiering" (deliberate restriction of output); rather than being intrinsically motivated, workers responded primarily to monetary incentives and external control. Third, due to the large variability in how to do one's job (e.g., which methods, which tools), scientific management focused on reducing the variations and finding the one best way to perform the work in order to maximize productivity.

This school presaged several recent movements in management thinking. The emphasis on decomposing tasks into their constituent elements and worker training anticipated the early work on job design; later efforts to amend this approach included the job redesign approach (Hackman, 1975, 1983), human factors engineering (Herzberg, Mausner, and Snyderman 1959), and the quality of work life movement. These topics are taken up in Chapters 3 and 5. The emphasis on reducing variations in work anticipated the later work of W. Edwards Deming and total quality management movement in the United States of the 1980s—a topic taken up in Chapter 9. And the emphasis on specialized tasks and productivity anticipated the focused factories of the 1980s and 1990s (Herzlinger, 1997).

# Classical School of Administration

The writings of Gulick (1937), Gulick and Urwick (1937), and Fayol (1949) took many of the concepts developed by Weber and Taylor and formulated them into general principles of management—essentially continuing Taylor's view of "one best way" to manage. These principles included unity of command (i.e., one boss), unity of direction (one objective, one plan, one boss), subordination of individual interest to general interest, centralization, authority, span of control (optimal number of people to supervise), and departmentalization (Fayol, 1949). Such principles directed managerial practice for much of the twentieth century.

Departmentalization has been one of the most enduring principles articulated by this school. These writers identified two principal models for the firm's division of labor: process departmentalization and purpose departmentalization. These have since been relabeled functional and divisional organization: organizing by functional area versus organizing by product line, customer, or geographic area. Alfred Chandler (1962) depicted the large-scale shift in the organization of American enterprise from the former to the latter. Twenty years later, Goldsmith (1981) described a similar transformation taking place among U.S. hospitals. Efforts to commingle the two forms of management gave rise to matrix structures utilized both in industry and in health care (Burns, 1989; Galbraith, 1973). Alternative forms of departmentalization comprise the core of thinking on organization design and coordination, the topic of Chapter 3.

# Human Relations School

The **human relations school** developed a model of worker motivation that sharply differed from the Taylorist approach, and thus suggested a different way of management. Work conducted by Elton Mayo (1945) and Roethlisberger and Dickson (1947) at the Hawthorne plant of the Western Electric Company ironically began as a Taylorism project to assess the impact of lighting changes on worker productivity. In contrast to Taylor's focus on individual workers and their jobs, their research anticipated Kurt Lewin's (1951) insight about the primacy of the group in structuring individual behavior.

The findings implied that to improve productivity, management must attend to a new set of considerations beyond monetary incentives and top-down control of work. Managers must instead understand the informal organization of workers (groups, group sentiments, team work), the need of workers to be listened to and participate in the design of their work (participation, self-governance), and the importance of morale and satisfaction as motivators of worker effort. Group structure and process are considered in Chapter 5; communication skills are discussed in Chapter 6.

Mayo's work suggested that workers are less rational than Taylor believed, guided less by financial incentives and more by human sentiments. Workers were also motivated to be accepted by their peer groups and achieve social solidarity. Finally, workers had an array of goals and needs that did not necessarily coincide with, or were subordinated to, the firm's interests. This insight led to an entirely new managerial approach called "organization development," which recognized the interdependence of the organization and groups of employees, and sought ways to simultaneously achieve both the firm's goals and those of its workers. By extension, this school paved the way for later recognition of the employee as the firm's key asset.

Subsequent research and writing expanded the human relations school's approach. Douglas McGregor (1960) contrasted this school and its emphasis on managing human resources (Theory Y) with scientific management and its emphasis on control and coercion (Theory X). For McGregor, human relations management sought ways to integrate the firm and the worker, as well as ways to harness the worker's creativity and imagination. Taking account of Maslow's (1943) hierarchy of needs, McGregor argued that satisfying the worker's higher-order needs of belongingness, esteem and self-actualization was critical. Herzberg refined Maslow's approach and suggested that such intrinsic motivation was inherently satisfying, while extrinsic factors were merely dissatisfying if not met. These approaches led to the entire field of job-redesign (Hackman, 1981) and self-managing work teams. The topics of motivating people and developing teams are considered in Chapters 4 and 5.

## Contingency Theory of Leadership

By the mid-twentieth century, two schools of management thought had been established. One argued for greater structure, control, top-down decision making, and reliance on extrinsic rewards (Theory X); the other argued for more participative management, self-governance, bottom-up decision making, and reliance on intrinsic rewards (Theory Y). For decades these schools were often (but erroneously) viewed as polar opposites. Subsequent research conducted during the 1960s and 1970s (summarized in Bass, 1981) suggested the choice of leadership style is not either-or. Instead, the effectiveness of specific management approaches depends on key situational factors (see Chapter 2).

## Decision-Making School

The **decision-making school** of management—also labeled the "Neo-Weberian" model (Perrow, 1986)—developed during the 1950s and 1960s, spearheaded by researchers at Carnegie Mellon University (Cyert and March, 1963; March and Simon, 1958; Simon, 1947). This school focused as much on how decisions were made and goals were set as on the structure of the firm—but all within a context with which Weber and scientific managers were comfortable: control of the work process and the worker.

In contrast to both scientific management and human relations, the decision-making school focused neither on top executives or lower-level workers, but rather on the large cadre of middle managers that had developed inside the large firms of the mid-twentieth century. Such managers and their decisions needed to be controlled. Because of limits on managers' cognition—known as **bounded rationality**—decision making needed to be guided by "satisficing" behavior (limited search among alternative options, and selection of first acceptable solution) and the use of "programs" and "routines" (e.g., solutions or problem-solving paths used before) (cf. Simon, 1947; March and Simon, 1958). Such approaches served as points of stability and biases against innovation by narrowing the strategic choices available to managers. Decision making was also organized and controlled through means-ends hierarchies, in which the goal (ends) of one layer of management (e.g., increase profits) became translated into sub-goals (means) pursued by the subordinate layer of management (e.g., raise revenues, decrease costs). They also presaged the "garbage can model" of decision making, in which solutions have a life of their own distinct from the problems they are called on to solve, and may behave as answers looking for questions to solve (March, 1994).

The decision-making school had entirely different views of worker motivation as well. Rather than viewing workers as extrinsically or intrinsically motivated, or having goals that were shared or divergent from the firm, researchers described "inducements-contributions contracts" through which the firm and the worker engaged in exchange (Barnard, 1938). This had implications for the goals pursued by the firm. There was no necessary harmony or consistency in the goals pursued. Instead, firms could have multiple coalitions, each in pursuit of their own sub-goals. Conflict could thus exist internally, and conflict resolution was never complete. Agreement on firm goals was thus accomplished through bargaining and negotiation. This school of thought thus presaged more political theories of the firm, which viewed organizations not as unified hierarchies but as competing coalitions pursuing self-interests (see Chapter 7).

Finally, the decision-making school introduced several new themes in organization theory and analysis. Rather than overt supervision and control espoused in Taylorism and scientific management, this school emphasized more unobtrusive controls over managerial decisions and behaviors. These controls included: standard operating procedures (SOPs), decision-making routines, socialization and training, organizational vocabularies and communication, and uncertainty absorption strategies (e.g., techniques to filter, process, edit, classify, and restrict the flow of information inside the firm).

## Institutional Theory

In contrast to the scientific management and classical administration schools, which viewed organizations as rational tools for achieving purposive goals, **institutional theory** viewed organizations as organisms that adapt to pressures from without and within. What are these pressures? Similar to the decision-making school, firms here are limited in their degree of rationality by both the environment (which can deflect the firm's purposes) and internal members (who bring their own goals and interests that may vary from those of the firm's).

According to Selznick (1957), the early proponent of this perspective, firms develop a distinctive character through a process of institutionalization: they take on a distinctive set of values, structures, and capacities as part of a natural history of development. Selznick's (1949) history of the Tennessee Valley Authority (TVA) illustrates its strategy of cooptation of local leaders to ensure the agency's survival long after its initial goals were met, but at the expense of some of the agency's own goals. In this manner, the firm becomes endued with values and goals from its environment as well as its initial charter. The history of hospitals shows how board members initially endowed and financed many facilities in the late nineteenth century to support charity care. They then broadened the medical staff in the early twentieth century to include many community practitioners to attract paying patients. However, by virtue of their control over patient access and medical knowledge, the medical staff came to dominate decision making within the institution and broadened its goals from charity care to provision of quality care to the middle class and supporting the physician's private practice (Perrow, 1963). Indeed, Pauly and Redisch (1973) argued that hospitals became the de facto workshop of physicians during much of the twentieth century.

The institutional view received further impetus from the work of Meyer and Rowan (1977) and DiMaggio and Powell (1983). They outlined the normative pressures in the environment that constrained the choice of organizational form and other structural elements adopted by the firm, leading to similarities across firms. Such structural similarities were not enacted for efficiency reasons but rather for sake of conformity with prevailing norms and values of what represented appropriate modes of organizing. Burns and Wholey (1993) documented the impact of local networks of influence in promoting the diffusion of matrix management among hospitals; Arndt and Bigelow (2000b) documented the impact of such normative ideologies and pressures on hospital management during the past century; D'Aunno, Sutton, and Price (1991) described the impact of such forces on the organization of drug abuse treatment centers; and Ruef and Scott (1998) examined the characteristics affecting hospital legitimacy over a 55-year period.

## Open Systems and Resource Dependence Theories

The idea that organizations exist within an environmental context, from which it must secure resources, support, and legitimacy in order to survive and operate, received a more complete explication in **open systems theory** (Katz and Kahn, 1966). The institutional theorists described one set of (normative) constraints on the firm's structures and behaviors imposed by environmental forces. Thompson (1967) extended the decision-making view and its attempt to deal with bounded rationality by describing organizations as "open systems, hence indeterminate and faced with uncertainty, but at the same time as subject to criteria of rationality and hence needing determinateness and certainty" (1967). At lower levels in the organization, managers would seek to seal off the firm from its environment through a host of "uncertainty absorption" techniques. At higher levels, the firm embraced and actively sought to manage its interdependence with the environment.

Additional research conducted during the 1960s suggested that the effectiveness of specific management and structural approaches depended on the firm's environment, technology, and critical tasks. Thus, a more bureaucratic or "mechanistic" approach is suitable when the environment is stable and the tasks are routine and well understood, while a less bureaucratic or "organic" approach is more suitable when the environment is turbulent and the tasks are complex and less well understood (Burns and Stalker, 1961; Woodward, 1967; Lawrence and Lorsch, 1967). Later researchers went further to suggest the bureaucratic and participative structures are neither opposites, nor a one-dimensional linear continuum, but rather two different dimensions on which firms and their management approaches may rest. That is, the most effective approaches are not "either or" but "both and" (Blake and Mouton, 1964; Misumi and Peterson, 1985; Collins and Porras, 1994; Johnson, 1996). Indeed, recent research emphasizes the importance of **ambidexterity** in organizational performance: e.g., firms that are both centralized and decentralized, firms that have units that are both mechanistic and organic in structure, etc. (Quinn, 1988; Tushman and O'Reilly, 1997; Beer and Nohria, 2000).

The open-system view of organizations (Katz and Khan; Thomson 1967) contained within it the seeds of **resource dependence theory**. In this model, organizations depend on other firms for critical resources and engage in strategies to protect themselves. Thompson described four elements in the firm's task environment (customers, suppliers, competitors, and regulators) and the firm's interdependence with its task environment and technology. Subsequent scholars (Pfeffer and Salancik 1978) described the firm's effort to manage or strategically adapt to this task environment. This research suggested that organizations were not passive recipients of environmental change but actively sought to change their environments. Inter-organizational relationships (IORs) constitute one key adaptive strategy for managing this interdependence. IORs have become a major focus of corporate activity, and can take many forms, including horizontal mergers

and vertical integration (see Chapter 10), strategic alliances (see Chapter 11), lobbying and managing regulatory demands (see Chapter 12), and managing community physicians (see Chapters 4 and 11). In this manner, organization theory began to confront the emerging field of corporate strategy and the strategic management perspective.

## Strategic Management Perspective

The field of strategic management has evolved considerably since the 1960s, when it was dominated by the logic of top-down decision making, deliberate corporate rationality, and environmental stability. The field now encompasses at least three main schools of thought, many of which have their precursors in the schools discussed above. One school of thought emphasizes industry structure and competitive forces (Porter, 1980), similar to Thompson's articulation of the task environment. A second school of thought emphasizes the firm's distinctive capabilities and resources, building upon the decision-making school's discussion of organization programs and routines (March and Simon, 1958; Barney, 1991). A third school emphasizes the firm's relational capabilities and collaboration with upstream suppliers and downstream distributors and customers (Dyer and Singh, 1998). Such relationships can be developed with other constituents as well, including competitors, regulators, or other firms in the task environment. These schools are covered in depth in Chapter 10.

## Organizational Ecology

The school of organizational ecology, or **population ecology**, is typically associated with the work of Hannan and Freeman (1977) and Aldrich (1979) but developed out of early sociological work conducted by Amos Hawley (1950) and his mentor Roderick McKenzie (1968) on organizational forms, competition among forms for resource space, and organization-environment covariation. Borrowing from a biological metaphor, organizational ecology principles suggest that the environment selects out and retains the most appropriate organizational form from an existing population of various forms (Baum and Amburgey, 2005). Such forms are selected out due to their superior ability to compete for and acquire scarce resources. In this school, the emphasis is on (a) the population of firms rather than the individual firm, and (b) changes in organizational populations due to variation, selection, retention, and competitive forces. In contrast to the institutional school, organizational ecology focuses on diversity rather than isomorphism. It also suggests that environmental forces make managerial choice and discretion very important for organizational survival and growth.

Research on organizational ecology has tended to focus on the economic and social conditions that affect the number and diversity of organizations, and their changing composition over time (Baum and Amburgey, 2005). Thus, some common themes studied include conditions that explain organization foundings (entries) and failures (exits), organizational inertia versus momentum, and changes to organizational niches (generalist versus specialist firms).

This perspective has been quite helpful in understanding the transition among competing organizational forms in certain sectors of the health care industry. Researchers have identified the environmental conditions under which generalist and specialist hospitals will survive (Alexander et al., 1986), the environmental selection pressures in the hospital industry (Alexander and Amburgey, 1987), the impact of size on the failure rates of health maintenance organizations (HMOs) (Wholey et al., 1992), the transition from the original group-model and staff-model HMOs to the more prevalent IPA model (Wholey and Burns, 1992), and the transition of the hospital industry from a cottage industry to a more organized industry of 600 systems and networks (Bazzoli et al., 1999).

## Social Network Perspective

Sociologists have long taken the **social network approach** in describing the embeddedness of human behavior in social relationships (Granovetter, 1985). As noted by the human relations school, these social networks can operate within formal and informal work groups to shape and constrain individual behavior. As noted by the institutional theorists, they can also operate at the inter-firm level to exert normative pressures on managerial choice and organizational structure.

Social network structure can be analyzed in two ways: in terms of interaction patterns and in terms of structural similarity (Knoke, 1990). The interaction approach emphasizes the consequences of interaction and the ability to control interactions because of a central role in the network. Actors who have relationships with one another are grouped together in a network. This network has certain dimensions. "Network centrality" refers to the actor's linkage to others within the network who themselves are connected. "Strength of ties" refers to the frequency and intensity of interaction with others in the network; such ties can be direct or indirect (mediated by another). "Network density" refers to the number of different

linkages between two or more actors (Uzzi, 1999); the greater the number of linkages, the more dense the network, and the more embedded the network's actors. Such networks may have a greater capacity for transferring knowledge and facilitating learning across network members (Gulati, 1995; Uzzi, 1997). For example, opinion leaders on the medical staff have often been utilized by hospitals to influence adoption of new practices by their colleagues, just as manufacturers have used them to sway adoption of new products.

The structural approach, on the other hand, groups actors by the similarity in their relations with others. "Structural equivalence" refers to two actors who have no direct connection but have similar ties with others. "Structural holes" refer to networks of actors who are interdependent but are not interacting; the presence of such holes has been shown to retard innovation (Ahuja, 2000). Structural holes can become filled by a third party who mediates their exchange (Burt, 1992). For example, foundation grants established "community care networks" during the late 1990s to bring a variety of local health agencies and providers together to promote primary care and health promotion activities (Bazzoli, Stein, Alexander et al., 1997). Similarly, integrated delivery networks (IDNs) can fill the structural hole between independent physician groups who can jointly develop and implement care management practices (Shortell and Rundall, 2003).

Social networks are also important for understanding team functioning and performance. Medical clinics exhibit varying levels of information provision among their professionals depending on network centrality, density, and homophily (Wholey et al., 2009). Similarly, strength of ties with academic researchers and centrality in research and development collaboratives furthers the access of biotechnology companies to labor expertise and capital as well as to promising projects and future collaborations (Powell, Koput, and Smith-Doerr, 1996). Finally, research on innovation within medical device firms suggests that new ideas are more likely to emerge from heterophilous networks with weak ties (to generate variations) but are more likely to be widely adopted in homophilous networks with strong ties (Van de Ven, Polley, Garud et al., 1999).

## System Perspectives

In recent years, management theory and health care professionals have developed a host of new **system perspectives**, focused on the broader system in which individual and organizational behavior occurs. Some of these perspectives have focused on health systems broadly conceived. Hsiao and the World Health Organization have both developed models linking the major inputs, throughputs, and outputs of health care (see Figure 1.2). The Centers for Disease Control (CDC) has likewise developed their "Health Run" model of the determinants of health outcomes (Figure 1.3). Other models have been developed to encapsulate the delivery system portion of the health care industry. During the 1990s and the rise of IDNs, Shortell and colleagues described a conceptual model of system integration based on functional, physician-system, and clinical integration. Nelson et al. (2008) described the embeddedness of patients and clinical micro-systems that treat them within a larger network of mesosystems (collection of clinical microsystems treating a shared patient population) and the larger macrosystem.

Other system analogies rest on biological metaphors. For example, interactions of insects (e.g., termites or ants) can result in self-organized, coordinated teamwork characterized as "swarm intelligence" (Bonabeau and Meyer, 2001). Such interactions promote robustness, flexibility, and adaptability without the need for central control or local supervision. More

broadly, firms can employ the "wisdom of crowds" (Surowiecki, 2004) via social networks with customers and innovators, collaborative software, wikis, and other information markets to develop collective intelligence and make better decisions (Bonabeau, 2009).

Such approaches are referred to as **complex adaptive systems** (or, alternatively, complexity science). They are complex in that they are composed of multiple, diverse, interconnected elements; they are adaptive in that they have the capability to change and learn from their experience (see Chapter 9). Thinking on complex adaptive systems has been applied to health care in the study of clinical pathway development (Priesmeyer et al., 1996), the nursing profession's resistance to change (Begun and White, 1999), medication errors in hospitals (Dooley and Plsek, 2001), and innovations in health care delivery such as HIV/AIDS prevention and treatment and the structure and performance of IDNs (Begun, Zimmerman, and Dooley, 2003). In the broader management literature, thinking on complex adaptive systems has been widely applied to strategic change and implementation.

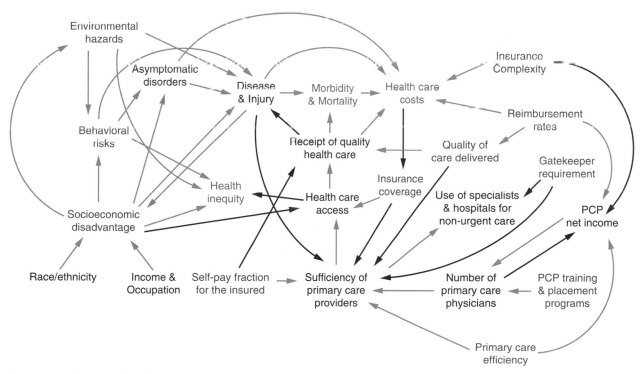

**Figure 1.3** Centers for Disease Control (CDC) "Health Run."
SOURCE: Adapted from the Centers for Disease Control.

# SUMMATIVE VIEWS OF ORGANIZATION THEORY

The various theoretical schools reviewed above should be viewed not as competing but rather as complementary approaches for understanding and managing organizational behavior. Collectively, they provide the practitioner as well as the researcher with a rich, diverse set of lenses or frames. Some schools clearly operate at distinct *levels* of analysis: e.g., Taylorism focuses on structuring the tasks of individual workers, the human relations and social networks schools focus on groups, the decision-making school focuses on middle managers, the Weberian and classical administration schools focus on top executives who structure the firm and its activities, while the resource dependence, population ecology, and institutional schools focus heavily on the **external environment**.

In addition to the different levels of analysis, the schools also suggest different *strategies* for changing organizations and different *competencies* that managers need to develop. Thus, Weber, the neo-Weberians, and the classical administration theorists focus on how to design organization structures and control (worker and managerial) behavior. Researchers in the human relations school focus heavily on motivating workers, satisfying employee needs, promoting quality of life at work, and managing conflict. Resource dependence focuses on the development of interorganizational relationships and market strategies the firm can use to control its environment, while the population ecologists and institutional theorists highlight the environmental forces (both ecological and normative) that constrain such use. Finally, the network and complex adaptive system perspectives highlight the importance of social networks—especially network structure and interactions—for generating and diffusing new ideas, forming bonds of solidarity, and promoting adaptability.

## Applying Organizational Theory to Practices: Hospital-Physician Relationships

How might the perspectives and insights of these different schools be used together? We can illustrate this with a concrete example: executives' efforts to foster improved **hospital-physician relationships** (HPRs). In what ways are these relationships tied to the delivery of value in health care? Studies from the 1990s suggest that excellent HPRs are tied to hospital profitability under the Medicare program (Bray, Carter, Dobson et al., 1994; ProPAC, 1992). The Health Systems Integration Study suggests that economic integration of hospitals and physicians forms part of the bedrock for improving clinical integration (Shortell, Gillies et al., 2000). Empirical evidence suggests that a handful of models of economic integration help to control cost and improve quality (Bazzoli et al., 2000; Burns and Muller, 2008; Shortell, Gillies, and Anderson, 1994).

From the Weberian perspective, executives might seek to resolve the dual-hierarchy in hospitals that has long divided the medical staff from administration, perhaps by creating a more unified organization. For example, in many academic medical centers, the two lines of authority over (a) the medical school and its faculty and (b) the hospital and its professional and ancillary departments have been consolidated under one individual—the medical school dean. Alternatively, there are calls today to reorganize the hospital medical staff and improve its governing structure to promote greater accountability for quality of care.

From a scientific management perspective, hospitals might more vigorously pursue efforts at clinical integration, such as developing and disseminating clinical guidelines, and monitoring their physicians' adherence to them. Such efforts are believed to promote higher quality of care. They also serve to reduce unwanted variations in clinical practice, and to promote **evidence-based medicine**, in which health care professionals identify and apply scientific information in order to make clinical decisions.

Classical administration's focus on organization design orients hospital executives to develop the most appropriate structures within which their clinicians work. As an illustration, during the 1990s executives erected multiple vehicles for partnering with physicians and contracting with managed care organizations. These included the physician-hospital organization (PHO), the independent practitioner association (IPA), the management services organization (MSO), and the integrated salary model (ISM). Each model offered a different level of professional autonomy and hospital financial support that catered to the individual physician's needs and desires. More recently, hospitals have shifted away from their process/functional structures and developed new organizational designs based on purpose departmentalization. These are alternatively called service line management models, hospitals within hospitals, and centers of excellence. Following the dictates of the classical school, they decentralize authority for a clinical area, along with supporting personnel and/or ancillary functions, to physicians in that specialty area.

Following the human relations approach, hospitals have long engaged in efforts to include physician representatives on their board and give them the opportunity to express their voice in governing the institution. In addition, they have long conducted surveys of the medical staff to understand trends in physician morale, to identify sources of physician satisfaction and dissatisfaction with the hospital, and to elicit physician suggestions for change. More recently, some medical schools have begun training future physicians in areas such as teamwork and analysis of the health care system, partly to satisfy new requirements from the AMA's Committee on Graduate Medical Education (COGME).

The decision making school emphasizes the importance of unobtrusive controls to reduce discretion and shape the premises of decisions made by managers. Leading IDNs in the United States, such as the Mayo Clinic and the Kaiser Permanente Medical Groups, have long utilized an internally developed and inculcated corporate culture of teamwork to promote collaborative medicine. During the 1990s, some community-based hospital systems sought to emulate this approach by developing questionnaires to evaluate prospective new members of the medical staff in terms of their orientation to quality and efficient health care delivery. Other hospitals utilized clinical databases to develop practice profiles of their physicians; such profiles were then disseminated to the practitioners with the aim of steering them to more cost-effective practice patterns. Some went so far as to perform "economic credentialing" for prospective or current members of the medical staff.

HPRs are a domain in which strong professional forces (e.g., the logics, values, norms, and beliefs of the medical profession) confront a host of institutional and market forces (Alexander and D'Aunno, 2003). At one extreme, medical profession desires for open medical staffs have long competed with hospitals' financial interests to exclusively contract with one group to cover hospital ancillary services (Burns, Goldsmith, and Muller, 2010). HPRs have also been shaped by strong institutional forces such as government reimbursement systems (e.g., diagnosis related groups or DRGs, bundled payment) that have led hospitals to engage their medical staffs in more cooperative decision making. Since the 1990s, the physicians' professional interests have been subsumed under a series of market-based arrangements—in effect, reducing the

traditional loose-coupling between the hospital and medical staff. These reflect "heteronomous professional organizations" (Scott, 1982) such as the PHO, IPA, and ISM models.

Open systems theory has been applied to hospital-physician relationships in several ways. During the 1990s, hospitals located in markets subject to intense managed care pressures (or the anticipation of managed care) were encouraged by consultants and academics to develop vertically integrated delivery networks; these could include the acquisition of primary care physician practices, medical groups, or specialist practices. Conversely, hospitals in markets characterized by low managed-care penetration were encouraged to focus on more traditional activities to work with their medical staffs (APM/University HealthSystem Consortium, 1995). Later thinking suggested that hospitals develop ambidextrous approaches for dealing with their medical staffs—in effect, being both hospital centric and physician-centric at the same time. Some IDNs in the 1990s aspired to hospital systems that were organizations of physicians, or to promote clinical autonomy through the collectivization of physicians (Burns, 1999).

Following resource dependence theory, HPRs can be characterized as external strategies engaged in by hospitals to control inputs critical to their survival. Hospitals have traditionally depended on community physicians to refer patients to their specialists, to admit patients to their inpatient areas, and to provide specialty coverage in the emergency room. More recently, they have depended on physicians to assist in the provision of efficient care (to manage under DRGs or bundled payments) and quality care (e.g., under pay for performance programs). HPRs can be viewed as efforts to partner with community physicians in strategic alliances—in effect, developing interorganizational relationships—and co-opt the desired behaviors in a variety of economic exchanges. Alexander et al. (1996) described a host of physician-organization arrangements developed by hospital systems in the 1990s to ensure these critical physician inputs.

From the strategic management perspective, some types of HPRs reflect not only a strategy of securing critical inputs (similar to resource dependence) but also a deliberate effort to foreclose competitors' access to those inputs. Thus, during the 1990s, hospitals engaged in a bidding war with one another and with physician practice management companies to acquire the primary care physicians in the local area. This acquisition strategy was viewed as a zero-sum gain: i.e., the physicians my hospital acquired would be loyal to my institution and direct all of their referrals and admissions to my institution (rather than yours). HPRs thus represented a classic vertical integration strategy (Porter, 1980). A smaller number of hospitals and IDNs viewed HPRs as a platform for developing strategic capabilities and resources (e.g., cooperation with the medical staff, physician teamwork, physician leadership, etc) that could be applied to solving other business problems or pursuing other economic ventures.

Ecological analysis has not been widely applied to the analysis of HPRs. Nevertheless, the health care reform debates of 1993 and 2009 pointed to particular models of delivery as being the most efficient mode of organizing. In 1993, the Clinton health plan called for accountable care plans (consortiums of providers) to contract with state-based health insurance purchasing cooperatives in risk-bearing contracts. The 2010 health reform encourages pilot demonstration projects for accountable care organizations (again, consortiums of local providers—this time, community hospitals and the physicians that utilize them) to deliver on both cost and quality metrics in contractual, risk-based agreements with the Medicare program. Tightly coupled HPRs—such as the Cleveland Clinic, the Mayo Clinic, Kaiser Permanente Medical Groups, and the Geisinger Clinic—have been touted as the model for other providers to emulate.

Research applying social network analysis to HPRs has developed several important hypotheses (Shortell and Rundall, 2003). The "strength of strong ties" among physician organizations is associated with the success of HPRs in developing economic exchange and altruism. Moreover, as social linkages (both direct and indirect) increase in a network, the network becomes more embedded, thus facilitating more weak ties and the spread of information and cost-effective opportunities for learning. Centrality in HPR networks, the presence of organizations that can fill structural holes in the network, and the strength of ties linking the physician organization to the network will facilitate adoption and implementation of clinical process innovations.

Finally, Begun et al. (2003) utilize the complex adaptive perspective to analyze the Minneapolis-based merger of HealthSpan and Medica into the Allina Health System in 1994. Rather than focus on the explicit merger strategy and intent, the researchers analyze how the merger actually unfolded and how Allina's strategy and structure co-evolved over time. They suggest that integration of entities would be more effective if they were allowed to "e-merge" rather than "be-merged."

In a similar vein, Cappelli et al. (2010) attribute the ascendance of Indian firms in a number of industries, including health care, to managerial practices of improvisation and adaptability. Emergent business practices and models, rather than explicit strategies or even Western theories, have enabled Indian firms to develop solutions such as micro-insurance and low-cost hospital care for the poor to address the needs of the "bottom of the pyramid." The researchers characterize these practices and models as "the Indian way" of learning by doing, and suggest they may serve as sources of learning and reverse innovation for Western organizations.

# ORGANIZATION THEORY AND BEHAVIOR: A GUIDE TO THIS TEXT

The challenge for managers is to understand the complexity of the health care system (e.g., Figures 1.1 and 1.2), and the interests and roles of the different actors within it, and then determine which managerial perspectives discussed above can be usefully applied, at what level of analysis, and using what levers to address the value equation. Table 1.5 attempts to summarize this and describe where the book's chapters tackle these issues.

The book is divided into three parts. This chapter and the next introduce the reader to the issues of leadership and management in health care. The next part considers the **micro perspective**: the internal environment of organizations. Topics taken up here include organization design, motivation, groups and teams, communication, power/politics/conflict, organization learning and innovation, and organizational performance, improvement, and change management. The last part of the book considers the *macro perspective*: the external environment of organizations. Topics here include strategy, strategic alliances, policy and regulation, information technology, consumerism, and forces shaping health care throughout the rest of the world.

**TABLE 1.5  Organization Theory and Behavior: A Guide to the Text**

| Health Care Organizations and Their Managers | |
|---|---|
| Organization Theory and Management of Health Care Firms (Chapter 1) | |
| Leadership, Management, and Culture in Health Care Firms (Chapter 2) | |
| **Micro Perspective: Manage the Internal Environment** | **Macro Perspective: Manage the External Environment** |
| Organization Design (Chapter 3) | Achieving Competitive Advantage (Chapter 10) |
| Motivating People (Chapter 4) | Managing Strategic Alliances (Chapter 11) |
| Managing Groups and Teams (Chapter 5) | Health Care Policy & Regulation (Chapter 12) |
| Communication (Chapter 6) | Managing Information Technology (Chapter 13) |
| Managing Power, Politics, and Conflict (Chapter 7) | Consumerism (Chapter 14) |
| Organization Learning and Innovation (Chapter 8) | Globalization & Health Management (Chapter 15) |
| Organization Performance, Improvement, and Change Management (Chapter 9) | |

# CASE: Can Organization Theory Inform Efforts to Improve Health Care Quality?

Improving the quality of health care has proven to be an elusive and difficult task. Health care organizations have experienced considerable difficulty in grasping all of the individual-level, team-level, organization-level, and system-level factors that shape quality. They have also been challenged to measure quality, to motivate providers to change their practices, and to implement quality improvement projects. The problems have been manifest in high rates of hospital readmission, high rates of preventable deaths and medical errors, uneven quality of care for people with inadequate insurance, and the introduction of new and expensive medical technologies without concomitant gains in life expectancy.

**Questions**

1. Does theory and research in management offer *any* guidance for practitioners seeking to improve quality of care?
2. What does *each* school of thought reviewed in this chapter suggest about what to do?
3. Which of the schools of thought seem to offer the *most* useful advice?

# REFERENCES

Aaron, H., & Ginsburg, P. (2009). Is health spending excessive? If so, what can we do about it? *Health Affairs, 28,* 1260–1275.

Ahuja, G. (2000). Collaboration networks, structural holes, and innovation: A longitudinal study. *Administrative Science Quarterly, 45*(3), 425–455.

Aldrich, H. E. (1979). *Organizations and environments.* Englewood Cliffs, NJ: Prentice-Hall.

Alexander, J. A., Kaluzny, A. D., & Middleton, S. C. (1986). Organizational growth, survival and death in the U.S. hospital industry: A population ecology perspective. *Social Science and Medicine, 22*(3), 303–308.

Alexander, J. A., & Amburgey, T. (1987). The dynamics of change in the American hospital industry: Transformation or selection? *Medical Care Research and Review, 44*(2), 279–321.

Alexander, J. A., Burns, L. R., Zuckerman, H. S., Vaughn, T., Andersen, R., Torrens, P., & Hilberman, D. (1996). An exploratory analysis of market-based physician-organization arrangements. *Hospitals and Health Services Administration,* 311–329.

Alexander, J. A., & D'Aunno, T. A. (2003). Alternative perspectives on institutional and market relationships in the U.S. health care sector. In S. Mick & M. Wyttenbach (Eds.), *Advances in health care organization theory* (pp. 45–77). San Francisco: Jossey-Bass.

Altman, S., & Rodwin, M. (1988). Halfway competitive markets and ineffective regulation: The American health care system. *Journal of Health Politics, Policy and Law, 13*(2), 323–339.

Altman, D., & Levitt, L. (2002). The sad history of health care cost containment as told in one chart. *Health Affairs,* 23, W83–W84.

Altman, S. (2010). Is it possible for the U.S. to control health care costs? Presentation to the Leonard Davis Institute, University of Pennsylvania. January 29, Philadelphia.

APM/University HealthSystem Consortium. (1995). How markets evolve. *Hospitals and Health Networks, 69,* 60.

Arndt, M., & Bigelow, B. (2000a). The transfer of business practices into hospitals: History and implications. In *Advances in health care management* (Vol. 1, pp. 339–368). New York: Elsevier.

Arndt, M., & Bigelow, B. (2000b). Presenting structural innovation in an institutional environment: Hospitals' use of impression management. *Administrative Science Quarterly, 45,* 494–552.

Arrow, K. (1963). Uncertainty and the welfare economics of medical care. *American Economic Review, 53*(5), 941–973.

Bacharach, S., Bamberger, P., & Conley, S. (1990). Work processes, role conflict, and role overload. *Work and Occupations, 17*(2), 199–228.

Barnard, C. (1938). *The functions of the executive.* New York: Oxford University Press.

Barney, J. (1991). Firm resources and sustained competitive advantage. *Journal of Management, 17,* 99–120.

Bass, B. (1981). *Stogdill's handbook of leadership.* New York: Free Press.

Bazzoli, G. J., Stein, R., Alexander, J. A., Conrad, D. A., Sofaer, S., & Shortell, S. M. (1997). Public-private collaboration in health and human services delivery: Evidence from community partnerships. *Milbank Quarterly, 75*(4), 533–561.

Bazzoli, G. J., Shortell, S. M., Dubbs, N., Chan, C., & Kralovec, P. (1999). A taxonomy of health networks and systems: Bringing order out of chaos. *Health Services Research, 33*(6), 1683–1717.

Bazzoli, G. J., Chan, B., Shortell, S. M., & D'Aunno, T. (2000). The financial performance of hospitals belonging to health networks and systems. *Inquiry, 37,* 234–252.

Baum, J., & Amburgey, T. (2005). Organizational ecology. In J. Baum (Ed.), *The Blackwell companion to organizations* (pp. 304–326). Blackwell Business.

Beer, M., & Nohria, N. (2000). *Breaking the code of change.* Cambridge, MA: Harvard Business School Press.

Begun, J. W., & White, K. R. (1999). The profession of nursing as a complex adaptive system: Strategies for change. In J. J. Kronenfeld (Ed.), *Research in the sociology of health care* (pp. 189–203). Greenwich, CT: JAI Press.

Begun, J. W., Luke. R. D., & Pointer, D. D. (1990). Structure and strategy in hospital-physician relationships. In S. Mick (Ed.), *Innovations in health care delivery: Insights from organization theory.* San Francisco: Jossey-Bass.

Begun, J. W., Zimmerman, B., & Dooley, K. J. (2003). Health care organizations as complex adaptive systems. In S. Mick & M. Wyttenbach (Eds.), *Advances in health care organization theory* (pp. 253–288). San Francisco: Jossey-Bass.

Berlin, I. S. (1953). *The hedgehog and the fox: An essay on Tolstoy's view of history*. New York: Simon & Schuster.

Berwick, D. M., Nolan, T. W., & Whittington, J. (2008). The triple aim: Care, health, and cost. *Health Affairs, 27*, 759–769.

Blake, R., & Mouton, J. (1964). *The managerial grid*. Houston, TX: Gulf Publishing Co.

Bogue, R., Antia, M., Harmata, R., & Hall, C. (1997). Community experiments in action: Developing community-defined models for reconfiguring health care delivery. *Journal of Health Politics, Policy and Law, 22*, 1051–1076.

Bonabeau, E. (2009). Decisions 2.0: The power of collective intelligence. *Sloan Management Review, 50*, 45–52.

Bonabeau, E., and Meyer, C. (2001). Swarm intelligence: A whole new way to think about business. *Harvard Business Review, 79*(5): 107–114.

Bray, N., Carter, C., Dobson, A., Watt, J., & Shortell, S. M. (1994). An examination of winners and losers under Medicare's prospective payment system. *Health Care Management Review, 19*, 44–55.

Braverman, H. (1974). *Labor and monopoly capital*. New York and London: Monthly Review Press.

Burns, T., & Stalker, G. M. (1961). *The management of innovation*. London: Tavistock.

Burns, L. R. (1989). Matrix management in hospitals: Testing theories of matrix structure and development. *Administrative Science Quarterly, 34*, 349–368.

Burns, L. R. (1999). Polarity management: The key challenge for integrated health systems. *Journal of Healthcare Management, 44*, 14–33.

Burns, L. R. (2002). *The health care value chain*. San Francisco: Jossey-Bass.

Burns, L. R. (2005). *The business of healthcare innovation*. Cambridge, UK: Cambridge University Press.

Burns, L. R., & Wholey, D. (1993). Adoption and abandonment of matrix management programs: Effects of organizational characteristics and interorganizational networks. *Academy of Management Journal, 36*, 106–138.

Burns, L. R., & Wholey, D. R. (2000). Responding to a consolidating healthcare system: Options for physician organizations. In *Advances in health care management* (Vol. 1, pp. 273–335). New York: Elsevier.

Burns, L. R., & Pauly, M. V. (2002). Integrated delivery networks: A detour on the road to integrated health care? *Health Affairs, 21*(4), 128–143.

Burns, L. R., D'Aunno, T. D., & Kimberly, J. R. (2003). Globalization and its many faces: The case of the health care sector. In H. Gatignon and J. R. Kimberly (Eds.), *The INSEAD-Wharton alliance on globalizing: Strategies for building successful global businesses* (pp. 395–421). Cambridge, UK: Cambridge University Press.

Burns, L. R., Nicholson, S., & Evans, J. (2005). Mergers, acquisitions, and the advantages of scale in the pharmaceutical sector. In L. R. Burns, *The business of health care innovation* (pp. 223–268). Cambridge, UK: Cambridge University Press.

Burns, L. R., & Muller. R. (2008). Hospital-physician collaboration: Landscape of economic integration and impact on clinical integration. *Milbank Quarterly, 86*, 375–434.

Burns, L. R., Goldsmith, J. C., & Muller, R. (2010). History of physician-hospital collaboration: Obstacles and opportunities. In J. Crosson and L. Tollen (Eds.), *Partners in health: How physicians and hospitals can be accountable together*. Oakland, CA: Kaiser Institute for Health Policy.

Burt, R. S. (1992). *Structural holes: The social structure of competition*. Cambridge, MA: Harvard University Press.

Cappelli, P., Singh, H., Singh, J., & Useem, M. (2010). *The India way*. Cambridge, MA: Harvard Business School Press.

Chandler, A. D. (1962). *Strategy and structure*. Cambridge, MA: MIT Press.

Chen, L., Jha, A., Guterman, S., Ridgway, A., Orav, E., & Epstein, A. (2010). Hospital cost of care, quality of care, and readmission rates: Penny wise and pound foolish? *Archives of Internal Medicine, 170*(4), 340–346.

Centers for Medicare and Medicaid Services (CMS). (2010, April 22). *Estimated financial effects of the "Patient Protection and Affordable Care Act" as amended.* Washington, DC: CMS.

Collins, J. C., & Porras, J. (1994). *Built to last: Successful habits of visionary companies.* New York: Harper Business.

Commonwealth Fund. (2007a). *Bending the curve: Options for achieving savings and improving value in U.S. health spending.* New York: The Commonwealth Fund. December.

Commonwealth Fund. (2007b). *Slowing the growth of U.S. health care expenditures: What are the options?* New York: The Commonwealth Fund. January.

Congressional Budget Office. (2008). *Technological change and the growth of health care spending.* Washington, DC: CBO. January.

Congressional Budget Office. (2008). *Geographic variation in health care spending.* Washington, DC: CBO. February.

Cyert, R. M., & March, J. G. (1963). *A behavioral theory of the firm.* Englewood Cliffs, NJ: Prentice-Hall.

D'Aunno, T. D., Sutton, R., & Price, R. (1991). Isomorphism and external support in conflicting institutional environments: A study of drug abuse treatment units. *Academy of Management Journal, 34,* 636–661.

Deloitte. (2009). *2009 survey of health care consumers: Key findings, strategic implications.* Washington, DC: Deloitte Center for Health Solutions.

DiMaggio, P. J., & Powell, W. W. (1983). The iron cage revisited: Institutional isomorphism and collective rationality in organizational fields. *American Sociological Review, 48,* 147–160.

Dooley, K., & Plsek, P. (2001). A complex systems perspective on medication errors. Working paper, Arizona State University.

Dranove, D. (2008). *Code red.* Princeton, NJ: Princeton University Press.

Dyer, J. H., & Singh, H. (1998). The relational view: Cooperative strategies and sources of interorganizational competitive advantage. *Academy of Management Review, 23,* 660–679.

Enthoven, A. C. (2009). Integrated delivery systems: The cure for fragmentation. *American Journal of Managed Care, 15,* S284–S290.

Esty, D. C., et al. (1999, Summer). State failure task force report: Phase II findings. *Environmental change and security project report.* No. 5 (pp. 49–72). Washington, DC: Woodrow Wilson Center.

Fayol, H. (1949). *General and industrial management.* London: Sir Isaac Pitman & Sons.

Federal Trade Commission and Department of Justice (FTC/DOJ). (2004). *Improving health care: A dose of competition.* Washington, DC: FTC and DOJ.

Field, R. (2007). *Health care regulation in America: Complexity, confrontation, and compromise.* New York: Oxford University Press.

Freidson, E. (1970). *Professional dominance.* Chicago: Aldine.

Fuchs, V. (1986). *The health economy.* Cambridge, MA: Harvard University Press.

Galbraith, J. (1973, February). Matrix organization designs. *Business Horizons, 14*(1): 29–40.

GAVI Alliance. (2010). *Saving lives and protecting health: Results and opportunities.* Geneva, Switzerland: The GAVI Alliance.

Gelijns, A., & Rosenberg, N. (1994). The dynamics of technological change in medicine. *Health Affairs, 13*(3), 28–46.

Goldsmith, J. C. (1981). *Can hospitals survive?* Homewood, IL: Dow Jones-Irwin.

Granovetter, M. (1985). Economic action and social structure: The problem of embeddedness. *American Journal of Sociology, 91*, 481–510.

Gulati, R. (1995). Does familiarity breed trust? The implications of repeated ties for contractual choice in alliances. *Academy of Management Journal, 38*, 85–112.

Gulick, L. (1937). *Notes on the theory of organization*. Memorandum prepared for the President's Committee on Administrative Management.

Gulick, L., & Urwick, L. (1937). *Papers on science of administration*. New York: Columbia University Press.

Hackman, J. R., Oldham, G. R., Janson, R., & Purdy, K. (1975). A new strategy for job enrichment. *California Management Review, 17*(4), 57–71.

Hackman, J. R. (1981). Work redesign for organization development. In H. Meltzer (Ed.), *Making organizations humane and productive* (pp. 373–387). New York: John Wiley & Sons.

Hannan, M. T., & Freeman, J. H. (1977). The population ecology of organizations. *American Journal of Sociology, 82*, 929–964.

Hansmann, H. (1987). Economic theories of nonprofit organizations. In W. W. Powell (Ed.), *The nonprofit sector: A research handbook* (pp. 27–42). New Haven, CT: Yale University Press.

Hawley, A. (1950). *Human ecology*. (New York: Ronald Press).

Herzberg, F., Mausner, B., & Snyderman, B. (1959). *The motivation to work*. Second edition. New York: John Wiley & Sons.

Herzlinger, R. E. (1997). *Market-driven health care*. Reading, MA: Addison-Wesley.

Herzlinger, R. E. (2006). Why innovation in health care is so hard. *Harvard Business Review, 84*(5): 58–66

Hsiao, W. C. (2003). What is a health system? Why should we care? In M. Roberts, W. Hsiao, P. Berman, & M. Reich (Eds.), *Getting health reform right: A guide to improving performance and equity*. New York: Oxford University Press.

Institute for Health Care Improvement. (2009). How do they do that? Low-cost, high-quality health care in America. Retrieved February 12, 2010, from http://www.IHI.org/IHI/Programs/StrategicInitiatives/HowDoTheyDoThat.htm?TabId=4

Institute of Medicine (2001). *Crossing the quality chasm: A new health system for the 21st century*. Washington, DC: National Academy Press.

Johnson, B. (1996). *Polarity management: Identifying and managing unsolvable problems*. Amherst, MA: HRD Press.

Katz, M. (2010). Decreasing hospital costs while maintaining quality: Can it be done? *Archives of Internal Medicine, 170*(4), 317–318.

Katz, D., & Kahn, R. L. (1966). *The social psychology of organizations*. New York: Wiley.

Kimberly, J. R., de Pouvourville, G., & D'Aunno, T. D. (2009). *The globalization of managerial innovation in health care*. Cambridge, UK: Cambridge University Press.

Kissick, W. L. (1994). *Medicine's dilemmas*. New Haven, CT: Yale University Press.

Knoke, D. (1990). *Political networks: The structural perspective*. Cambridge, UK: Cambridge University Press.

Lawrence, P., & Lorsch, J. (1967). *Organization and environment*. Cambridge, MA: Harvard University Press.

Lewin, K. (1951). *Field theory in social science*. New York: Harper.

Lindenauer, P. K., Remus, D., Roman, S., Rothberg, M. B., Benjamin, E. M., Ma, A., & Bratzler, D. W. (2007, February 1). Public reporting and pay for performance in hospital quality improvement. *New England Journal of Medicine, 356*(5), 486–496.

Lydon, P., Levine, R., Makinen, M., Brenzel, L., Mitchell, V., Milstien, J., Kamara, L., & Landry, S. (2008). Introducing new vaccines in the poorest countries: What did we learn from the GAVI experience with financial sustainability? *Vaccine, 26,* 6706–6716.

March, J. G. (1994). *A primer on decision making: How decisions happen*. New York: Free Press.

March, J., & Simon, H. A. (1958). *Organizations*. New York: John Wiley & Sons.

Martin, J. F., & Marshall, J. (2003). New tendencies and strategies in international immunization: GAVI and the vaccine fund. *Vaccine, 21,* 587–592.

McKenzie, R. (1968). The scope of human ecology. In A. Hawley (Ed.), *Roderick D. McKenzie: On human ecology* (pp. 19–32). Chicago: University of Chicago Press.

Maslow, A. (1943). A theory of human motivation. *Psychological Review, 50,* 370–396.

Mayo, E. (1945). *The social problems of an industrial civilization*. Boston, MA: Harvard University Press.

McGregor, D. (1960). *The human side of enterprise*. New York: McGraw-Hill.

Meyer, J., and Rowan, B. (1977). Institutionalized organizations: Formal structure as myth ceremony. *American Journal of Sociology, 83,* 340–363.

Milstien, J., Kamara, L., Lydon, P., Mitchell, V., & Landry, S. (2008). The GAVI financing task force: One model of partner collaboration. *Vaccine, 26,* 6699–6705.

Mintzberg, H. (1994). *The rise and fall of strategic planning*. New York: Free Press.

Misumi, J., & Peterson, M. (1985). The performance-maintenance (PM) theory of leadership: Review of a Japanese research program. *Administrative Science Quarterly, 30,* 198–223.

Murashkin, W. (2004). The global alliance for vaccines and immunization: Is it a new model for effective public-private cooperation in international public health? *American Journal of Public Health, 94*(11), 1922–1925.

Nelson, E. C., Godfrey, M. M., Batalden, P. B., Berry, S. A., Bothe, A. E., McKinley, K. E., Melin, C. N., Muething, S. E., Moore, G., Watson, J. H., & Nolan, T. W. (2008). Clinical microsystems, part I: The building blocks of health systems. *Joint Commission Journal on Quality and Patient Safety, 34,* 367–378.

Parsons, T. (1951). *The social system*. Glencoe, IL: Free Press.

Pauly, M. V., & Redisch, M. (1973). The not-for-profit hospital as a physicians' cooperative. *American Economic Review, 63,* 87–99.

Perrow, C. (1963). Goals and authority structures: A historical case study. In E. Freidson (Ed.), *The hospital in modern society* (pp. 112–146). New York: Free Press.

Perrow, C. (1986). *Complex organizations: A critical essay* (3rd ed.). Glenview, IL: Scott Foresman & Co.

Pfeffer, J., & Salancik, G. R. (1978). *The external control of organizations*. New York: Harper & Row.

Pfeffer, J., & Sutton, R. (2006). *Hard facts, dangerous half-truths and total nonsense; Profiting from evidence-based management*. Cambridge, MA: Harvard Business School Press.

Pool, J. (1991). Hospital management: Integrating the dual hierarchy. *International Journal of Health Planning and Management, 6*(3), 193–207.

Porter, M. E. (1980). *Competitive strategy: Techniques for analyzing industries and competitors*. New York: Free Press.

Porter, M. E. (1985). *Competitive advantage: Creating and sustaining superior performance*. New York: Free Press.

Porter, M. E., & Teisberg, E. O. (2006). *Redefining health care*. Boston, MA: Harvard Business School Press.

Powell, W. W., Koput, K., & Smith-Doerr, A. (1996). Interorganizational collaboration and the locus of innovation: Networks of learning in biotechnology. *Administrative Science Quarterly, 41*, 116–145.

Premier. (2009). Model hospital value-based purchasing program continues to improve patient outcomes. August 17. Retrieved from http://www.premierinc.com/p4p/hqi/

Priesmeyer, H. R., Sharp, L. F., Wammack, L., & Mabrey, J. D. (1996). Chaos theory and clinical pathways: A practical application. *Quality Management in Health Care, 4*, 63–72.

ProPAC. (1992). *Evaluation of winners and losers under Medicare's prospective payment system*. Washington, DC: Prospective Payment Assessment Commission.

Quinn, R. (1988). *Beyond rational management: Mastering the paradoxes and competing demands of high performance*. San Francisco: Jossey-Bass.

Roberts, M. J., Hsiao, W., Berman, P., & Reich, M. R. (2003). *Getting health reform right*. New York: Oxford University Press.

Roemer, M. (1961, November 1). Bed supply and hospital utilization: A natural experiment. *Hospitals*, 36–42.

Roethlisberger, F. G., & Dickson, W. (1947). *Management and the worker*. Cambridge, MA: Harvard University Press.

Ruef, M., & Scott, W. R. (1998). A multidimensional model of organizational legitimacy: Hospital survival in changing institutional markets. *Administrative Science Quarterly, 43*(4), 877–904.

Ryan, A. M. (2009). Effects of the Premier hospital quality incentive demonstration on Medicare patient mortality and cost. *Health Services Research, 44*(3), 821–842.

Sachs, J. (2001). *Macroeconomics and health: Investing in health for economic development*. Geneva, Switzerland: World Health Organization.

Sager, A., and Socolar, D. (2005). *Health costs absorb one-quarter of economic growth, 2000–2005*. Data Brief No. 8. Health Reform Program. Boston University School of Public Health. Boston, MA.

Scott, W. R. (1982). Managing professional work. Three models of control for health organizations. *Health Services Research, 17*, 213–240.

Searcey, D., & Goldstein, J. (2009, September 3). Tangible and unseen health care costs. *The Wall Street Journal*, p. A13.

Selznick, P. (1949). *TVA and the grass roots*. New York: Harper & Row.

Selznick, P. (1957). *Leadership in administration*. New York: Harper & Row.

Senge, P. (2006). *The fifth discipline*. New York: Doubleday.

Shakarishvili, G. (2009). Building on health systems frameworks for developing a common approach to health systems strengthening. Paper prepared for the World Bank, the Global Fund, and the GAVI Alliance Technical Workshop on Health Systems Strengthening. Washington, DC, June 25–27.

Shortell, S. M., Gillies, R. R., & Anderson, D. (1994). The new world of managed care: Creating organized delivery systems. *Health Affairs, 13*, 46–64.

Shortell, S. M., Gillies, R. R., Anderson, D. A., Morgan-Erickson, K. & Mitchell, J. B. (1996). *Remaking health care in America: Building organized delivery systems*. San Francisco: Jossey-Bass.

Shortell, S. M., & Rundall, T. G. (2003). Physician-organization relationships: Social networks and strategic intent. In S. Mick & M. Wyttenbach (Eds.), *Advances in health care organization theory* (pp. 141–173). San Francisco: Jossey-Bass.

Simon, H. A. (1947). *Administrative behavior*. New York: MacMillan.

Sloan, F., Picone, G., Taylor, D., & Chou, S. Hospital ownership and cost and quality of care: Is there a dime's worth of difference? *Journal of Health Economics, 20*(1), 1–21.

Studdert, D. M., Mello, M. M., Sage, W.M., DesRoches, C. M., Peugh, J., Zapert, K., & Brennan, T. A. (2005). Defensive medicine among high-risk specialist physicians in a volatile malpractice environment. *Journal of American Medical Association,293*(21), 2609–2617.

Surowiecki, J. (2004). *The Wisdom of Crowds*. New York: Doubleday.

Taylor, F. W. (1911). *The principles of scientific management*. New York: W. W. Norton.

Thompson, J. D. (1967). *Organizations in action*. New York: McGraw-Hill.

Towers Perrin. (2008). 2008 update on U.S. tort cost trends. Retrieved July 31, 2010, from http://www.towersperrin.com/tp/ge twebcachedoc?webc=USA/2008/200811/2008_tort_costs_trends.pdf

Tushman, M. L., & O'Reilly, C. (1997). *Winning through innovation: A practical guide to leading organizational change and renewal*. Cambridge, MA: Harvard Business School Press.

Ulrich, D., Kerr, S., and Ashkenas, R. (2002). *GE Work-Out*. New York: McGraw-Hill.

Uzzi, B. (1997). Social structure and competition in interfirm networks: The paradox of embeddedness. *Administrative Science Quarterly, 42*, 35–67.

Uzzi, B. (1999). Embeddedness in the making of financial capital: How social relations and networks benefit firms seeking financing. *American Sociological Review, 64*, 481–505.

Van de Ven, A., Polley, D. E., Garud, R., & Venkataraman, S. (1999). *The innovation journey*. New York: Oxford University Press.

Weber, M. (1964). *The theory of social and economic organization*. Glencoe, IL: Free Press.

Weisbrod, B. A. (1991). The health care quadrilemma: An essay on technological change, insurance, quality of care, and cost containment. *Journal of Economic Literature, 29*, 523–552.

Wennberg, J. E., Fisher, E. S., & Skinner, J. S. (2002). Geography and the debate over Medicare reform. *Health Affairs* Web Exclusive, W96–W114.

Westphal, J. D., Gulati, R., & Shortell, S. M. (1997). Customization or conformity: An institutional and network perspective on the content and consequences of TQM adoption. *Administrative science quarterly, 42*(2), 366–394.

Whitley, M. A. (2009, June 4). Cleveland Clinic praised by President Barack Obama for efficiency, control of costs. *The Plain Dealer* (Cleveland, OH). Retrieved July 31, 2010, from http://www.cleveland.com/medical/index.ssf/2009/06/cleveland_clinic_praised_by_pr.html

Wholey, D. R., Christianson, J. C., & Sanchez, S. (1992). Organization size and failure among health maintenance organizations. *American Sociological Review, 57*, 829–842.

Wholey, D. R., & Burns, L. R. (1993). Organizational transitions: Form changes by health maintenance organizations. In S. Bacharach (Ed.), *Research in the sociology of organizations* (pp. 257–293). Greenwich, CT: JAI Press.

Wholey, D. R., Wilson, A. R., Riley, W., & Knoke, D. (2009). Work and talk: Information provision in informal consulting in medical clinics. Unpublished manuscript.

Woodward, J. (1965). *Industrial organization: Theory and practice*. London: Oxford University Press.

World Health Organization. (1996). *The world health report 1996: Fighting disease, fostering development*. Geneva, Switzerland: WHO.

World Health Organization. (2000). *The world health report 2000: Health systems: Improving performance*. Geneva, Switzerland: WHO.

# Chapter 2

# Leadership and Management: A Framework for Action

**Jane Banaszak-Holl, Ingrid Nembhard, Lauren Taylor and Elizabeth H. Bradley**

## CHAPTER OUTLINE

- **Introduction**
- **Leadership versus Management**
- **Leadership in Organizations**
- **Theories of Leadership**
- **Leadership Roles**
- **Leadership in Health Care Organizations**
- **Sustaining Leadership**

## LEARNING OBJECTIVES

**After completing this chapter, the reader should be able to:**

1. Differentiate between leadership and management
2. Define leadership as a relational concept
3. Describe the evolution of leadership theory from trait theory to contingency theory
4. Describe contemporary conceptions in leadership
5. Solve problems according to the Eight-Step Strategic Problem Solving Method
6. Appreciate current research findings in leadership literature
7. Understand how to sustain successful leadership

# KEY TERMS

| | |
|---|---|
| **Administrative Leadership** | **Objectives** |
| **Behavioral Theories** | **Organizational Culture** |
| **Clinical Leadership** | **Performance Outcomes** |
| **Competencies** | **Self-Care** |
| **Contingency Theories** | **SMART** |
| **Followership** | **Strategic Problem Solving** |
| **Front-Line Managers** | **Senior Management** |
| **Goals** | **Trait Theories** |
| **Leadership** | **Transactional Leadership** |
| **Management** | **Transformational Leadership** |
| **Middle Managers** | |

---

**IN PRACTICE:** The Case of Paul Levy, CEO of Beth Israel Deaconess Medical Center[1]

Paul Levy is an unusual leader in health care because his first job in health services was as CEO of Beth Israel Deaconess Medical Center (BIDMC). Immediately prior to taking the job at BIDMC, Mr. Levy was executive dean for administration at Harvard Medical School, and prior to that, he directed the Massachusetts Water Resources Authority (1987–1992) and worked in public utilities. Mr. Levy became the CEO at BIDMC as it struggled to become financially stable, and he successfully turned the health system around. His success illustrates how individuals can succeed as leaders across multiple situations and that the challenges at BIDMC required a leader with new ideas about how to meet the medical center's challenges.

BIDMC is a large medical center associated with Harvard University. In 2001, the year Paul Levy became CEO of BIDMC, the medical center had 1,200 physicians on its staff; 4,500 full-time employees; and 513 licensed beds.[2] It also experienced total losses of $28 million and losses in the operating budget were as high as $58 million.[3] These losses were attributed to limited integration of duplicative and costly operations after BIDMC was created from the merger of two large hospitals and a number of other smaller community hospitals in the extremely competitive Boston area. Mr. Levy forced change to happen quickly after taking office; within a year of becoming CEO, BIDMC experienced several months of positive financial status relative to budget and subsequently experienced steady improvement in financial health.

---

[1] The topic and historical timeline in this case are based roughly on the Harvard Business School Case # 9-303-008, "Paul Levy: Taking Charge of the Beth Israel Deaconess Medical Center (A)," written by Professors David A. Garvin and Michael A. Roberto, 2002.

[2] These data are taken from the Harvard Business School Case # 9-303-008, "Paul Levy: Taking Charge of the Beth Israel Deaconess Medical Center (A)," written by Professors David A. Garvin and Michael A. Roberto, 2002.

[3] Ibid.

---

**IN PRACTICE:** The Case of Paul Levy, CEO of Beth Israel Deaconess
Medical Center *(Continued)*

---

How did he implement change so quickly? Both he and others argue that it came not from making quick decisions about how to make cuts within the health system but from empowering others to make these decisions more efficiently. He changed the culture to emphasize staff-driven change. Partly, this was and still is done by more clearly outlining both the positive and negative consequences of the situation, setting expectations for what should come from organizational change, and repeatedly communicating how change is going and whether expectations are met, which includes being transparent about the organization's operations, successes, and failures. Today, Paul Levy blogs regularly on the Internet and you will find on his blog forthright discussions of both positive aspects of BIDMC's health care and the financial troubles the institution now faces again.

The mechanisms of Paul Levy's leadership are visible today as BIDMC again confronts financial trouble. In 2009, BIDMC had the worst financial year since 2001, and these problems are expected to continue at least through 2010 as the economic downturn persists and the health care environment in Boston changes. Indeed, all the hospitals in Boston have been facing a similar situation. Levy though has insisted that his staff will contribute to the solution. In his communication to staff, Mr. Levy writes, "Our task, it seems to me, and the one with which you have been so helpful in your comments [via e-mail and other mechanisms], has been to come up with alternatives that dramatically reduce this number of layoffs [set at 600]."[4] while achieving our cost-cutting goals. Mr. Levy received these suggestions after asking employees for help in identifying options. Now, his challenge is to determine which suggestions to use and to convey to staff the value of all the recommendations received. How would you weigh the multitude of options employees suggest? Who should contribute ultimately to decisions about where the biggest cuts in hospital operations occur? What values would you commit to maintaining through periods of cost cutting and economic downturn? All these questions reflect hard decisions about the process by which a leader both inspires followers and maintains the organization's culture and mission.

# CHAPTER PURPOSE

The purpose of this chapter is to define and distinguish the concepts of leadership and management, identify theoretical traditions through which leadership has been analyzed, consider the role of organizational culture, explain the larger set of roles leaders may play in health care organizations, and summarize recent research on healthcare and leadership.

# INTRODUCTION

Individuals placed in management positions are often expected to exhibit leadership through directing others in the work setting. Consequently, it is common to study managers in order to understand what leadership is. Unfortunately, this tendency has created some confusion over what leadership is as compared with management. A full understanding of leadership extends well beyond an understanding of traditional managers, as leadership includes additional skills and responsibilities than management alone, and, at the same time, can be demonstrated by individuals in nonmanagement positions within an organization. The person in the leadership role at the beginning of this chapter, Paul Levy, represents both some of the best personal qualities of leadership and the authority of a top management position from which he can use his skills to impact organizational change.

In this chapter, we distinguish the concepts of leadership and of management, identify theoretical traditions through which leadership skills in health case provision have been analyzed, consider the role of developing organizational culture, explain the larger set of roles leaders may take in health care organizations, and summarize the most current research within the health care sector on leaders and leadership.

---

[4] See http://www.bidmc.org/GivetoBIDMC/NewsRoom/CommunicationFromPaulLevy.aspx, accessed on 1/24/2010.

# LEADERSHIP VERSUS MANAGEMENT

**Leadership** can be defined as the process in which one engages others to set and achieve a common goal, often an organizationally defined goal (Robbins & Judge, 2010). In contrast, **management** can be defined as the process of accomplishing predetermined objectives through the effective use of human, financial, and technical resources (Longest Jr., Rakich, & Darr, 2000). Although these two ideas are often conflated, it is important to note at least one key distinction: Leadership is concerned with setting large goals, while management is concerned with the execution of actions to achieve these goals.

Those in leadership roles vary substantially in the approaches used to influence employee behaviors, and consequently may have very different effects on an employee's response to a work issue. For example, one can take several tactics when dealing with an employee whose performance drops over several months. A person in a leadership role may act in her official role as supervisor and indicate that job security depends on turning performance around; this tactic may instill such fear in the employee that the employee seeks to hide further performance problems. Alternatively, the person in the leadership role may first approach the employee using personal influence and discuss the problems that led to performance dropping, which may leave the employee more open to considering what to change. The choice of actions has a substantial impact on the employee's subsequent behavior.

Individuals can also use leadership skills to design organizational structures and cultures that outlast their tenure in the organization and that influence employees for years to come (Hooijberg, Hunt, Antonakis, Boal, & Lane, 2007). For example, the responsibility of refining the organization's goals often falls to middle managers and frontline managers, who have a firm grasp on organizational realties that the top management may not understand. In this way, these managers may be called upon to exhibit leadership by proactively feeding information back to the organization's top managers in addition to their traditional management functions.

In sum, one person may be called upon to perform both leadership and management functions within an organization, thus allowing for overlap in the leadership and management processes. For example, people in the leadership role may influence people to act from managerial positions of authority that give them the information, resources, and tools to control and direct others to accomplish the organization's goals (Kotter, 2001).

# LEADERSHIP IN ORGANIZATIONS

The managerial positions from which individuals lead have become increasingly complex in modern health care organizations as these organizations have evolved to become large bureaucracies requiring managers at multiple levels. In many health organizations, it is possible to distinguish three levels of management: (1) **Front-line managers** provide supervision directly to care providers, (2) **middle managers** have responsibility for entire units within the health care organization, and (3) **top managers** include those who are responsible for managing the entire organization and hence have responsibility for all of the units within the organization. Top managers are often referred to as the "C-suite" because their formal job titles include chief executive officer, chief financial officer, chief information officer, chief nursing officer, and chief medical officer.

In any organization, governance, or decisions regarding the strategic direction, mission, and values of the organization, is conducted by both the C-suite and external governing board or board of trustees. The governing board's role takes on special importance within nonprofit organizations, which have a legal obligation to provide community benefit as defined by the governing board. It is the responsibility of the C-suite managers to ensure effective board communication as well as effective communication with other critical stakeholders. C-suite managers are also responsible for defining and communicating organizational mission and vision, for providing priorities in strategic decision making, and for leading organizational culture. All three of these activities affect the daily routines of each and every employee within the organization.

Middle management makes up the majority of managers within any organization, and these managers face the double bind of managing up or reporting to their own manager while managing down or supervising a group of subordinates. Some authors refer to them as the "linking pins" within organizations because of their fundamental role in communication and coordination (Floyd & Woolridge, 1992; Likert, 1961), although the flattening of organizational hierarchies and increased availability of outcomes data today has reduced the number of middle managers within the workforce. Strategically, middle managers are critical as organizational champions of new ideas about work practices and for innovation and change within work design (Floyd & Woolridge, 1992). Furthermore, it is within these positions that managers learn critical lessons about how to set organizational agendas, handle formal relationships, and personally, how to handle the toughness and uncertainty of management jobs while maintaining perspective (McCall, Lombardo, & Morrison, 1988). Within frontline management positions, individuals gain exposure to managing teams, directly integrating clinical professionals and improving quality and reducing inefficiencies in clinical care, frequently by addressing quality problems routinely.

# THEORIES OF LEADERSHIP

The people in leadership roles represented in media images and within heroic stories of success in organizational turnarounds or dramatic business successes evoke personalities that often take on larger-than-life characteristics. These images are not false. These are often individuals with extraordinary personalities and skills, working in a context where their capacities are most effective. Take, for example, Paul Levy, whom we described at the start of this chapter and who is seen as largely responsible for the turnaround of Beth Israel Deaconess Medical Center. Early in his tenure at Beth Israel Deaconess, the *Boston Globe* reported, "The turnaround of Beth Israel Deaconess is as much about management as health care. By most accounts Levy's predecessor, Dr. James Reinertsen, understood well the hospital's problems. But every time he pushed, the institution pushed back and little got done. Levy, best known for running the Massachusetts Water Resources Authority got things done, big and small."

In studying leadership, however, we must remember that these individuals are examples of leadership and understanding the full range of leadership qualities requires examination of a range of individuals in diverse leadership roles. Furthermore, leadership theories should not focus only on select elements of leadership stories, such as within the individual's story, but should examine a range of important factors that affect leadership selection and performance. Leadership theories can be categorized by the key factors used to explain leadership success and can be categorized in

three types: (1) **trait theories** that examine personality traits associated with leadership success, (2) **behavioral theories** that examine how those in leadership roles act towards those they are influencing, and (3) **contingency theories** that examine how those in leadership roles are influenced by their surrounding environment and the subsequent performance within specific contexts.

## Trait Theories, 1920s–1950s

Over the years, researchers have examined the importance of a range of personality traits in predicting leadership success, although research on critical traits reached its heyday during the last century and has since declined in use and is more likely currently to be used in conjunction with other models of leadership. Trait researchers have had only limited success in connecting personality to performance despite the fact that research has evaluated the role of more than 40 different individual traits and personality characteristics (Landy & Conte, 2004). Robbins and Judge (2010) argue that the extant literature indicates that extraversion is the most common trait of successful leaders; however, as they speculate, extraverted individuals may be more likely to find themselves in leadership roles and to be involved in the types of activities necessary to make those in leadership roles successful. In other words, the trait itself may be less important than the activities that extraverted leaders are likely to choose and the behaviors that a person with that trait is likely to use when on the job (Judge, Bono, & Locke, 2000).

Gender, along with other demographic traits, has also been studied extensively for its connection to leadership and performance as a leader. Gender is significantly associated with women's more limited mobility into health care leadership roles (Lantz, 2008) and lower incomes within those roles (Bradley, White, Anderson, Mattocks, & Pistell, 2000; Dey & Hill, 2007; Suter & Miller, 1973). This leads to the question of whether women exhibit different leadership styles and whether women's styles may be less effective, and consequently serve as a barrier to their achieving higher leadership within health organizations. Contrary to such expectations, women have very effective leadership styles. Some studies have found that women are more likely to use a transformational style of leadership that encourages intellectual stimulation of subordinates and that has been linked to higher performance in leadership roles (Eagly & Carli, 2007).

## Behavioral Theories, 1960s–1970s

Leadership theories subsequently evolved into a much stronger focus on the behaviors that those in leadership roles both use consistently across situations and on the ways in which those behaviors can be taught to future leaders. A behavioral approach to leadership emphasizes the actions that the person in the leadership role takes on the job; these are readily observable by another party as well as teachable through both education and on-the-job training. Furthermore, behaviors can be more easily connected to the roles that leaders take within organizations.

Some of the earliest studies to map leadership behaviors, coming from Ohio State University and the University of Michigan in the late 1940s, identified several dimensions to encompass a range of behaviors consistently separating people skills from behaviors targeting goal achievement in the organization. The Ohio State studies, for example, differentiated initiating from consideration behaviors. While initiating behaviors include the ability to define reasonable goals and develop individual roles among employees that effectively enable achievement of goals (Robbins & Judge, 2010), consideration behaviors include the ability to gain trust from your employees, demonstrating interest in their ideas and regard for their feelings (Robbins & Judge, 2010). Similarly, in the model developed at the University of Michigan, behaviors were identified as either production-oriented or employee-oriented. In this case, production-orientation is very similar to the dimension of *initiating structure* found in the Ohio State model, in its focus on tasks that lead to goal attainment, and employee-orientation is similar to the dimension of consideration. These behavioral perspectives on leadership readily link to more current theories that identify those in the leadership role as using either transformational or transactional styles of leadership.

## Contingency Theories, 1970s–1990s

Contingency theories describe further how leadership behaviors contribute to the individual's success in a leadership role with the recognition that the success of a specific behavior depends on the organizational context. One of the first extensive descriptions of contingency factors in leadership came from Fiedler in 1967 who argued that a leader's success depends not just on the leader's behaviors, but also on the leader's relationship to his or her followers and on the types of tasks followers are expected to undertake (Fiedler, 1967).

Even greater elaboration of how the work environment affects success in leadership is explored in the path-goal model, which argues that those in the leadership role must identify the strongest barrier to a follower achieving their goal and target their leadership style and actions to address those needs for the employee. Subsequently, those in the leadership role may either direct followers to specific goals, challenge them to set higher goals, draw the followers more into participation in setting goals, or support followers through times when goals are emotionally or physically stressful.

Another contingency model, which has been central in theories of leadership, is the leader-member exchange (LMX) theory. Leader-follower exchanges become more complicated when social interests and relationships of the person in the leadership role are considered. LMX theories argue that those in the leadership role react differently to their trusted and limited "in group," who are given more autonomy and flexibility in tasks than the "out group," who may also report to or work with the person in the leadership role, but among whom clearly defined roles and greater formality is the norm. LMX theories have also considered the potential movement of individuals from "out group" to "in group" as individuals gradually become trusted and tasked with the in-group activities.

In conclusion, all three theoretical perspectives—the trait, behavioral, and contingency—have influenced modern research in leadership and resonate with the types of situations that modern health care leaders confront. The theoretical context is critical to self-reflection not only on how one develops leadership expertise, but also equally important to strategically understanding the conditions in which one acts as a leader, which has been a focus of contemporary theories of leadership.

## Contemporary Theories of Leadership

Models of leadership behavior have become more complex in order to fit the reality that those in leadership roles often respond to a situation with a set of behaviors rather than a single response. An influential model of leadership style in contemporary theories is that of **transformational leadership**. Table 2.1 lists the four key behaviors demonstrated by transformational leaders: (1) influence through a vision, (2) motivating through inspiration, (3) stimulating the intellect of subordinates, and (4) individualized consideration. Theories of transformational leadership argue it is effective because it changes the attitudes, values, and behaviors of staff in ways

**TABLE 2.1  Defining Characteristics in Transactional and Transformational Leadership**

| Transactional Leadership | Transformational Leadership |
|---|---|
| Contingent rewards | Idealized influence |
| Management by exception (active) | Inspirational motivation |
| Management by exception (passive) | Intellectual stimulation |
| Laissez-faire | Individualized consideration |

that align with organizational goals. Empirical research indicates that transformational leadership may be more effective in some situations. The finding that people-oriented leadership styles are correlated with better current performance outcomes is largely based on studies of transformational leadership. Although this style of leadership is positively associated with a variety of performance outcomes, there is evidence that it is insufficient for successful organizational change.

Theoretically, transformational leadership is contrasted to **transactional leadership**, which uses more direct appeals for performance through explicit reward structures. Transactional leadership is composed of these four behavioral elements, (1) making rewards contingent on performance, (2) correcting problems actively when performance goes wrong, (3) refraining from interruptions of performance if it meets standards (i.e., passive management of exceptions), and (4) a laissez-faire approach to organizational change. While initial conceptualizations of transformational leadership argued that leadership within a specific situation can be defined as either a transformational *or* a transactional approach, some researchers would argue that the same individual can choose between these approaches, and that those who are most successful in leadership roles use both approaches.

Current theoretical models have also focused on emotional intelligence (EI) as a necessary and defining element of leadership, where EI is defined as a person's ability to "1) be self-aware (to recognize her own emotions when she experiences them), 2) detect emotions in others, and 3) manage emotional cues and information" (Robbins & Judge, 2010). EI may be closely related to transformational leadership because both theories focus on the social needs of followers as a critical target of interpersonal interactions between those in leadership roles and their subordinates. This issue is also highlighted by contingency models that argue those in leadership roles must adapt their interpersonal style to the needs of specific individuals, which is discussed in the next section.

Most recently, researchers have also begun to explore how individuals acquire the knowledge and ability to use leadership behaviors. Education within graduate professional programs is the first step and a natural place to focus on building behavioral skills. This has required graduate business programs to evaluate their use of pedagogical methods (Calhoun et al., 2009), as is discussed later in this chapter. On-the-job training offers a second and critical method for acquiring leadership behaviors. As some argue, there is no better way to learn than to do something. Particularly at the management level, there are leadership lessons about managing under uncertainty and through persuasion that can be very difficult to learn outside the right conditions (DeRue & Wellman, 2009; McCall et al., 1988). Assuming then that leadership can be taught suggests that individuals can adopt different leadership styles, and ultimately, that they may choose to adopt a specific leadership style contingent upon the situation in which they find themselves.

Current models of team leadership have also noted that those in leadership roles may support the team's members with more attention and latitude and also should adapt leadership styles to the unique nature of team leadership (DeRue & Wellman, 2009; Morgeson, DeRue, & Karam, 2010). In particular, teams require substantial autonomy in completing group tasks but require additional political support to protect them from conflicting demands within the workplace and to allow them flexibility in balancing group tasks with other job tasks. These days, the demands of team leadership need not be taken on by a single individual, but may require specific processes for addressing group needs that can be taken on by a number of individuals within the organization (Klein, Ziegert, Knight, & Xiao, 2006). This leads us to shift attention to the roles of leadership, which we discuss next.

## DEBATE TIME: Leadership and Management: Any Differences?

1. Many leadership experts argue that leadership is a role rather than a personal or professional trait. Is this a distinction worth making?
2. Many people, even those well acquainted with the two concepts, confuse management and leadership. Some argue that management is simply one skill that a leader may or may not possess. Others depict leadership as enlightened management, saying "Management is doing things right. Leadership is doing the right things." Are they really two separate ideas?
3. Many professional development courses are available for building leadership skills and competencies. Courses differ substantially, but most presuppose that leadership can be taught or developed within a person. Is this presupposition valid? Based on what you know of your peers and the leaders you consider to be great, can anyone demonstrate leadership?

# LEADERSHIP ROLES

## Goal Setting

A critical role of leadership is goal setting. The terms goals and objectives have different, although related, uses. **Goals** refer to the larger aspirations of the organization, whereas objectives refer to the subordinate goals that must be accomplished to meet the larger aspirations. Research suggests that goal achievement is most likely when the goals are broadly shared in the organization, perceived to be challenging but feasible, include a time element, and are aligned with reward systems (Bogardus, Bradley, & Tinetti, 1998; Locke & Latham, 1990; March & Simon, 1958). **Objectives**, which are subordinate goals that must be achieved to accomplish the overall organizational goal, are often many and comprise a fundamental place in strategic problem solving.

The approach to organizational leadership termed "Management by Objectives" (MBO) (Drucker, 1954) is the most commonly discussed method of using goals and objectives to align organizational action toward achieving organizational goals. The MBO school of thought argues that objectives should be designed to be what is termed **SMART** (Doran, 1981). The acronym means specific, measurable, achievable, realistic, and time bound. Specific means that the objective is concrete and well defined with adequate detail. Measurable means that there are metrics that can be assessed that will determine if the objective has been met. Achievable and realistic mean that the objective has been defined in a way that can be accomplished if prioritized with the resources available and time given. Time bound means providing target times when the objective will be achieved. Theoretically, managing by SMART objectives (George T. Doran. "There's a S.M.A.R.T. way to write managements's goals and objectives." Management Review, Nov 1981, Volume 70 Issue 11) makes explicit the process of goal setting and facilitates shared expectations about what is to be accomplished, how, and by when. Such a process can enhance motivation and, with clear metrics, organizational units can be held accountable for progress toward the shared objectives and goals.

## Strategic Problem Solving

**Strategic problem solving** is an approach to integrating the strategic function of leadership involving goal and objective setting with the subsequent organizational action required to achieve the set objectives. Strategic problem solving uses an eight-step approach, outlined in Figure 2.1. The steps, while sequenced in the description, are in reality completed in a

1. Define the problem,
2. Set the overall objective,
3. Conduct a root cause analysis,
4. Generate alternative strategies to interventions,
5. Perform a comparative analysis of alternatives,
6. Select the best strategy and address its limitations,
7. Develop an implementation plan and implement, and
8. Develop an evaluation plan and evaluate.

**Figure 2.1** The Eight-Step Strategic Problem Solving Process.
SOURCE: Delmar, Cengage Learning.

more iterative fashion with feedback loops and adjustments throughout the process.

The eight steps in the strategic problem-solving model are designed to help an organization (or organizational unit) move from a current state to a desired future state, where strategy is viewed as the road map for the trip between where the organization presently is and where the organization would like to be. Therefore, the eight steps are: define the problem, set the overall objective, conduct a root cause analysis, generate alternative strategies that could be used to address the problem given the root causes identified, perform a comparative analysis of the alternative strategies, select the strategy, develop an implementation plan and implement, and develop an evaluation plan and evaluate.

## Step 1: Define the Problem.

The first step to strategic problem solving is to define the problem in a way that allows us to find solutions. Writing down the problem in a clear "problem statement" is one way to clearly define what one is trying to fix. Consistent with the principles of achievability and realism, it is helpful to define single problems. While people in leadership roles face complex circumstances with multiple facets, strategic problem solving identifies an important but single problem in order to focus attention. Ideally, there are many strategic problem-solving efforts ongoing throughout organizations; however, in each, there is clarity about the specific problem being addressed, and the problem is one that can be realistically addressed with the potential resources available. The best problem statements are short, widely shared by key constituents, and include not the solution to the problem, but rather the problem itself. Table 2.2 shows weak problem statements and how they may be strengthened to foster more effective strategic problem solving.

## Step 2: Set the Overall Objective.

Once the problem is clearly defined, the problem statement can be translated into an overall objective. Good overall objectives address the problem defined in the problem statement and are SMART objectives as shown in Figure 2.2. For instance, an organization with a poor inventory control system might define the problem statement as "Supply stockouts are common." An overall SMART objective that addresses that problem might be "Reduce supply stock out events by 25 percent by the end of the quarter."

## Step 3: Conduct a Root Cause Analysis.

In order to design strategies, a root cause analysis can help identify the causal factors associated with the problem. With clarity about the problem causes, a more effective set of alternative strategies to address the problem can be designed. Finding the root cause requires careful analysis. Several management tools can help people in leadership roles find the root causes of the problem, including but not limited to: Ishakawa (fishbone) diagramming, flow charting, Pareto charts, histograms, scatter plots, and regression analyses.

## TABLE 2.2 Writing Problem Statements

| Weak Problem Statements | Suggestions for Improvement | Strong Problem Statements |
| --- | --- | --- |
| "We need more regular delivery of supplies." | Focus on a problem, rather than the solution. In this case, why is more regular delivery important? | "Stock-outs of essential supplies are common in our organization." |
| "Due to understaffing, nurses are overworked." | Focus on a single problem, rather than the cause of the problem. | "Nurses are overworked." |
| "Our budgets are too small; we have a rundown building, and our medical director is leaving the organization soon, along with several key nurses and paraprofessionals." | Focus on a single problem; keep the problem statement short. | "There is not sufficient revenue to cover costs." |

**S**pecific—What exactly are we going to do, with or for whom? The program states a precise outcome to be accomplished. This outcome is often stated in numbers, percentages, or frequencies.

**M**easurable—Is the target of the objective measureable? How will it be measured, including the metrics to be tracked and the methods for data collection and analysis?

**A**chievable—Can the objective be accomplished in the proposed time frame given the economic and political environment?

**R**ealistic—Will this objective realistically bring the organization closer to accomplishing our goal or overall objective?

**T**ime bound—Is a time frame for achieving the objective provided?

**Figure 2.2** Is Your Objective Statement SMART?
SOURCE: Delmar, Cengage Learning.

## Step 4: Generate Alternative Interventions.

Based on the results of the root cause analysis, alternatives to address the key causes and hence reduce the problem and fulfill the objective can be designed. The list should be tractable in number, and each strategy can include multiple interventions, although as a full strategy, each should be mutually exclusive with the other strategies listed. For instance, one strategy might include doing A and not B. An alternative might be to do B and not A, and a third alternative might be to do both A and B. In addition, each strategy should be reasonable for addressing the problem; hence potential strategies that are known to be unrealistic or ineffective should not be considered in the alternative strategy list. Because it cannot address the problem, typically, the strategy to do nothing is not typically included in such an exercise. An effective set of alternative strategies then are clearly described, comprehensive but not overwhelming in number (try to identify 3–4 strategies), feasible to implement, and mutually exclusive so they can be compared as alternatives.

## Step 5: Perform Comparative Analysis of Alternatives.

Once several alternative strategies have been generated, it is important to perform a side-by-side comparison of the strategic alternatives using evaluative criteria to rate and choose among the alternative strategies. Evaluative criteria are characteristics that are important to the organization and by which the potential merit of each alternative can be judged. Illustrative evaluative criteria are the degree to which the strategy under consideration is (1) effective to addressing the problem, (2) cost-effective, (3) consistent with the organization's overall strategy, (4) timely in effect, or (5) politically feasible. Alternative strategies can then be rated either with quantitative measures (using a single scoring system or natural units) or with qualitative scales using a matrix as shown in Table 2.3 and Table 2.4 If the matrix is quantitative, scores can be summed or weighted and summed to identify the most desired strategy. If the matrix is

## TABLE 2.3  Qualitative Rating Matrix for Comparative Analysis

| Options | Evaluative Criteria | | | |
|---|---|---|---|---|
| | Impact on Productivity | Annual Expense | Political Feasibility | Time Required |
| 1: Increase Staff | Very Good | High | Low | 3 Months |
| 2: Increase Pay | Unclear | High | Very Low | 1 Year |
| 3: Improve Supervision | Fairly Good | Low | High | 1 Month |

**TABLE 2.4  Quantitative Rating Matrix for Comparative Analysis**

| Options | Evaluative Criteria | | | | |
|---|---|---|---|---|---|
| | Impact on Productivity | Annual Expense | Political Feasibility | Time to Effect | Total Score |
| 1: Increase Staff | 5 | 1 | 2 | 4 | 12 |
| 2: Increase Pay | 3 | 1 | 1 | 1 | 6 |
| 3: Improve Supervision | 3 | 4 | 4 | 4 | 15 |

qualitative, ratings can be integrated to discuss the merits and disadvantages overall of each alternative strategy. Sensitivity analysis, taking into account the riskiness of alternative outcomes from a single strategy, can be conducted as desired to understand the impact of alternative scoring or weighted on the choice of alternatives to pursue. This type of analysis is shown in Table 2.5. Importantly, such matrices are merely guides to frame collective discussions and arguments; they cannot provide a definitive answer that will always be a right answer, as strategy has substantial flexibility and judgment involved. However, the approach is useful for organizing much information and communicating about the decision-making criteria and process in ways that make ultimate strategic choices more explicit and generally easier to then describe to the organization and external stakeholders.

To get the weighted value, multiply the raw score by the percentage (as a decimal). Then add the weighted values across the row to get the total weighted score.

Example:

Increasing staff has a raw score of 5 in "impact on productivity," and the criterion, impact on productivity, is weighted by 50 percent. The weighted value is therefore the raw score (5) multiplied by the weighting percent as a decimal (5 x 0.50 = 2.5; the weighted value is 2.5). Summing the weighted values across the row provides the total weighted score for the strategy listing in that row (i.e., the total weighted score for the strategy "increasing staff" is 3.6). Based on the raw score (without weighting), the strategy "improve supervision" has the highest total score; based on the total weighted score, the strategy, "increase staff" has the highest score.

### Step 6: Select the Best Intervention and Explain Your Decision.

Based on the results of the comparative analysis, select the best intervention. As part of this, describe the potential limitations to the selected alternative and, ideally, address

**TABLE 2.5  Quantitative Rating Matrix with Weighting for Comparative Analysis**

| Implementation Options | Evaluative Criteria | | | | |
|---|---|---|---|---|---|
| | Impact on Productivity | Annual Expense | Political Feasibility | Time to Effect | Total |
| Weighting: | 50% | 20% | 15% | 15% | 100% |
| 1: Increase Staff | 5 (2.5) | 1 (.2) | 2 (.3) | 4 (.6) | 12 (3.6 weighted) |
| 2: Increase Pay | 3 (1.5) | 1 (.2) | 1 (.15) | 1 (.15) | 6 (2 weighted) |
| 3: Improve Supervision | 3 (1.5) | 4 (.8) | 4 (.6) | 3 (.45) | 14 (3.35 weighted) |

these limitations, recognizing that managerial problem solving involves tradeoffs and nearly all management decisions have limitations. The strongest approach to problem solving identifies and refutes the limitations of the managerial choices. The ability to foster support for a strategic direction, despite its recognized drawbacks, is an important skill for leadership.

### Step 7: Develop Implementation Plan and Implement.

Implementation plans identify the steps to take in order to put the selected strategy into action. A strong implementation plan specifies major tasks to be completed, timelines for each task, and the people or groups accountable to complete each task. Implementation plans often include a work plan, which organizes the various tasks, timelines, and resources involved in the implementation. To be complete, implementation plans might include early tasks related to fostering key stakeholder support for subsequent strategies and tasks. An example work plan, also known as a Gantt chart, is included in Figure 2.3. An implementation plan is critical to strategic problem solving as it provides a clear timeline for the overall project, a sequencing of steps to complete a larger strategy, a method of assigning responsibility to individuals and groups for accomplishing tasks, and a vehicle for communicating expectations and monitoring progress toward meeting objectives.

### Step 8: Develop Evaluation Plan and Evaluate.

Although evaluation is listed as the last step of strategic problem solving, the conceptualization of the evaluation should begin at the start of the problem-solving process. Often, evaluation includes both monitoring of progress in planned activities relative to the work plan or budget as well as evaluation, which encompasses examining the degree to which the overall objective was met in addition to whether the planned activities were accomplished. A strong monitoring and evaluation plan creates a transparent process for understanding how a project's progress and outcomes will be assessed and can motivate staff to work toward a common target.

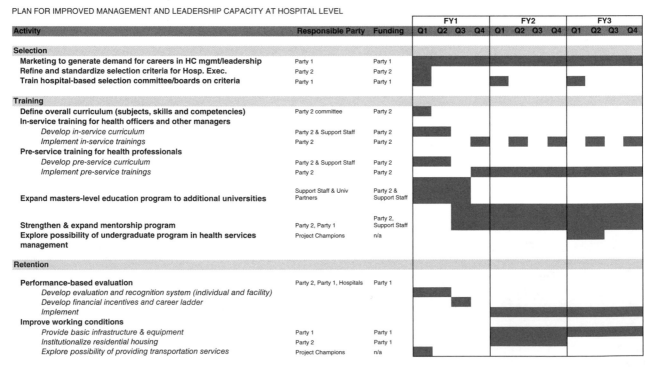

**Figure 2.3** Example of a Gantt Chart.

SOURCE: Delmar, Cengage Learning.

Central to evaluation is the selection of indicators of performance. Indicators, sometimes termed metrics, are the items measured to determine performance (e.g., profit, mortality rates, adherence to medications). Many evaluation plans also include targets, or the level one wants to reach in the indicator. For instance, the indicator might be "reduce mortality rates after acute myocardial infarction," and the target might be "reduce mortality rates after acute myocardial infarction by 1 percent in the next year."

Indicators may be process or outcome indicators. Process indicators measure whether specific activities needed to achieve the objective have been accomplished (e.g., number of staff trained; whether or not a workshop was held; amount of new equipment purchased). Outcome indicators, in contrast, measure whether or not the overall objective was achieved. Gathering data can be costly and difficult if indicators are not chosen correctly. To make sure that your indicators are meaningful and realistic, be sure to consider who will use the data, how it will be collected and verified, how it will be analyzed, and how it will be reported. As a cautionary note, data collection, analysis, and reporting can be expensive and overwhelming for organizations. It is important, therefore, to select a modest number of indicators that are viewed as most meaningful. Tracking a few indicators consistently and accurately is more useful than tracking many indicators that are measured or analyzed imperfectly.

## Managing External Stakeholders

Strategically, one of the key roles of the C-suite is to interact with key external stakeholders, including the board of directors, who are not immersed in the daily activities of the organization and often look to the top managers to keep them informed about the organization's activities. Particularly, the board of directors should play a critical role both in setting the strategic agenda for the organization and in establishing accountability within the organization. Yet, these individuals may be chosen not just for their business expertise or knowledge of the organization's services, but also for their role as leaders in the community or more generally as representatives of community interests. Consequently, communicating with the board is a challenging activity.

Experts have provided a few simple rules for making communication with the board and other external stakeholders go more smoothly (Letts et al., 1999). Most critical is the understanding that organizational performance cannot be reduced to financial profits. Particularly in the nonprofit sector, the organization's overall performance depends on a balanced scorecard of outcome measures, and that must be communicated effectively to external stakeholders. Second, external stakeholders do not have the same bureaucratic incentives to contribute to the organization's performance, and hence, people in leadership positions must strive to enhance the motivation of external stakeholders to contribute positively to performance. Finally, external stakeholders must be viewed as champions of the organization within the community, and hence, their communication skills must be enhanced through their involvement in the organization. Overall, as those in leadership positions manage the external relationships for the organization, they learn to depend on their strategic partners and governance board as critical allies.

## Managing the Internal Workforce: Leadership and Followership

A major role for people in leadership roles is managing the workforce to accomplish organizational goals together. This involves managing people as team members and as individuals simultaneously (Smith & Berg, 1997). Current conceptions of leadership suggest that leadership may best be understood as being born of the relationship between a leader and follower. In this way, organizational leadership can be thought of as a relational concept (Berg, 1998).

Before exploring the relationship between these two roles, it is first important to clarify what is meant by each. Leadership is classically defined as influencing a group of people towards the achievement of a goal; however, more recent conceptualizations of leadership consider this definition incomplete because it does not acknowledge followership. **Followership** has been defined as those who "share a common purpose with the leader, believes in what the organization is trying to accomplish, and wants both the leader and the organization to succeed" (Chaleff, 1995; Kelley, 1988). Much like leadership, then, followership is a critical role in an organization. Furthermore, leadership and followership roles are mutually dependent (Berg, 1998). Leadership cannot exist without followership, and followership cannot exist without leadership. Most people in an organization play both roles at varying times and in varying assignments within their position responsibilities (Kellerman, 2008).

Given the interdependence of leadership and followership, the effectiveness of people in the leadership role may be measured by the extent to which they are able to leverage and manage the capacities and motivation of those in followership roles. This kind of leveraging and managing is best done through the cultivation of relationships, which can enable the group to draw upon the depth and breadth of the group's collective skill to achieve its task. In order to effectively cultivate these intra-group relationships, both the person in the leadership role and those in the followership role must recognize cognitively and emotionally the value of relationships (and of managing relationships) in accomplishing organization goals.

Despite the importance of the leader-follower relationship, people in leadership roles are often uncomfortable managing people who report to them in a way that fosters genuine, participatory followership. Instead, people in leadership roles often misconstrue their role as a source of information and power, thereby failing to fully incorporate people in followership roles in agenda- and priority-setting processes and decision making. Such failures come with enormous opportunity costs, as the participation of energetic people in the followership role has been consistently shown to strengthen group performance. Similarly, managing people in leadership roles may seem similarly uncomfortable for people in followership roles. Many fear "overstepping" their professional boundaries or being seen as either overly eager or overly critical of their supervisor's plans or actions. Nevertheless, it is often a willingness to actively engage with the person in the leadership role in an enthusiastic, intelligent, and self-reliant manner that distinguishes traditional from effective followership.

The relationship between the people in leadership roles and people in followership roles can potentially provide the organization with a greater range of leadership capacities to draw upon in pursuit of organizational goals. When this relationship is weak or nonexistent, the person in the leadership role is apt to overtax themselves, resort to rigid role boundaries or hierarchical structures, and be unreceptive to the input of followers (Kelley, 1988). Those in followership roles in these cases are apt to participate in a more limited, dogmatic fashion and to keep potentially useful perspectives to themselves. This leaves the organization limited in the scope of its functioning and slow to react in the face of changing circumstances. In contrast, when the relationship between those in leadership and those in followership roles is strong—that is, built on a history of trust and mutual appreciation—people can fearlessly contribute their unique skills and perspectives as needed to the accomplishment of the goal (Berg, 1998; Weick, 1993). Strong relationships between those in the leadership and followership roles thus provide durability to an organization, allowing it to have collaborative connections across the hierarchy (Berg, 1998) and to adapt and respond to changing circumstances and challenges.

## Influencing Organizational Culture

A key role of leadership is the ability to understand and influence organizational culture (Kotter, 1996; Longest Jr. et al., 2000; Schein, 1985; Senge, 1990). Johnson and Johnson is an excellent example of a company whose founders left a legacy through their development of organizational culture. The organization's values statement ("Our Credo"), written in the 1940s, is retained today and can still be found posted on the walls throughout the Johnson and Johnson companies (Collins & Porras, 1998). Modern leadership literature would describe the Johnson and Johnson founders as transformational leaders (Tichy & Ulrich, 1984) because they were able to establish an organizational culture that effectively guided the company's operations. A comprehensive review of the concept of organizational culture is beyond the scope of this chapter. We refer the reader to Chapter 3 for greater detail. Here we focus on the aspects most central to the leadership role of influencing organizational culture.

What is organizational culture? According to Schein (1985), **organizational culture** is the deepest level of basic and shared assumptions and beliefs that are shared by members of an organization. These assumptions and beliefs are learned responses to organizations' efforts to survive within the external environment. The culture survives because it solves problems for the organization, and hence it is de facto considered valid. Additionally, the organizational culture is thought to operate unconsciously and defines the "way we do things around here." Schein (1985) proposes the following definition:

> A pattern of basic assumptions—invented, discovered, or developed by a given group as it learns to cope with its problems of external adaptation and internal integration—that has worked well enough to be considered valid and, therefore, to be taught to new members as the correct way to perceive, think and feel in relation to those problems.

Although the essence of organizational culture is basic assumptions and beliefs shared in the organization, these are nonetheless manifest in more visible levels of organizational life, including tangible artifacts and expressed values that operate at more superficial levels of the organization. Although the more surface levels of artifacts and values may not be the essence of culture, they do signal the essence of culture and are therefore important to understand, interpret, and use as part of the leadership role of influencing organizational culture.

Artifacts are signs of the physical, psychological, or social environment. This might include the physical space, modes of communication both written and verbal, signage in the organization, language used, and other overt behaviors. In the health care setting, artifacts might include the terms used to describe the people served by the organization. Consider the difference between, for example, "diabetic patients" and "patients with diabetes." This simple wording change shifts the focus from the disease to the person, who happens to have a disease. In another example, consider the artifact of referring to "mental health patients" to "clients with mental health issues." Other artifacts might include the way in which an organization uses e-mail, the approach to staff meetings, physical layout of offices or patient care areas, the use or nonuse of uniforms for staff, and so on.

Values are what groups and individuals think ought to be and is distinct from what does exist. For instance, organizational values might include patient-centeredness. In reality, some activities may suffer from inadequate patient-centeredness, but the organization might still hold the value, and its value would be a sign of the culture. Such values are often semi-visible to the degree they are expressed in communication of all kinds. People seeking to influence organizational culture, therefore, can start with discussions of values in forums where they can be debated and challenged, and gradually, if successful, transformed into the basic beliefs about the organization. Such embedding of the values into the basic beliefs will occur only if the values are viewed to solve the fundamental problems of organizational life: survival in the external environment and internal integration of activities.

Table 2.6 illustrates the relationships among basic assumptions and beliefs, values, and artifacts illustrated in a health care organization. Identifying these levels of organizational culture is important for effective leadership, as organizations that are able to align basic assumptions, values, and artifacts foster effective power within organizational members to work together towards common objectives and goals. As organizational change is a critical role of leadership,

individuals in leadership roles can use organizational culture to affect true changes that become embedded as routine practice. For more on the role organizational culture plays in the success of an organization, see the In Practice section on South Essex Partnership University NHS Foundation Trust's experience.

# LEADERSHIP IN HEALTH CARE ORGANIZATIONS: EVIDENCE FROM RESEARCH

## Overview

Leadership in health care organizations is a popular topic for empirical researchers in health services and general management. A simple search for "leadership" in PubMed, the electronic bibliographic database of health care–related articles, produces over 27,000 citations. Most of these citations reference articles that review theories of leadership, provide anecdotes of great leaders, or hypothesize that their study results may be explained by leader behavior. A relatively small number of the citations reference articles that report on data-driven, original research studies of leadership in health care. In these studies, researchers largely have sought to answer five questions: (1) Does leadership matter in health care? In other words, does leadership contribute to desired performance outcomes? (2) Are there individual or setting characteristics that predict leadership effectiveness? (3) What competencies are required for leadership in health care organizations? (4) What are the primary challenges facing those in leadership positions in health care organizations? and (5) What role does leadership play in successful organizational change? While research has not provided definitive answers to these questions, it has found patterns that are suggestive. We review key findings in this section. More extensive reviews of research on leadership can be found in several systematic reviews (Altieri & Elgin, 1994; Cummings et al., 2008; Cummings et al., in press; Gilmartin & D'Aunno, 2007; McCloskey & Molen, 1987). Much of this review relies on these more extensive reviews.

## Leadership and Performance

A key research and practical question is whether leadership contributes to performance. **Performance outcomes** in health care are classified into three major categories: (1) patient-related, (2) staff-related, and (3) management-related

**TABLE 2.6  Elements of Organizational Culture: Assumptions and Beliefs, Values, and Artifacts**

| Basic Assumptions and Beliefs | Values | Artifacts |
|---|---|---|
| The organization has patients' best interests at heart | Patient safety and patient-centeredness | Employee orientation includes patient safety |
| | | Board reporting on patient safety indicators |
| | | Reading library for patients and families |
| | | Satisfaction surveys reviewed by senior management |
| | | Customer relations programs |
| Health is multifaceted | Interdisciplinary care | Interdisciplinary care teams and rounds |
| | | Matrix reporting relationships |
| | | Interdisciplinary quality teams |
| | | Green programs to sustain environment |
| | | Social support groups with patients and families |
| High quality care is essential | Quality of care | Quality metrics defined, measured, and reported |
| | | Incentive systems (monetary and nonmonetary) for quality |
| | | Performance reviews include quality-of-care goals |
| | | Public reporting of quality outcomes |
| | | Quality improvement committee structure |
| Health care is a human right | Equity and ethics | Free clinic partnerships |
| | | Outreach to low-income communities |
| | | Staff voluntarism in community |
| | | Ethical review boards |
| | | Medical ethics training for staff of all levels |
| Health care resources are limited | Efficiency | Process improvement efforts to reduce redundancy |
| | | Pay scales within range |
| | | Physical plant is cost-efficient |
| | | Limit staffing to what is necessary |
| | | Clear travel and conference rules |

(Schofield & Amodeo, 1999). Patient-related outcomes are those that indicate quality of patient care, such as prevalence of adverse events, patient mortality, and patient satisfaction. Staff-related outcomes are those that indicate staff satisfaction with the organization, such as reported job satisfaction, retention rates, and staff commitment to the organization. Lastly, management-related outcomes are the remaining indicators of organizational performance for which management is responsible, such as productivity, effectiveness (i.e., goal achievement), and financial performance. Researchers have found links between leadership and performance outcomes in each of the three categories.

**IN PRACTICE:  South Essex Partnership University NHS Foundation Trust**

Thameside Community Healthcare NHS Trust (now South Essex Partnership University NHS Foundation Trust) merged with another health care organization in April 2000. At the time, there were few remaining Executive Directors from the other trust, it had a track record of weaker performance, and there was a history of competition between the two providers. At the front line, there was a perception among staff that the term "merger" had been used to manage any potential "political" opposition to the change, and in fact it was a "takeover."

At the same time as there were some excellent clinical and nonclinical services in both trusts there were as well as a number of serious weaknesses in clinical service delivery and a faltering hospital closure program in the other trust. These included pockets of negativity in some teams and services, an overreliance on bed-based services, fragmentation of community services, and a belief that community care was unlikely to succeed as a high-quality alternative in the longer term.

In addition to these issues, the local health and social care economy was facing serious financial challenges, reductions in funding were on the horizon, and one of the local authority areas served was on enhanced monitoring for mental health services. Initial analysis of the situation revealed poor and inconsistent leadership, poor communication and morale in many services, and a lack of clarity regarding strategic direction and the desired state in terms of service model. Considering the sensitivity and overt resistance of some of the staff remaining in the other trusts services, the situation needed incisive but well-planned and sensitive intervention.

In order to free up the capacity to move matters forward quickly, interim local management arrangements were put in place for the Thameside operational services and the executive team was freed up to focus their attention on the other trusts services. Initial actions included:

- Face-to-face open and honest staff briefings outputs were undertaken as well as diagnostic and planning sessions involving staff from both trusts. The outputs from these sessions were used to review the service strategy and plans. These were worked through and agreed with local authority partners, commissioners and other stakeholders. Revised plans were jointly published.

- Regular all-staff communication against the revised plans regarding service modernization and service improvement activity were introduced;

- The executive team relocated to a building in the long-stay hospital, to signal that direct attention would be given to the closure program and problem service areas.

A change program of this scale required a challenging multilayered approach to organizational development and service transformation. Ultimately, however, the approach proved successful. The outcomes of this process have been tremendous, and have included:

- Successful closure of the long-stay hospital into world-class accommodation

- Modernization of services with significantly improved delivery as a result

- As staff gained confidence that there was strong management support for improvement, the incidence of "whistle-blowing" poor clinical practices increased; where this was proven, very clear action was taken to reestablish acceptable standards of practice and drive out poor practice

- Public confidence in the ability of the system to deliver safe services and transformation plans increased

Ten years later, a SEPT (South Essex Partnership NHS foundation Trust) is consistently a top performer in the delivery of mental health services. It has been selected to acquire another mental health trust and help transform local services in another locality. As such, SEPT's experience highlights real-world applications of several concepts discussed in this chapter. For example, note how the SEPT leadership team made use of artifacts and feedback loops to change the culture. What other tactics did the leadership team use that may have contributed to their success? What, if anything, was the key to their success?

## Leadership and Patient-Related Outcomes.

Despite the importance of patient outcomes as a measure of quality in health care, few studies have examined the relationship between leadership and patient-related outcomes. A systematic review of these studies (Wong & Cummings, 2007) found that leadership style is highly correlated with key indicators of quality of care, such as the prevalence of adverse events (e.g., patient fractures) and complications for patients (e.g., pneumonia). Negative outcomes are significantly reduced when leaders use people-oriented leadership styles. The use of these styles also correlates with the achievement of clinical goals for patients (e.g., appropriate hemoglobin A1c levels for diabetic patients [Xirasagar, Samuels, & Stoskopf, 2005] and timely receipt of beta blockers for heart attack patients [Bradley et al., 2004]).

The contribution of leadership to other important patient-related outcomes such as patient mortality and satisfaction is less clear. While some studies show no effect of leadership on patient mortality (Boyle, 2004; Pollack & Koch, 2003), others show a significant effect (Cummings, Midodzi, Wong, & Estabrooks, 2009; Houser, 2003). For example, a study of over 21,000 patients in 90 hospitals found that people-oriented leadership was significantly associated with a lower 30-day mortality rate (Cummings et al., 2009). Additionally, leadership explained 5.1 percent of the variance in mortality, after adjusting for patient demographics, co-morbidities, and hospital and nursing factors. Published studies of the effect of leadership on patient satisfaction provide more mixed results about the magnitude and direction of any effect. Some studies find no effect (Larrabee et al., 2004; Raup, 2008), others find a positive effect of people-oriented leadership, and yet others find a positive effect of task-oriented leadership. In sum, current research suggests that the leadership's relationship to patient-related outcomes depends on the outcome measured.

## Leadership and Staff-Related Outcomes.

One of the most robust findings in health care leadership research is that a significant link exists between leadership style and staff-related outcomes. Studies consistently show that the use of people-oriented leadership styles is positively associated with staff job satisfaction, satisfaction with the leader, retention, intention to stay with the organization, and staff commitment to the organization (Cummings et al., in press). Even emotionally exhausted staff members report job satisfaction, if their managers use emotionally intelligent leadership (Cummings, Hayduk, & Estabrooks, 2005). Conversely, research shows that task-oriented leadership styles are negatively associated with staff-related outcomes. The data suggest that the positive effect of people-oriented leadership styles stems from their effect on intermediate staff outcomes. These styles have been linked to workgroup cohesion, reduced stress, empowerment over decisions, and self-efficacy—all of which are associated with increased job satisfaction and retention (Gilmartin & D'Aunno, 2007). Furthermore, when staff work with managers who use people-oriented leadership styles, staff health, anxiety, and stress are improved (Cummings et al., in press).

## Leadership and Management-Related Outcomes.

People-oriented leadership styles also have been associated with several management-related outcomes, including productivity, effectiveness, and staff effort to meet organizational goals. A systematic review of 18 studies of nursing leadership found individual, team, and workgroup effectiveness and productivity were higher in association with people-oriented leadership styles in 13 of the studies (Cummings et al., in press). Six of the 18 studies also found significantly reduced effectiveness and productivity associated with task-oriented styles. These relationships may be explained by the influence of leadership style on workgroup processes. People-oriented styles are positively associated with interdisciplinary teamwork, collaboration, role clarity, innovation, and the use of evidence-based practices—all of which contribute to management-related outcomes.

## Leadership Styles and Organizational Performance.

Despite the many performance benefits associated with people-oriented leadership styles, research suggests that health care leaders as a group rely more on task-oriented styles (Gilmartin & D'Aunno, 2007; Institute of Medicine, 2004). However, the research also shows differences in leadership style by position. Specifically, those who are higher in the organizational hierarchy use more transformational, people-oriented behaviors than those lower in the hierarchy (Gilmartin & D'Aunno, 2007). Their use of one style does not preclude their use of other styles. Those in leadership positions often use a combination of styles. Researchers found that 50 percent of nurses worked in settings in which their manager's leadership styles were mixed, as opposed to people- or task-oriented. Additionally, studies consistently have shown that individuals who use people-oriented, transformational leadership also use contingent reward systems, a behavior associated with task-oriented, transactional leadership (Lowe, Kroeek, & Sivasubramanian, 1996). Researchers hypothesize that staff view the use of contingent rewards as transformational because such rewards have not been used by health care leaders historically (Garman, Davis-Lenane, & Corrigan, 2003).

## Predicting Leadership Effectiveness

Guided by key leadership theories, empirical researchers have sought to determine whether leadership effectiveness can be predicted from three sets of factors: leader traits and characteristics, leader behavior and practices, and the context or practice setting. Their research provides evidence linking aspects of all three sets of factors with leadership effectiveness (Cummings et al., 2008).

### Leader Traits and Characteristics.

Studies of nursing leaders' traits and characteristics find that the most effective managers have personality traits of openness, extroversion, and motivation to manage (Hansen, Woods, Boyle, Bott, & Taunton, 1995). Additionally, age is positively related to leadership effectiveness such that, for example, older nurses demonstrate greater leadership skill. The highest quality studies show no relationship between gender and leadership effectiveness (Cummings et al., 2008). Evidence on the influence of individual work experience is less straightforward. One study found a negative relationship between length of time in position and effectiveness; however, other studies show that having previous leadership experience is positively associated with greater leadership skill (Cummings et al., 2008). These findings related to work experience suggest that greater experience enhances performance, but maintaining the same position for a prolonged period contributes to less effectiveness due to apathy and burnout. More research is needed to identify how much experience is required for leadership effectiveness.

### Leader Behavior and Practices.

Relative to research on traits and characteristics, ample research has been conducted on the influence of individual behavior and practices on leadership effectiveness. Studies have found that increased effectiveness is associated with several behaviors, including practicing and modeling leadership skills, initiating facilitative work structures, providing resources, establishing systems for staff accountability and reward, expressing consideration for staff, being responsive to staff and issues, and using relationship-based competencies (Cummings et al., 2008). One study of nurses in leadership roles found that practicing leadership skills not only increased the leadership effectiveness of the individual, but also the skills

of nurses who worked with the individual (Jenkins & Ladewig, 1996). Additionally, key to a supervisor's effectiveness is using a variety of practices. Staff members perceive supervisors who use a variety of behaviors and practices to be more effective than those who use a more limited set of behaviors (Blankenship, Wilhoit, & Blankenship, 1989).

Only a handful of studies have examined whether specific leader behaviors and practices are more effective in certain situations than others, as suggested by situational and contingency theories. The findings from these studies are mixed. Those examining the effect of matching supervisor behaviors to staff characteristics have largely found no evidence that such matching contributes to leadership effectiveness (Norris & Vecchio, 1992). However, recent studies find that leadership effectiveness depends on individuals in leadership roles matching their behavior to other situational characteristics (e.g., patient severity, team experience, and resources). For example, a study of trauma resuscitation teams found that an empowering leadership style was more effective when patient trauma severity was low and team experience was high, while a directive leadership style was more effective when trauma severity was high or team experience was low (Yun, Faraj, & Sims, 2005). Thus, the evidence suggests that individuals with situational awareness and ability to tailor their behavior to the situation may be more effective.

### Context and Practice Setting.

Research based on nursing practices shows that a key feature of context and practices settings—organizational climate—is associated with the use of leader behaviors critical for effectiveness in a variety of clinical practice settings (e.g., inpatient, outpatient, nursing homes, etc.) (Jones, Guberski, & Soeken, 1990). Specifically, the data show that organizational climates characterized by support for risk-taking, the feeling of being rewarded for a job well done, rules and regulations, and belief in the importance of implicit and explicit goals and performance standards are positively associated with the use of important leadership activities. The finding that organizational climate can influence leadership does not undermine the notion that leadership shapes culture; rather, it suggests that a reciprocal relationship may exist.

## Competencies for Leadership in Health Care

The complexity and difficulty of leading health care organizations (HCOs) in a dynamic world has spurred interest in identifying the **competencies**—defined as knowledge, skills, and abilities—needed to be an effective leader of such organizations. Consortia of major professional organizations such as the Healthcare Leadership Alliance (HLA), leadership development organizations such as National Center for Healthcare Leadership (NHCL), accrediting organizations such as the Commission on the Accreditation of Healthcare Management Education (CAHME), and other researchers have conducted studies to identify core competencies for those in leadership positions in HCOs. These studies (Bradley et al., 2008; Calhoun et al., 2008; Griffith, Warden, Neighbors, & Shim, 2002; Robbins, Bradley, & Spicer, 2001; Stefl, 2008; Stoller, 2008) consistently point to four competency areas for effective leadership: (1) knowledge of the health care industry, (2) technical skills, (3) analytic/conceptual skills, and (4) interpersonal/communication skills. Table 2.7 describes these competencies. The competencies viewed as most critical by people in leadership roles varies with their years of experience. Researchers have found that new nurse managers value interpersonal/communication skills the most, while more experienced nurse managers value technical business skills, particularly negotiation skills, the most (Dienemann & Shaffer, 1993; Kleinman, 2003).

With the identification of core competencies for leadership effectiveness, greater attention has been given to designing and evaluating competency-driven educational programs. Such programs are now offered by universities, medical societies, and HCOs. HCO-sponsored programs are often called "leadership development programs." Conger and Benjamin (1999) observed that such programs often have four aims: develop leadership skill, socialize company vision and values, contribute to strategic leadership initiatives, and foster action learning. To achieve these aims, HCOs rely on a variety of practices such as skill-based training, 360-degree feedback, targeted job assignments, and formal mentoring programs (McCall et al., 1988; McCauley, Moxley, & Van Velson, 1998; Revans, 1980).

The handful of studies on the effectiveness of educational programs provides support for the notion that such programs enhance the leadership capability of individuals. A systematic review of 24 studies of nursing leadership found that participation in educational activities had the most positive effect on leadership practices (Cummings et al., 2008). This review also examined studies that evaluated the effects of individual leaders' traits and characteristics, their behaviors and practices, and characteristics of the context or setting in which individuals work. Not only did the studies find that participation in educational programs contributed to leadership effectiveness immediately, but also a handful of studies found that the effects were sustained. Two studies of nurse leadership development programs found that improved leadership skills remained three months after program participation (Jenkins & Ladewig, 1996; Wessel-Krejci & Malin, 1997) and a third study found positive effects remained at both six and 12 months after program participation (George et al., 2002). Sustained effects appear to exist for graduate education programs as well. A longitudinal study of graduates

## TABLE 2.7  Leadership Competencies in Health Care

| Core competency | Description |
| --- | --- |
| Knowledge of the health care industry | Knowledge of the health care system and the environment in which health care organizations operate (e.g., internal and external stakeholders, reimbursement systems, regulations, etc.) |
| Technical skills | The ability to apply principles from core management disciplines (e.g., accounting, finance, operations, marketing, human resources, information management, negotiation, strategic planning) in the health care environment |
| Analytic and conceptual skills | The ability to organize, manipulate, and use data and knowledge to assess situations, identify alternative courses of action, investigate hypotheses, and accomplish goals |
| Interpersonal and communication skills | The ability to establish, maintain, and facilitate constructive interactions with individuals, within teams, and between groups. Critical to constructive interactions is the ability to communicate clearly and persuasively in verbal and written forms with diverse audiences (e.g., staff, patients, regulators, etc.) |

of one master's-level health care management program found that competencies acquired during the program were retained and improved five years after graduation (Bradley et al., 2008). The graduates—who held positions in a variety of health care organizations (e.g., hospitals, consulting firms, etc.)—reported that the most important competencies for successful job performance in their current position were interpersonal/communication skills, analytic/conceptual skills, and knowledge of the health care industry.

Notably, most of the studies of leadership competency that report a positive effect of education or development programs are based on participants' self-ratings of learning, ability or behavior. Few studies have used objective measures of competency or compared the competency of participants and non-participants. Thus, the question remains whether the effect of such programs is truly positive. Reviewers of this body of work (e.g., Bradley, 2003; Cummings et al., 2008) warn that the positive data on the effect of leadership development programs should be viewed cautiously given the lack of objective data and the tendency for journals not to publish studies that show no significant effects.

## Primary Challenges

People in leadership roles may hold a variety of positions in health care organizations – board member, **senior management** team member (e.g., CEO), department manager, team leader, etc. Each position requires the management of a particular set of challenges. However, a seminal analysis of the U.S. health care system conducted by the Institute of Medicine (IOM) (Institute of Medicine, 2001) indicates *all* individuals in leadership roles face six challenges. According to the IOM, these individuals must develop, implement, and sustain systems that improve the (1) safety, (2) timeliness, (3) efficiency, (4) cost-effectiveness, (5) equity and (6) patient-centeredness of care delivered in their organizations. The IOM explained that these six aims need to be met for the health care system to "cross the chasm" between current practice, which often results in patient harm and waste, and best practice, which the system is capable of delivering to patients.

Little research has examined the extent to which the aims or challenges identified by the IOM overlap with those leaders—in various positions across the spectrum of HCOs—believe they face. However, two surveys of leaders in hospitals—CEOs and board members—offer insight into the challenges confronting those in leadership positions in hospitals. According to the American College of Healthcare Executives'

(ACHE, 2008) annual survey of top issues confronting hospital CEOs, CEOs are most concerned about financial challenges, patient safety and quality, care for the uninsured, and physician-hospital relations. Table 2.8 provides a list of the specific concerns related to each of these issues. The list of CEOs' top concerns has remained consistent since the 2006 survey. A separate survey suggests that hospital board members share CEOs' perceptions of the challenges facing people in hospital leadership roles. The survey results show that board members rate financial performance, quality of care, operations, and business strategy among the top priorities for hospital board oversight (Jha & Epstein, 2009). Thus, there appears to be some consensus about the challenges facing people in senior leadership roles in hospitals. More research is needed to understand whether the perceived leadership challenges are the same for those in other positions and those in other types of HCOs.

## Leadership's Role in Organizational Change

To address the challenges in health care, experts argue that organizational change is required (Institute of Medicine, 2001). Unfortunately, change and implementation efforts frequently fail in health care (and in other industries too) (Nembhard, Alexander, Hoff, & Ramanujam, 2009). This observation has prompted researchers to investigate potential explanations for failed efforts as well as contributors to successful efforts. Much of their investigation has focused on the role of leadership. Based on this investigation, we draw three conclusions about the role of leadership in successful organizational change.

### Conclusion 1: Transformational Leadership Is Important, but Insufficient.

Of all the leadership styles, transformational leadership has received the most attention, in part because it is believed that it is positively associated with current performance and the ability to implement organizational changes that lead to better future performance. The underlying theory is that transformational leadership is effective because it changes the attitudes, values, and behaviors of staff in ways that align with organizational goals. Empirical research supports the positivity of transformational leadership. The finding that people-oriented leadership styles are correlated with better current performance outcomes is largely based on studies of transformational leadership. Although this style of leadership is positively associated with a variety of

## TABLE 2.8 Specific Concerns of Hospital CEOs in Order of Importance

| Financial Challenges |
|---|
| Medicaid reimbursement |
| Bad debt |
| Increasing costs for staff, supplies, etc. |
| Medicare reimbursement |
| Inadequate funding for capital improvements |
| Managed-care payments |
| Other commercial insurance reimbursement |
| Revenue cycle management |
| Emergency Department |
| Competition from specialty hospitals |
| Other |

| Patient Safety and Quality |
|---|
| Redesigning care processes |
| Redesigning work environment to reduce errors |
| Compliance with accrediting organizations |
| Medication errors |
| Nosocomial infections |
| Nonpayment for "never events" |
| Pay-for-performance |
| Leapfrog demands |
| Public reporting of outcomes data |
| Surgical mistakes |
| Other |

| Care for the Uninsured |
|---|
| Medicaid |
| Advocacy for funding |
| Underwriting costs |
| Reaching out to all community members |
| Other |
| Response to other hospital closings |

SOURCE: http://www.ache.org/Pubs/Releases/2009/CEOTopIssues_2008.pdf

performance outcomes, there is evidence that it is insufficient for successful organizational change. A study of nurse managers found managers who received high scores for transformational leadership, yet received low scores from peers and subordinates for effectiveness in leading organizational change (Kan & Parry, 2004). This finding has lead scholars to conclude that additional factors—beyond transformational leadership—are required for successful change in health care (Gilmartin & D'Aunno, 2007).

### Conclusion 2: Supportive Leadership Is Critical to Success.

A large body of work theorizes and shows that leadership support for change efforts greatly impacts the success of such efforts (Bradley et al., 2003; Bradley, Webster, Schlesinger, Baker, & Inouye, 2006; Greenhalgh, Robert, Macfarlane, Bate, & Kyriakidou, 2004; Lukas et al., 2007). Furthermore, this work has identified two types of support that those in leadership roles must provide for successful change: instrumental support, and interpersonal support (Yukl, 2006). Instrumental support refers to various forms of tangible assistance such as providing resources, removing organizational barriers such as existing institutional policies, developing structures to facilitate change efforts, and information sharing. Interpersonal support refers to often intangible actions that contribute to individuals' feeling valued and appreciated, such as providing encouragement, offering feedback, and being inclusive. Inclusive leadership invites and appreciates others' words and deeds, collaborates with others across the professional hierarchy, shares power with others, frames tasks as a team effort, and generally facilitates a positive work climate for all staff members, regardless of profession and position (Nembhard & Edmondson, 2006). In theory, the combination of instrumental and interpersonal support fosters intrinsic motivation within staff, which increases staff commitment and effort in support of change. In turn, staff commitment and effort—in conjunction with a compelling vision and staff accountability—has contributed to successful organizational change.

### Conclusion 3: Successful Change Requires Administrative and Clinical Leadership.

Studies have shown that the support of administrative leadership and clinical leadership is needed for successful organizational change (Bradley et al., 2001; Greenhalgh et al., 2004). **Administrative leadership** support refers to the instrumental and interpersonal support provided by those who hold senior positions in the organization, such as chief executive officer, chief operating officer, and vice president for performance improvement. **Clinical leadership** support refers to instrumental and interpersonal support provided by those who hold clinical positions, such as physicians and nurses. Research on organizational change efforts consistently shows that the support of physicians, and in particular a respected physician champion (of change), is critical to the success of change efforts (Greenhalgh et al., 2004).

## Summary of the Research

While much remains to be learned about the leadership in HCOs, the existing research does offer insights. First, it shows that people-oriented leadership styles (more than task-oriented styles) positively contribute to patient-, staff-, and management-related performance outcomes. Second, it suggests that leaders' traits and characteristics, leaders' behavior and practices, and attributes of the context or practice setting influence leadership effectiveness. Third, it consistently identifies five competencies for leadership of health care organizations. Fourth, it shows that people in leadership roles in health care organizations face a clear set of challenges that have been relatively stable. Finally, it affirms that leadership support—administrative and clinical—is critical for successful organizational change.

These findings have largely been found in studies of nurse leaders, in which a leader was generally defined by holding a formal position in the organization (e.g., dean, administrator, or manager). Relatively few studies have examined the development of informal leadership by professionals with other disciplinary backgrounds (e.g., physicians, administrators, etc.), although there is a growing research stream on physician leadership particularly with respect to change efforts as noted above. As with much research, the extent to which causal inferences can be made based on existing research is limited due to study design issues—e.g., sample selection, variable measurement and data analytic choices (Cummings et al., 2008). Nevertheless, the descriptive and statistical findings support the notion that leadership plays a critical role in influencing performance in health care (Wells & Hejna, 2009).

# SUSTAINING LEADERSHIP

## Succession Planning

Organizations are successful in achieving their goals because, although individuals can come and go, the organizational structure provides a way for activities to continue across such transitions. Unfortunately, turnover in leadership has high costs, which include the search for a suitable replacement; and at senior management levels, searches require substantial consideration of the fit between the applicant and the organizational culture. Subsequently, effective succession planning can make transitions go smoothly and keep the costs of transitions low.

Succession planning is not limited to planning for how to replace any particular individual, but should also include review and codification where possible of organizational cultural elements, work practices, and job design. Furthermore, succession planning includes developing a plan for how remaining staff can provide both context and leadership. It is critical to insure that productivity does not cease or even falter when leadership transitions occur within organizations, and this becomes more difficult the higher the managerial position and the selectivity of the selection process.

Formally, succession planning recognizes cyclical change that involves (1) identifying individuals with the potential for greater responsibility, (2) preparing them to take on those responsibilities through both mentoring and training, and (3) moving them into the higher-level positions, which then leads to identifying new individuals with potential, and the cycle starts again (Garman & Tyler, 2004). A key element of preparing new people for leadership positions includes giving them the opportunity to take on critical developmental assignments that provide the opportunity to develop leadership skills. This cannot be done without allowing them a role in decision making. McCall et al. (1988) asked CEOs to identify elements of developmental experiences critical to their own success and identified five critical abilities that should be developed through early leadership experiences: (1) the ability to set and implement agendas, (2) to handle complex relationships, (3) to promote basic organizational values, (4) to manage the personal demands of top management positions, and (5) to maintain a critical self-awareness, especially in terms of performance. Succession planning should include ways to provide individuals with opportunities to develop these abilities.

## Self-Care

Leadership roles confer substantial personal stress. Although managing both internal and external environments are core responsibilities of leadership, **self-care**, or managing oneself, is also fundamental to sustaining leadership. Managing self is particularly difficult because leadership stresses can be overwhelming and because limited time is available to ensure adequate pause and reflection during the execution of the many responsibilities of those in leadership roles.

Key approaches to managing oneself involve the recognition, analysis, and processing of stressful situations regardless of what can be changed in the situation. Recognition begins with perspective on the larger picture of what might be occurring in one's environment while not losing track of the engagement with the core activities. Holding both perspectives, that of the larger picture and that of the more immediate situation, has been suggested as fundamental to sustained leadership (Bradley et al., 2006a; Heifetz, 1994; Johnson, 1992). As Heifetz has described (1994), people in their leadership role must "get on the balcony" to see the pattern of the dance below, while still also being part of the dance. This metaphor illustrates well the ability to see both the larger system and yet being engaged with the action itself. An additional aspect of recognition is distinguishing the role of the leadership from oneself. Consistent with viewing leadership as a role not only a person, the approach of viewing the failures, conflicts, and setbacks as attributed to the role being played rather than one's personal actions can help address undue stress of leadership.

Analysis of the situation can also be helpful in addressing personal stress and allowing for sustained leadership despite challenges. Analysis might include focused efforts to understand the origins of conflict and to avoid internalizing conflicts as one's own problem when such conflicts may be among or between others (Heifetz, 1994). Such analysis is only possible with adequate listening to the evidence around oneself. Therefore, the ability to listen, hear, and absorb potentially difficult or ambiguous information as part of analyzing sources and solutions to stress is a critical skill for people in leadership roles to practice in order to sustain their personal balance.

Finally, processing the stress related to leadership action is recommended as a routine approach to self-care in leadership positions. Methods of processing stress vary depending on the individual but typically include finding partners and alliances that understand and share values and finding a sanctuary that can provide the reflective space to express and come to terms with stresses of leadership positions. Such reflective time might include relaxation provided by time spent in various hobbies or by more structured coaching or therapy directed at preserving oneself and one's sense of purpose even within the turbulent and sometimes conflicting aspects of executing the leadership function within an organization.

## SUMMARY AND MANAGERIAL GUIDELINES

1. Leadership and management are complementary, but distinct fields of study. Leadership can be defined as the process in which one engages others to set and achieve a common goal, often an organizationally defined goal. In contrast, management can be defined as the process of accomplishing predetermined objectives through the effective use of human, financial, natural, and technical resources.

2. Management and leadership are neither exhaustive not mutually inclusive. A person may occupy a management role but not a leadership role, a leadership role but not a management role, or both roles at the same time.

3. Leadership is born of the relationship between the person(s) in the leadership role and the person(s) in the followership role. Just as followership cannot exist without leadership, leadership cannot exist without followership.

4. Transformational leadership can create changes in organizational culture, but it is important to consider the reasons why a given organization gave rise to the culture. Organizational culture survives because in one way or another, it solves problems for the organization.

5. Strategic problem solving is a useful approach by which those in leadership and management positions may integrate the strategic functions of their roles with the subsequent organizational action required to achieve the set objectives.

# DISCUSSION QUESTIONS

1. Where do leadership and management overlap in definition and responsibilities? Where do they diverge?

2. How have theories of leadership evolved over the course of the twentieth century and into the twenty-first century? When compared with the trait theories of the early 1900s, have modern theories of leadership been simplified, or grown more complex?

3. How does emotional intelligence differ from traditional conceptions of intelligence? What is the relationship between emotional intelligence and leadership?

4. How do transformational and transactional leadership differ? Give an example of each type of leadership and when it might be preferable to the other.

5. What is organizational culture?

6. What are artifacts, and how might they play a role in organizational change?

7. What is a "SMART" objective? Give an example that lays out how the objective meets each of the "SMART" requirements.

8. How might one compare a series of alternative strategies? What are the concerns in using a purely quantitative scale of evaluation?

9. What are the responsibilities of the engaged follower?

10. What kind of actions might an organization take in order to ensure sustained leadership?

# CASE: The New Department Director

As a new director of ambulatory care at the Kennedy Medical Center, Dr. Grant, started to review issues in the hospital, it was clear that something was wrong. Every day, a large crowd of patients and families waited for hours in the emergency department. Although the outpatient ambulatory practices seemed to be running smoothly, the emergency department, which was within Dr. Grant's responsibility, seemed to be a mess. The hospital was typically going "on divert," meaning they would divert ambulances from the emergency room sending them to another hospital in the city because Kennedy Medical Center did not have the beds and staff to accept more patients. Dr. Grant was embarrassed by the situation and was surprised that no one higher up in the administration had noted this as a concern. When he asked about it, his boss, the chief operating officer of the hospital, said it had been this way for a while.

Dr. Grant approached Ms. Downs, the nurse manager of the emergency department and a nurse with 25 years of experience at the hospital, about the issue. She also reported that the situation was no worse than usual and, while it was not ideal, Kennedy Medical Center did better than other hospitals in the area. Still, the situation bothered Dr. Grant, and he made a promise to himself that he would fix it, setting a goal of having 90 percent of the emergency department outpatients in and out of the emergency department in four hours and having the emergency department be on divert no more than once per month. He was not sure what the current percentage meeting this goal was, but given his previous experience at other hospitals, he aimed to accomplish these objectives in six months.

With his problem identified and clear objectives set, Dr. Grant set out to implement a new strategy, which involved (1) teaching the staff about root cause analysis, (2) reengineering the triage work flow to speed access to a clinician, and (3) making what he viewed as a minor fix to the current electronic registration system to improve team communication. This approach had worked well in his former hospital, reducing wait times by more than 30 percent within six months.

After much planning, Dr. Grant held a staff meeting of the nurse manager and the three emergency department supervisors who reported to her to discuss the new strategy. He described the new processes, which were supposed to smooth out redundancies and save time. The staff seemed to like the reengineering process ideas best, so Dr. Grant decided to start with those. He suggested that they could begin the new work flow in two weeks, after staff education and training. The staff meeting was friendly, and no one said much. Ms. Downs had to leave slightly early to pick up her son from school, but the supervisors said that training should be no problem and that two weeks gave them plenty of time. They agreed as a group to start two weeks from Monday.

On the "go live" Monday, Dr. Grant had a morning of meetings outside the hospital but was comforted that Ms. Downs was there and in charge. Unfortunately, two clerks had days off requested months earlier, and the charge nurse for the day had a family emergency over the weekend and was late to work. The staff members remaining were thankfully the most efficient.

When Dr. Grant returned to the hospital after his outside meeting, Ms. Downs was waiting in his office and upset. She said that the new work flow process had fallen apart and that the crowds were worse than ever. She raised her voice and then turned quickly away to go back to her work area, saying, "You have not fixed anything. You have made it worse here. Look at the mess we have today. And it will be just as bad tomorrow. We need to go back to the way it used to be."

Dr. Grant was surprised at how angry Ms. Downs seemed to be. He looked in at the emergency department triage area, and it did look very crowded. The efficient registration clerks were there working, but they could not keep up with the crowds. The beds in the emergency department were already full, and the medical director was suggesting it was time to divert ambulances already even though it was only Monday at noon. Dr. Grant went back to his office and wondered what he should do.

### Questions

1. What problem(s) does Dr. Grant face?

2. Consider individual-level, team-level, and system-level problems. For each, set an objective that is SMART.

3. Could Dr. Grant have avoided the current situation? How?

4. Use concepts of leadership and management from this chapter to recommend what Dr. Grant should do going forward.

# REFERENCES

Altieri, L. B., & Elgin, P. A. (1994). A decade of nursing leadership research. *Holistic Nursing Practice, 9*, 75–82.

American College of Healthcare Executives (ACHE). (2008). American College of Healthcare Executives Announces "Top Issues Confronting Hospitals: 2008" (Press Release). Retrieved November 1, 2008, from http://www.ache.org/Pubs/Releases/2009/CEOTopIssues_2008.pdf

Berg, D. N. (1998). Resurrecting the muse: Followership in organizations. In E. Klein, F. Gabelnick & P. Herr (Eds.), *Psychodynamics of Leadership*. Madison, CT: Psychosocial Press.

Blankenship, M., Wilhoit, K., & Blankenship, C. (1989). Leadership: Do it with style. *Nursing Management, 20*, 81–82.

Bogardus, S. T., Jr., Bradley, E. H., & Tinetti, M. E. (1998). A taxonomy for goal setting in the care of persons with dementia. *Journal of General Internal Medicine, 13*(10), 675–680.

Boyle, S. M. (2004). Nursing unit characteristics and patient outcomes. *Nursing Economics, 22*(3), 111–123.

Bradley, E. H. (2003). Use of evidence in implementing competency-based teaching. *Journal of Health Administration, 20*, 287–304.

Bradley, E. H., Cherlin, E. J., Busch, S. H., Epstein, A., Helfand, B., & White, W. D. (2008). Adopting a competency-based model: Mapping curricula and assessing student progress. *Journal of Health Administration Education, 25*, 37–51.

Bradley, E. H., Curry, L. A., Webster, T. R., Mattera, J. A., Roumanis, S. A., Radford, M. J., et al. (2006a). Achieving rapid door-to-balloon times: How top hospitals improve complex clinical systems. *Circulation, 113*(8), 1079–1085.

Bradley, E. H., Herrin, J., Mattera, J. A., Holmboe, E. S., Wang, Y., Frederick, P., et al. (2004). Hospital-level performance improvement: beta-blocker use after acute myocardial infarction. *Medical Care, 42*(6), 591–599.

Bradley, E. H., Holmboe, E. S., Mattera, J. A., Roumanis, S. A., Radford, M. J., & Krumholz, H. M. (2001). A qualitative study of increasing beta-blocker use after myocardial infarction: Why do some hospitals succeed? *Journal of the American Medical Association, 285*(20), 2604–2611.

Bradley, E. H., Holmboe, E. S., Mattera, J. A., Roumanis, S. A., Radford, M. J., Krumholz, H. M., et al. (2003). The roles of senior management in quality improvement efforts: What are the key components? . *Journal of Healthcare Management, 48*(1), 15–28.

Bradley, E. H., Webster, T. R., Schlesinger, M., Baker, D. W., & Inouye, S. K. (2006). The roles of senior management in improving hospital experiences for frail older adults. *Journal of Healthcare Management, 51*, 323–337.

Bradley, E. H., White, W., Anderson, E., Mattocks, K., & Pistell, A. (2000). The role of gender in MPH graduates' salaries. *Journal of Health Administration, 18*, 375–390.

Calhoun, J. G., Dollett, L., Sinioris, M. E., Wainio, J. A., Butler, P. W., Griffith, J. R., et al. (2008). Development of an interprofessional competency model for healthcare leadership. *Journal of Healthcare Management, 53*(6), 375–390.

Calhoun, J. G., Wainio, J. A., Sinoris, M. E., Decker, M., Hearld, L. R., & Brandsen, L. E. (2009). Outcomes-based health management education: Baseline findings from a national curriculum development project. *Journal of Health Administration, 26*(3), 171–192.

Chaleff, I. (1995). *Courageous follower: Standing up to and for our leaders*. San Francisco, CA: Berrett-Koehler.

Collins, J. C., & Porras, J. L. (1998). Organizational vision and visionary organizations. In G. R. Hickman (Ed.), *Leading organizations: Perspectives in a new era*. Thousand Oaks, CA: Sage.

Conger, J. A., & Benjamin, B. (1999). *Building leaders: How successful companies develop the next generation*. San Francisco: Jossey-Bass.

Cummings, G., Hayduk, L., & Estabrooks, C. (2005). Mitigating the impact of hospital restructuring on nurses: The responsibility of emotionally intelligent leadership. *Nursing Research, 54*(1), 2–12.

Cummings, G., Lee, H., MacGregor, T., Davey, M., Wong, C., Paul, L., et al. (2008). Factors contributing to nursing leadership: a systematic review. *Journal of Health Services Research and Policy, 13*(4), 240–248.

Cummings, G. G., MacGregor, T., Davey, M., Lee, H., Wong, C. A., Lo, E., et al. (in press). Leadership styles and outcome patterns for the nursing workforce and work environment: A systematic review. *International Journal of Nursing Studies*.

Cummings, G. G., Midodzi, W. K., Wong, C. A., & Estabrooks, C. A. (2009). *A multilevel analysis of the impact of hospital nursing leadership styles on 30-day mortality*. Technical Report: University of Alberta Small Faculties Grant Programs. University of Alberta, Edmonton, Canada.

DeRue, D. S., & Wellman, N. (2009). Developing leaders via experience: the role of developmental challenge, learning orientation, and feedback availability. *Journal of Applied Psychology, 94*(4), 859–875.

Dey, J. G., & Hill, C. (2007). *Behind the Pay Gap*. Washington, DC: American Association of University Women Educational Foundation.

Dienemann, J., & Shaffer, C. (1993). Nurse manager characteristics and skills: Curriculum implications. *Nursing Connections, 6*, 15–23.

Doran, G. T. (1981). There's a S.M.A.R.T. way to write management's goals and objectives. *Management Review, 70*, 35–36.

Drucker, P. F. (1954). *The practice of management*. New York: Harper.

Eagly, A. H., & Carli, L. L. (2007). *Through the labyrinth: The truth about how women become leaders*. Boston: Harvard Business School Press.

Fiedler, F. E. (1967). *A theory of leadership effectiveness*. New York: McGraw-Hill.

Floyd, S. W., & Woolridge, B. (1992). Middle management involvement in strategy and its association with strategic type: A research note. *Strategic Management Journal, 13*, 153–167.

Garman, A., Davis-Lenane, D., & Corrigan, P. (2003). Factor structure of the transformational leadership model in human service teams. *Journal of Organizational Behavior, 24*, 803–812.

Garman, A. N., & Tyler, J. L. (2004). CEO succession planning in freestanding U.S. hospitals: Final report. A report submitted to the American College of Healthcare Executives Retrieved from http://www.ache.org/PUBS/Research/SuccessionRpt04.pdf

George, V., Burke, L. J., Rodgers, B., Duthie, N., Hoffmann, M. L., Koceja, V., et al. (2002). Developing staff nurse shared leadership behavior in professional nursing practice ... three studies. *Nursing Administration Quarterly, 26*(3), 44–59.

Gilmartin, M. J., & D'Aunno, T. A. (2007). Leadership in research in health care: A review and roadmap. *Academy of Management Annals, 1*, 387–438.

Greenhalgh, T., Robert, G., Macfarlane, F., Bate, P., & Kyriakidou, O. (2004). Diffusion of innovations in service organizations: Systematic review and recommendations. *Milbank Quarterly, 82*(4), 581–629.

Griffith, J. R., Warden, G. L., Neighbors, K., & Shim, B. (2002). A new approach to assessing skill needs of senior managers. *Journal of Health Administration Education, 20*(1), 75–98.

Hansen, H. E., Woods, C. Q., Boyle, D. K., Bott, M. J., & Taunton, R. L. (1995). Nurse manager personal traits and leadership characteristics. *Nursing Administration Quarterly, 19*, 23–25.

Heifetz, R. A. (1994). *Leadership without easy answers*. Cambridge, MA: Belknap Press of Harvard University Press.

Hooijberg, R., Hunt, J. G., Antonakis, J., Boal, K. B., & Lane, R. (2007). Introduction. In R. Hooijberg, J. G. Hunt, J. Antonakis, K. B. Boal & R. Lane (Eds.), *Being there when you are not: Leading through strategy, structures, and systems* (pp. 1–9). Amsterdam: Elesvier Science.

Houser, J. (2003). A model for evaluating the context of nursing care delivery. *Journal of Nursing Administration, 33*(1), 39–47.

Institute of Medicine. (2001). *Crossing the quality chasm: A new system for the 21st century*. Washington, DC: National Academy Press.

Institute of Medicine. (2004). *Keeping patients safe: Transforming the work environment of nurses*. Washington, DC: National Academy Press.

Jenkins, L. S., & Ladewig, N. E. (1996). A self-efficacy approach to nursing leadership for shared governance. *Nursing Leadership Forum, 2*, 26–32.

Jha, A. K., & Epstein, A. M. (2009). Hospital governance and the quality of care. *Health Affairs, Web Exclusive*. Retrieved July 31, 2010, from http://content.healthaffairs.org/cgi/content/abstract/hlthaff.2009.0297v1

Johnson, B. (1992). *Polarity management: Identifying and managing unsolvable problems*. Amherst, MA: HRD Press.

Jones, L. C., Guberski, T. D., & Soeken, K. L. (1990). Nurse practitioners: leadership behaviors and organizational climate. *Journal of Professional Nursing, 6*, 327–333.

Judge, T. A., Bono, J. E., & Locke, E. A. (2000). Personality and job satisfaction: the mediating role of job characteristics. *Journal of Applied Psychology, 85*(2), 237–249.

Kan, M. M., & Parry, K. W. (2004). Identifying paradox: A grounded theory of leadership in overcoming resistance to change. *Leadership Quarterly, 15*, 467–491.

Kellerman, B. (2008). *Followership: How followers are creating change and changing leaders*. Boston: Harvard Business School Press.

Kelley, R. E. (1988). In praise of followers. *Harvard Business Review, 66*(6), 142–148.

Klein, K. J., Ziegert, J. C., Knight, A. P., & Xiao, Y. (2006). Dynamic delegation: Shared, hierarchical and deindividualized leadership in extreme action teams. *Administrative Science Quarterly, 51*, 590–621.

Kleinman, C. (2003). Leadership roles, competencies and education: How prepared are our nurse managers? *Journal of Nursing Administration, 33*(9), 451–455.

Kotter, J. (2001). What leaders really do. *Harvard Business Review, 79*(11), 85–96.

Kotter, J. P. (1996). *Leading change.* Boston: Harvard Business School Press.

Landy, F. G., & Conte, J. M. (2004). *Work in the 21st century: An introduction to industrial and organizational psychology.* Boston: McGraw-Hill.

Lantz, P. M. (2008). Gender and leadership in healthcare administration: 21st century progress and challenges. *Journal of Healthcare Management, 53*(5), 291–301; discussion, 302–303.

Larrabee, J. H., Ostrow, C. L., Withrow, M. L., Janney, M. A., Hobbs, G. R., & Buran, C. (2004). Predictors of patient satisfaction with inpatient hospital nursing care. *Research in Nursing & Health, 27*, 254–268.

Letts, C. W., Ryan, W. P., & Grossman, A. (1999). *High performance nonprofit organizations. Managing upstream for greater impact.* New York: John Wiley.

Likert, R. (1961). *New patterns of management.* New York: McGraw-Hill.

Locke, E. A., & Latham, G. P. (1990). *The theory of goal-setting and task performance.* Englewood Cliffs, NJ: Prentice Hall.

Longest Jr., B. B., Rakich, J. S., & Darr, K. (2000). *Managing health services organizations and systems* (4th ed.). Baltimore: Health Professions.

Lowe, K. B., Kroeek, K. G., & Sivasubramanian, N. (1996). Effectiveness correlates of transformational and transactional leadership: A meta-analytic review of the MLQ literature. *Leadership Quarterly, 7*, 385–425.

Lukas, C. V., Holmes, S. K., Cohen, A. B., Restuccia, J., Cramer, I. E., Shwartz, M., et al. (2007). Transformational change in health care systems: An organizational model. *Health Care Management Review, 32*(4), 309–320.

March, J. G., & Simon, H. A. (1958). *Organizations.* New York: John Wiley.

McCall, M. W., Lombardo, M. M., & Morrison, A. M. (1988). *The lessons of experience: How successful executives develop on the job.* New York: Free Press.

McCauley, C. D., Moxley, R. S., & Van Velson, E. (1998). *The Center for Creative Leadership handbook of leadership development.* San Francisco: Jossey-Bass.

McCloskey, J. C., & Molen, M. T. (1987). Leadership in nursing. *Annual Review of Nursing Research, 5*, 177–202.

Morgeson, F. P., DeRue, D. S., & Karam, E. P. (2010). Leadership in teams: A functional approach to understanding leadership structures and processes. *Journal of Management, 36*, 5–39.

Nembhard, I. M., Alexander, J. A., Hoff, T. J., & Ramanujam, R. (2009). Why does the quality of health care continue to lag? Insights from management research. *Academy of Management Perspectives, 23*(1), 24–42.

Nembhard, I. M., & Edmondson, A. C. (2006). Making it safe: The effects of leader inclusiveness and professional status on psychological safety and improvement efforts in health care teams. *Journal of Organizational Behavior, 27*(7), 941–966.

Norris, W. R., & Vecchio, R. P. (1992). Situational leadership theory: a replication. *Group & Organization Management, 17*(3), 331–342.

Pollack, M. M., & Koch, M. A. (2003). Association of outcomes with organizational characteristics of neonatal intensive care units. *Critical Care Medicine, 31*(6), 1620–1629.

Raup, G. H. (2008). The impact of ED nurse manager leadership style on staff nurse turnover and patient satisfaction in academic health center hospitals. *Journal of Emergency Nursing, 34*(5), 403–409.

Revans, R. W. (1980). *Action learning*. London: Blond and Briggs.

Robbins, C. J., Bradley, E. H., & Spicer, M. (2001). Developing leadership in healthcare administration: A competency assessment tool. *Journal of Healthcare Management, 46*(3), 188–202.

Robbins, S. P., & Judge, T. A. (2010). *Essentials of organizational behavior* (10th ed.). Upper Saddle River, NJ: Pearson Prentice Hall.

Schein, E. H. (1985). *Organizational culture and leadership. A dynamic view*. San Francisco: Jossey-Bass.

Schofield, R. F., & Amodeo, M. (1999). Interdisciplinary teams in health care and human services settings: Are they effective? *Health & Social Work, 24*(3), 210–219.

Senge, P. (1990). The leader's new work: Building learning organizations. *Sloan Management Review, 32*(1), 7–23.

Smith, K. K., & Berg, D. N. (1997). Cross cultural groups at work. *European Management Journal, 15*, 8–15.

Stefl, M. (2008). Common competencies for all healthcare managers: The healthcare leadership alliance model. *Journal of Healthcare Management, 53*(6), 360–373.

Stoller, J. K. (2008). Developing physician-leaders: Key competencies and available programs. *Journal of Health Administration Education, 25*(4), 307–328.

Suter, L. E., & Miller, H. P. (1973). Income differences between men and career women. *American Journal of Sociology, 78*(4), 962–974.

Tichy, N. M., & Ulrich, D. O. (1984). The leadership challenge—a call for the transformational leader. *Sloan Management Review, 26*(1).

Weick, K. E. (1993). The collapse of sensemaking in organizations: The Mann Gulch disaster. *Administrative Science Quarterly, 38*(4), 628–652.

Wells, W., & Hejna, W. (2009). Developing leadership talent in healthcare organizations. *Healthcare Financial Mangement, 63*(1), 66–69.

Wessel-Krejci, J. W., & Malin, S. (1997). Impact of leadership development on competencies. *Nursing Economics, 15*, 235–241.

Wong, C. A., & Cummings, G. G. (2007). The relationship between nursing leadership and patient outcomes: A systematic review. *Journal of Nursing Management, 15*, 508–521.

Xirasagar, S., Samuels, M. E., & Stoskopf, C. H. (2005). Physician leadership styles and effectiveness: An empirical study. *Medical Care Research and Review, 62*, 720–740.

Yukl, G. A. (2006). *Leadership in organizations* (6th ed.). Upper Saddle River, NJ: Pearson Prentice Hall.

Yun, S., Faraj, S., & Sims, J. H. P. (2005). Contingent leadership and effectiveness of trauma Resuscitation Teams. *Journal of Applied Psychology, 90*(6), 1288–1296.

# PART TWO

# Micro Perspectives

# Chapter 3

# Organization Design and Coordination

Martin P. Charns and Gary Young

## CHAPTER OUTLINE

- **Why Is Organization Design Important?**
- **Twin Structural Issues: Differentiation and Integration**
- **Coordination at the Macro Level**
- **Line and Staff Positions**
- **Integrated Delivery Systems**
- **Service Lines**
- **Centralization and Decentralization**
- **Parallel Organization**
- **Hybrid Structures**
- **Organizations with Multiple Goals**
- **Governance and the Three-Legged Stool of Administration, Medical Staff, and Board**
- **Micro-Level Coordination**

## LEARNING OBJECTIVES

1. Describe the variants of organization structure found in health care organizations

2. Describe the facilitating and hindering effects of organization structure on coordination

3. Provide a framework for determining what organization design is most appropriate for a given health care organization

4. Describe the mechanisms and processes of coordination at the micro level and their effects on quality of care

# KEY TERMS

| | |
|---|---|
| Centralization | Planning and Goal Setting |
| Communication | Pooled Interdependence |
| Coordination | Program Organization Structure |
| Decentralization | Programmable Work |
| Differentiation | Programming Approaches to Coordination |
| Direct Contact | Reciprocal Interdependence |
| Feedback Approaches to Coordination | Relational Coordination |
| Functional Structure | Relationships |
| Governance | Rules and Procedures |
| Group Coordination | Sequential Interdependence |
| Hierarchy of Authority | Service Line |
| Hybrid Organization | Simultaneous Interdependence |
| Integrated Delivery Systems | (Team Interdependence) |
| Integration | Specialization |
| Integrators | Standardization of Output |
| Interconnected | Standardization of Skills |
| Interdependence | Standardization of Work |
| Liaison Roles | Supervision |
| Matrix Organizations | Task force |
| Mutual Adjustment | Task Uncertainty |
| Organization Design | Team |
| Organization Structure | Vertical Information Systems |
| Parallel Organization | |

---

## IN PRACTICE: A Tale of Two Units

Unit A, a general medical unit in a major Eastern teaching hospital, is characterized by high dissatisfaction among the nursing staff and is the target of frequent complaints from residents and attending physicians. Communication among the nurses, therapists, social workers, residents, and attending physicians regarding patient care is poor, and relationships among them are strained.

The unit generally appears to be in a state of chaos. Patients and their families seek information about their status from physicians, nurses, and other staff, and frequently complain that they receive conflicting information from the medical and nursing staffs. At the same time, lengths of stay are unacceptably long due to poor communication among the staff rather than due to unique patient needs.

---

**IN PRACTICE: A Tale of Two Units** *(Continued)*

The organization of the hospital is similar to that of most major teaching facilities, with the major departments representing professional (nursing, social service, dietary) and nonprofessional (housekeeping, security, transportation) functions.

On Unit A, care paths—protocols specifying the sequence and timing of tasks for patients with particular routine conditions—have been introduced to streamline delivery of care. However, they frequently are not followed. Unit A staff stopped holding interdisciplinary rounds several years ago on the belief that these meetings consume too much valuable staff time. Because many different internal medicine physicians admit patients to the unit, unit staff found it difficult to conduct rounds with the physicians.

Unit B is a general medical unit in a different Eastern teaching hospital. It has a reputation for quality care and responsiveness to both patients and their families. Nurses and other staff express high satisfaction about their work. Communication between nurses, therapists, social workers, residents, and attending physicians is said to be frequent, timely, and accurate, and relationships among them appear to be strong. In general, the unit runs smoothly and responds well to routine situations as well as unusual cases.

Unit B differs from Unit A in several ways. Nursing staff on the unit are organized into teams, with each team responsible for assigned patients from admission to discharge. The house staff in medicine in the hospital also are organized into teams, and except when beds are not available, each team admits patients to one patient care unit. Two house staff teams admit to unit B, and each works primarily with one nursing team. Other health professionals in the hospital, such as social workers, clinical pharmacists, physical therapists and occupational therapists, care for patients primarily on one unit.

Nurses, physicians, and other health professionals on unit B conduct interdisciplinary rounds daily. Unit B patients are assigned to care paths, and patients' progress on the care paths is reviewed in the interdisciplinary rounds. In addition, the nurse manager and chief resident meet regularly to review unit performance measures, such as patient satisfaction, hospital-acquired infections, and pressure ulcers, and to plan actions to improve care.

---

# CHAPTER PURPOSE

Differences between the effectively functioning Unit B and the chaotic Unit A are seen by many administrators and health care professionals as arising from differences in leadership or staff competence. Others attribute the differences in unit performance to Unit A having been "chaotic" as long as anyone remembers. But is the chaos on Unit A inevitable? The concepts presented in this chapter provide a perspective that illuminates how the effective functioning of Unit B and the chaotic functioning of unit A are affected by both the organizational structures of the two hospitals and the differences in the mechanisms and process of **coordination** in the two units.

**Organization design** is the arrangement of responsibilities, authority, and flow of information within an organization, resulting in its **organization structure**. The structure of an organization is analogous to human anatomy, with the caveat that an organization's structure can be changed. The

two closely interrelated parts to organization design are (1) how to divide the work and responsibilities and allocate them to units in an organization, and (2) how to coordinate the work of those units to perform the organization's overall work effectively. These two parts of organization design are intimately related, because the division of labor and grouping of responsibilities directly affect the ease of achieving coordination. It is especially important in large organizations, where the arrangement of individuals into separate groupings results in the facilitation of some flows of information and coordination while simultaneously hindering others.

There is no one universally best organization design. What design is best for a given organization depends on characteristics of its environment, work, and technologies, and its strategy. For example, a large hospital pursuing a strategy of providing the best care in a number of different patient conditions and diseases (e.g., heart disease, cancer, women's health, mental health) might organize into different mini-hospitals, each containing all of the professional and nonprofessional staff required to deliver care to its particular patients. This would facilitate the coordination among staff within each mini-hospital and focus the organization's resource allocation on each mini-hospital. On the other hand, a teaching hospital emphasizing its graduate medical education and educational programs in other professions might best organize along the traditional lines of different medical specialties and professions. (Why these are appropriate organization designs for different strategies will be explained later in the chapter).

# WHY IS ORGANIZATION DESIGN IMPORTANT?

Many people, including many senior leaders of major health care organizations, are not fully aware of the effects of organization design. Similar to the physical design of buildings, many health care organizations reflect the incremental addition of new activities in the organization, without rethinking how the organization would be best structured. What results is a design that may no longer fit the organization's strategy or contribute to organization performance. The reference to "silos" in health care organizations has become commonplace and is a reflection of a dysfunctional organization design where the different parts function autonomously and do not communicate or coordinate well with each other. Because there is strong empirical evidence that coordination is related to patient outcomes (Gittell et al., 2000; Young, 1997), organization design and its effect on coordination should be important for health care leaders.

At the most micro level in an organization, people are grouped together into work units having a common supervisor. What we call these smallest work units varies from organization to organization. For example, faculty in a medical school may be organized into divisions (e.g. cardiology, medical oncology, infectious diseases), each led by a division chief. These are part of larger units, which in the medical school example typically are departments (e.g., medicine, surgery, pathology), led by department chairs. Nurses in hospitals typically are organized into nursing units (here we are using the term "unit" to refer to generic "nursing units" or "patient care units" and not just to "intensive care units"), each led by a nurse manager. In small hospitals, the nurse managers may report directly to the vice president for nursing or vice president for patient care services. In larger hospitals, there is typically an intermediate level of organization in nursing, with several nurse managers being accountable to each associate director of nursing, who in turn is accountable to the vice president. Because there is so much variation in the position titles used in practice, it is difficult to discuss through example, but what is key is understanding that the building blocks of units aggregate hierarchically into larger and larger entities.

Through their hierarchies, organizations allocate resources and conduct planning and hold people accountable for performance and the use of those resources. For example, the nursing department in a hospital has an annual budget, most of which is for staff salaries, and the vice president of nursing is held accountable for effective management of that budget. The authority and responsibility for staff supervision and budget is typically delegated down the hierarchy to the lowest level managers, in our example the nurse managers. Different organizational units also have different goals, the achievement of which are planned to aggregate into achievement of the overall organizational goals. Usually, people with a common supervisor are located in the same physical proximity to facilitate supervision. Both the reporting relationship and physical proximity of people affects the frequency of their interactions, and this in turn affects the ease or difficulty of coordinating their work.

A "table of organization" or "organizational chart," consisting of boxes and lines, provides a shorthand for describing structure. Organizations are complex. No one chart, diagram, or perspective of any organizational model will provide total understanding of all organizational phenomena, nor is taking any single perspective sufficient to manage an organization effectively. Considering structure, however, is an important approach to understanding the complexity of organizations. It helps us understand why some things seem to "fall through the cracks" all too often and not get done properly or at all, even when they are supposed to be the responsibility of capable and motivated people. It also helps us to understand and predict where conflict will occur in an organization and to manage it better. Knowledge of the effects of organization structure can pinpoint areas where conflict can occur without even considering the people involved. This is not to say that the characteristics of individuals are not important; it is to say that by taking a structural perspective on the dynamics of organizational phenomena, an even deeper understanding can be developed and used to manage more effectively.

In complex organizations, every way of dividing work and responsibilities to be performed by different units has both advantages and disadvantages. The problems of any structure accompany its benefits. In a large organization it is always necessary to partition the organization into units. One of the most critical design choices is determining where to place the boundaries between units. Wherever they are placed, they encourage people within work units to work closely together, but at the same time they make it more difficult for people in different units to work with each other. People within work units tend to develop a common set of goals and perspectives on their work, but the different goals, as well as competition for resources, contributes to conflict among units. When organization design is done well, those tradeoffs are made in a way that most facilitates and least hinders the accomplishment of an organization's work. The problems inherent in a good design are the ones an organization can live with and the ones that interfere as little as possible with its most important work.

# TWIN STRUCTURAL ISSUES: DIFFERENTIATION AND INTEGRATION

Every organization design has both functional and dysfunctional characteristics. The key question, then, is whether there is any way to determine what is the best design for a given organization? Structural contingency theory (Lawrence and Lorsch, 1967) is one framework that helps in considering the complex tradeoffs in organization design. Structural contingency theory is based on the premise that there is no one best universal way to organize, but that the best way to structure and manage an organization depends on its unique work, environment, and strategy. While today this is well accepted, for much of the twentieth century organization researchers were searching for the one best way. Only in the 1960s did researchers begin to see that the highest-performing organizations in different industries (performing different types of work and having different technologies) were organized and managed differently (Thompson, 1967; Woodward, 1965).

## Differentiation

Lawrence and Lorsch (1967) extended earlier findings relating organizational performance to the "fit" between organization design and the characteristics of an organization's task (and

associated technology) and environment. The environment of an organization includes not only its physical environment, but also the political, financial, technological, scientific and regulatory conditions that are outside of the organization but affect it. Environment consists of other organizations such as suppliers, competitors, regulatory bodies, professional societies, labor unions, and customers or clients, individually and collectively. Environment also includes the information and resources needed by an organization. Different units in an organization perform different tasks, using different technologies, and face different sub-environments from each other. The original research on industrial firms noted that the tasks and sub-environments differ among research, engineering, manufacturing, marketing, and sales departments. Not only do these departments do different work, but they require different interpersonal, time, and goal orientations to do their work most effectively. For example, researchers need relatively long time horizons, whereas manufacturing staff need relatively short time horizons because those match the nature of their work.

Similarly, different departments face and interact with different sub-environments. The researchers have to keep up with scientific advances in their field and interact with a scientific sub-environment. The marketing staff, in contrast, needs to keep in touch with what their customers are looking for, what competitors are doing, and what market trends are; they have to focus on a market sub-environment. Thus, Lawrence and Lorsch found that the highest performing industrial firms encouraged each subunit in the organization to develop staff cognitive and emotional orientations and operating practices that were tailored to their particular tasks and sub-environments. This means that they had different goals, and recruited and developed staff with different time and interpersonal orientations. Since generally people in the same workgroup interact more frequently with each other than with people in other workgroups, have similar goals, and are evaluated on similar objectives, they tend to develop a common way of thinking and viewing their work and their sub-environment.

Building on work of earlier researchers (Burns and Stalker, 1961; Miller and Rice, 1967; Woodward, 1965) they also noted that the internal structures and management styles also appropriately varied among organization units. Thus, units with tasks that were highly uncertain (such as research), largely staffed by highly educated professionals, should not be closely supervised or expected to produce results in short time periods. The organization structure that is most appropriate for supervising researchers is one in which each supervisor has a large span of control—i.e. many subordinates—and there are few levels in the hierarchy. In contrast, manufacturing, with its shorter time frames (you do not want a manufacturing process to be out of control for very long, lest you have much waste and inefficiency), requires a closer level of supervision and control. This would generally require a smaller span of control and more levels in the hierarchy. Lawrence and Lorsch referred to these needed differences in both structure and employee orientations among different organization units as **differentiation**.

One way of looking at differentiation is as **specialization**. Each part of an organization performs a specialized function. It does this best if it is organized and managed to meet the unique requirements of its specialty work. Different specialties relate to different sub-environments, and different specialists have different personal characteristics. For example, comparing internists and surgeons, internists are often referred to as being more cerebral with somewhat longer time orientations, whereas surgeons are more action-oriented with shorter time spans. Psychiatrists are more people-oriented, and radiologists focus more on technology. Different specialties also relate to different professional and accrediting organizations and read different journals, reflecting the different scientific bases of their work. Similarly, nurses, doctors, social workers, and physical therapists also have different characteristics (nurses focused on caring and doctors on curing) and have different professional and accrediting organizations, and journals.

## Integration

In addition to the relationship between differentiation and organizational performance, Lawrence and Lorsch also found a strong relationship between integration and organizational performance. **Integration** is the coordination of activities among organizational units, including the management of conflicts among the units. They also found that differentiation and integration were antagonistic to each other. The greater the differences among units, the more difficult it is for them to integrate their efforts. This is both because of the differences among units, such as in the orientation of staff in the different units, and the tendency to be focused on the unit's goals and activities to the exclusion of the larger organizational goals and activities. However, the highest-performing organizations

in this line of research were those that achieved both differentiation and integration. How they did so, we will address below.

# COORDINATION AT THE MACRO LEVEL

Coordination needs to be considered at two levels in the organization: the macro level, where the focus of analysis is on the overall coordination needs and structural approaches to address those needs, and the micro level, where the focus is more on the actual processes used to achieve coordination in specific situations. To understand coordination at the macro level, we first have to address needs for coordination, or **interdependence** among organizational units.

## Interdependence

If different units in an organization could work independently of each other, there would be little need for coordination. However, in complex organizations this total independence is never the case. One way to start to examine interdependence is to ask questions such as, "For what reasons, and how often, do various people or organizational units need to work together?" "How critical is it that they coordinate their efforts?" and "To what extent can the work of one unit affect the work of another?" In answering these questions, it is helpful to consider the flow of work in the organization. In examining the flow of work, the most critical work to focus on is that work which directly contributes to the central goals of the organization. In health care organizations, this is the direct delivery of patient care. Secondarily, it is important to examine work that is conducted in support of direct patient care, such as performance of diagnostic tests. Third in importance is the work to support the functioning of the overall organization, such as accounting, finance, and human resource management.

As a first broad assessment of the needs for coordination, three elements should be considered:

1. Interconnectedness of the work of the units
2. Uncertainty of the tasks
3. Size of the organization

As Galbraith (1973) noted, as each of these increases, so do the information-processing requirements within the organization, and this is a major part of the need for coordination.

## Interconnectedness of Work

Interconnectedness is an attribute of work itself. To the degree that different elements of work need to fit together, we refer to them as being **interconnected**. This consideration is quite separate from whether one person, several people, a group, a unit, or several units in the organization perform the different work elements. To the extent that an organization structure separates elements of work that are highly interconnected, the work efforts must be coordinated for successful task accomplishment. A few examples ranging from low to high interconnectedness will illustrate this point. At the low end of the scale, consider hospital outpatient clinics. To the extent that the clinics have different staff and serve different patient populations, the work of any one clinic inherently has little connection with the work of other clinics. Their need to coordinate stemming from interconnectedness in delivering care is low. (Among these same clinics, there might be a greater interconnectedness in education of medical and nursing students and house staff where the various clinical experiences need to "mesh.") To the extent that the clinics serve the same patient population having multiple diseases, the potential interconnectedness of the clinics' work is greater. At the other end of the continuum, where medical staff, nurses, and therapists together serve a patient population in a particular clinical area, the work of these different groups is highly interconnected. Similarly, the elements of work performed by different members of a surgical team are highly interconnected.

## Task Uncertainty

As **task uncertainty** increases, so does the need for coordination. This theme is central in the writing of the early contingency theorists (Burns and Stalker, 1961; Duncan, 1972; Galbraith, 1973; Lawrence and Lorsch, 1967; Perrow, 1967, 1972). Quite simply, where there is a high degree of certainty in a task, few things arise that cannot be planned in advance. Different units in an organization can perform their work in a predetermined manner, with few exceptions that require redirecting efforts to assure coordination. For example, most of the work done by clinical laboratories in performing tests for patients has little inherent task uncertainty, so the work contributes little to the need for coordination between clinical units and laboratories. Uncertainty is introduced when a patient's condition is changing rapidly, and it is necessary to perform laboratory tests at unanticipated times and to perform them quickly. Unreliable equipment in the laboratory also increases uncertainty. Accompanying this uncertainty is a somewhat greater need for coordination between a clinical unit and clinical laboratories. Uncertainty related to changes in a patient's condition can also be seen to increase needs for coordination among the different providers caring for that patient and between a patient care unit and support services.

Although greater than in the example above, relatively little uncertainty exists in the task of postoperative care for simple surgical procedures. Thus, there is a low need for coordination between surgeons and nursing personnel providing postoperative care. On the other hand, the very nature of medical diagnosis reflects high uncertainty, which contributes to the need for coordination between nursing and medical staff on an inpatient medical unit. Interconnectedness and uncertainty are conceptually distinct; they interact in contributing to the need for coordination.

## Size

Size also contributes to the need for coordination. As more parts of an organization have a role in performing a particular task, the problem of coordinating these parts increases in complexity. Usually in larger organizations, work is more specialized than in smaller organizations, and interconnected elements are in different units. Thus, size is related to the need for coordination both directly by complicating coordination in specific instances, and indirectly by contributing to placement of interconnected work in different units.

When needs for coordination deriving directly from an organizational task are not adequately addressed, performance of that task is reduced, and overall organizational performance suffers. Examples are reduced quality of care, complications of treatment, and extended length of hospital stays.

## Sharing Resources

Interdependence among organizational units also stems from *sharing of resources* such as space, people, and equipment. Greater efficiency in use of resources can be attained by sharing among units, but at a cost of requiring coordination. If the strategy of sharing resources is chosen but coordination needs are not effectively met, both efficiency and effectiveness can suffer. For example, if a social worker shares time among several clinical areas and needs to attend clinical conferences on each and if the conferences are not coordinated so that no time conflict exists for the social worker, that person's contribution to the delivery of care to patients on one or more units will be compromised.

Slack resources and duplication of resources can also be used to reduce information-processing requirements. One of the best examples of this in a health care setting is having excess capacity in support services. Scheduling would be less critical and all requests could be met rapidly, but at the cost of having to invest in and maintain additional equipment and personnel. (The concept of slack resources is discussed in greater detail in Chapter 9.)

### Types of Interdependence

Another classical view of interdependence was presented by Thompson (1967), who defined three types of interdependence: **pooled interdependence**, **sequential interdependence**, and **reciprocal interdependence**. He saw them as presenting increasing coordination costs for an organization. The least costly to address is pooled interdependence, a situation in which the work of different units has low interconnectedness. The elements of work in the different units simply do not need to fit together directly. The outpatient clinics treating different patient populations described earlier have pooled interdependence. With both sequential and reciprocal interdependence, there is a greater interconnectedness among the work of the different units than with pooled interdependence. Thompson argued that needing a direct link between the work of two units (sequential) was more difficult and therefore more costly to coordinate than needing only indirect links (pooled), and that needing direct links in two directions (reciprocal) was even more difficult to coordinate. Van de Ven and Delbecq (1974) later

added **team interdependence** (also called **simultaneous interdependence**) as a fourth category, where the reciprocal tasks need to be performed simultaneously; for example, the work in a surgical team. (For more on interdependence, please refer to Chapter 5.)

## Structural Approaches to Coordination

In designing the structure of an organization, it is necessary to consider both the benefits of differentiation (specialization) and those of integration. Galbraith (1973, 1977) argued that organizations apply a series of approaches to meet the needs for coordination at a macro level. These are:

1. Hierarchy of authority
2. Rules and procedures
3. Planning and goal setting
4. Vertical information systems
5. Lateral relations

### Hierarchy of Authority

In the simplest of situations, the **hierarchy of authority** itself acts as an adequate coordinating device to ensure that the work of different units meshes together. In such situations, different units are able to conduct their work relatively independently of other units. Often the need to coordinate stems primarily from the sharing of resources. For example, consider the nursing department hierarchy in Figure 3.1. On the

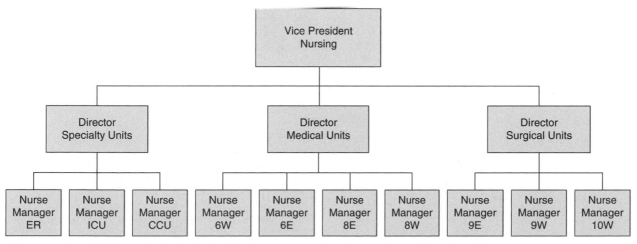

**Figure 3.1** Partial Organization of Nursing Department in a Large Acute Care Hospital.
SOURCE: Delmar, Cengage Learning.

few occasions when disagreements among units arise, issues can be referred for resolution to the first common supervisor in the hierarchy. To minimize the number of levels, issues need to be referred up the hierarchy, units that have more occasions to refer issues should be placed as close together as possible in the hierarchy. These are units that have greatest interdependence. For example, consider the organizational units labeled A through F in Sample Organization I in Figure 3.2. If A and D were more interdependent than any other units, placement of A and D under the same supervisor, as shown in Sample Organization II in Figure 3.2, would allow the hierarchy to function more effectively as a coordinating device than the grouping shown in Sample Organization I. For the classical organization theorists, the hierarchy was the primary coordinating mechanism. However, few health care organizations have coordinating needs that can be met solely by the hierarchy. Furthermore, since physicians often are not employees of many health care organizations such as community hospitals and long-term care facilities, no common supervisor exists in these health care organizations. Other approaches must be used to achieve coordination.

## Rules and Procedures

Frequently, use of the hierarchy of authority is augmented by organizational **rules and procedures** specifying how things are to be done and what things should not be done. Examples range from "food is not to be taken from the cafeteria," to procedures for ordering supplies, to complex protocols for delivering care. As long as the work is programmable, rules and procedures can be developed and applied to facilitate coordination. When predictable exceptions arise, the rules themselves may call for application of additional rules. When unanticipated exceptions arise, an issue may require referral up the hierarchy.

Such use of the hierarchy and rules and procedures is the basis of bureaucratic organizations. Their efficiency lies in the development of optimal procedures, eliminating the need to

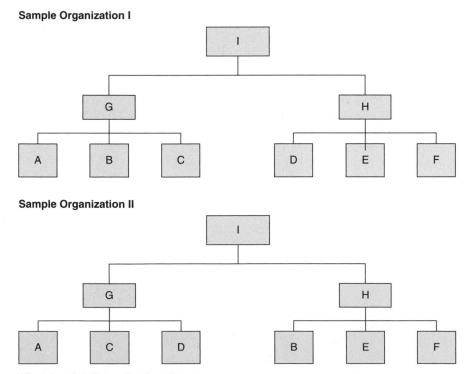

**Figure 3.2** Simplified Partial Organization Structures.
SOURCE: Delmar, Cengage Learning.

"reinvent the wheel" each time a situation is encountered. They can be used in two different ways. First, they can provide certainty for people at the top by delineating and controlling the behavior of others lower in the organization. Their weakness, however, lies in the difficulty in fully controlling behavior, which is a special problem in professional organizations, and the inability to respond to unprogrammable tasks. Second, they can be used to provide guidance in performing work and to promote codification of agreements on how work is to be done, determined by the individuals responsible for interconnected elements. More on use of rules and procedures will be discussed below in the section on the micro level of coordination.

## Planning and Goal Setting

In utilizing **planning and goal setting**, the degree of control is reduced over that inherent in the use of rules and procedures, since only outcomes are specified and not the procedures to reach those outcomes. These techniques allow for adaptability in addressing new or unforeseen circumstances, so they can be used in situations that are less programmable than those that can be handled by rules and procedures. Planning and goal setting will also be discussed in more detail in the section below on the micro level of coordination.

## Vertical Information Systems

The approaches described above can be enhanced through the use of **vertical information systems**, such as planning and budgeting systems, computer-based and manual information systems, and assistants to various managers. Such approaches increase the information-processing capacity of the hierarchy by facilitating information flow up and down the hierarchy and by increasing the capabilities of various managers to handle more information. Vertical information systems allow managers to control the units under them better by providing more and also more timely information about what is happening in the units. These systems augment use of the hierarchy, rules and procedures and planning, but they rely upon vertical—up and down—interactions among people in the organization and are built on the hierarchy itself.

## Lateral Relations

A qualitatively different approach to coordination is the use of lateral relations, where members of different units interact directly with other units and laterally across internal boundaries. Use of lateral relations is most appropriate if there

is both high interdependence and high uncertainty. Usually, members of the units must interact frequently to ascertain what is happening and to plan actions to respond jointly—for example, in diagnosis and treatment involving more than one specialist or health care provider. Several different types of lateral relations can be used in response to differing needs for coordination. Among these are direct contact, liaison roles and integrators, teams and task forces, and a matrix organization. The most extreme approach to use of lateral relations is a complete reorganization in which the previously existing organizational units are eliminated and the organization is restructured placing the most interdependent activities and people into new organization units. This "program structure" will be described in more detail below.

Building on the work of Galbraith (1973), Charns and Tewksbury (1993) developed a continuum of organizational forms representing increasingly greater emphasis on coordination across traditional specialized departments in health care organizations. An elaboration of their continuum of organizational forms is displayed in Figure 3.3. On the far left of the continuum is the traditional **functional structure**, where the organization design emphasizes each profession and discipline independently. This is graphically indicated in Figure 3.3 by the vertical expense of top triangle, "emphasis on differentiation/specialization" being at its greatest size. On the far right of the continuum in Figure 3.3 is the complete organization design by programs. "Program organization" is the generic term for the structure on the far right end of the continuum, but in health care it is often called a "service line" organization. This organization design emphasizes each program independently as well as coordination across disciplines within programs. This is graphically indicated by the height of bottom triangle, "Program/Service Line Integration" being at its greatest size at the right end of the continuum. Using the continuum to compare different organization designs, we will first describe these contrasting organizational structures, and second, we will describe alternative forms starting with augmentations to enhance coordination across disciplines by building on the functional structure.

*Functional Structure (1)*: In this structure, segmentation is based on specialty departments. The structure emphasizes each specialty department functioning relatively independently of the other departments. The functional structure appears on the far left side of the continuum to indicate its extreme emphasis on differentiation by specialty departments and

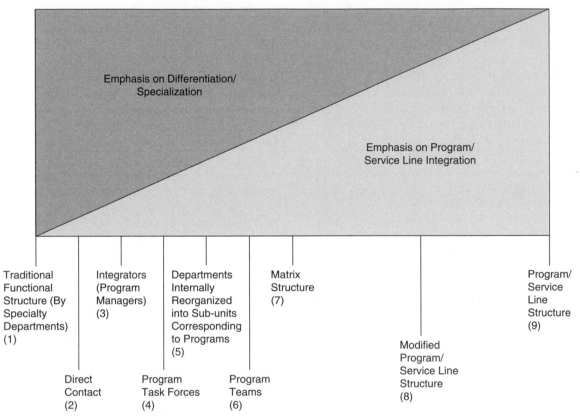

**Figure 3.3** Continuum of Organization Structures.
SOURCE: Delmar, Cengage Learning.

lack of any emphasis on integration across the specialties. In health care, the departments typically correspond to different professional functions (e.g., medical specialties and subspecialties, nursing, social work, etc.) and nonprofessional functions (e.g., environmental services, transportation). These are displayed as the "boxes" in the organization chart in Figure 3.4.

*Program Structure (9)*: At the extreme other end of the continuum is the program structure (or "service line" structure). In this structure, the emphasis is on individual programs, such as heart, cancer, women's health, and mental health. There may be up to 20 such programs in a large hospital, but we have shown only two, for heart and cancer, in Figure 3.5 due to limitations of space. Each program contains all of the key staff from different professions and disciplines needed to deliver services to its patient population. The program manager has authority over the staff who work in

that program. Where there are several staff from any particular profession, they typically report to a supervisor from that profession, who in turn reports to the program manager. For example, nursing staff on the cardiology unit report to a nurse manager for the cardiology unit, who in turn reports to the heart program manager. Similarly, in Figure 3.5, medical and surgical subspecialties of cardiology and cardiac surgery, social work and clinical pharmacy are shown in addition to nursing as subunits within the heart program; and medical oncology, surgical oncology, radiation oncology, nursing, social work, and clinical pharmacy for the cancer program are shown as subunits of the cancer program. These professional subunits are representative, and others such as physical therapy and occupational therapy may also be subunits within their respective programs. These are not shown in Figure 3.5 only due to limitations of space. Note that no nursing department is shown in Figure 3.5, as all components of nursing are

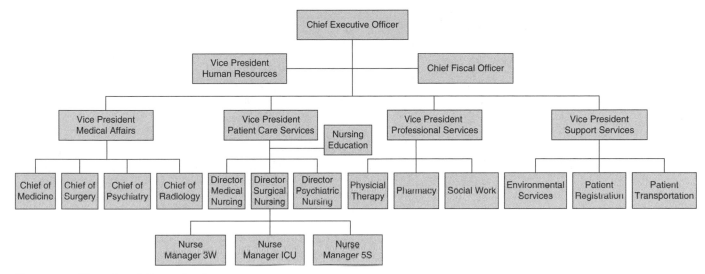

**Figure 3.4** Functional Organizations.
SOURCE: Delmar, Cengage Learning.

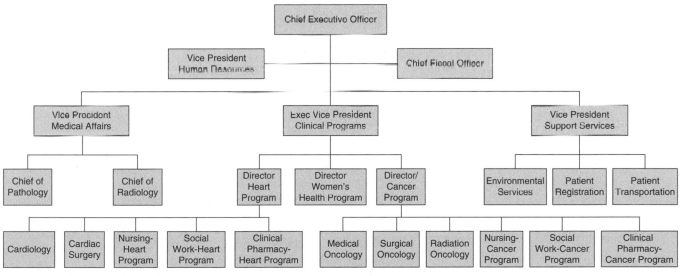

**Figure 3.5** Program Organization.
SOURCE: Delmar, Cengage Learning.

located within respective programs. However, medical specialties of pathology and radiology are shown because it is not practical to completely divide these up and include them in different programs, radiation oncology being an exception. These specialties must provide services to patients cared for by different programs. Thus, at the highest level of the pure program organization, there is no differentiation by profession or discipline; this differentiation by profession and discipline only occurs *within* each program. For each program, the program manager can determine staffing mix and levels that are most appropriate for the particular program. This contrasts with the functional structure, where staffing decisions are made by each department independently. Note also that in large hospitals, the programs function as "mini-hospitals," having all staff needed to provide care for their patients and sometimes even having their own buildings. The program structure is shown at the extreme right end of the continuum of organizational structures in Figure 3.3 because it places total emphasis on integration of disciplines and professions within each program, and no emphasis on managing the professions and disciplines individually.

Neither the pure functional structure nor the pure program structure meets all the needs of a typical health care organization, and in its completely pure form, the program organization (9) is not feasible except in extremely large organizations. In the functional structure (1), no formal mechanism other than the hierarchy exists to facilitate coordination of professionals from different departments, yet there is interdependence among these professionals in delivery of care. Conversely, in the program structure (9), each program unit facilitates the coordination of professionals within the program, but there is no mechanism other than the hierarchy to facilitate coordination of like professionals (e.g., nurses) across programs or to facilitate coordination of care for patients whose illness requires care of more than one program (e.g., a patient with heart disease and diabetes). Although the hierarchy (a vertical coordinating mechanism, as described above) can be effective for decisions such as resource allocation, it is too limited for addressing high levels of interdependence, such as those inherent in the delivery of complex patient care. It is common, then, to find that health care organizations implement various other mechanisms to facilitate coordination across functional departments. These are shown as alternatives (2) through (8) in Figure 3.3 and are discussed below.

*Direct Contact (2):* The **direct contact** form is structurally the same as the functional structure but differs in that staff in one functional department may directly contact members of other departments. This is relatively simple and consumes few organizational resources. On the other hand, it is not as powerful as other lateral relations, which is why it is displayed only slightly to the right of the functional structure on the continuum in Figure 3.3, indicating a small degree of integration across departments. Direct contact occurs very frequently in health care and other organizations, especially where it is facilitated by having the people who need to interact most frequently

located physically close to one another. Factors that limit its effectiveness are:

- The people contacted may be occupied with other issues and not motivated to contribute to solving a problem they see as belonging only to the initiator of the contact. This is not unusual, and often is exacerbated by an organization's reward system. Thus, what is a high priority for a contacting unit may be a low priority for a unit being contacted.

- In responding to the request of another unit, the work flow of the contacted unit may be interrupted, resulting in reduced efficiencies and thus a cost to the organization. The more a unit is pressed for performance on a particular set of goals unique to itself, the less willing members will be to assist other units. For example, if a maintenance department is held closely to its budget, it will be reluctant to meet the requests of other departments if such requests might jeopardize achievement of the maintenance department's budget objectives. Thus, it is not unusual to find a maintenance department responding more slowly than is desired by nursing or other staff members to a request they see as urgent, even when all parties agree that that is maintenance's responsibility. Often maintenance sees the request as one that would require either interruption of other activities or use of overtime, both of which would negatively affect its ability to meet its budget.

- Members of one unit may not know whom to contact in a second unit to initiate their requests.

Note that in some organizations, direct contact is discouraged by managers in functional departments for reasons of maintaining control over their personnel, but historically, the prohibitions on direct contact have diminished. In health care, direct contact among providers from different disciplines and professions is commonplace in the direct delivery of care.

*Integrators and Liaison Roles (3):* Added to the functional structure are individuals who have responsibility for coordination of program issues across the traditional professional specialty departments. Sometimes these integrators are called "program managers" even though, by definition, they do not have formal authority. Without formal authority for staff in any of the specialty departments, **integrators** must rely upon their interpersonal skills, association with senior managers to whom they report who do have formal authority, and the perception of the value they add to the organization as the sources of their influence with other staff and departments. Integrators are more effective when they have good interpersonal skills and when they are seen by those they are integrating as being able to understand their points of view. Characteristics of effective integrators is well described in Lawrence and Lorsch (1967) and Charns and Tewksbury (1993). **Liaison roles** are created within departments to facilitate coordination between that department and others. For example, the clinical laboratories may appoint individuals to answer calls from patient care units trying to locate test results. Note that while the liaison role can facilitate coordination, it is typically not a highly influential position. Because it is located within a department, the individuals in those roles have loyalties to their departments, are not as likely to understand the needs of other departments, and do not fulfill a neutral position among parties being coordinated.

*Program Task Forces (4):* Program **task forces** are groups constituted of members from different professional departments to address a program-related task, such as planning for new services or improving a care process. They may be led by the program manager, but not necessarily. By definition, a task force is a temporary structure, and it disbands once its task is completed. Its strength as an integrating mechanism derives from its bringing together people from different departments so that they can work directly together.

*Departments Restructured Internally (5):* Reorganizing departments so that their subunits correspond to programs facilitates coordination. It does so by establishing a consistent pattern of interaction among staff in different departments performing activities for the same program. An example is organizing nursing into specialized units (e.g., cardiology, oncology, etc), rather than having general medical-surgical units. This would facilitate the coordination between specialist physicians and nursing staff on the corresponding specialty units. Assigning patients to social workers, physical and occupational therapists, and other professionals based on the patient condition and treating medical specialty (which correspond to different programs) is another example of reorganizing departments by specialty program and results in facilitating coordination among all staff working in each program. Note that staff continue to be accountable to their professional departments, but the departments lose some influence over these personnel as they are influenced by others from other departments working together in the same program.

*Program Teams (6):* This structural alternative formalizes the interactions among staff from different professional departments and forms them into **teams**. Two types of such

teams frequently seen in health care are multidisciplinary patient care teams organized around specialized patient care units or ambulatory care clinics or practices, and program management teams. The latter might consist of one or more physicians, a nurse manager and an administrator, mutually responsible for managing a program. For example, a team of the chief of cardiology, chief of cardiac surgery, nurse manager for the cardiology unit, and an administrator can have joint responsibility for a heart program. In contrast to task forces, teams are enduring over time with ongoing responsibility for their mutual work. Often, the program managers have input, but not responsibility, for performance evaluations of staff who work in the program.

*Matrix Structure (7):* The **matrix organization** is two organization structures—the traditional functional structure and the program structure—overlaid on each other. The two dimensions of the matrix are the specialty departments and the programs, and it is shown in the middle of the continuum of Figure 3.3 to represent its balance between the functional and program organizations. Typically a small portion of the personnel are in "matrixed" positions—i.e., they have two bosses of equal authority. Other staff have a single supervisor. A matrix organization for an acute care hospital is shown in Figure 3.6. To simplify the drawing, only a few departments, programs and positions are shown. An example of a

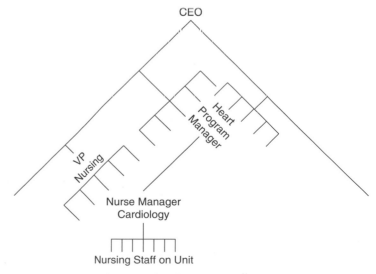

**Figure 3.6** Matrix Organization.
SOURCE: Delmar, Cengage Learning.

"matrixed" position is the nurse manager of cardiology, who is jointly responsible both to the nursing department and the heart program. Staff nurses who work in the cardiology unit are responsible only to the nurse manager.

Matrix structures have all of the advantages of both the traditional functional structure and program structure, providing management and coordination of both functions and programs simultaneously. The matrix, however, is the most complex organizational form and is costly to manage, having two complete hierarchical structures and bringing conflicts between them out to a manifest level in the organization. This requires a high level of conflict management skills, which few organizations have.

*Modified Program Structure (8)*: While the pure program structure (9) is theoretically possible, it is not practical in any but the largest organizations where there are sufficient numbers of staff in each profession in each program to use resources effectively and have needed coverage, and to address the maintenance of professional competence and other professional issues (this is the "mini-hospital" described above). Therefore, organizations that adopt a program structure typically modify it by establishing coordinating mechanisms that cross the programs and address professional needs.

A modified program structure for a teaching hospital is shown in Figure 3.7. Note the position of vice president for nursing and nursing education, and that there are no lines of authority from the nursing VP to the nurse managers in the various programs. The VP for nursing and/or a Nursing Council are responsible for professional issues in nursing. The VP of nursing would not have formal authority over the nurses in the programs, however. S/he, in conjunction with the Nursing Council (if one is established), would set policy for professional practice, and assist in recruitment and professional education. Note also the addition of chiefs of medicine and surgery in the modified program structure (Figure 3.7), as compared to the pure program structure (Figure 3.5). They or their subordinates would be responsible for professional development of physicians in internal medicine and surgery, respectively, and also for educational activities, such as the residency programs, within each of these specialties. Without these or similar positions, there would be no mechanism to coordinate the specialty physicians who organizationally are in different programs (heart, cancer, etc.). The pure program structure (9) and modified program structure (8) can be thought of as mirror images of structural alternatives (1) through (6), with alternatives (2) through (6) providing

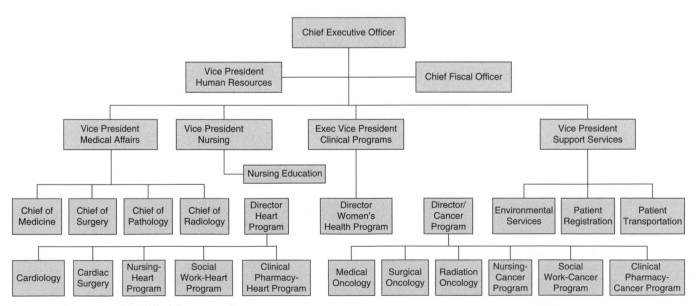

**Figure 3.7** Modified Program Structure.
SOURCE: Delmar, Cengage Learning.

coordination across functional departments and alternative (8) providing coordination across programs. In practice, there are fewer variations of coordinating mechanisms across programs (8) than there are coordinating mechanisms across departments (2–6).

Until the 1980s, few health care organizations were structured in matrix or program forms, with most following traditional structures with task forces and sometimes with teams. In the 1980s a number of health care organizations adopted program structures, with the programs representing families of services, as described above. Some of these organizations returned to traditional structures and others have maintained their program structures. Some organizations have adopted program structures to mimic apparent trends or at the suggestion of consultants. There is little evidence in the organizational literature to support the benefits of a program structure as compared to a traditional functional structure, although some health care leaders have very strong feelings about the benefits of their service line structures (Byrne et al., 2004; Charns and Tewksbury, 1993; Greenberg et al., 2003; Young et al., 1994).

## Line and Staff Positions

Managers who have authority and responsibility for activities and decisions that directly contribute to the provision of goods and services are referred to as "line managers." In the functional structure in health care, these are the managers and their subordinates in supervisory positions of the various professional and nonprofessional departments, as shown in the organization chart in Figure 3.4. In the program organization, the program managers and their subordinates who are supervisors are the "line managers." Units that provide support services to the organization, such as human resources, finance, and information systems, are referred to as "staff departments." Individuals in staff departments do not directly provide care to patients. This is sometimes confusing in health care because we use the term "staff" also to refer to providers of care (e.g., medical staff, nursing staff). In the functional organization in Figure 3.4 and the program organization and modified program organizations in Figure 3.5 and Figure 3.7, the staff departments are shown with a horizontal line connecting to the side of the box (cf. human resources, finance, nursing education).

## Integrated Delivery Systems

The organization structures described above have focused on single health care organizations, such as an individual hospital. The concepts can also be applied to multiple locations in an integrated delivery system (IDS). The two dimensions discussed above, profession and program, are augmented by consideration of geography in IDSs. Traditionally, IDSs are organized into one or more regions, with each region consisting of all of the health care organizations—hospitals, long-term care facilities, rehabilitation facilities, ambulatory care facilities, and home health agencies—in that geographic region. A large IDS may have several regions, and the regional hierarchical structure in which each facility is accountable to regional management provides for a management perspective of each region as a whole. This allows for resource allocation that considers all of the needs in each region and a perspective that is greater than that of any single facility. This is important to minimize competition among facilities in each region and avoid unnecessary duplication of services. The regional management structure can also provide some coordination among facilities within each region. For example, it can contribute to transfer of patients among locations. This structure is similar to the traditional functional structure described above, in that the primary focus is on each facility independently.

To augment coordination across facilities or across regions, lateral coordinating mechanisms can be used. For example, establishing a senior-level nurse executive to coordinate and set policy for professional practice and disseminate best practices at the highest level of the IDS is conceptually similar to position 3 in Figure 3.3, except that what is being coordinated across the regions and facilities is professional practice. The individual high-level nurse executive can be further augmented with task forces or teams, for example by having a systemwide nursing council to discuss professional practice issues across the system. Similarly, within a region, program managers can have program oversight for each of several clinical programs, such as those discussed above (heart, cancer, women's health, etc.). This will provide greater management focus on each program and help to coordinate policy and resource allocation decisions from a regional perspective as well as assist in disseminating best practices for each program among the facilities within each region. This can also be done for the IDS as a whole, but the broader focus of the program manager will be a limiting factor in how much attention can be placed on operational, as contrasted with policy, issues. The position of individual program managers also can be augmented with teams and task forces, as described above. In some IDSs, a matrix or program structure is implemented. To implement a program structure for an

IDS would require organizing each facility into a program structure. Comprising each program in each region would be the respective programs at each facility in the region (for example, mental health programs in each facility). Because of the practical need for local management of the facility as a whole, it is difficult to carry this to the extreme program form (9), in which case the facility leadership responsibilities would be limited to maintaining the facility, and staff in each program would report first to a local program manager, who in turn would report to the regional program manager.

## Service Lines

In the section above, we have used the term "program" and indicated that the term "service line" is often used in health care instead of the generic term "program." **Service lines** are programs that are organized around diseases or conditions, patient populations or "technologies" (such as transplant). Service lines can be established for any combination of three purposes: to monitor expenses, to facilitate marketing, or to manage a service as a business entity, including coordinating delivery of patient care. Each of these purposes carries with it different interdependencies among departments, and therefore different coordinating needs. Coordination needs are highest for delivery of patient care and are substantially less for monitoring expenses and for marketing. The structures on the right side of the continuum in Figure 3.3 are needed only for achieving high levels of coordination across professional departments. Therefore, the matrix and program structures are needed only when the intent is to address coordination of patient care and not for marketing or monitoring expenses alone. A detailed discussion of service lines is presented in Charns and Tewksbury (1993).

## Centralization and Decentralization

Within a given organization structure, responsibilities and authority for various actions and decisions can be located at different levels vertically and shared horizontally in the hierarchy. For example, in a hospital, decisions on equipment purchases can be made at the level of department managers or at the level of the chief officers (i.e., chief operating officer, chief executive officer, chief financial officer). They can be made by an individual or by a committee. The degree to which decisions are made lower in the organization is referred to as vertical **decentralization**, and conversely the degree to which decisions are made at the higher levels of the organization is referred to as **centralization**. In fact, some

decisions may be centralized and others decentralized within the same organization. Department managers may make equipment purchases up to a fixed amount, while having to refer larger purchase decisions to higher levels. They may also have authority for hiring decisions but not for financial decisions (or vice versa).

In general, the important question to ask is whether decisions are being made at the level in the organization at which the relevant information resides. In high-technology industries such as health care, greater vertical decentralization is expected because of the expertise at lower levels in the organization. As a general rule, decisions should be made at the lowest possible levels, especially when the majority of workers are professionals. In addition, decentralization has positive benefits for motivation of lower level managers. That is, having authority to make decisions for their departments provides motivation to make those decisions wisely.

Greater decentralization also leads to less uniformity and standardization in the organization, as each department or unit can make its decisions independently of others. Thus, with greater decentralization of personnel policies and equipment purchases, an organization will find greater variation in personnel policies and practices and in the equipment purchased. This may be good or bad for organizational performance. Thus, many organizations use a combination of centralization and decentralization, with organization-wide policies that operating units have to follow, but local authority in making the specific operating decisions.

In **program organization structures**, the full advantage of managing programs is achieved when decisions are decentralized to the program managers. This way, each program (or mini-hospital) has the overall perspective of its program and can act to set policy and make operational decisions most appropriate for each program. However, full decentralization of decision making to programs contributes to greater variation among programs in their policies and practices.

In multi-institutional systems (or integrated delivery systems), decisions can be centralized in the corporate office or decentralized to the regions or further to the individual operating organizations (hospitals, long-term care facilities, etc.). When the majority of decisions are centered at the corporate office, the organization is said to be vertically centralized. In the design of a health care system, for example, an important design factor is deciding upon the extent to which individual operating units can develop their own strategic plans separately from those developed by the corporate office. Typically, major policies are determined at the corporate office to provide for uniform approaches across the whole system. A major part of the activities at the decentralized level are concerned with the direct delivery of care, implementation of policies and ensuring quality.

## Parallel Organization

The concept of **parallel organization** refers to a part of an organization structure that is parallel to and distinct from the main part of the organization. The concept is used in two different ways. First, a parallel structure of committees and task forces accountable to an oversight committee is often used for large change programs. In this case, the parallel organization is usually temporary, although "temporary" may last for several years. The task forces are multidisciplinary and usually are comprised of individuals from different levels in the organization. The purpose of this type of parallel organization is to bring people together, while avoiding the negative effects of differences in power of different participants and of limits in perspectives of each department and level in the hierarchy. It facilitates openness, creativity, and problem solving for the purpose of organizational improvement. Second, the organizational forms from "addition of program managers" through "teams," depicted as forms (3) through (6) on the continuum in Figure 3.3, are sometimes referred to as parallel structures (Charns and Tewksbury, 1993). More commonly, however, they are referred to as "integrating mechanisms."

## Hybrid Structures

One other variation on the organization designs described above is the **hybrid organization** structure. In this case, organizations maintain their traditional functional structures and create program structures for just one or two programs. For example, they may develop a freestanding heart center or cancer center (or both), each with all the key personnel required to provide those services. Thus, the organization is a hybrid, with most of it following a functional design but with a few distinct programs organized as completely separate entities from the main part of the organization. The advantages of this structure are the focus it places on the activities of the freestanding center(s) and the facilitation of coordination within each center. It also maintains the advantages and disadvantages of the functional structure for the main part of the organization. However, this structure introduces a barrier between each freestanding center and the rest of the organization.

## Organizations with Multiple Goals

The literature on organization structure has been developed primarily in industrial organizations, whose primary goal is to effectively and efficiently produce products or services. Although in multiproduct firms, the organization design problem is more complex than in single-product firms, the goal of effectiveness and efficiency in producing the products remains. Health care organizations, however, often have the multiple goals of patient care, research, and education. Designing a structure to meet one of these goals often conflicts with designs to meet others. Using teaching hospitals as their primary example, Stoelwinder and Charns (1981) wrote about structuring organizations that have multiple goals. They noted that organizing for patient care would result in segmenting the organization into multidisciplinary units, each aligned with a disease or patient population (i.e., a program structure). They also noted that in contrast, organizing for maintaining state-of-the-art competence in each profession and discipline and recruiting and developing new members of each profession and discipline would result in an organization segmented into units, each representing a different profession or discipline. Note that the discipline-based organization structure places greatest emphasis on differentiation, as shown on the left in Figure 3.3 and discussed earlier in the chapter. The program organization structure emphasizes integration, or coordination, across professions and disciplines in the delivery of care, as shown on the right in Figure 3.3. These conflicts among goals and among organization designs are often resolved by the differential power among different stakeholders.

## Governance and the Three-Legged Stool of Administration, Medical Staff, and Board

Hospitals also differ from other types of organizations because of the unique position of their medical staffs. Whereas professionals in other types of organizations are typically employed by the organizations, this is not true in the majority of hospitals. In community hospitals, physicians are organized into a voluntary medical staff, governed by bylaws and a set of committees. All other hospital personnel are organized hierarchically within clinical and administrative units. The coexistence of separate lines of authority for hospital administration and medical staff has long been a distinguishing feature of community hospitals. The medical staff is ultimately accountable to the board of trustees, as is the chief executive officer (CEO) and the other staff of the hospital who ultimately report to the CEO. Throughout much of the twentieth century, this type of **governance** structure was quite viable for community hospitals, as the reimbursement and competitive environment for hospitals generally imposed few pressures for greater integration between hospital and medical staff leadership. However, during the last 20 years, significant changes in reimbursement policies and market competition within the industry have forced hospitals to develop stronger linkages between administration and medical staff that include placing medical staff members on the hospital governing board (Young, 1997). In most academic health centers, the medical staff are faculty of the affiliated medical school. An affiliation agreement is the vehicle that binds the medical school and teaching hospital. Traditionally there have been stronger linkages between medical staff and hospital administration in academic health centers than has been the case with community hospitals.

# MICRO-LEVEL COORDINATION

The macro-level approaches to coordination discussed above provide the vehicles for achieving coordination, but it is the micro-level processes through which coordination actually is achieved. In analyzing micro-level needs for coordination, it is helpful first to ask whether the work is **programmable work**. Can specific activities be detailed and assigned to different individuals and groups so that if each piece is performed correctly and according to plan, different people's and units' efforts will mesh together? If so, then the work is programmable. Tasks having inherently high uncertainty, where one cannot fully anticipate the events that might possibly occur, do not lend themselves to detailed rules and procedures and are largely not programmable. Neither are tasks for which relationships between causes and effects are not well understood. Examples of unprogrammable work are

diagnosing complex or unusual diseases, developing research hypotheses, and designing programs for educating the public in new health practices.

The second question to ask in assessing micro-level needs for coordination is how familiar the people involved are with a particular action or decision. What is familiar to an experienced worker may be unfamiliar to an inexperienced one. Familiarity with an issue affects understanding of cause-and-effect relationships and of how to perform required activities, as well as the chances for successful completion of the work. Thus, although an appendectomy is a fairly programmable surgical task, coordination among members of a surgical team who have never performed this procedure would be more complicated than for a team experienced in the procedure.

Coordination of work at the micro level has been the subject of considerable research. This research has shown, in health care and other settings, that coordination affects organizational performance (e.g., Argote, 1982; Duncan, 1973; Georgopoulis and Mann, 1962; Shortell et al., 1994; Van de Ven and Delbecq, 1974). Knaus et al. (1986) found that variations in mortality in critical care units were related to the level of coordination in the units. With the development of more refined measurement tools, this line of work continues to be advanced (Shortell et al., 1991). In one of the largest empirical studies, Young et al. (1998) found the pattern of coordination among nurses, surgeons, and anesthesiologists to be related to risk-adjusted rates of postsurgical complications. In addition to clinical outcomes, some studies have found a link between coordination and outcomes such as greater patient satisfaction and shorter lengths of stay (Gittell et al., 2000). These performance outcomes are increasingly relevant in a more cost-conscious, patient-centered health care environment.

But research also shows that the most effective way of achieving coordination varies with the characteristics of the work performed, primarily its certainty or uncertainty.

## DEBATE TIME: Service Lines

Many health care leaders are proponents of service line organization structures. What are the reasons why hospitals should adopt a service line structure? What are the reasons why hospitals should organize by a functional structure? When do you think task force and team structures, augmenting the functional structure, are most appropriate?

Duncan (1973) for example, provided one of the first empirical studies of variation in coordination within work units, finding that work units change their patterns of interaction in response to differing levels of task uncertainty. Building upon the theoretical work of March and Simon (1958), Van de Ven and Delbecq (1974) found variations in patterns of coordination among units facing different levels of task uncertainty.

Charns et al. (1981) and Charns and Schaefer (1983) extended the findings of Van de Ven and Delbecq (1974) and the theoretical writings of Mintzberg (1979) to suggest that work groups use two primary approaches to coordination: **programming** and **feedback**; and that the use of these approaches is related to the effectiveness of patient care units. This work was the basis for the study by Young et al. (1998) on coordination and surgical outcomes.

## Programming Approaches to Coordination

The set of **programming approaches to coordination** includes three ways of standardizing the performance of work that are most effective when the work is well understood and programmable. These approaches may also be called "standardized approaches".

**Standardization of work** processes is the use of rules, regulations, schedules, plans, procedures, policies, and protocols to specify the activities to be performed. Included are care plans and multidisciplinary clinical critical paths, which specify for any particular patient condition the interventions required and anticipated results at various times.

**Standardization of skills** is the specification of the training or skills required to perform work. Often this is achieved through specification of minimum levels and types of education, certification as evidence of meeting minimum qualifications, or on-the-job training.

**Standardization of output** specifies either the form of or specifications for intermediate outcomes of work as they are passed from one job to another. It can also set specifications and goals for the service or product being provided.

## Feedback Approaches to Coordination

In situations of high uncertainty, programming approaches alone cannot provide the needed coordination. Exchange of information and feedback is needed. **Feedback approaches to coordination** (also called "personal approaches"), which facilitate the transfer of information in unfamiliar situations, include the following:

**Supervision** is the basis for coordination through an organization's hierarchy. It is the exchange of information between two people, one of whom is responsible for the work of the other.

**Mutual adjustment** is the exchange of information about work performance between two people who are not in a hierarchical relationship, such as between two nurses, between a nurse and a physician, or between a case manager and other care providers.

**Group coordination** is the exchange of information among more than two people, such as through meetings, rounds, and conferences.

Feedback approaches to coordination are more time consuming and require more effort than programming approaches. However, they are needed to achieve effective decisions and actions in situations characterized by high levels of uncertainty.

Evidence indicates that higher-performing patient care units in teaching hospitals differ from lower-performing units in their greater use of all six types of coordinating mechanisms (Charns, 1981; Young, 1998). High-performing units utilize plans, rules, procedures, and protocols not as constraints and organizational "red tape," but as guidelines for routine work. Contrary to earlier writings, effective use of programming approaches actually allows staff—especially nurses—greater discretion in their work.

Often, new roles (a macro-coordination approach) are created in health care organizations to facilitate coordination, and these rely upon both programming and feedback approaches to achieve coordination at the micro level. Case management is one example. There has been an explosion of case-management jobs in health care, employed by hospitals, health maintenance organizations, and physician groups, specifically to improve the coordination of care. Case managers use both predetermined plans for guiding their work (programming) and interpersonal contacts with other providers and organizations (feedback). Case managers play the role of "boundary spanners," helping to facilitate handoffs and helping the patient negotiate the boundaries between different members of the care provider team. Like boundary spanners, more generally, case managers play an information-processing role within organizations (Galbraith, 1977) and between organizations (Aldrich and Herker, 1977). Organizational scholars have learned that boundary spanners are most successful when they not only process information, but also read contextual clues (Tushman and Scanlan, 1981), build trust (Currall and Judge, 1995), and build shared goals, shared knowledge, and mutual respect across boundaries (Gittell, 2002). However, to play these multiple roles effectively is time consuming. Research in both airlines and health care shows that case managers are more effective in coordinating work when they are responsible for a relatively small number of flights (Gittell, 2003) or patients (Gittell, 2002). Smaller caseloads for case managers can allow other participants to use their time more efficiently, therefore reducing overall resource utilization.

Similarly, one programming approach that has become increasingly prevalent—clinical pathways (Bohmer, 1998)—has the potential to increase the quality of communication and the quality of working relationships, rather than replace the need for them, as earlier theory would have predicted. A nine-hospital study of care coordination for surgical patients showed that clinical pathways that included greater numbers of the relevant clinical functions led to higher levels of relational coordination among clinical staff, as well as higher quality and more efficient patient outcomes (Gittell, 2002). Faraj and Xiao (2006) showed that even in the high-velocity environment of trauma units, programming in the form of trauma protocols plays an important role in the coordination of care. Like clinical pathways that are used for surgical patients, these protocols take the form of a standard operating procedure whereby roles, decision points, and event sequences are specified. These programming approaches appear to improve coordination across different members of the patient care team even when actions cannot be fully prespecified, because above all, they provide a shared cognitive framework of the task. Both studies show, however, that these programming approaches do not diminish the need for informal, feedback forms of coordination. Rather, they provide a context within which feedback forms of coordination can more effectively occur.

In addition, when faced with unfamiliar situations, high-performing units increase their use of feedback approaches to a greater extent than the low-performing ones. This result is consistent with findings from an earlier study of emergency rooms that nonprogrammed approaches to coordination were more effective under conditions of high uncertainty (Argote, 1982). Other feedback approaches help to improve coordination

and patient outcomes. For example, in a study of joint replacement surgery, more inclusive team meetings predicted higher levels of coordination among clinical staff, as well as more efficient and higher-quality patient outcomes (Gittell, 2002).

Taken together with the findings about clinical pathways, these findings suggest that even relatively straightforward procedures benefit from using feedback approaches in addition to programming approaches. Consistent with previous findings, feedback approaches to coordination have an even stronger impact on outcomes as the uncertainty in patient conditions increases.

Feedback and programming approaches to coordination can both be designed to help strengthen working relationships, but there are many practices in health care organizations that work in the opposite direction. Nursing staff turnover and rotation, house staff rotation, and limited physicians' and other professionals' involvement in a patient care unit greatly hinder the development of such relationships and can prevent full use of feedback approaches to coordination. Working relationships are also undermined by the professional identities of health care workers (Abbott, 1988) and by the occupational communities that tend to grow up around those professional identities (Van Maanen and Barley, 1984). Coordinating mechanisms, as discussed in the section on macro-level coordination above, can be used to counteract these divisive tendencies and to strengthen key working relationships. Physician job design also has large and highly significant effects on coordination between the physician and other clinicians, and on patient outcomes (Gittell, 2008). Physician job design can be changed to foster physicians who specialize in hospital-based care (i.e., hospitalists), giving them the opportunity to focus on the delivery of care for a particular type of patient and to become familiar with the staff and routines of a particular hospital. This specialization improves coordination rather than increasing the challenge of coordination, because it is specialization around type of patient, rather than further splitting up the work involved in caring for a given patient. (Using hospitalists does, however, fragment the care of patients between the hospital and ambulatory care settings, thus creating a different coordination challenge).

To summarize, coordination affects both the quality and efficiency of organizational performance. Second, the types of coordinating approaches that can be used effectively depend somewhat upon the nature of the work of the unit. Greater advantage can be taken of programming approaches when the work of the unit is limited in scope and uncertainty, though even then programming appears to work better in tandem with feedback approaches. Similarly, programming approaches complement, but do not replace, feedback approaches in situations of higher uncertainty. It should be noted that people with greater experience in a particular job will encounter fewer unfamiliar situations than people with less experience. The people with less experience, therefore, need to use feedback approaches to a greater extent than do highly experienced people. This is typically reflected in their greater reliance on discussions with their manager or peers. Finally, feedback approaches require trust and understanding among people, which in turn requires organizational practices such as consistency in working together, conflict-resolution processes, or selection of staff members who are skilled at teamwork.

## Relational Coordination

A new perspective has emerged in recent years, called **relational coordination**, which captures aspects of both the programming and feedback approaches to coordination. Relational coordination encompasses technical concerns with information flow and task interdependence, as well as psychosocial concerns with relational interdependence (or the quality of working relationships). Coordination is not seen as a mechanical process of information exchange, but rather as a relational process involving a network of communication and relationship ties among people whose tasks are interdependent (Faraj and Xiao, 2006; Gittell, 2002; Weick and Roberts, 1993).

Relational coordination takes account of the work itself, but also the process of people working together and its affective aspects. Often the two have been disconnected in conceptualizing processes of coordination. Relational coordination is comprised of two interacting components: **relationships** and **communication**. Relationships can be seen as consisting of shared goals, shared knowledge, and mutual respect. Communication can be viewed in terms of its frequency, timeliness, accuracy and focus on problem solving. Relational coordination tends to be weakest among people who carry out different jobs in the same work process, especially when those people are part of different work units and have different professional backgrounds, such as doctors, nurses, and social workers (note how this reflects the discussion above of differentiation at the macro level). This need for effective coordination across disciplines in health care is most critical to delivery of effective care, yet is most challenging to achieve. To achieve the quality and efficiency outcomes that health care organizations are striving for, managers must invest in relationships where they are hardest to build—among people with distinct, competing professional identities, whose work is highly interconnected.

Relational coordination and programming and feedback approaches to coordination are complementary ways of looking at coordination at the micro level. Some scholars argue that relational coordination provides in depth detail to the feedback approach to coordination. Other scholars argue that both programming and feedback are mechanisms to achieve relational coordination, which they see as the overarching concept regarding coordination at the micro level. Both conceptual frameworks have shown strong relationships to clinical outcomes. In addition, since effective coordination contributes to task performance, staff receive greater satisfaction from their work when their contributions to care are effective. This, in turn, has a positive effect on their motivation.

---

### IN PRACTICE:  The Veterans Healthcare System

The Veterans Healthcare System (formally, the Veterans Health Adminstration, VHA), the largest fully integrated health care system in the United States, began a redesign effort in 1995 (Kizer, 1999; Young, 2000). The overall goal in redesigning was to systematize quality management (QM) to ensure the provision of consistent and predictable high-quality care and access by patients to the entire system. The decision to redesign the organization structure of the VHA came about for a number of reasons, including pressures from the external environment such as the market-based restructuring of health care in general, growth of scientific and biomedical knowledge, general dissatisfaction with health care (especially VHA), consumer expectations for quality, and many managerial and operational problems.

## IN PRACTICE:  The Veterans Healthcare System  *(Continued)*

Because of these factors, the VHA embarked on an ambitious process to redesign the health system in order to improve effectiveness and efficiency in day-to-day operations and bring about a quality transformation. During 1994 and 1995, various planning efforts and consensus-building activities were carried out to design and begin to implement a new operating structure. Prior to the redesign, VHA had 172 hospitals and four regions. Approximately 40 to 45 hospitals were accountable to each regional manager. The large span of control in each region allowed the hospitals to function relatively autonomously, with a high degree of decentralization of operations within the system and a low level of supervision and actual accountability. Resources were allocated to hospitals based on the amount of services provided in previous years. The hospitals competed with each other for resources, and had a duplication of services in facilities located close to each other.

The structure changed the basic operating unit within the system from individual hospitals and medical centers to 22 regional networks called Veterans Integrated Service Networks (VISNs). Funding of operations was then allocated to VISNs on the basis of their populations, and care patterns began to shift away from acute hospitals. Decisions were centralized from the hospitals to the regions, and simultaneously they were decentralized from headquarters in Washington, D.C., to the regions. These changes were a fundamental shift from the VHA's former disease-oriented, hospital-based, and professional discipline-based paradigms to ones that are patient-centered, prevention-oriented, community-based, and premised on universal primary care. In the new system, multidisciplinary teams had shared responsibility and accountability for patient care.

## Results

Results suggest that VHAs transformation contributed to a remarkable level of achievement. Between 1994 and 1998 (approximately), some of the successes were:

- Fifty-two percent (27,319 of 52,315) of all VHA acute-care hospital beds were closed.

- VHA's bed-days of care per 1,000 patients decreased 62 percent. The current VHA rate is now about 5 percent lower than the projected Medicare rate for the same time period.

- Universal primary care has been implemented, and by March 1998, 80 percent of patients could identify their primary caregiver.

- Annual inpatient admissions were 32 percent (284,596), while ambulatory care visits per year increased 43 percent (from 25.0 million to 35.8 million per year).

- The management and operation of 50 hospitals has been merged into 24 locally integrated health care systems.

- By 2010 nearly 800 new community-based outpatient clinics were established to improve access to care. The clinics were funded from redirected savings—that is, no "new" funds have been provided for these clinics.

- Surgeries performed on an outpatient basis increased from 35 percent to 75 percent of all surgeries. This change was accompanied by increased surgical productivity and reduced mortality.

- Systemwide staffing was decreased by 11 percent (23,112 of 206,578 full-time employee equivalents), whereas the number of patients treated per year increased by 18 percent. This included 8 percent more psychiatric/substance-abuse treatment patients, 19 percent more homeless patients, and 53 percent more blind rehabilitation patients.

- Telephone-linked care ("call centers") has been implemented at all VA medical centers, as well as temporary lodging ("hotel") beds.

- Over 2,700 VHA forms were eliminated (67 percent of the total), and all remaining forms and directives were put into electronic form.

- A pharmacy benefits management program has produced an estimated cumulative savings of $347 million.

---

**IN PRACTICE:** The Veterans Healthcare System *(Continued)*

Jha et al. (2003) reported on an assessment of changes in quality of care indicators at VHA from 1994 through 2000 and compared these results for the VHA with the quality of care afforded by the Medicare fee-for-service system using the same quality indicators. Results showed VA patients were receiving appropriate care at 90 percent or greater for 9 of 17 quality indicators. Quality indicators exceeded those for not only the average community hospital but also the average academic health center.

In addition, VHA had implemented:

- A national medication administration system (bar coding for medication administration)
- A national electronic medical record
- Computerized drug interaction system
- Computerized physician order entry

These findings suggest that changing an organizational design that matches the characteristics of the external and internal environments and is in keeping with the vision and missions of the organization can increase the outcomes of the organization in terms of quality of services.

---

# SUMMARY AND MANAGERIAL GUIDELINES

1. Organization design is a key factor in affecting behavior, and thus outcomes, of organizations. It operates in several ways. These include focusing people's attention on the work and goals of their units to the relative exclusion of work and goals of other units; and facilitating coordination among people in the same unit, while hindering coordination of work across units.

2. All organization designs have both beneficial and dysfunctional characteristics. The functional structure yields benefits of specialization by profession and medical specialties and subspecialties, contributing to high levels of competence and professional development in each profession individually. This structure, however, impedes coordination among different professions. To address the needs for coordination across departments, structural integrating mechanisms can be used.

3. Program structures provide the strongest structures for integrating across professions within each program, but they have the dysfunctional characteristic of a lesser focus on professional specialization and professional development. In addition, the program structure hinders coordination across programs. With a large number of possible ways to structure an organization, it is important to choose a structure that is the best fit for a given organization's purpose and strategy.

4. Within the context of an organization's structure, micro-level process and mechanisms of coordination can facilitate the achievement of coordination.

5. Programming approaches to coordination can be used best when work is predictable and cause-and-effect relationships are well known.

6. Feedback approaches, which rely upon the relationships among people, are most needed when the work is relatively uncertain.

7. Since much clinical work is highly uncertain but much is also predictable and routine, a combination of programming and feedback approaches to coordination yields more effective and efficient delivery of care.

# DISCUSSION QUESTIONS

1. In the tale of two units, Unit B functioned much more smoothly that Unit A. Identify the macro-level coordination mechanisms being used in Unit B that were not used in Unit A. What is the nature of task interdependence among staff in the patient care units in the "tale of two units"?

2. Identify the micro-level coordination mechanisms used in Unit B that were not used in Unit A.

3. In the VA case study, reorganizing this integrated delivery system into regional networks (VISNs) and decentralizing authority to the VISN directors seemed to have contributed to a substantial improvement in organization performance. What are the negative aspects of the reorganized structure and decentralization?

4. Describe alternatives for a service line structure internal to each VISN in the VA case.

5. Why is the hierarchical structure limited in its capability to facilitate coordination in health care organizations?

# CASE

The vice president for patient care services (VP-PCS) and the vice president for medical affairs (VP-MA) at Northeast Medical Center (NMC) were very concerned about coordination between Medicine and Nursing in the inpatient medical/surgical units. NMC was a large tertiary-care teaching hospital, affiliated with the Northeast Schools of Medicine (NSOM) and Nursing (NSON). NMC participated in a joint residency program with three other hospitals affiliated with NSOM. Most residents spent six weeks at NMC.

The VPs had observed that coordination sharply decreased after restrictions on resident hours were implemented. The VP-PCS noted, "The residents rotate through our hospital so quickly that the nurses hardly get to know their names, much less establish a working relationship." The VPs also observed that handoffs of patients from one resident team to another were problematic and had become more so, they believed, as a result of the shorter shifts worked by the residents.

The VP-MA suggested expanding NMC's hospitalist program to address the coordination problems. He argued that hospitalists would provide a consistent medical coverage that would compensate for what he called "fragmented" coverage by residents. However, the chief of medicine was opposed to this proposal. He argued that it would negatively affect the educational experience of residents by reducing their responsibilities. He was backed in this argument by the chairman of medicine at NSOM. As was common in academic centers, the chief of medicine reported to the VP-MA at NMC and also to the chairman of medicine at NSOM.

## Questions

1. Is it consistent with organizational theory to expect that coordination between nurses and residents would suffer as a result of the change in resident working hours?

2. Would the addition of hospitalists improve coordination?

3. What other changes could improve coordination?

4. What are counterarguments to the position held by the chief of medicine and chairman of medicine that the hospitalists would negatively affect the educational experience of residents?

# REFERENCES

Abbott, A. (1988). *The system of professions: An essay on the division of expert labor*. Chicago: University of Chicago Press.

Aldrich, H., & and Herker, D. (1977). Boundary spanning roles and organization structure. *Academy of Management Review, 2*(2), 217–230.

Argote, L. (1982). Input uncertainty and organizational coordination in hospital emergency units. *Administrative Science Quarterly, 27*, 420–434.

Bohmer, R. (1998). Critical pathways at Massachusetts General Hospital. *Journal of Vascular Surgery 28*, 373–377.

Burns, T., & Stalker, G. M. (1961). *The management of innovation*. London: Tavistock.

Byrne, M., Charns, M. P., Parker, V. A., Meterko, M. M., & Wray, N. (2004). The Effects of Organization on Hospital Performance: An Analysis of Service Line Organization. *Medical Care*.

Charns, M. P., & Tewksbury, L. S. (1993). *Collaborative management in health care: Implementing the integrative organization*. San Francisco: Jossey-Bass.

Charns, M. P., & Schaefer, M. J. (1983). *Health care organizations: A model for management*. Englewood Cliffs, NJ: Prentice-Hall.

Charns, M. P., Stoelwinder, J. U., Miller, R. A., & Schaefer, M. J. (1981). *Coordination and patient unit effectiveness*. Academy of Management Annual Meetings, San Diego, CA.

Currall, S. C., & Judge, T. A. (1995). Measuring trust between organizational boundary role persons. *Organizational Behavior and Human Decision Processes, 64*(2), 151–170.

Duncan, R. B. (1972). Characteristics of organizational environments and perceived environmental uncertainty. *Administrative Science Quarterly, 17*, 313–327.

Duncan, R. B. (1973). Multiple decision-making structures in adapting to environmental uncertainty: The impact on organizational effectiveness. *Human Relations, 26*(3), 273–291.

Faraj, S., & Xiao, Y. (2006). Coordination in Fast Response Organizations. *Management Science 52*(8), 1155–1169.

Galbraith, J. R. (1973). *Designing complex organizations*. Reading, MA: Addison-Wesley.

Galbraith, J. R. (1977). *Organization design*. Reading, MA: Addison-Wesley.

Georgopoulis, B. S., & F. C. Mann (1962). *The community general hospital*. New York: Macmillan.

Gittell, J. H. (2002). Coordinating mechanisms in care provider groups: Relational coordination as a mediator and input uncertainty as a moderator of performance effects. *Management Science, 48*(11), 1408–1426.

Gittell, J. H. (2003). *The Southwest Airlines way: Using the power of relationships to achieve high performance*. New York: McGraw-Hill.

Gittell, J. H., Fairfield, K., Bierbaum, B., Head, W., Jackson, R., Kelly, M., Laskin, R., Lipson, S., Siliski, J., Thornhill, T., & Zuckerman, J. (2000). Impact of relational coordination on quality of care, post-operative pain and functioning, and length of stay: A nine hospital study of surgical patients. *Medical Care, 38*(8), 807–819.

Gittell, J. H., Weinberg, D., Bennett, A., Miller, J. A. (2008). Is the doctor in? A relational approach to job design and the coordination of work. *Human Resource Management 47*(4), 729–755.

Greenberg, G., Rosenheck, R. A., & Charns, M. P. (2003). From professional dominance to service line management in the Veterans Health Administration: Impact on mental health care. *Medical Care, 41*(9), 1013–1023.

Jha, A. K., Perlin, J. B., Kizer, K. W., & Dudley, R. A. (2003). Effect of the transformation of the Veterans Affairs Health Care System on the quality of care. *New England Journal of Medicine, 348*(22), 2218–2227.

Kizer, K. W. (1999). The "new VA": A national laboratory for health care quality management. *American Journal of Medical Quality, 14*(1), 3–20.

Knaus, W. A., Draper, E. A., Wagner, D. P., & Zimmerman, J. E. (1986). An evaluation of outcome from intensive care in major medical centers. *Annals of Internal Medicine, 104*, 416–418.

Lawrence, P. R., & Lorsch, J. W. (1967). *Organization and environment: Managing differentiation and integration.* Boston: Division of Research, Harvard Business School.

March, J. F., & Simon, H. A. (1958). *Organizations.* New York: John Wiley & Sons.

Miller, E. J. & A. K. Rice (1967). *Systems of organization.* London: Tavistock.

Mintzberg, H. (1979). *The structuring of organizations.* Englewood Cliffs, NJ: Prentice-Hall.

Perrow, C. B. (1967). A framework for the comparative analysis of organizations. *American Sociological Review, 32*(2), 194–208.

Perrow, C. B. (1972). *Complex organizations: A critical essay.* Glenview, IL: Scott, Foresman.

Shortell, S. M., Rousseau, D. M., Gillies, R. R., Devers, K. J., & Simons, T. L. (1991). Organizational assessment in intensive care units (ICUs): Construct development, reliability, and validity of the ICU nurse-physician questionnaire. *Medical Care, 29*(8), 709–727.

Shortell, S. M., Zimmerman, J., Rousseau, D., Gillies, R., Wagner, D., Draper, E., Knaus, W., & Duffy, J. (1994). The performance of intensive care units: Does good management make a difference? *Medical Care 32*(5), 508–525.

Stoelwinder, J. U., & M. P. Charns (1981). A task field model of organization design and analysis. *Human Relations 34*(9), 743–762.

Thompson, J. D. (1967). *Organizations in action.* New York: McGraw-Hill

Tushman, M. L., & T. J. Scanlan (1981). Characteristics and external orientations of boundary spanning individuals. *Academy of Management Journal, 24*(1), 83–98.

Van de Ven, A. H., & Delbecq, A. L. (1974). A task contingent model of work unit structure. *Administrative Science Quarterly, 19*(2), 183–197.

Van Maanen, J., & Barley, S. R. (1984). Occupational communities: Culture and control in organizations. *Research in Organizational Behavior,6*, 287–365. Greenwich, CT: JAI Press.

Weick, K. E., & Roberts, K. (1993). Collective mind in organizations: Heedful interrelating on flight decks. *Administrative Science Quarterly, 38*, 357–381.

Woodward, J. (1965). *Industrial organization: Theory and practice.* London: Oxford University Press.

Young. G. (1997). Insider representation on the governing boards of nonprofit hospitals: Trends and implications for charitable care. *Inquiry, 33*, 352–362.

Young, G. (2000). Managing organizational transformations: Lessons from the Veterans Health Administration. *California Management Review, 43*(1), 66–82.

Young, G., Charns, M., & Hereen, T. (1994). Product line management and employee assessments of their work environments: A study of hospitals. *Academy of Management Journal, 47*(5), 723–734.

Young, G., Charns, M., Desai, K., Khuri, S., Forbes, M., Henderson, W., & Daley, J. (1998). Patterns of coordination and clincial outcomes: A study of surgical services. *Health Services Research, 33*(5), 1211–1236.

# Chapter 4

# Motivating People

## Thomas A. D'Aunno and Mattia J. Gilmartin

## CHAPTER OUTLINE

- **Motivation and Management**
- **The What and How of Motivation**
- **Process Perspectives**
- **Motivating Health Care Professionals**
- **Motivational Problems**

## LEARNING OBJECTIVES

**After completing this chapter, the reader should be able to:**

1. Define motivation and distinguish it from other factors that influence individuals' performance
2. Recognize popular but misleading myths about motivation
3. Understand that motivation depends heavily on the situations in which individuals work
4. Understand managers' roles in motivating people
5. Identify key characteristics of the content of peoples' work that motivates them
6. Identify important processes involved in motivating people
7. Assess and deal with motivational problems

## KEY TERMS

| | |
|---|---|
| **Empowerment** | **Hygiene Factors** |
| **Equity** | **Job Redesign** |
| **Expectancy** | **Motivation** |
| **Feedback** | **Motivators** |
| **Goal Setting** | **Pay-for-Performance** |
| **Hierarchy of Needs** | **Self-Actualization** |

---

## IN PRACTICE: Dr. Intimidation

If hospitals want to reduce medication errors, one challenge is to get their physicians and other medication prescribers to react without condescension and intimidation to questions and concerns from the professionals charged with carrying out the orders. That is the conclusion reached by the Institute for Safe Medication Practices after a survey it conducted showed that such intimidation contributes to medical errors by preventing nurses and pharmacists from voicing concerns about the correctness or safety of medications.

In a survey of 2,099 health care practitioners, 40 percent of respondents assumed a prescription was correct at least once during the previous year rather than raise the matter with a physician or other prescribing professional with a reputation for reacting with intimidation. When they did speak up, 49 percent said they felt pressure to give the medication despite their concerns. Often no harm resulted, but 7 percent of all respondents said they were involved in a medication error during the past year "in which intimidation clearly played a role," according to the institute. Some 10 percent of pharmacists reported intimidation-related medical errors.

Hospitals are trying to change their culture to head off medical errors by encouraging caregivers to report errors without fear of sanction and enable everyone to learn from them, said Hedy Cohen, the institute's vice president. Good working relationships among those caregivers are crucial to the effort. "Part of this culture change is working as a team, which will prevent errors," Cohen said.

Often, however, pharmacists and nurses were left to huddle with colleagues or do research on their own to assuage fears about orders. Among pharmacists, 23 percent said they attempted to clarify the safety of an order themselves at least 10 times during the year rather than interact with a prescriber.

Physicians were more likely to use condescending language or be impatient with requests from nurses rather than pharmacists, but more than 20 percent of both groups reported such incidents happened at least 10 times in the past year. Nearly half of all respondents said past experiences with intimidation had altered how they handle questions or clarifications.

The experiences sometimes included strong verbal abuse, mentioned by 48 percent, but subtle expressions of exasperation may be all it takes to throw cold water on communication, Cohen said. "It's like with your spouse," she said. "If every time you ask a question they look at you derisively and they put their hands on their hips, you're not going to ask more questions."

For additional information on the Institute for Safe Medication Practices, visit: http://www.ismp.org.

SOURCE: Morrissey, J. (2004, April 5). Dr. Intimidation: Surly prescribers increase risk of errors: Survey. *Modern Healthcare, 34*(14), 10.

---

# CHAPTER PURPOSE

The objective of this chapter is to develop in readers the understanding and ability needed to effectively motivate individuals in health care organizations. Results from the Institute for Safe Medication Practices survey (Morrissey, 2004) illustrate the profound implications that motivation and relationships among health care professionals can have for patient safety and quality of care (see "In Practice: Dr. Intimidation").

This chapter consists of four major sections. The first section defines motivation and distinguishes it from other factors that can affect performance. This section also describes common but misleading myths about motivation. As antidotes to these myths, we emphasize that motivation is situational. There are several characteristics of individuals and the settings in which they work that managers should take into account in trying to motivate people. The section concludes by examining the role that managers can play to maintain or increase motivation.

The next section identifies several important factors that managers can influence to improve or maintain the motivation of employees and coworkers. The focus is on those approaches that seem most useful, and we refer readers to more extensive reviews (Higgins and Kruglansky, 2000; Locke and Latham, 2004). The third section of the chapter discusses motivational issues that are particular to professionals, especially physicians and nurses, who are central to providing health care. This section also briefly discusses motivational issues that are particular to nonprofessional occupations, which are common in health care organizations. Finally, the last section examines common motivational problems and discusses how to assess them. We explore alternative approaches for dealing with motivational problems.

# MOTIVATION AND MANAGEMENT

Motivation is a central topic for health care managers, but it also can be an especially difficult one. The types of workers managers might be expected to motivate can range from highly educated professionals, such as physicians and nurses, to minimum-wage workers such as nurse's aids in long-term care settings.

The environment of health care continues to change rapidly, requiring regular improvements in productivity and quality of care, while simultaneously requiring cost containment. The principles and practices of motivation that we describe in this chapter are excellent tools for making health care's most expensive resource, staff members, its most valuable asset. Empirical evidence indicates that human resource practices, such as those that improve motivation, can positively influence an organization's performance, including its financial performance (Huselid, 1995; Pfeffer, 1998a). Consequently, a highly motivated workforce can serve as a difficult-to-replicate competitive advantage (Zigarelli, 1996).

In addition to motivating individuals to improve productivity and efficiency, managers may wish to motivate workers to reduce absenteeism and tardiness (Mercer, 1988); to improve problem-solving ability; to promote creativity and innovativeness (Colvin, 1998); to work interdependently and cooperatively as team members; to develop consumer-oriented attitudes and behaviors (O'Connor and Shewchuk, 1995); to reenergize those who no longer feel challenged (Kennedy, 1997); to remotivate following layoffs (McConnell, 1996); to get people to take on added responsibilities (Nordhaus-Bike, 1997); to recruit hard-to-find workers such as information

technology professionals (Appleby, 1998); and to motivate moral and ethical behavior (Vidaver-Cohen, 1998).

# Defining and Distinguishing Motivation

The beginning of wisdom in motivating people is to recognize what motivation is and is not (Mohr, 1982). We define **motivation** as a state of feeling or thinking in which one is energized or aroused to perform a task or engage in a particular behavior (Steers and Porter, 1987). This definition focuses on motivation as an emotional or cognitive state that is independent of action. This focus clearly distinguishes motivation from the performance of a task and its consequences. Notice, too, that motivation can be a state of either feeling or thinking, or a combination of the two. For some individuals, motivation is more a matter of feeling than thinking, while for others, the reverse is true.

# Myths about Motivation—and Some Antidotes

There are several popular but misleading myths about motivating people. Our view is that these myths are more harmful than helpful and, as a result, need to be confronted early in this chapter. Four particular myths are addressed below.

### Myth 1: Motivated Workers Are More Productive

To illustrate this myth, consider this conversation (Muchinsky, 1987).

> Supervisor: George just isn't motivated any more!
> Foreman: How can you tell?
> Supervisor: His productivity has fallen off by more than 50 percent.

Motivation should not be confused with performance. People can be highly motivated but still perform poorly. Performance depends not just on motivation but also on ability and a host of situational factors such as the availability of resources needed to perform a job well (Locke and Latham, 2004). Motivation is just one of several factors that managers need to consider in trying to improve or sustain individuals' performance. Nonetheless, it is often a critical factor.

### Myth 2: Some People Are Just Motivated and Others Are Not

This myth is based on the view that motivation is a personality trait or characteristic that remains relatively stable from time to time and place to place. If this view were taken to its extreme, it would suggest that managers should carefully select only those employees who have the trait of motivation, for managers could otherwise do little to influence motivation and behavior.

In contrast, we take the view that motivation is more specific to situations (i.e., influenced by factors in an individual's environment) than it is a stable personality trait or characteristic (Kanfer, 1990). There is strong empirical support for the view that situations significantly shape individual behavior (Davis-Blake and Pfeffer, 1989). For example, as illustrated in the case of "Dr. Intimidation," if the situational environment is poor (e.g., condescension, intimidation, verbal abuse, and disrespect), it is difficult for people to remain motivated. This de-motivation can have a direct impact on patient care and safety.

We argue that, even if motivation were a somewhat stable personality trait, it would still be important for managers to ensure that employees have work conditions that reinforce their tendency to be motivated or change their tendency to be unmotivated. In short, situational and individual factors interact to produce motivation and behavior.

## *Myth 3: Motivation Can Be Easily Mass Produced*

A major myth about motivation is that it can be easily mass produced (for example, in speeches by charismatic leaders to large groups of people or by placing motivational posters throughout the workplace). Though these approaches sometimes work, most often they do not (Laurinaitis, 1997). Typically, to motivate people effectively, managers need to treat them as individuals. Contrary to the myth of mass production, we assert that individuals vary widely from each other in many ways. As a result, it is a central and recurring theme of this chapter that managers must motivate employees and coworkers on an individual basis, taking each person's situation into account.

---

## IN PRACTICE: A Cry for Help

*Working and keeping motivated on a busy 24-bed general intensive care unit, a charge nurse tells her story:*

ICU nursing is becoming frustrating. It is frustrating to always be there, to work so closely with patients, to do so much to keep them going, and then have someone else get all the credit. The nurses do the work, they act as the eyes and ears monitoring and responding to the patients' condition, but it is always the physician who saves them and gets the accolades.

The ICU is also becoming a more dangerous and scary place to work. In addition to tuberculosis, HIV, and hepatitis, there are more bloodborne and communicable diseases than ever before. Patients who come here are often under the influence of drugs or alcohol. They often react badly to pharmaceuticals we administer to them. Because the atmosphere is unfamiliar, they frequently get violent. Even old people can get violent.

Consumerism is rampant in health care. Everyone is an expert. The families continually remind me to wash my hands. Administration has recently been demanding more consumer-friendly behavior from the ICU nurses. They recently instituted wide open, 24-hour visiting hours. They told us, "You will tolerate someone being here 24 hours a day as long as there is no bonafide reason that they shouldn't be there." For the most part this is fine with us. We are part of a very family- and community-oriented health system, and families can really help out. Spending time in the ICU allows families to reassure kids that all is well, make certain their elderly parents or grandparents don't fall out of bed and are comfortable. In some cases, if a family member is not available, we have to hire sitters for $12 an hour to keep an eye on the patient. Generally, the sitters are unskilled people who can't participate in the patient care process. Usually they knit, eat chips, read, listen to the radio, or sleep.

**IN PRACTICE:  A Cry for Help**  *(Continued)*

Although the presence of family members can assist us, more often than not, they can also impede our ability to do our work. We have one "frequent flyer" who is in here all the time. His wife will not leave. She insists on doing his care. The husband has severe diabetes, and she insists on doing the glucose monitoring and dressing changes. We can't get rid of her. She makes the nurses very uncomfortable. Sometimes you have to take care of the entire family, not just the member in the bed. Many families are already dysfunctional to begin with; they don't usually function any better in the ICU setting.

People who go into ICU nursing go into it because they are more comfortable working with technology than with people. They are peak performers in the unfortunate circumstances when a patient is paralyzed, sedated, and ventilated. Those nurses who enjoy more patient interaction go into oncology or the other so-called "touchy-feelies," not ICU.

Our system has been restructuring lately, and administration has been trying to focus less on financial rewards and more on nontangible rewards. The ICU nurses do receive a higher pay differential, because the work is more demanding and specialized. However, administration wants to get away from differentials because, as they say, "Everything is getting to be a specialty." But believe me, money still talks! A year ago, administration cut back ICU staffing in an effort to save money. Shortly after that time, we went into a 10-month period of very high census and very high acuity. The highest anyone could ever remember, and we were understaffed! Work became horrible. I didn't want to go. Every time it would be hellish. The 24 ICU beds were always full of seriously ill people.

As the demands and stresses became greater, the necessary ICU "community behaviors" were just put aside. The nurses weren't motivated to work as a team anymore; they began focusing on "their" patients only. But we all have to keep watch on the telemetry banks and the arrhythmia alarms. Phones ring that have to be answered. The pneumatic tubes [which transport lab results, blood samples, and pharmaceuticals] need to be attended to. These activities are not assigned, but need to be done as a team.

Often, nurses that were scheduled to work eight hours would have to stay for 12. For a while, we had to work every weekend and holiday. To help ease the staffing void, the hospital began to rely on external agency, pool nurses at a higher wage. When the pool nurses come here, they are not 100%. They might be totally unfamiliar with our environment, and we don't necessarily know their skill level. Naturally, these nurses take a lot of orientation and maintenance time. Furthermore, because pool nurses are not given computer passwords, we have to do their computerized charting, which creates more work for us. The pool nurses are hired guns who are paid about $12 more per hour than we are. They also work whenever they want to.

Although we are a nonprofit, we have a gain-sharing plan. Administration thinks money is not an issue with us. They played with the equations. We worked very hard—all out—for 10 months in a very difficult and understaffed environment. We did receive our gain-share checks, but it was practically nothing. Because of the high patient census and acuity, coupled with staff cutbacks, the external agency pool was used heavily. They are paid a premium. Apparently, that is where most of our gain-share went. We didn't feel that the gain-share checks rewarded us at all. In the end, it had nothing to do with all the extra effort. That was our reward for being full-time, committed, extremely hard working, and concerned for quality.

I can go down to the agency tomorrow and make $12 an hour more than I do now.

For additional information, see American Association of Colleges of Nursing, Information about the nursing workforce and labor shortage in the United States. Retrieved August 15, 2010, from http://www.aacn.nche.edu

At least three important types of individual and situational differences should be considered:

1. *Job Position or Occupation:* One of the most distinctive features of health care organizations is the number of different occupational groups and job categories involved. These groups range from nurse's aides and porters to nurses, physical therapists, and physicians. Health care occupations vary along dimensions such as the amount and type of training they require, their power and status, and what types of individuals are attracted to them. Managers should understand how their ability to motivate individuals may vary according to their occupation or job category. For example, union contracts often prohibit certain types of changes in job design and responsibilities; managers need to know what occupational groups are covered by such contracts and how they affect certain approaches to motivation.

2. *Career Stage:* A second important way in which individuals vary is their career stage. To illustrate, consider a recent graduate of a health care management program. She may be highly motivated by assignments that provide opportunities for learning about the different divisions of her new organization. In contrast, her colleague, who has more experience, may wish to work on a single project from start to completion. Managers need to be sensitive to such career stage needs, motives, and values (Kanfer and Ackerman, 2004).

3. *Personal Factors:* Perhaps more than we generally recognize, a variety of factors from their personal lives influence people at work. For example, personal factors sometimes parallel career stages. A recent graduate may have few family ties that would limit his interest in work that involved travel, whereas a manager with young children may be less motivated by opportunity for travel on the job. Other important personal influences that can affect motivation include family illness, divorce, substance abuse, health problems, child care, and financial stress. These are clearly delicate areas for managers to tread yet, managers need to be aware that such personal factors can affect work motivation. On the one hand, it may be harmful to pry into the personal lives of employees and coworkers. On the other hand, it may be very helpful to be sensitive to needs at work that stem from their personal lives.

### Myth 4: Money Makes the World Go 'Round

We do not deny that many, if not most, individuals care about and are motivated by money (Stajkovic and Luthans, 2001). But too often managers think only of money when trying to motivate people. Unfortunately, money is likely to be in short supply for health care managers, at least in the next several years. Fortunately, money is not always the most important motivator; indeed, it seldom is for those who choose careers in health care (World Health Organization, 2008). In the next sections, the importance of several other factors in motivating people that do not require cash will be discussed.

## The Manager's Role

The situational perspective described above implies that managers should take an active role in systematically assessing the motivation of their employees and coworkers. Individuals' motivation can vary over time and with the kind of work they are performing. Thus, managers need to periodically assess motivation and performance, taking into account the occupational, career-stage, and personal factors discussed above. Such assessments should include informal interviews with employees and coworkers in which open-ended questions are asked about individuals' needs, motives, perceptions, and values. These assessments need not be lengthy. What matters more is that they are timely; employees feel comfortable in openly expressing their concerns; and managers use the opportunity to do problem solving and goal setting. In short, managers can play a critical role not only by assessing their employees' motivation, but by taking initiative to alter conditions to promote motivation.

## THE "WHAT" AND "HOW" OF MOTIVATION

What factors energize people to work? How are people energized? How can managers enable individuals to build and maintain high levels of energy for their work? Based on results from studies conducted in the past 60 years, as well as insights from management practice, several principles and practices have emerged to guide managers as they seek to effectively motivate people at work. We now turn to these.

## Needs as the Foundation for Motivation

We begin with a simple but important observation: many people are energized to work in order to meet particular needs. A common need, for example, is the need for social interaction and feeling that one is part of a social group (Maslow, 1943; McClelland, 1961). More generally, needs are physical or psychological deficiencies that make specific outcomes or goals attractive. A need, in turn, stimulates individuals' internal drives that direct them toward those goals that have the capacity to satisfy the need. In this view, motivation is a goal-directed, internal drive aimed at satisfying needs.

The motivation framework in Figure 4.1 is a good starting point for understanding how needs can motivate people. The motivation process often begins with needs that reflect some deficiency within the individual. For example, an employee might feel underpaid or lacking in recognition vis-à-vis other employees. In response to these unsatisfied needs, she searches for ways to satisfy them. She may ask for a raise or promotion, work harder to try to earn either, or seek another position outside the organization. Next, she chooses one or more options. After implementing the chosen option or options, she then evaluates her success. If her hard work resulted in a pay raise or a promotion, she will probably continue to work hard. If neither has occurred, she will probably try another option.

The need-based view of motivation raises a key question: Can managers identify individuals' needs and design their work so as to maximize motivation? We summarize below a few of the most prominent efforts to address this question and then draw some conclusions for management practice.

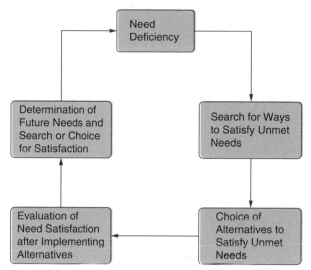

**Figure 4.1** A Framework for Employee Motivation.
SOURCE: Delmar, Cengage Learning.

## *Hierarchy of Needs*

Maslow's (1943) **hierarchy of needs** is one of the earliest, most well-known, and most influential models of motivation. He proposed that people want to satisfy various needs that can be arranged in a hierarchy of importance, as shown in Figure 4.2.

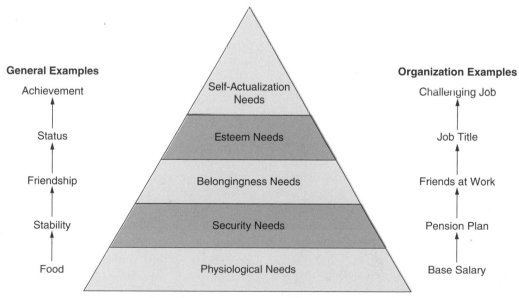

**Figure 4.2** Maslow's Hierarchy of Needs.
SOURCE: Adapted from Maslow, A.H. (1943), A theory of human motivation. *Psychology Review 50*, 370–396.

Maslow argued that there are five need levels that must be satisfied sequentially. The *physiological* needs include such things as air, water, food, warmth, shelter, and sex. They represent basic issues of survival and biological function. In work organizations, such needs are generally satisfied by adequate wages and a satisfactory work environment that provides adequate lighting, temperature, and ventilation.

The *security* needs include a secure physical and emotional environment. Examples include the need to be free from worry about money and job security. In the workplace, security needs are satisfied by job continuity (no layoffs), a grievance system (to protect against arbitrary action), and an adequate health insurance and retirement package (for security against illness and eventual retirement). Because health care organizations have the potential to be fairly hazardous places to work, security needs are frequently important in these settings. The ICU nurses (see "In Practice: A Cry for Help") for example, feared being subject to violence or of contracting conditions such as tuberculosis, hepatitis, or HIV.

*Belongingness* needs involve social processes. They include the need for love and affection and the need to be accepted by one's peers. For most people, they are satisfied by a combination of family and community relationships outside the job and friendships on the job. A manager can promote the satisfaction of these needs by encouraging social interaction and by making employees feel part of a team or workgroup. Sensitivity to an employee's family problems can also help employees meet this need.

*Esteem* needs are actually composed of two different sets of needs: the need for a positive self-image or self-respect, and the need for recognition and respect from others. For example, the ICU nurses felt they did not receive adequate recognition for what they did on the job. They believed that physicians were getting all the credit. Managers can help address esteem needs by providing signs of accomplishment such as job titles, public recognition, and praise (i.e., extrinsic rewards). They may also provide more challenging job assignments and other opportunities for employees to feel a sense of accomplishment.

**Self-actualization** needs, at the top of the hierarchy, involve realizing one's potential for continued growth and individual development. These are most difficult for a manager to identify and meet due to individual differences in goals. However, allowing employees to participate in decision making and the opportunity to learn new things about their work may promote self-actualization.

## Two-Factor View of Needs

Another well-known perspective on needs and motivation is Herzberg's (1987) two-factor theory, which, surprisingly, argues that entirely different sets of factors are associated with satisfaction and high motivation and with dissatisfaction and low motivation. Herzberg's research found that the key factors in satisfaction and motivation were achievement, recognition, the work itself, responsibility, and advancement. He labeled these factors **motivators** because their presence increases job satisfaction and motivation, but their absence does not lead to dissatisfaction. Herzberg also found that if a second group of factors, **hygiene factors**, were negative or absent, dissatisfaction results. These hygiene factors included company policy, supervision, salary, interpersonal relations, and working conditions. The presence of positive hygiene factors, by themselves, prevents dissatisfaction but does not lead to satisfaction and motivation.

Note that the factors influencing the satisfaction dimension—motivation factors—are specifically related to the work content (i.e., intrinsic factors). The factors presumed to cause dissatisfaction—hygiene factors—are related to the work environment. According to Herzberg, changing the environment alone will not enhance employee motivation.

## Learned Needs

The theories of Maslow and Herzberg and others (e.g., Alderfer, 1968, 1972) identify a number of individual needs and then attempt to arrange them in some order of importance. Other views of employee motivation focus on the important needs themselves without concern for ordering them. The three needs most often discussed are the needs for *achievement, power,* and *affiliation* (Atkinson, 1961; McClelland, 1961, 1975). Importantly, this perspective argues that individuals can learn these needs as well as the behaviors associated with the efforts to satisfy them.

The first basic drive is the need for achievement and refers to an individual's need to accomplish complex tasks, compete, and resolve problems. It reflects the desire to achieve a goal more effectively than in the past. People with a high need for achievement are assumed to have a desire for personal responsibility, a tendency to set moderately difficult goals, a need for specific goals and immediate **feedback** (defined as exchange of information between employees and managers), and a preoccupation with their task.

The second basic drive, a need for power, refers to the individual's desire to influence or control others' behavior. It also represents the desire to control one's environment. Individuals high in power needs are thought to be more suited to management than achievers. In this view, "power" implies being responsible for control of others and for influencing behavior in complex situations (McClelland and Burnham, 1976).

The third drive, the need for affiliation, reflects an individual's desire to associate with others in friendly circumstances. It is similar to Maslow's belongingness need. Those high in affiliation prefer friendly, participative work environments in which the quality of group interaction with coworkers is more highly valued than achievements or influence. People with a strong need for affiliation are likely to prefer (and perform better in) a job that entails a lot of social interaction. As teamwork becomes increasingly necessary to manage health care organizations effectively, needs for affiliation may be a welcome characteristic of health care managers. By being more accommodating and cooperative, those managers maintaining greater needs for affiliation may benefit a team-based work setting by reducing dysfunctional conflict and bringing together diverse groups of workers.

## From Concept to Practice: Using Need-Based Views to Motivate People

It is well accepted that motivation has important origins in human needs. Need theories of motivation assume that people attempt to satisfy such needs. A simplistic view is that all a manager or supervisor has to do to release his or her employees' motivation potential is to identify their needs and then take steps to satisfy them. Unfortunately, there is no simple set of needs and need satisfiers that would be universally applicable.

First, as noted above, people differ on the basis of age, gender, race, and other demographic and background characteristics. No one set of motivators is likely to be appropriate for all employees because their needs will be different.

Second, the context and culture of work differ both across organizations and within organizations. The learned needs of a given individual may vary depending on the incentives present in his or her organization.

Third, for a given individual, needs change over time. Because the relative importance of various needs changes, managers must aim at a moving target (Fried and Slowik, 2004).

Fourth, employees in different positions in an organizational hierarchy will likely differ in terms of their configuration of needs and potential motivators. Fifth, resource constraints or lack of such constraints may also affect the relative importance of various needs.

Despite these caveats, need-based theories provide useful insights into factors that may promote motivation in a given situation (e.g., Herbst, 2006; Weick, 2007). Moreover, they are not separate and discrete views of motivation but share much in common with one another. Figure 4.3 compares the needs identified by three prominent theories described in this section. It should be noted that some of their basic concepts are similar and overlap with one another.

Managers can identify employees' needs using attitude surveys and frequent face-to-face communication with both individuals and various subgroups. When possible, managers also should attempt to recognize what needs are important in the motivation of each individual employee and to match those needs to the requirements of positions to which those individuals are assigned.

Based on identified needs, effective managers will alter their leadership and communication style, economic rewards, noneconomic rewards, job assignments, training and development programs, and feedback to maximize the need fulfillment of as many subordinates as possible. For example, some will need to be left alone to work independently. Others will need more structure, goals, and feedback. Because employees have different needs, they must be managed in different ways. The Managerial Guidelines (see page 113) provide a convenient summary of the managerial implications of need-based theories.

Though need-based views provide useful insights into motivational factors, they do not constitute a complete approach to employee motivation. They do not shed much light on the "how" of motivation. For example, they do not explain why employees might be motivated by one factor rather than by another at a given level, or how their different needs might be satisfied. These questions involve behaviors or actions, goals, and feelings of satisfaction that are addressed by various perspectives on the processes involved in motivation. It is to these perspectives that we now turn.

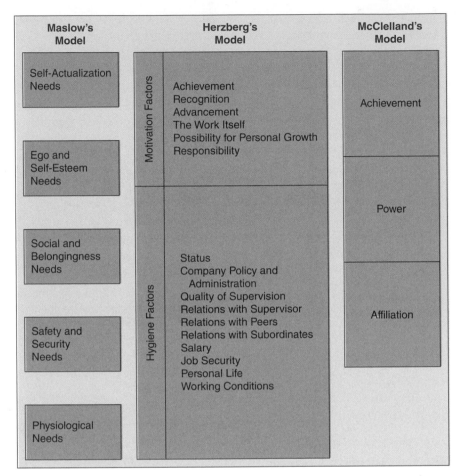

**Figure 4.3** A Comparison of Needs Theories of Motivation.
SOURCE: Delmar, Cengage Learning.

# PROCESS PERSPECTIVES

In this section, we examine three approaches to motivation that, though they differ from each other, share a focus on the processes involved in motivation. In contrast to the approaches examined in the previous section that concern the content of work and its influence on motivation, these approaches attend to the context in which work is done as well as individuals' reactions—especially thoughts and feelings—to work.

## Equity: The Importance of Fairness

Adams proposed a theory of work motivation that assumes that individuals value and seek fairness, or **equity**, in their relationships with employers (Adams, 1963, 1965). Relationships are fair when people perceive that their outcomes (e.g., pay) are proportionate to their perceived contributions or inputs (e.g., task performance). Further, people evaluate fairness by comparing themselves to others. In other words, people contrast their perceived inputs and outcomes with their perceptions of others' inputs and outcomes. To the extent that this ratio is seen as unequal, individuals experience tension.

Adams also proposed that people are motivated to reduce tensions that result from perceived inequity: the greater the perceived inequity and resulting tension, the greater the motivation to reduce it.

Depending on the magnitude of the perceived injustice and individual as well as situational circumstances, people may use one of several approaches to reduce inequity and restore balance in their relationships with employers. These approaches include altering their perceptions of their own or others' inputs or outcomes, changing their inputs or outcomes, getting others to change their inputs or outcomes, and leaving the inequitable situation altogether (Campbell and Pritchard, 1976).

We believe that the equity perspective provides some useful guidelines for health care managers. First, it is important to note that people compare themselves to others in many situations and in many ways. Such comparisons affect not only their motivation, but other aspects of their behavior as well. When people experience uncertainty, they are especially likely to turn to others, consciously or unconsciously, to provide them with cues about what to do. The equity perspective would be useful even if its only contribution were to remind us of the importance of social comparison. The case of the ICU nurses (see "In Practice: A Cry for Help") is a good example of this. The ICU nurses compared themselves to the external pool nurses who worked alongside them. From this comparison, they felt that they earned $12 per hour less and contributed substantially more.

Second, managers need to directly address perceptions of inequities so that individuals are not motivated to reduce their contributions or inputs or to leave their jobs. It may be that managers can change perceptions of inequity simply by explaining differences between jobs or other conditions that make it necessary to reward or treat people differently (Kim and Mauborgne, 2003). In other cases, managers may need to consider pay raises or increases in other non-financial rewards. In still other cases, there may be nothing that a manager can do to restore perceptions of equity. But, if such concerns are not addressed, it is clear that they can be a source of motivational problems (Brockner, 2006).

Finally, though we have argued that it is important to motivate people on an individual basis, equity theory reminds us that even this approach has limits. To the extent that people are treated as individuals, perceptions of inequity are likely to increase because people will be comparing themselves to others who are being treated differently, and such differences can trigger perceptions of inequity.

---

## IN PRACTICE: Motivating a Primary Care Physician in a Community Health Center

Susan Smith, MD, a primary care physician, is employed by an urban community health center. Because such a large proportion of her patients are diabetic, she has been intimately involved in the development of a new, long-term diabetic disease-management program for the center. The center wants the disease to be managed in such a way that it is kept under control so that patients can maintain a higher quality of life and longer-term costs do not rise as a result of the need for more extensive medical interventions.

Dr. Smith is very confident that between her own ability and the detailed guidelines for managing the disease developed by the center, she will be able to do a good job of keeping her diabetic patients' disease under control. The disease-management guidelines require her to get patients to test their blood sugar levels four times per day using testing strips, and to frequently order laboratory tests, glaucoma screenings, and podiatric referrals throughout the course of a year.

The center uses financial incentives to motivate primary care physician behavior, primarily through the use of a bonus pool of dollars from which the physicians can share at the end of the year. The more productive a physician is over the course of the year (as measured by the number of patients that physician sees), the bigger the bonus check at year's end. Although the disease-management guidelines recently went into effect, the center's financial incentive system for its primary care physicians has not changed in any way. Dr. Smith realizes that since a large percentage of her patients are diabetic, if she is to vigorously adhere to the guidelines, she may not receive any bonus at year's end because following the guidelines will require her to take more time with each patient, thus reducing the number of patients she sees overall.

# The Power of Expectations

Another early, prominent, and useful view of motivation, termed expectancy theory (Georgopoulos, Mahoney, and Jones, 1957; Vroom, 1964), begins by assuming that people make rational calculations about how to expend effort on work, and they make choices that will lead to desired rewards. Further, this view assumes that people know what rewards they want from work and understand that their performance will determine the extent to which they attain the rewards they value.

Building on these assumptions, expectancy theory has four central components (Mitchell, 1982). First, there are **job outcomes**. These include both rewards (e.g., pay raises, promotions, recognition) and negative experiences (e.g., job loss, demotion).

Second, there are **valences**. These are individuals' feelings about job outcomes. Like the job outcomes themselves, they can range from positive to neutral to negative, and they vary in strength as well as direction. The third component is **instrumentality**, which is the extent to which individuals believe that attaining a job outcome depends on, or is conditional on, their performance. For example, if a nurse thought that an outcome (pay raise) depended highly on his performance rather than some other factor (hospital patient volume), the instrumentality for the outcome would be high. Finally, **expectancy** is the perceived link between effort and performance. To what extent do individuals believe that there is a relationship between how hard they try and how well they do?

Using expectancy theory, we can illustrate the degree to which the primary care physician described in "In Practice: Motivating a Primary Care Physician in a Community Health Center" will be motivated to vigorously adhere to the community health center's disease-management guidelines. This physician is confident that by following the guidelines, she will be able to do a reasonably good job of controlling the disease among her patients. However, the physician knows that due to the additional time required to effectively manage her patients, there also is a high probability that she will not share in any financial bonuses paid out at year's end. Because this is a job outcome she does not favor, it receives a negative valence. Instrumentality, or the probability that performance will lead to outcomes, is fairly high, but the outcome has a forceful negative valence. Because the outcome (no end-of-year bonus) is not related to performance, the physician's motivation to carry out high-quality diabetes disease management has been substantially reduced.

Motivation is the end product of valence, instrumentality, and expectancy. People are motivated when a combination of factors occurs: They value an outcome (i.e., valence is high and positive), they believe that good performance will be rewarded with desired outcomes (i.e., instrumentality is high), and they believe that their efforts will produce good performance (i.e., expectancy is high). In contrast, motivation is likely to be low if the components of expectancy theory have low values. If people do not care about their job outcomes, then they have less reason to work for them. Or, if organizations do not link outcomes to performance (e.g., pay raises are linked to seniority rather than performance), then people have less reason to care about their performance. Similarly, if effort and performance seem unrelated, then there is less reason to try hard.

Each of these factors can decrease motivation, and if all are present, it is improbable that motivation will be high. The manager of the community health center from the "In Practice" may improve the linkage between outcomes and performance by placing greater emphasis on quality indicators as a condition of participating in the bonus incentive pool.

In sum, expectancy theory (Figure 4.4) provides useful guidelines for managerial action (Pritchard, De Leo, and Von Bergen, 1976). These include:

1. Incentives, rewards, or job outcomes should be chosen so that they are attractive to employees. Perhaps the best way to do this is to ask employees directly about their preferences using surveys or interviews.

2. The rules for attaining incentives or rewards must be clear to all involved. For example, expected levels of performance should be spelled out in as much detail as possible. Such rules should be stated in job descriptions and employee orientations. These rules should also be reviewed periodically, both informally and formally. We add here a note from equity theory: The rules should be perceived as fair.

3. People must perceive that their efforts will lead to the desired level of performance.

At the same time, there are practical limitations on using the expectancy model simply because several factors can intervene to weaken the link between effort and performance. For example, people may be trying hard but lack the resources (e.g., equipment) to do well, or as is often the case in health

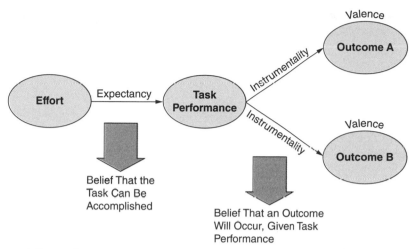

**Figure 4.4** Expectancy Theory Process.
SOURCE: Delmar, Cengage Learning.

care, there is a great deal of interdependence between people so that performance depends on all their efforts. Work done in groups or teams often has this feature. When this is the case and coworkers' efforts are lacking, an individual's perceptions of the link between their efforts and group or unit performance can be easily diminished. In any case, managers need to make it clear that, insofar as they are able, they will not hold people accountable for performance problems that stem from factors not in their control.

## Goal Setting and Feedback

Locke (1968) proposed a motivation theory that focuses on the role of goals and **goal setting**. He and his colleagues define a *goal* as something that an individual is consciously attempting to attain (Latham and Locke, 2006; Locke and Latham, 2004). Goals are powerful because they direct people's attention, focus effort on tasks related to goal attainment, and encourage people to persist in such tasks. Further, Locke proposed that the more difficult and specific the goal, the greater the motivation will be to attain it. In short, a goal provides guidelines for how much effort to put into work.

Several conditions must be met for goals to have a positive influence on performance. First, people must be aware of goals and know what must be done to attain them. Second, individuals must accept goals as something that they are willing to work for. People must be committed to goals. Goals

can fail to motivate people if they are seen as too difficult (Sherman, 1995; Tully, 1994) or too easy or if an individual does not know what tasks are required for goal attainment (Muchinsky, 1987). The empirical support for key parts of goal-setting theory is impressive. Nearly 400 studies—mostly experimental—show that specific, difficult goals lead to better performance than specific, easy, vague goals, such as "do your best" or no goals at all (Locke and Latham, 1990a).

Research also shows that goal setting is more effective, and usually only effective, when feedback is given to individuals so that they can monitor their performance in relation to goals. Indeed, goal setting without feedback seems to have little long-term effect on performance (Becker, 1978). On the other hand, feedback without goal setting is also ineffective. People need both goals and feedback on progress toward goals to be motivated. Furthermore, self-created feedback appears to exert a greater effect on motivation than feedback from external sources (Ivancevich and McMahon, 1982). Finally, for goal setting to be effective, people must have the ability to reach or approach the goals (Locke, 1982). Once again, this result is consistent with the expectancy theory.

The implications for managers are relatively straightforward:

1. Set or encourage people to set goals that are difficult and specific; revise and update goals as necessary. Prompts such as daily, weekly, or monthly "to do" lists are examples of useful techniques.

2. Provide timely and specific feedback to people on their progress toward goals.

3. Build commitment to goals by helping people believe they can attain goals and by selecting goals that are congruent with their values.

4. Rewards should be given contingent on goal attainment. Results from many studies show that performance is better when rewards are given contingently—that is, when individuals receive rewards or incentives based directly on performance.

5. Make sure that individuals have the ability to achieve goals they or you set.

## From Concept to Practice: Using Process Approaches to Motivate People

Taken together, the process approaches to motivation offer a powerful set of guidelines for health care managers (see "Summary and Managerial Guidelines"). Process models share the view that the content of work is often not enough to motivate people; they need reinforcement, expectations, fairness, and goals to be energized to perform their best. Indeed, process theories suggest a cycle of managerial action as indicated in the Managerial Guidelines.

# MOTIVATING HEALTH CARE PROFESSIONALS

Health care organizations typically have a varied and large number of professionals working within them, including, for example, clinical professionals (physicians, nurses, physical therapists, social workers), attorneys, and accountants. Professionals are distinct from other occupational groups in the extent to which (1) they control who may become a member of the group by means of rigorous selection and licensure (which typically results in a high degree of cohesion among members); (2) their work is based on codified, often scientifically based, knowledge and standards; (3) they adhere to a service-focused code of ethics; and (4) they are autonomous and control their own activities (O'Connor and Lanning, 1992). Autonomy is the most important of these defining characteristics (Haug, 1988).

Because professionals are educated and socialized to think and act with a great deal of individual discretion and autonomy in their day-to-day work, managers often find it difficult to motivate them to change their behavior; indeed, professionals generally resent managerial or organizational forays into their activities (O'Connor, 1996; Starr, 1982). Yet, because professionals, especially physicians and nurses, carry out so much of the day-to-day work in health care organizations, managers must be able to motivate clinicians to provide high-quality, cost-effective services, for example, by persuading clinicians to abandon detrimental behaviors such as excessive use of resources (e.g., unnecessary diagnostic testing).

## Physicians

Though there is not "one best way" to motivate physicians to improve their performance, research and practice suggest several important guidelines. First, it is clear that passive or "one-shot" approaches to behavior change will not work. Merely distributing guidelines, protocols, or other tools to improve clinical practice results in little or no change in behavior (Smith, 2000). Similarly, traditional medical education programs that do not involve follow-up also do not work well.

Further, as we discuss in more detail below, relatively little evidence shows that financial incentives or payment systems alone modify physician behavior (Rosenthal and Frank, 2006): "While compensation is as powerful an extrinsic motivator for physicians as it is for anyone, this incentive operates in the context of other powerful motivational resources, routinely underestimated and ignored by management" (Plume, 1995). For example, merely using a reward system such that physicians who use fewer resources receive more economic rewards is probably not a good idea. Such a system—exclusively rewarding reduced resource consumption—ignores other critical activities such as participating in quality improvement programs, complying with organizational policies, and exhibiting concern for patient satisfaction (Kongstvedt, 1996).

In contrast, more useful approaches include the use of reminders and feedback, especially data-driven feedback that provides benchmarks (AHRQ, 2010; Smith, 2000). Because of their professional socialization and strong achievement needs, most physicians want to deliver not only high-quality, but exceptional care to their patients. For them to know the extent to which they are achieving these objectives, they need to be able to assess how well they are doing with respect to peers; their own past performance; and to benchmark goals. One way of accomplishing this is to develop high-quality information systems that provide feedback on a regular basis. Such a system can allow medical professionals to know not only how well they are doing, but to also enhance their confidence that they are doing things right (Kongstvedt, 1996).

Though feedback can be a powerful tool to assist managers in motivating physician behavior, several factors should be considered to maximize the effectiveness of feedback. First, for feedback to be of value, physicians must recognize that their behavior needs to change. Second, feedback needs to be frequent, timely, and given at precise time intervals to sustain new behaviors. Third, feedback must be usable, consistent, correct, and of sufficient diversity. It should contain important and valid data, for example, on finances and quality of care. Otherwise, behavior problems can intensify as rewards flow to improvements based on flawed feedback data (Charns and Smith Tewksbury, 1993). Last, managers should not portray the feedback as "good" or "bad."

Finally, and perhaps most importantly, it is critical to involve physician leaders in efforts to change physician practices; indeed, physicians are likely to respond more favorably to projects in which they can participate heavily or control entirely. As Loewenhaupt (1997) observes (see In Practice), it is more effective to motivate physicians to change their behavior when they are partners who share in a project's mission, investment, and returns.

---

## IN PRACTICE:  The M.D. Factor

*Manuel Loewenhaupt, M.D. knows doctors. Thousands of them. For nearly a decade, he's been consulting with them, learning from them, and helping them to navigate the troubled waters of change. Now, he's a partner at Accenture. This is his take on changing physician behavior.*

**Q:** How important to population-based health is a change in the ways physicians practice?

**A:** It's the heart of the whole movement because the bottom line is the way that patient care is delivered. Population-based health is powered by doctors. Without the driver, you have nothing.

**Q:** In what ways does the relationship between health care organizations and doctors complicate change?

**A:** Health systems don't have true authority over doctors. If they don't own them, they can't fire them. In some ways, doctors are like high level programmers in the computer software industry. If they don't like where they are working, they pick up and find a better place. In health care, the incentives for change don't come through a relationship of control and authority.

**Q:** How does the physician mentality fit in?

**A:** We're trained not to think of teams or collaboration as an ideal way of working. We're trained to rely on our own independent judgment. I recently read a survey in which doctors were asked to list their fictional heroes. The most popular responses were Superman, the Lone Ranger and Maverick, the combat pilot in the movie *Top Gun*. I can't think of a tougher group of people to try to manage.

**Q:** How well do doctors respond to business management concepts?

**A:** Physicians don't work well with an authority model. In fact, most view themselves as artists, not managers or executives. There attitude often is, "Please don't bother me, please don't irritate me, and please don't try to manage me. Just leave me alone and let me do my thing."

**Q:** What mistakes do health care organizations make trying to motivate doctors to change?

**A:** Too often, administrators couch the message in the wrong terms. Telling a doctor that a new way of working will help the health system thrive may have little motivating effect. Few doctors are lying awake at night worrying about the financial well-being of a hospital or health system. In fact, many doctors may actually fear improved performance of a hospital, because in a reimbursement state of mind, a strong hospital may get that way by reducing its payment to doctors.

**Q:** Are you saying that the best strategy is motivating doctors financially?

**A:** Not necessarily. Most people's first guess is that doctors are motivated by money, and they wouldn't be completely wrong. When doctors rank their priorities, money is in the top five, but not always number one. There are other key motivators, too. Among them are the increased ability to provide excellent care, more time in which to do it, efficiency, and peer recognition. If you want to influence doctors, you need to look at these elements, too.

**IN PRACTICE:  The M.D. Factor  *(Continued)***

**Q:**  What misconceptions do physicians have about the business of running a health system?

**A:**  Most doctors have very little understanding of the way that care is delivered through a system. They view administrators as little more than bean counters. And they don't understand the complicated financial models that drive and influence health care delivery.

**Q:**  Specifically, which behaviors need to change?

**A:**  First, we have to move away from the solo model of practice to a more collaborative model. Second, we need to work toward eliminating inappropriate variations in care. Most variations are driven not by clinical science, but by a "this-is-the-way-I-was-trained" mentality. And third, we need to get away from reflexive medicine—the kind of medicine that's driven by tradition rather than by scientific evidence. We can no longer rely on the "way it's always been done here."

**Q:**  Are physicians beginning to "get it"?

**A:**  Many are. But there's still a great deal of resistance out there. In some of my meetings with physicians, I do an exercise in which I ask them to describe the ideal practice environment of the future. When I read their responses, I see a lot of descriptions that sound exactly the way things were 10 years ago. People want to turn back the clock. Then I find myself explaining repeatedly that there's probably not going to be a rewind like that.

**Q:**  Whose job is it to change the way that health care is delivered?

**A:**  It's going to take a real collaboration between health system leaders and physician leaders. Many smaller organizations haven't figured out how to build that collaborative piece, and that's where they're struggling. One of the big problems that they are facing is history. There is still a lot of leftover bad feelings from earlier moves. But everyone is going to have to get beyond all that.

**Q:**  What's the first step in moving physicians toward new ways of practicing?

**A:**  Awareness. Often, that comes not from a health system, but from the market. In Detroit, for example, when the Ford Motor Company declared that it is going to reduce its health care expenditures by 30 percent, it was a wake-up call. Ford got aggressive in its contracting, and everyone realized that business as usual was over. There was this instant awareness that it would be crazy to try to achieve different results by doing the same old thing.

**Q:**  What's your advice to health care organizations that are trying to influence physician behavior?

**A:**  It's a complicated process, and it's not necessarily linear. It's going to happen at a tempo that many business managers will see as too slow. At the same time, doctors are probably going to see it as too fast. But if you work toward a partnership with physicians, and you can achieve a sense of shared investment, shared returns, and shared mission, you can convert physicians from barriers to champions of the cause.

## Nurses

Unfortunately, high levels of job dissatisfaction and voluntary turnover among nurses have become a major and chronic problem that threatens quality of care in health care organizations across the United States (see "In Practice: A Cry for Help") (Aiken et al., 2002; American Association of Colleges of Nursing, 2007). An American Nursing Association study from 1962 reported a nurse turnover rate in excess of 40 percent. The situation is little changed today: more than 40 percent of hospital nurses are dissatisfied with their jobs, and the national average for voluntary nurse turnover is estimated to be 21 percent (Aiken et al., 2001; PricewaterhouseCoopers' Health Research Institute, 2007).

Of course, nurses, like others, voluntarily leave their jobs for many reasons. For some, life circumstances precipitate a job change (e.g., children, illness, relocation, or retirement). Many nurses, however, leave their jobs because they can no longer take the work pressure, long hours, ineffective managers and unhelpful colleagues, limited opportunities for advancement, or the lack of recognition for their accomplishments. As a leading nurse management researcher, Linda Aiken, put it in a commentary on the state of the nursing workforce crisis, "It's the poor work environment, stupid!" (2002). Indeed, results from research in both general management and health care settings show that job satisfaction and turnover are consistently and positively related to several characteristics of work environments, many of which we have discussed above (e.g., Kovner, Brewer, Wu, Cheng, and Suzuki, 2006).

In response to poor working environments for nurses, the American Nurses Credentialing Center founded the Magnet program in 1983 (see "In Practice: A Cry for Help"). This program, which has expanded significantly since its inception, aims to improve the work environment for nurses and thus increase their motivation, satisfaction and performance, while reducing turnover. The name "Magnet" conveys that good work environments will attract and retain nurses.

To achieve designation as a Magnet hospital, an organization must meet several criteria, including, for example, demonstrating that it has effective nurse leaders; substantial participation of nurses in organizational decision making; and collegial relationships between nurses and physicians. Recent studies show that hospitals that meet these criteria are more likely not only to have higher levels of job satisfaction among nurses (Manojlovich and Lashinger, 2007), but also to have better outcomes for surgery patients (Friese, Lake, Aiken, Silber, and Sochalski, 2007). The key lesson from the Magnet program seems clear: managers in health care need to focus attention and effort on improving the work environment for nurses.

## A Note on Support Staff

Methods of staff motivation may vary somewhat depending on the type of personnel. Whereas professionals may exhibit high levels of need for autonomy and control, achievement, and personal growth on the job, support personnel (i.e., clerical and service workers) may exhibit lower levels of these higher-order needs. Not all clerical and service employees respond to the same incentives as do professionals. For example, a manager who assumes that such needs are the same among all staff members might be surprised to learn that some support personnel will not respond to opportunities for autonomy and personal growth on the job. Rather, they may view their jobs as a means of providing income and seek various forms of personal fulfillment off the job through their families and leisure activities.

At the same time, one should not conclude that support personnel lack higher-level needs and necessarily need more structure and control. Consider the following episode that we witnessed. A university hospital used two attendants to maintain its school of nursing. Each attendant was responsible for his particular area with no supervision, and the facility was always spotless. They were commended verbally and in writing for the high quality of their work. The vice president for Human Resources attributed their motivation and good work to the pride and ownership they felt in what they viewed as "their" area.

When the School of Nursing was closed, the two attendants were transferred to the hospital. In the hospital, they were viewed as new employees, moved around on a regular basis, and no longer had autonomy and ownership of a specific area. The quality of their work suffered, and they were written up by supervisors for attitudinal problems, lack of motivation, and inadequate work performance. Even though there was no fault of their own, their job structure and environment had changed, and so too had their motivation.

These previously highly motivated employees became accustomed to autonomy, personal control, responsibility, and pride of ownership. All of these had been taken away when their jobs were restructured. Even though they were not professional staff members, they had responded positively to opportunities to fulfill their higher-level needs noted above and negatively when these opportunities were withdrawn.

The important point in motivating both professional and support personnel is that various methods of motivation noted in the "Managerial Guidelines" in this chapter should be viewed contingently. When it comes to managing staff, one size (i.e., style) typically does not fit all.

# MOTIVATIONAL PROBLEMS

## Nature and Causes

A major challenge for all health care organizations is to avoid employee motivation problems and to remedy such problems if they do occur. Despite their best efforts, most organizations do experience some problems of employee motivation. The symptoms may involve apathy, low-quality work, and complaints from supervisors and patients.

The causes of motivational problems often fall into three categories. First, there may be inadequate definition of the desired performance, including little or no ongoing orientation for employees about effective job performance. Symptoms of this problem include a lack of goals, inadequate job descriptions, inadequate performance standards, and inadequate performance assessment.

Second, there may be impediments to employee performance. Among the most important of these may be bureaucratic or environmental obstacles, inadequate support or resources, and a mismatch between the employee's skills and job requirements. An example is a hospital experiencing significant understaffing in nursing. Because the nursing staff is probably overworked and under stress, efforts to provide a motivating environment will fail unless and until adequate staffing is provided. Research shows that inadequate nurse staffing and consequent high workloads are major problems motivating nurse turnover (Fottler, Crawford, Quintana, and White, 1995).

Third, there may be inadequate performance-reward linkages. Symptoms of this problem are inappropriate rewards that are not valued by employees, inadequate rewards for performance, delay in receipt of rewards, a low probability of receiving rewards, and inequity in the distribution of rewards.

Determining the specific causes of a particular employee motivation problem is difficult. The most effective approach is for managers to develop interpersonal skills so that two-way communication with employees is effective. The emphasis is on listening and encouraging employees to speak frankly. As a result, the problems and frustrations of particular employees—both individuals and groups—are well understood by both their immediate supervisors and higher-level managers. Many organizations find that an upward communication system can have several benefits, including reduced absenteeism and turnover, increased productivity, and higher profits (Pfeffer, 1998a).

Employee surveys also can be useful in collecting information about beliefs and attitudes as long as the surveys are anonymous and there is assurance the results will be acted on (Fottler et al., 1995). First, such surveys are valuable for identifying the problems and impediments to performance that need to be reviewed and modified. Second, they are useful for learning the value that employees attach to a number of different outcomes such as money, recognition, autonomy, and affiliation. Discrepancies between employee

and management views provide a basis for exploring ways to modify employee beliefs or job conditions to create a better match of employee values and job attributes.

However, merely conducting attitude surveys is not sufficient by itself. The results need to be used in organizational decision making to address problem areas that employees identify (Fottler et al., 1995). Otherwise, employees may become angry and cynical if management fails to act on their comments, complaints, and suggestions.

## Potential Solutions

Table 4.1 outlines the three motivational problems discussed in the beginning of this section together with potential solutions. It is important to recognize that most motivational problems have more than one cause and more than one solution. In fact, successful employee motivation programs might include several integrated and mutually reinforcing approaches (Locke and Latham, 1990b, 2004). At a minimum, these approaches should include some combination of goal setting, with high-challenge or difficult goals; valued rewards contingent upon performance; clear and shared expectancy of success; employee feedback, employee involvement or participation; and job redesign. The long-run goal should be to develop and retain a "culture of performance" (see "Case: Staff Motivation at Sharp HealthCare").

Currently, an important and controversial approach to improving the link between performance and rewards is **pay-for-performance**, which links desired behaviors or outcomes to financial rewards or penalties. Pay-for-performance programs vary along several dimensions. The most important of these are: (1) the aspect of performance that is assessed (e.g., patient safety; cost-efficiency); (2) the level at which performance is measured—individual, group, or organization; (3) a focus on processes or outcomes (e.g., if the focus is on processes a hospital would be paid for providing appropriate antibiotic medicines to patients versus a focus on outcomes in which a hospital is financially penalized if a patient develops infections post-discharge); (4) the magnitude of payment that is linked to performance; (5) the use of penalties versus rewards (such as bonuses).

Pay-for-performance programs have increased substantially in number and importance in the past few years. More than 40 private sector hospital pay-for-performance programs now exist that focus specifically on inpatient hospital care

**TABLE 4.1  Common Employee Motivation Problems and Potential Solutions**

| Motivational Problems | Potential Solutions |
|---|---|
| 1. Inadequate performance definition (i.e., lack of goals, inadequate job descriptions, inadequate performance standards, inadequate performance assessment) | • Well-defined job descriptions<br>• Well-defined performance standards<br>• Goal setting |
| 2. Impediments to performance (i.e., bureaucratic or environmental obstacles, inadequate support or resources, poor employee-job matching, inadequate information) | • Feedback on performance<br>• Improved employee selection<br>• Job redesign<br>• Enhanced hygiene factors (i.e., safe and clean environment, salary and fringe benefits, job security, staffing, time off job, equipment) |
| 3. Inadequate performance-reward linkages (i.e., inappropriate rewards, inadequate rewards, poor timing of rewards, low probability of receiving rewards, inequity in distribution of rewards) | • Pay for performance<br>• Enhanced achievement or growth factors (i.e., employee involvement-participation, job redesign, career planning, professional development opportunities)<br>• Enhanced esteem or power factors (i.e., autonomy or personal control, self-management, modified work schedule, recognition, praise or awards, opportunity to display skills or talents, opportunity to mentor or train others, promotions in rank or position, information concerning organization or department, preferred work activities or projects, preferred work space)<br>• Enhanced affiliation (i.e., work teams, task groups, social activities, professional and community group participation, personal communication or leadership style) |

(Mehrotra, Damberg, Sorbero, and Teleki, 2009). Further, the Medicare Payment Advisory Commission and the Institute of Medicine have recommended that Medicare adopt a hospital pay-for-performance program. The Centers for Medicare and Medicaid Services have been experimenting with these programs since 2003, and, more recently, the experiments expanded to include physician practices.

The reason for the rising prominence of pay-for-performance programs is straightforward: payers, consumers, and other stakeholders believe that health care organizations are not providing services at a satisfactory level of quality or cost, and that strengthening the link between performance and financial rewards will produce better results. Nonetheless, it is not clear that these programs will meet their aims. To date, there is relatively little sound evidence that pay-for-performance programs meet their goals either in health care settings (e.g., Rosenthal and Frank, 2006; Glickman et al., 2007; Mehrota et al., 2009; Campbell, Reeves, Kontopantelis, Sibbald, and Roland, 2009) or in other industries (e.g., Tosi, Werner, and Katz, 2000; Barkema and Gomez-Mejiia, 1998).

Indeed, critics charge that pay-for-performance programs can have detrimental effects that outweigh their benefits. One concern is that individuals will focus narrowly on performance measures and associated rewards to the extent that they do not give adequate attention or effort to other important work that is not part of a pay-for-performance program (Campbell et al., 2009). Critics also argue that measures used in these programs may have fundamental flaws. For example, programs can emphasize clinical care processes that, in practice, are not strongly linked to patient outcomes (e.g., Krumholz et al., 2007). To the extent that this is the case, clinicians will work diligently to provide services that ultimately do not improve patients' health.

Further, the measures and standards that pay-for-performance programs use may not give clinicians enough autonomy to make decisions about patients whose problems do not fit well with a particular protocol. In the worst case, clinicians can be motivated to practice "cookbook" medicine that actually harms individual patients.

Another major concern is that pay-for-performance programs will hold individuals and organizations accountable for work processes or outcomes that are not under their control (Jones, Brown, and Opelka, 2005). For example, consider Dr. Smith from the In Practice section "Motivating a Primary Care Physician": under a pay-for-performance plan, she might receive a bonus if her patients' diabetes symptoms are under control. Even if she follows treatment guidelines very carefully, however, her patients may not do their part—for example, by eating a proper diet. Should Dr. Smith be penalized? In fact, much of the work that individuals do in health care organizations requires coordination with coworkers, patients, and their families, as well as community organizations. This high level of interdependence poses a challenge for pay-for-performance programs.

More generally, critics charge that pay-for-performance programs put too much emphasis on external rewards for work (termed extrinsic motivation) compared to rewards and motives that are more psychological and internal to individuals (intrinsic rewards) (Janus, 2010). In the extreme, extrinsic motivation to earn financial rewards may "crowd out" or undermine intrinsic motives for work (Pfeffer, 1998b; Deci and Koestner, 1999). As discussed above, a range of factors motivate individuals and, most often in health care, money is only part of the picture; but it is clearly possible that money can become too important.

Similar criticisms recently have been made of goal setting: critics argue that it can be overemphasized as a motivational tool, causing individuals to have a narrow focus on achieving particular goals, even to the extent that they engage in unethical behavior to attain rewards linked to goal achievement (Ordonez, Schweitzer, Galinsky, and Bazerman, 2009). Overzealous striving to attain goals and their associated financial rewards can undermine overall performance. There also is evidence that pay-for-performance programs fail for the opposite reason: the rewards are too small or criteria for receiving them conflict with each other, resulting in a weak signal and little impact on motivation (Rynes, Gerhart, and Minette, 2004).

Considering these potential weaknesses with pay-for-performance programs, are managers and policy makers wrong to increase reliance on them? Not necessarily. There also is some evidence that pay-for-performance programs can be effective if they are well designed and well implemented, thus avoiding or minimizing the major pitfalls discussed above (Gerhart, Rynes, and Fulmer, 2009).

To begin, it is critical to develop a set of well-balanced performance measures that takes into account several important aspects of a job (Kaplan and Norton, 1996). As noted, for example, it may be important to reward teamwork as well as individual performance, especially because good outcomes for patients typically require coordination among specialists (Gittell, 2009). Second, successful pay-for-performance programs follow many of the principles discussed above that characterize other approaches to motivation: they establish high standards of performance; develop accurate performance measurement systems; and train managers in the practices of effective feedback.

Third, it is important to recognize that individuals will vary in their reactions to pay-for-performance programs. For example, individuals with high need for achievement and those with a history of high achievement are more likely to prefer pay-for-performance programs (e.g., Trank, Rynes, and Bretz, 2002).

Finally, it is critical to take a well-balanced approach to rewards and incentives, relying on nonfinancial rewards as well as financial ones (WHO, 2008). Unlike many Wall Street bankers who are motivated primarily by money, many health care workers choose their profession for reasons other than salary. Consequently, health care organizations need to identify and respond to a wide variety of noneconomic needs that may motivate their employees (see Table 4.1). For example, simple recognition practices and programs offer another method of linking employee participation and rewards, including: informal public praise for good work; organizing a departmental gathering to honor achievements of one or more employees; and publishing employee accomplishments and complimentary letters from patients or visitors on the organization's Web site or in a newsletter (Huseman and Hatfield, 1989; McConnell, 1997).

One well-known example of an organization that has designed and implemented an effective pay-for-performance program is Lincoln Electric, a company that manufactures welding devices. Lincoln, founded more than 100 years ago, teaches some essential lessons about pay-for-performance. One is that developing an effective program takes years. Lincoln's approach has evolved over a period of decades through trial and error. This should serve as a warning to managers and policy makers in health care who expect pay-for-performance programs to produce quick results. Lincoln also clearly uses a balanced set of performance measures that assesses individuals' productivity, quality, teamwork, and contributions to innovations in work and products (Levin, 2003).

But, in our view, the most important lesson that health care organizations can learn from Lincoln is that its pay-for-performance system works well primarily because it is part of an approach to managing people that is characterized by several best practices: high levels of trust (Lincoln has never laid off workers when it faced financial problems); employee involvement in decision making (employees are well-represented on a management governing board); investment in employees (Lincoln promotes from within and provides many training and development opportunities); flat hierarchy and equality (there are very few layers of management and no management "perks"); and high levels of employee stock ownership in the company. Of course, making welding equipment is not the same as providing health care. Nonetheless, health care organizations can benefit substantially from using these practices, especially if they plan to rely on pay-for-performance programs (see "Case: Staff Motivation at Sharp HealthCare").

**Job redesign** is yet another strategy that can lead to increased motivation (see also Chapter 7). It is based on the premise that altering certain aspects of the job to satisfy employees' psychological needs will motivate them to exert more effort. According to Hackman and Oldham (1980), satisfaction of higher-order needs occurs when the employee experiences the following psychological states. First, the job allows the employee to feel personally responsible for a significant segment of his or her work outcomes. Autonomy or personal control is the key job dimension that contributes to feelings of personal responsibility for job outcomes. Second, the job involves doing something that is perceived as meaningful by the individual. The three core dimensions that can make jobs meaningful are task identity (i.e., completion of a whole task), skill variety (i.e., utilization of different skills), and task significance (i.e., substantial impact). Third, the job provides the employee with knowledge of results. Feedback from the job itself or from another individual is the core job dimension, which provides knowledge of results.

One study, for example, examined job redesign for nurses and nurses' aides employed in long-term care settings. The results showed that family members' satisfaction with the quality of services received was positively influenced by the nurses' level of organizational commitment, which, in turn, was positively correlated with autonomy, task identity, and skill variety. This study indicates that redesigning nursing and nurse's aides' jobs in long-term care settings can serve to motivate these employees to be more committed to the organization as well as to provide higher levels of service quality (Steffen, Nystrom, and O'Connor, 1996).

Job redesign is most appropriate when it is feasible given the structure of jobs, legal constraints, technological constraints, and the characteristics and values of employees. Job redesign in health care is certainly feasible, but may be subject to more legal and professional constraints than most other industries (Blayney, 1992).

Research in both non–health care and health care organizations generally supports the validity of the job characteristics model in enhancing employee motivation, especially for employees who strongly value personal feelings of accomplishment and growth (Alpander, 1990; Grant and Parker, 2009; Guzzo, Jette, and Katzell, 1985). However, the success of any job redesign effort is likely to depend on other reinforcing factors such as the reward system and top management support (Fried and Ferris, 1987).

Finally, many of the strategies discussed above depend on employee **empowerment**. Empowerment involves "directed autonomy" whereby individuals or teams are given an overall direction yet considerable leeway concerning how they go about following that direction. It also necessitates sharing information and knowledge with employees, which enables them to understand and contribute to organizational performance, and giving them the autonomy to make decisions that influence organizational outcomes (Ford and Fottler, 1995). It is the issue of power that differentiates empowerment from other approaches to employee participation (i.e., delegation, decentralization, and participatory management) that emphasize employee input, but perhaps no real change in the assignment of power and authority.

Obviously, empowerment is a matter of degree rather than an absolute (Ford and Fottler, 1995). Managers could choose to provide higher degrees of empowerment for some individuals and teams doing certain tasks than for others. He or she could empower subordinates in terms of any or all of the following: problem identification, alternative development, alternative evaluation, alternative choice, and implementation.

## Overall Assessment

Though there are many approaches to dealing with motivational problems among employees, none are foolproof. Whether a particular approach succeeds in a particular setting depends first on whether it was properly matched with the primary causes of low motivation. Second, it depends on if and how the program was introduced and implemented so that resistance was minimized and commitment maximized. For example, favorable reaction is likely to be greatest if the affected employees have some voice in choosing and implementing a particular motivation program. Third, it depends on whether the program is compatible with other aspects of the organization's culture (Hames, 1991; Mohrmann and Lawler, 1984). The simultaneous introduction of several mutually supportive and mutually reinforcing motivation programs is probably most effective in overcoming motivational problems, assuming they are all relevant to the causes of the problem. An example is the program at Sharp HealthCare (see "Case: Staff Motivation at Sharp HealthCare").

## DEBATE TIME: Pros and Cons of Pay-for-Performance

As noted above, pay-for-performance programs of various kinds have increased substantially in number and importance in the past few years. The reason for the rising prominence of pay-for-performance programs in both the private and public sectors is that payers, consumers, and other stakeholders believe that health care organizations are not providing services at a satisfactory level of quality or cost and that strengthening the link between performance and financial rewards will produce better results.

Nonetheless, critics of these programs argue that they will meet their aims for several reasons. First, critics charge that under pay-for-performance, individuals will focus narrowly on performance measures and associated rewards to the extent that they do not give adequate attention or effort to other important work that is not part of a pay-for-performance program. Second, critics argue that measures used in these programs may have fundamental flaws. For example, programs can emphasize clinical care processes that, in practice, are not strongly linked to patient outcomes. Third, the measures and standards that pay-for-performance programs use may not give clinicians enough autonomy to make decisions about patients whose problems do not fit well with a particular protocol. Fourth, pay-for-performance programs may hold individuals and organizations accountable for work processes or outcomes that are not under their control. Fifth, critics claim that pay-for-performance programs put too much emphasis on external rewards for work (termed extrinsic motivation) compared to rewards and motives that are more psychological and internal to individuals (intrinsic rewards). In the extreme, extrinsic motivation to earn financial rewards may "crowd out" or undermine intrinsic motives for work. Finally, there also is evidence that pay-for-performance programs fail for the opposite reason: the rewards are too small or criteria for receiving them conflict with each other, resulting in a weak signal and little impact on motivation.

Given these concerns, do you support pay-for-performance programs? How will you manage individuals and teams working under these programs?

# SUMMARY AND MANAGERIAL GUIDELINES

1. Health care managers can motivate people by determining what needs and rewards they view as most important. This can be accomplished through formal and informal means of communication.

2. Rewards may be both economic and noneconomic. They should be relevant to the priority needs of particular employees or employee groups. If at all possible, solicit employee views on rewards and involve them in developing and implementing reward and incentive systems.

3. Goals should be set at the time of hiring and at periodic performance evaluations. Set or encourage people to set goals that are difficult and specific; revise and update goals as necessary.

4. Expectations about goal attainment and consequences also should be set at the time of hiring and reviewed periodically. Build commitment to goals by helping people believe that they can attain them and by selecting goals that are consistent with their values.

5. Make sure that the rules for attaining rewards are clear to everyone.

6. Check employees' perceptions of the fairness of their work and rewards. Address perceived inequities as best as possible, given resource constraints. Note that perceptions of inequity are especially likely when managers try to take individuals' different needs into account.

7. Provide timely and specific feedback to people on their progress toward goals.

8. Reward people contingent on performance.

9. Redesigning jobs is another alternative for increasing the match between individuals' needs and motives and their work. Redesigning offers much potential for increased motivation to the extent that it involves building-in responsibility, decision making, control, autonomy, challenge, and opportunities for achievement.

# DISCUSSION QUESTIONS

1. How can managers distinguish a motivational problem from other factors that affect an individual's performance?

2. In situations such as the ICU faced in "In Practice: A Cry for Help," what role can managers and clinical leaders play to improve staff morale and motivation?

3. What approaches other than a productivity bonus could the management team at the community health center have used to change Dr. Smith's practice patterns (see "In Practice: Motivating a Primary Care Physician in a Community Health Center")?

4. If you wanted to implement a Must Haves program in your organization, what elements would you include in your implementation plan? What metrics would you use to measure the success of the initiative?

# CASE: Staff Motivation at Sharp HealthCare

Sharp HealthCare is an integrated, regional health care delivery system based in San Diego, California, serving a population of approximately three million. Sharp includes four acute-care hospitals, three specialty hospitals, and three medical groups plus a full-spectrum of other facilities and services. It operates 1,878 beds, has approximately 2,600 physicians on medical staffs, more than 1,000 physicians in two affiliated medical groups, and has more than 14,000 employees with $5.852 million in assets and $1.9 billion in annual income. It is San Diego's largest private employer.

Sharp's goal is to be the best place to work, the best place to practice medicine, and the best place to receive care in San Diego. In 2008 Sharp HealthCare ranked fifth in the California "best places to work program" in the large-employer category and was rated 47th out of the top 100 places to work in the United States by *Modern Healthcare*.

Since launching the healthcare experience in 2001, Sharp has dedicated itself to transforming the health care experience for employees, physicians, and customers. The focus on purpose, worthwhile work, and making a difference has led to increased employee, physician, and patient satisfaction, enhanced loyalty, and improved outcomes. In 2007 Sharp HealthCare won the prestigious Malcolm Baldrige National Quality Award.

### Pillars of Excellence

Since 2001, Sharp has adopted six pillars of excellence as the foundation for its vision of the health care experience. These six pillars are the basis for everything from strategic planning, organizational goal setting, priority setting, management performance evaluation, and other agendas. There are measures and targets set under each pillar that align each individual leader's goal with their department, division, and the entire Sharp system. With the pillars as a guide, communications and work planning are made more manageable and various outcomes measurement enhanced.

Of the six pillars, the three most relevant to staff motivation are Quality, Service, and People. A few of the measures used to determine performance targets under each of these three pillars are:

- Quality: Accreditation and licensing scores; infection control measures; patient safety
- Service: Overall patient and physician satisfaction in Sharp hospitals and medical groups
- People: Increased employee satisfaction and retention

### Model Behaviors and Scripts

To ensure Sharp is the best place to work, the best place to practice medicine, and the best place to receive care, all employees are required to exemplify the Must Haves, five essential behaviors and actions in the workplace:

- Greet people with a smile and "Hello," using their name when possible.
- Take people where they are going, rather than pointing or giving directions.
- Use key words (scripts) at key times: "Is there anything else I can do for you? I have time."
- Foster an attitude of gratitude and send thank-you notes to deserving employees.
- Make rounds in the hospital to better connect with staff, patients, family, and other customers.

### Employee Forums

In the spirit of a "no-secrets" culture, Sharp keeps the line of communication between management and employees open; each unit holds quarterly employee forums led by the entity CEO. The purpose is to share important updates and information and recognize and celebrate the work of Sharp employees. Up to 20 forums are held around the clock over a two-day period to attract as many employees as possible. The agenda for these forums is based on each of the six pillars of excellence. Sample topics include system or entity report cards, patient satisfaction scores, physician satisfaction scores, model behavior standards, facility openings, celebrations, and wins.

### Re-Recruiting Employees

High and increasing levels of employee satisfaction and retention are top priorities for both individuals and managers, as well as the entire system. One of the tools managers use to retain the employees is re-recruitment of current employees rather than new ones. Re-recruiting recognizes employees for their contributions, renews their sense of self-worth and loyalty, and ensures their longevity.

The following four steps are used in Sharp's re-recruiting technique:

- Identify the great, good, and low-performing employees in each department. Great performers are those who always have a positive attitude and take initiative to tackle projects and solve problems. Good performers are those who need help developing in some areas, but are generally reliable employees. Low performers are those who take no initiative to complete tasks and have a negative attitude.

- Meet with your great performers individually to let each of them know they are a valuable asset to your department and company. Let them know what they are doing right, cite specific examples, and ask them what you can do to ensure their longevity with Sharp.

- Meet with your good performers individually to let them know how much you value their contribution, provide specific examples, and let them know that you want them to stay with your organization. Be sure to also specify areas in need of improvement.

- Meet with your marginal performers individually to let them know that their behaviors or actions are not consistent with the organization's standards. Specify areas in need of improvement and let them know the consequences of not taking steps to change negative behaviors and actions.

## Employee Opinion Survey

Sharp also surveys its 14,000 employees annually through an online employee opinion survey using a password sent from an outside vendor to the employee's home. The survey asks for team members' opinions on many aspects of their work experience to ensure they feel adequately supported and have the tools, supplies, and training to provide the best health care possible. Results are provided to all Sharp managers and employees. The employee opinion survey forms the foundation for management improvement plans to align the specific needs for each category of worker to contribute to Sharp's overarching performance goals and objectives.

Each manager reviews the system, entity, and department results with their staff members at a dedicated staff meeting set aside to vote on the top three priorities they would like their department to address. The manager assigns action teams to address each of these priorities. The actionable items and the plan to address them are part of a 90-day action plan that each manager must share with his or her supervisor. Progress toward the top three goals is addressed in quarterly updates that are reviewed with and turned in to the supervisor. Once the first three priorities are addressed, the manager then addresses additional priorities with his/her team. Actions and results emanating from employee opinion surveys are reported back to staff at staff meetings. The top actions to address staff needs are then shared and celebrated at Leadership Development for Managers at the end of each fiscal year.

## Workforce Planning and Development

In addition to the employee opinion survey, Sharp's "People" pillar of excellence is supported with a systematic workforce engagement and development program. The goal of the program is to promote meaningful work among all employees.

- Leadership System: All members of the Sharp workforce have the opportunity to participate in multidisciplinary teams to set goals, deliver patient care, problem solve, identify performance-improvement projects, and effect change.

- Performance Evaluation System: Each person employed at Sharp completes an annual review where they receive feedback on their overall performance and have the opportunity to develop personal goals for skill improvement and career advancement within the system.

- The Sharp University provides on-site continuing professional education to facilitate learning and skill development for Sharp's workforce. Course content is linked with assessment data to target key areas for workforce development. Workforce development focuses not only on clinical knowledge and expertise, but also process improvement, team work and care coordination skills.

**Questions**

1. What are the key factors in Sharp's successful approach to motivation?

2. Do you see any weaknesses in the Sharp approach?

3. Can the Sharp approach be replicated in other health care organizations? What are some important barriers and facilitators to using the Sharp approach?

SOURCES:

Murphy, M. W. (2004, June 4). *Using evidenced-based management to transform health care.* Presentation at the annual meeting of the Association of University Programs in Health Administration, San Diego, CA.

Sharp HealthCare. Malcolm Baldridge Award application. Retrieved August 15, 2010, from http://www.sharp.com

Sharp HealthCare. Web site. http://www.sharp.com.

# REFERENCES

Adams, J. S. (1963, November). Toward an understanding of inequity. *Journal of Abnormal and Social Psychology, 67,* 422–436.

Adams, J. S. (1965). Inequity in social exchange. In L. Berkowitz (Ed.), *Advances in Experimental Social Psychology, II.* New York: Academic Press.

Aiken, L. H. (2002). Commentary. *Medical Care Research and Review 59*(2): 215–222.

Aiken, L. H., Clarke, S, P., Sloan, D. M., Sochalski, J. A., Busse, R., Clarke, H., Giovannetti, P., Hunt, J., Rafferty, A. M., & Shamian, J. (2001). Nurses report on hospital care in five countries. *Health Affairs, 20*(3): 43–53.

Aiken, L. H., Clarke, S. P., Sloan, D. M., Sochalski, J., & Silber, J. H. (2002). Hospital nurse staffing and patient mortality, nurse burnout and job dissatisfaction. *Journal of the American Medical Association, 288*(16): 1987–1993.

Alderfer, C. P. (1968). An empirical test of a new theory of human needs. *Organization Behavior and Human Performance, 16*(2), 42–175.

Alderfer, C. P. (1972). *Existence, relatedness, and growth.* New York: Free Press.

Alpander, G. G. (1990). Relationship between commitment to hospital goals and job satisfaction: A case study of a nursing department. *Health Care Management Review, 25*(4), 51–62.

American Association of Colleges of Nursing. Nursing shortage resource fact sheet. Retrieved December 10, 2009, from http://www.aacn.nche.edu/Media/shortageresource.htm.

American Nurses Association (2009). *Nursing administration: Scope and standards of practice.* Silver Springs, MD: ANA.

American Nurses' Association. (1962). Spot Check of Current Hospital Employment Conditions. Kansas City, MO: Research and Statistical Unit, American Nurses' Association.

Appleby, C. (1998). Braindrain. *H&HN: Hospitals and Health Networks, 72*(8), 41–43.

Atkinson, J. W. (1961). *An introduction to motivation.* New York: Van Nostrand.

Barkema, H. G., & Gomez-Mejia, L. R. (1998). Managerial compensation and firm performance: A general research framework. *Academy of Management Journal, 41*(2), 135–145.

Becker, I. J. (1978). Joint effect of feedback and goal setting on performance: A field study of residential energy conservation. *Journal of Applied Psychology, 63,* 428–433.

Blayney, K. D. (Ed.). (1992). *Healing hands: Customizing your health team for institutional survival.* Battle Creek, MI: W. K. Kellogg Foundation.

Brockner, J. (2006). Why it's so hard to be fair. *Harvard Business Review, 84*(3), 122–129.

Campbell, J. P., & Pritchard, R. D. (1976). Motivation theory in industrial and organizational psychology. In M. D. Dunnette (Ed.), *Handbook of industrial and organizational psychology* (pp. 63–130). Skokie, IL: Rand McNally.

Campbell, S. M., Reeves, D., Kontopantelis, E., Sibbald, B., & Roland, M. (2009). Effects of pay for performance on the quality of primary care in England. *New England Journal of Medicine, 361*, 368–378.

Charns, M. P., & Smith Tewksbury, L. J. (1993). *Collaborative management in health care: Implementing the integrative organization.* San Francisco: Jossey-Bass Publishers.

Colvin, G. (1998). What money makes you do. *Fortune, 138*(4), 213–214.

Davis-Blake, A., & Pfeffer, J. (1989). Just a mirage: The search for disposition effects in organizational research. *Academy of Management Review, 14*(3), 385–400.

Deci, E. L., & Koestner, R. (1999). A meta-analytic review of experiments examining the effects of extrinsic rewards on intrinsic motivation. *Psychological Bulletin, 125*(6), 627–669.

Ford, R. C., & Fottler, M. D. (1995). Empowerment: A matter of degree. *Academy of Management Executive, 9*(3), 21–29.

Fottler, M. D., Crawford, M. A., Quintana, J. B., & White, J. B. (1995). Evaluating nurse turnover: Comparing attitude surveys and exit interviews. *Hospital and Health Services Administration, 40*(2), 278–295.

Freid, Y., & Ferris, G. R. (1987). The validity of the job characteristics model: A review and meta-analysis. *Personnel Psychology, 40*(2), 287–322.

Fried, Y., & Slowik, L. H. (2004). Enriching goal setting theory with time: An integrated approach. *Academy of Management Review, 29*(3), 404–422.

Friese, C. R., Lake, E. T., Aiken, L. H., Silber, J. H., & Sochalski, J. (2008): Hospital nurse practice environments and outcomes for surgical oncology patients. *Health Services Research, 43*(4), 1145–1162.

Georgopoulos, B. S., Mahoney, B. S., & Jones, N. W. (1957). A path-goal approach to productivity. *Journal of Applied Psychology, 41*, 345–353.

Gerhart, B., Rynes, S. L., & Fulmer, I. S. (2009). Pay and performance: Individuals, groups and executives. *Annals of the Academy of Management, 3*(1), 251–315.

Glickman, S. W. Fang-Shu Ou, F-S., Elizabeth, R., DeLong, E. R., Roe, M. T., Lytle, B. L., Mulgund, J., Rumsfeld, J. S., Gibler, W. B., Ohman, E. M., Schulman, K. A., & Peterson, E. D. (2007). Pay for performance, quality of care, and outcomes in acute myocardial infarction. *Journal of the American Medical Association, 297*, 2373–2380.

Gittell, J. H. (2009). *High performance health care: Using the power of relationships to achieve quality, efficiency and resilience.* New York: McGraw-Hill.

Grant, A. M., & Parker, S. K. (2009). Redesigning work design theories: The rise of relational and proactive perspectives. *Academy of Management Annals, 3*(1), 317–375.

Guzzo, R. A., Jette, R. D., & Katzell, R. A. (1985). The effects of psychologically based intervention programs on worker productivity: A meta analysis. *Personnel Psychology, 38*(3), 275–291.

Hackman, J. R., & Oldham, G. (1980). *Work redesign.* Reading, MA: Addison-Wesley.

Hames, D. S. (1991). Productivity-enhancing work innovations: Remedies for what ails hospitals? *Hospital and Health Services Administration, 38*(4), 545–557.

Haug, M. E. (1988). A re-examination of the hypothesis of physician deprofessionalization. *Milbank Quarterly, 66*(Suppl. 2), 48–56.

Herzberg, F. (1987). One more time: How do you motivate employees? *Harvard Business Review, 65,* 109–120.

Higgins, E. T., & Kruglansky, A. W. (Eds.). (2000). *Motivational science: Social and personality perspectives.* Philadelphia: Psychology Press.

Huselid, M. A. (1995). The impact of human resource management practices on turnover, productivity, and corporate financial performance. *Academy of Management Journal, 38(3),* 635–672.

Huseman, R. C., & Hatfield, J. D. (1989). *Managing the equity factor.* Boston: Houghton-Mifflin.

Ivancevich, J. M., & McMahon, J. T. (1982). The effects of goal-setting, external feedback, and self-generated feedback on outcome variables: A field experiment. *Academy of Management Journal, 25(2),* 359–372.

Janus, K. (2010). Managing motivation among healthcare professionals. Working paper. Columbia University, Mailman School of Public Health, Department of Health Policy and Management.

Jones, R. S., Brown, C., & Opelka, F. (2005). Surgeon compensation: "Pay for performance," the American College of Surgeons national surgical quality improvement program, the surgical care improvement program, and other considerations. *Surgery, 138,* 829–836.

Kanfer, R. (1990). Motivation theory and industrial and organizational psychology. In M. D. Dunnette & L. M. Houghlin (Eds.), *Handbook of industrial and organizational psychology* (pp. 75–170). Palo Alto, CA: Consulting Psychologists Press, Inc.

Kanfer, R., & Ackerman, P. L. (2004). Aging, adult development and work motivation. *Academy of Management Review, 29(3),* 423–439.

Kaplan, R. S., & Norton, D. P. (1996). Using the balanced scorecard as a strategic management system. *Harvard Business Review, 74(1),* 75–85.

Kennedy, M. M. (1997). How to put new life into an old job. *Healthcare Executive, 12(5),* 44–45.

Kim, W. C., & Mauborgne, R. (2003). Fair process: Managing in the knowledge economy. *Harvard Business Review,* January, 1–10, reprint number RO301K

Kongstvedt, P. R. (1996). *The managed care health care handbook* (3rd ed.). Gaithersburg, MD: Aspen Publishers, Inc.

Kovner, C., Brewer, C., Wu, Y-W., Cheng, Y., & Suzuki, M. (2006). Factors associated with work satisfaction of registered nurses. *Journal of Nursing Scholarship, 38(1):* 71–79.

Krumholz, H. M., Normand, S-L. T., Spertus, J. A., Shahian, D. M., & Bradley, E. H. (2007). Measuring performance for treating heart attacks and heart failure: The case for outcomes measurement. *Health Affairs, 26,* 75–85.

Latham, G. P., & Locke, E. A. (2006). Enhancing the benefits and overcoming the pitfalls of goal setting. *Organizational Dynamics, 34(5),* 332–340.

Laurinaitis, J. (1997). Actions speak louder than posters. *Psychology Today, 30(3),* 16.

Levin, J. (2003). Relational incentive contract. *American Economic Review, 93(3),* 835–857.

Locke, E. A. (1968). Effects of knowledge of results, feedback in relation to standards, and goals on reaction-time performance. *American Journal of Applied Psychology, 81,* 566–574.

Locke, E. A. (1982). Relation of goal level to performance with a short work period and multiple goal levels. *Journal of Applied Psychology, 67,* 512–514.

Locke, E. A., & Latham, G. P. (1990a). *A theory of goal setting and task performance.* Englewood Cliffs, NJ: Prentice-Hall.

Locke, E. A., & Latham, G. P. (1990b). Work motivation and satisfaction: Light at the end of the tunnel. *Psychological Science, 1(4),* 240–246.

Locke, E. A., & Latham, G. P. (2004). What should we do about motivation theory? Six recommendations for the twenty-first century. *Academy of Management Review, 29*(3), 388–403.

Manojlovich, M., & Laschinger, H. (2007). The nursing worklife model: Extending and refining a new theory. *Journal of Nursing Management, 15,* 256–263.

Maslow, A. H. (1943). A theory of human motivation. *Psychological Review, 50,* 370–396.

McClelland, D. C. (1961). *The achieving society.* Princeton, NJ: Van Nostrand.

McClelland, D. C. (1975). *Power: The inner experience.* New York: Irvington.

McClelland, D. C., & Burnham, D. H. (1976). Power is the great motivator. *Harvard Business Review, 54*(2), 100–110.

McConnell, C. R. (1996). After reduction in force: Reinvigorating the survivors. *Health Care Supervisor, 14*(4), 1–2.

McConnell, C. R. (1997). Employee recognition: A little oil on the troubled waters of change. *Health Care Supervisor, 15*(4), 83–90.

The M.D. Factor. (1997). *Crossroads: New directions in health management* (Supplement to *Hospitals and Health Networks*).

Mehrotra, A., Damberg, C. L., Sorbero, M. E. S., & Teleki, S. S. (2009). Pay for performance in hospital settings: What is the state of the evidence? *American Journal of Medical Quality, 24*(1), 19–28.

Mercer, A. A. (1988). Commitment and motivation of professionals. In M. D. Fottler, S. R. Hernandez, and C. L. Joiner (Eds.), *Strategic management of human resources in health services organizations* (pp. 181–205). New York: John Wiley and Sons.

Mitchell, T. R. (1982). Motivation: New directions for theory, research, and practice. *Academy of Management Review, 7,* 80–88.

Mohr, L. B. (1982). *Explaining organizational behavior.* San Francisco: Jossey-Bass.

Mohrmann, S. A., & Lawler, E. E. (1984). Quality of worklife. *Research in Personnel and Human Resources Management, 2,* 219–260.

Morrissey, J. (2004). Dr. Intimidation: Surly prescribers increase risk of errors: Survey. *Modern Healthcare, 34*(14), 10.

Muchinsky, P. M. (1987). *Psychology applied to work: An introduction to industrial and organizational psychology* (pp. 341–378). Belmont, CA: Wadsworth, Inc.

Nordhaus-Bike, A. M. (1997). Cutting with kindness. *Hospital and Health Networks, 71*(2), 62–63.

O'Connor, S. J. (1996). Who will manage the managers? In A. Lazarus (Ed.), *Controversies in managed mental health care* (pp. 383–401). Washington, DC: American Psychiatric Press.

O'Connor, S. J., & Lanning, J. A. (1992). The end of autonomy? Reflections on the post-professional physician. *Health Care Management Review, 17*(1), 63–72.

O'Connor, S. J., & Shewchuk, R. M. (1995). Service quality revisited: Striving for a new orientation. *Hospital and Health Services Administration, 40*(1), 535–552.

Ordonez, L. D., Schweitzer, M. E., Galensky, A. D., & Bazerman, M. H. (2009). On good scholarship, goal setting and scholars gone wild. *Academy of Management Perspectives, 23*(3), 82–87.

Pfeffer, J. (1998a). *The human equation: Building profits by putting people first.* Boston: Harvard Business School Press.

Pfeffer, J. (1998b). Six dangerous myths about pay. Harvard Business Review, May–June, 109–119.

Plume, S. (1995). Redesigning physician compensation mechanisms: A fool's errand. *Motivation & Emotion, 19*(3), 205–210.

Porter, L. W. (1987). *Motivation and work behavior.* New York: McGraw-Hill.

PricewaterhouseCoopers' Health Research Institute. (2007). What works: Healing the healthcare staffing shortage (Report). Retrieved October 15, 2007, from http://www.pwc.com

Pritchard, R. D., De Leo, P. J., & Von Bergen, C. W. (1976). A field experimental test of expectancy—valence incentive motivation techniques. *Organizational Behavior and Human Performance, 15*, 355–406.

Rynes, S. L., Gerhart, B., & Minette, K. A. (2004). The importance of pay in employee motivation: Discrepancies between what people say and what they do. *Human Resources Management, 43*(4), 381–394.

Rosenthal, M. B. & Frank, R. G. (2006). What is the empirical basis for paying for quality in health care? *Medical Care Research and Review, 63*(135), 135–157.

Sherman, S. (1995). Stretch goals: The dark side of asking for miracles. *Fortune, 132*(10), 231–232.

Smith, W. R. (2000). Evidence for the effectiveness of techniques to change physician behavior. *CHEST, 118*(Suppl. 2), 8S–17S.

Stajkovic, A. D., & Luthans, F. (2001). Differential effects of incentive motivators on work performance. *Academy of Management Journal, 4*(3), 580–590.

Starr, P. (1982). *The social transformation of American medicine*. New York: Basic Books.

Steffen, T. M., Nystrom, P. C., & O'Connor, S. J. (1996). Satisfaction with nursing homes: The design of employees jobs can ultimately influence family members' perceptions. *Journal of Health Care Marketing, 16*(3), 34–38.

Tosi, H. L, Werner, S., Katz, J. P., & Gomez-Mejia, L. R. (2000). How much does performance matter? A meta-analysis of CEO pay studies. *Journal of Management, 26*(2), 301–339.

Trank, C. Q., Rynes, S. L., & Bretz, R. D. (2002). Attracting applicants in the war for talent: Differences in work preferences among high achievers. *Journal of Business Psychology, 17*, 331–345.

Tully, S. (1994). Why go for the stretch targets? *Fortune, 130*(10), 145–158.

Vidaver-Cohen, D. (1998). Motivational appeal in normative theories of enterprise. *Business Ethics Quarterly, 8*(3), 385–407.

Vroom, V. (1964). *Work and motivation*. New York: Wiley.

World Health Organization (2008). *Guidelines: Incentives for health professionals*. Geneva, Switzerland: World Health Organization.

Zigarelli, M. (1996). Human resources and the bottom line. *Academy of Management Executive, 10*(2), 63.

# Chapter 5

# Teams and Team Effectiveness in Health Services Organizations

**Bruce Fried, Sharon Topping, and Amy C. Edmondson**

## CHAPTER OUTLINE

- **Introduction**
- **Types of Teams in Health Care**
- **A Typology of Teams in Health Care**
- **Understanding Team Performance**
- **A Model of Team Effectiveness**
- **Conclusions**

## LEARNING OBJECTIVES

**After completing this chapter, the reader should be able to:**

1. Describe the role and value of teams in health care organizations

2. Distinguish among different types of teams in health care organizations and how these differences affect team processes and performance

3. Understand the factors associated with high-performing teams

4. Describe the potential impact of team characteristics, nature of the work, environmental context, and team processes on team performance

5. Explain alternative methods of decision making in teams, including both functional and dysfunctional decision-making processes

6. Describe the importance of psychological safety to effective team decision making and performance

7. Discuss how factors external to the team may affect team processes and performance

8. Understand the multiple impacts of team cohesiveness on team performance

9. Describe key aspects of group process including leadership, the communication structure, decision making, and stages of team development

# KEY TERMS

Accountabilities in Teams

Ambassador Activities

Behavior Norms

Boundary Permeability

Boundary-Spanning Roles

Communication Networks

Communication Technology

Decisional Authority

Delphi Technique

Diversity

Environmental Context

Formal Leadership

Formal Groups

Free Rider

Groupthink

Informal Leadership

Informal Groups

Intergroup Relationships

Management Teams

Membership Fluidity

Nominal Group Technique

Organizational Culture

Parallel Teams

Performance Norms

Project Teams

Pooled Interdependence

Psychological Safety

Reciprocal Interdependence

Sequential Interdependence

Scout Activities

Skill-Based Pay

Social Capital

Social Loafing

Stages of Team Development

Status Differences

Support Teams

Task Coordinator Activities

Task Interdependence

Team-Based Rewards

Team Cohesiveness

Team Composition

Team Goals

Team Interdependence

Team Leadership

Team Learning

Team Norms

Team Performance

Team Processes

Team Size

Temporal Nature of Teams

Tenure Diversity

Work Teams

---

**IN PRACTICE:** Improving Preventive Services in a Pediatrics Practice:
A Less-Than-Successful Team

Glendale Pediatrics is a nine-clinician pediatric group practice. The practice serves a largely middle-class suburban population and prides itself on the provision of preventive services. One of the physicians recently attended a continuing medical education program on preventive services. Upon her return, she decided to assess the practice's performance in this area. She and the other physicians were surprised when she distributed the results. Among the findings were:

- Sixty percent of children were behind schedule in at least one immunization
- Vision screening was conducted and recorded for only 15 percent of children

## IN PRACTICE:  Improving Preventive Services in a Pediatrics Practice: A Less-Than-Successful Team  (Continued)

- Fifty percent of children were screened for anemia
- Twenty-five percent of children had their blood pressure recorded in the patient record
- Thirteen percent of children were screened for lead

While the pediatricians were bewildered by these findings, the medical record and nursing staff found them consistent with their impressions. The findings were presented and discussed at the monthly staff meeting. Two physicians who together saw about 40 percent of all patients were adamant that their patients were current in their preventive services, and there was no need for a practice-wide effort to improve their preventive service rates. Unfortunately, the data were not linked to individual physicians and thus there was no way to verify their claim. Nonetheless, it was agreed that staff, including the two reluctant physicians, work as a team to address the problem.

The first meeting was scheduled over the noon hour. One of the physicians arrived at 12:20 while two others left early, at 12:45. One of the nurses was out sick. No decisions were made, and the entire meeting was spent attempting to find a date and time for follow-up meetings.

At the next meeting, one physician stated that during an acute visit, physicians do not have time to go through the medical record to determine if a patient was behind on any preventive services. The other physicians agreed and decided that a form should be developed listing all preventive services, and this should be attached to the medical record. The nurses worked together after the meeting to design the form, known as the Preventive Services Chart (PSC).

Three thousand copies of the PSC were printed. When the physicians saw the form, they indicated that it was poorly designed. All relevant services and immunization schedules were not included. The forms were destroyed, and the physicians asked the nurses to redesign the form. The nurses consulted with the physician who attended the continuing education seminar to obtain information on the recommended preventive protocols. Based on this information, the form was redesigned with the immunization schedule and other information added. Confident that this was the right form, 3,000 copies were again printed. When presented to the physicians, it was discovered that there was little agreement among the physicians and an argument broke out at the next meeting about the immunization schedules and protocols for screening.

After this meeting, one of the nurses in consultation with two physicians developed yet another form with separate columns for each physician's preventive services preferred protocol. The medical records staff, hearing about this new procedure informally over lunch, was skeptical about its feasibility. Moreover, when one of the nurses asked a physician when nurses would record this information, she was told that "nurses have it too easy in this practice ... you have a great deal of down time and you certainly can find time to prepare charts for the next day's patients."

During the next three weeks, the following events transpired:

1. Nurses complained to the physicians that medical records staff were not making records available to them in time to do the preventive services review.

2. Medical records staff complained to the physicians that nurses were unrealistically requesting the next day's charts at 9:00 a.m. so they could spend the day preparing for the next day's patients. They also reported that nurses were rude in their requests.

3. Physicians complained among themselves that preventive services information was absent for almost half of the patients, and they suspected that the information was inaccurate for a significant number of cases for which information was provided.

4. Nurses were spending an additional 1–2 hours in the office preparing the next day's files. They complained that the medical records were very hard to decipher. They requested, and were denied, overtime pay.

---

**IN PRACTICE: Improving Preventive Services in a Pediatrics Practice:
A Less-Than-Successful Team** *(Continued)*

---

5. Confusion was rampant when files were prepared for one physician, but another physician ended up seeing the patient. An even more difficult problem was caused by drop-in patients, for whom record reviews were not prepared. Nurses spent up to 30 minutes looking over these drop-in charts and recording the information on the PSC.

6. Two weeks after the system was implemented, one nurse quit abruptly at 3:00 and walked out.

7. One physician gave each parent the PSC and asked parents to record preventive services themselves since the physicians were "too busy to keep track of this."

After a month, the team met again. The physicians decided that the "solution" caused more problems than it solved. They decided to disband the team and work on the preventive services problem individually.

---

# CHAPTER PURPOSE

Teams represent the bedrock of health care organizations, whether we are talking about delivering clinical care or preventive care services, teaching health professionals, or conducting all manner of clinical and health services research. The effectiveness of teams can have a direct impact on the effectiveness of the entire organization. A highly skilled professional may be unable to apply her training and skills without an effective team to support her work. Similar to the need to manage information, financial resources, and people, teams also need to be managed. They rarely function to their full potential without appropriate leadership. The purpose of this chapter is to help managers to draw on the full potential of teams and to overcome the most common obstacles to optimal **team performance**. The chapter presents evidence about team effectiveness and team management strategies that may be applied by managers to strengthen their competency in managing and improving teams.

# INTRODUCTION

The Glendale Pediatrics case illustrates the variety of ways that teams can run into difficulty. Nonetheless, teams are a mainstay of life in health care, and can be useful vehicles for improving quality—if they are organized and managed in an effective manner.

The use of teams is common in organizations, and this is particularly true in health care. In fact, teams represent the dominant way that work gets done in organizations. When working effectively, teams have the potential to improve organizational effectiveness while also having a positive impact on morale, job satisfaction, and commitment to the organization. The key, of course, is that teams need to be highly functional for us to reap the rewards that teams potentially bring. When teams suffer from dysfunctional processes or work relationships, productivity and effectiveness can be seriously jeopardized.

The use of teams in health care is no longer an option; teams and teamwork are a necessity. Clinical and management work both require teams, although there are many different types of teams. Work is simply too complex for it to be dependent on a single individual. The model for innovation and invention is no longer the solo scientist; the Thomas Edison model of innovation is long gone. One need only look at articles in such medical journals as the *New England Journal of Medicine* or the *Journal of the American Medical Association* (*JAMA*) to understand that advances in medicine are made and reported by teams. Furthermore, the composition of teams is usually multidisciplinary because innovation is dependent upon people with multiple skill sets. Successfully sending a man to the moon was the work of an effective team, while the *Challenger* disaster was, in part, due to a team with multiple communication and coordination problems.

In the clinical realm, effective patient care and management are dependent upon teams. This is the case whether we are dealing with a patient undergoing a surgical procedure in an operating room or a frail elderly person with multiple chronic medical conditions living at home. In clinical situations, teams are required to not only provide effective medical solutions but also recognize and take action to solve problems that may lead to medical errors. In fact, the entire quality improvement movement—whether in automobile manufacturing or hospital infection control—is dependent upon teams. Team training and effective team management are central to quality improvement initiatives. In reality, there are few, if any, individual heroes or heroines in organizations saving the day. In fact, even the most gifted and talented people need a supportive team to sustain their performance. In most situations in health care, the organization will not reap the full benefits of a talented person unless he or she is supported by, or part of, a strong, competent, highly functional team.

The goal of this chapter is to improve the reader's understanding of what makes teams effective. To do this, we provide background on the many types of teams that exist in health care, how teams differ in their functions and processes, the common pathologies facing teams, and strategies for improving team performance. We note as well that with globalization and advances in technology and communication have come new approaches to team organization, such as the use of virtual teams in which team members may never actually have face-to-face contact. For example, the authors of this chapter rarely interact in person; our collaboration is mediated by information technology. The use of virtual teams challenges organizations to develop new ways to manage such teams.

For many decades, teams have been the focus of extensive research, therefore, much has been learned about team effectiveness. Some of this research has been conducted in health care organizations, but the vast majority has been carried out in other settings, ranging from sports teams to product development teams to airline pilot crews. A remarkable aspect of this research is that lessons learned from one type of team are often applicable to other types of teams. This provides the opportunity to use the results of research carried out in diverse settings to inform this discussion of teams in health care. Thus, this chapter will present some of the most important research findings related to high-performing teams. The discussion will begin with a description of the types of teams found in health care organizations.

# TYPES OF TEAMS IN HEALTH CARE

Teams are groups, but not all groups are teams. Teams have a defined purpose, membership or composition, structure, specific processes, and leadership. Groups (that are not teams) may possess some characteristics of teams, but lack one or more key elements. A basketball team is, of course, a team. It has a purpose, defined members (composition), structure (team members are assigned positions and have roles), processes (how the team will work together), and formal leaders (captain and coaches). Often there are informal leaders as well. A surgical team clearly meets the characteristics of a team; it has a purpose, defined members, structure, processes, and leadership. However, one surgeon on the team may have more influence on team members than the second surgeon— even with all factors being equal. A group of nurses who go out to dinner together would likely not be a team, although meeting some of the characteristics of a team. While we can quibble about what is and what is not a team, our focus in this chapter is on work teams in health care organizations whose purpose is directly related to the goals of the organization. While this definition may seem narrow, we will show that even within this definition, there is a very wide range of teams in health care that differ along many different dimensions.

First, it is important to acknowledge that although not all groups are teams, groups that are not teams can have a substantial influence in an organization, often wielding considerable power. The importance of informal work groups and group processes has been recognized for at least 50 years. The Hawthorne experiments firmly established the proposition that an individual's performance is determined, in large part, by informal relationship patterns that emerge within work groups (Roethlisberger and Dickson, 1939). The work group has a pervasive impact on individual behaviors and attitudes because it controls so many of the stimuli to which the individual is exposed in performing organizational tasks (Hasenfeld, 1983). Thus, in addition to formally sanctioned teams, we need to be aware of informal groups and their influence on the organization. Some discussion of informal groups is therefore warranted.

## Informal Groups

**Informal groups** are those that are not formally established or sanctioned by the organization, but often form naturally by individuals in the organization to fill a personal or social interest or need. Informal groups can have high motivational value for individuals. A group of employees in different parts of an organization may serve a number of functions, such as social support and sharing of information. Such groups may be viewed positively by the organization because they may improve morale and communication in the organization. For example, an informal group of administrative support personnel may share valuable information about organizational procedures that may lead to increased efficiency.

Informal groups can also have a negative impact on an organization. Groups may become overly exclusionary and lead to interpersonal conflict. In some instances, informal groups can become so powerful so as to undermine the formal authority structure of the organization. Consider Etzioni's (1961) classic description of the role of informal groups in factories:

> The workers constituted a cohesive group which had a well developed normative system of its own. The norms specified, among other things, that a worker was not to work too hard, lest he become a "rate-buster"; nor was he to work too slowly, lest he become a "chiseler" who exploited the group (part of the wages were based on group performance). Under no condition was he to inform or "squeal." By means of informal social control, the group was able to direct the pace of work, the amount of daily and weekly production, the amount of work stoppage, and allocation of work among members. In this instance, informal groups of employees were able to maintain social control as well as control over the pace of work through the imposition of informal, though well enforced, rules of behavior.

Informal groups can also assume a change agent role. Such groups may initiate changes to improve working conditions and, as such, may evolve into formally sanctioned groups. In addition, informal groups may emerge to deal with a particular organizational problem or to work toward changes in organizational policies and procedures. Such groups may, in fact, initiate action against a corrupt manager or supervisor.

In sum, informal groups can play an important role in organizations. However, it is important that managers be aware of the existence of informal groups in the organization and the roles they play, whether positive or negative.

## Formal Groups

In the remainder of this chapter, we focus almost exclusively on teams in health care organizations. That is, the focus is limited to **formal groups**, or teams that are formally recognized, organizationally based, social systems. Extending the earlier definition, we view teams as intact social systems with boundaries, interdependence among members, and differentiated member roles or structure. Organizationally based teams are task-oriented with a specific purpose. They generally have one or more tasks to perform and produce measurable outcomes. Finally, they operate within an organizational context and interact with a larger organization or organizational subunits (Hackman, 1990a). This approach is consistent with the following definitions:

> A group is defined as two or more persons who are interacting with one another in such a manner that each person influences and is influenced by each other person (Shaw, 1976).

> A team is a collection of individuals who are interdependent in their tasks, who share responsibility for outcomes, who see themselves and who are seen by others as an intact social entity embedded in one or more larger social systems, and who manage their relationships across organizational boundaries (Cohen & Bailey, 1997).

We include in our discussion teams that are time-limited, such as project or product development teams, as well as those that are more permanent in nature. It is important to note that in addition to the permanence dimension, teams vary across many other dimensions as well. The most important of these are discussed below.

---

### IN PRACTICE:  Can We Create a Team Culture?

As Chair of a subspecialty department in a medical school, Dr. Rideout understands that patients are treated not just by individual physicians, but by teams of people in the department. For example, when a patient enters the clinic, she confronts a team of individuals—a desk clerk, nurse, technician, physician, a patient business associate, and so forth. He has found, however, that these teams have dysfunctional characteristics and result in low levels of patient satisfaction and poor morale. He has consulted with his staff and is struggling to create a department that is supportive of teamwork. Consider the following comments:

*From a Physician:* *"They're typical state employees. When I need a technician to prep a patient in the clinic, they're nowhere to be found. What do these people do all day? It's my job to treat patients, and since we're now paid partially on the basis of patient satisfaction scores, when a patient is left waiting, this brings down our scores and we all suffer. These state employees*

## IN PRACTICE: Can We Create a Team Culture? *(Continued)*

don't realize that we're in a teaching hospital, and I have responsibilities for research and teaching, not to mention being part of all of these hospital committees. These technicians have no sense of accountability. And don't even ask me about the patient business associates and the schedulers. We should fire them all and start from scratch."

*From a Technician:* "Many of these physicians treat the clinic as if it is their private practice. They think that all they have to do is snap their fingers and a technician will magically appear. Never mind that each technician works for three or four physicians and, when a physician needs me to prep a patient, I am usually in the process of prepping another patient for someone else. The physicians are worried about patient waiting time. Most of them show up around 8:45 in the morning for their 8:00 appointment, so we're already behind schedule by 8:01. Then they disappear midday without telling us where they are or when they'll be back. And they're blaming us for our dismally low patient satisfaction scores."

*From a Patient Business Associate:* "This is a difficult job. I do everything from answering phones, registering new patients, dealing with payment and insurance issues with patients, communicating with patients in person and by phone, and solving or trying to solve problems. When a patient is angry, it's my job to diffuse her anger. When a physician gets angry with me or someone else, I grin and bear it. The worst situation is when physicians argue with staff in front of patients. We provide excellent quality care, but patients do have other options. We need to think of the patient in customer terms. My days are filled with multitasking and being accountable to physicians and the clinic directors—and also advocating for patients. I must be focused, attentive to details and friendly. This is a stressful and unpleasant place to work. I've been here five years, and last week I started sending my resume out."

*From the Clinic Director:* "I am caught right smack in the middle. Everyone complains to me. The technicians complain about the physicians and schedulers, the patient business associates complain about the physicians, and they probably all complain about me. My co-director and I have worked hard to get some team spirit around here. We have social events on holidays and birthdays, but only the Chair and one or two physicians ever attend. As I see it, everyone here has turned into a caricature. Physicians and staff don't speak to each other as individuals, but as stereotypes. 'Technicians are lazy, schedulers are incompetent, patient business associates are do-gooders who try to get patients seen even if they can't pay, and physicians are arrogant.' The only thing positive here is the Chair. Everyone likes Dr. Rideout, but he doesn't like confrontation and has let things go too far. He should have been stronger and gotten these people into line long ago. We're a teaching hospital, and these people behave like they're 6-year old brats. I love the mission of this hospital, but I could get a job in a private medical practice for better pay and far less stress."

As the chair of the department in a Midwestern medical school, Dr. Rideout realizes that this situation has gone from bad to worse. The department is among the lowest in the health system in patient satisfaction scores, and staff morale is at its lowest point in the 10 years that he has been chair. "Our employees are loyal, but we scare away many good potential employees. On several occasions, new staff members have left after two weeks here."

Dr. Rideout is a firm believer in teamwork, but he has become exceedingly frustrated because of deterioration in whatever teamwork there may once have been. This was a tough place when he came 10 years ago and has not improved. He is skeptical of all of the complaining, and thinks they are all to blame—or no one is to blame. He is a good listener, and has hoped that his listening will diffuse the anger felt by physicians and staff. This has not worked. He is planning on retiring in two years and wants to leave the department in better shape than it was when he arrived.

Dr. Rideout is sincere and well meaning, but does not know where to turn. He feels he is dealing with some very difficult personalities, and perhaps this is just the way of the world. Dr. Rideout has consulted with other department heads, his wife, a psychiatrist, and with his clinic directors. He has even spoken with his minister. These people were kind and supportive, but could provide no real help. However, at the Christmas party two weeks ago, he happened to be talking with a student working on her MHA. Being in the holiday mood, he shared some of his problems with her. She had some interesting comments and observations. Most memorable were two specific comments: The first was: "*Many health care organizations are filled with good people working in bad processes.*" The other comment, which really caught his attention, was: "*Every system is perfectly designed to achieve the results that it produces.*"

# A TYPOLOGY OF TEAMS IN HEALTH CARE

A discussion of team characteristics can be confusing because of the multiple ways teams have been described over time. Using a typology (i.e., grouping by dimensions) generally facilitates this type of discussion; therefore, in this chapter, we use the subsequent typology along with a description of each element:

1. Function or purpose
2. Decisional authority
3. Temporal nature
4. Time and space
5. Diversity
6. Accountabilities
7. Membership fluidity and boundary permeability

## Function or Purpose: Why a Team?

The first element in our typology is function or purpose. Teams are used for multiple purposes in health care and have become the norm for getting work done. An important question worthy of attention is whether it is desirable to have a team, rather than an individual, accomplish a particular task. In many settings, it is routine for a manager, faced with a difficult decision, to assign a team to analyze the options and make a recommendation. That is, if a complex task is to be accomplished, a team is the most appropriate vehicle for accomplishing the work. It is not an exaggeration to say that teams are the building blocks of organizations.

There are many potential advantages to teamwork. Assuming that teams are functioning effectively, they have the potential to create synergy among its members—when the productivity of a team exceeds that of the sum of individual members. This is because innovation can result from the interplay of ideas among team members, especially when members build on and critically evaluate the work and ideas of others on the team during the decision-making process. In this way, if one member of a team misses an important factor, other members can supplement such gaps with the information necessary to make an effective decision. In addition, teams can be a source of empowerment and satisfaction for employees, which, in turn, may lead to lower turnover and absenteeism, and greater commitment to the goals of the organization. Perhaps of greatest importance is that teams bring together

diverse expertise and perspectives from multiple disciplines (Galbraith, 1977; Kanter, 1988). As a result, this knowledge is brought to bear on a particular problem, decision, or task.

This chapter focuses on the use of teams and emphasizes their advantages; however, it also is important to note that drawbacks exist, and managers should exercise caution in the use of teams. For example, instances exist where the use of teams may diffuse talent in an organization. Is the organization asking its most talented people to spend time on a team when their time could be better spent addressing important organizational concerns? Teams also require a level of infrastructure and processes to function effectively. Is an organization that is not team-focused prepared to make the infrastructure and process changes required for team performance? For example, most organizations are organized under traditional unity of command principles. That is, each person is accountable to one person. However, when an organization moves to cross-functional teams, employees may have multiple **accountabilities**, perhaps to a project team manager as well as their functional manager. As a result, the organization must be prepared to train managers to supervise teams, while also training employees to work in a team-focused environment. Following from this, individuals within the organization must have **team leadership** skills pertaining to conflict resolution, overcoming communication obstacles, and effective structure techniques, among other issues facing teams. Although teams have the capability to boost productivity and improve quality, they also have the potential to increase costs and stress if they are initiated in an organization unprepared to meet the challenges of working with teams.

In determining if the use of a team is appropriate for a particular task or decision, it is important to understand the multiple purposes of teams. We describe work teams, support teams, parallel teams, project teams, and management teams in the following paragraphs.

**Work teams** are groups of people responsible for producing goods or providing services. These teams are directed at the primary mission and objectives of the organization: treating emergency department patients, providing immunizations and other preventive services to children, and developing a new pharmaceutical product, among others. These teams may be directed by supervisors or manage themselves. In the health care environment, work teams include treatment teams, research teams, home care teams, and community-based crisis intervention teams. Work teams are usually ongoing and relatively permanent in nature, although membership and leadership of these teams may vary. Work teams can consist of members of the same discipline, or they can be multidisciplinary. They may also involve people at multiple levels in the organization, and people with significantly different levels of education. Some people have used the term "microsystems" to describe small groups of people who work together on a regular basis to provide care to patient sub-populations (Nelson, et al., 2002). These are freestanding clinic units with both clinical and business aims designed to maximize performance outcomes (Batalden, et al., 2003). We can say that work teams do the fundamental work of the organization, whether this means providing services, producing a product, or producing knowledge.

Other types of teams provide support for the primary functions of the organization. Such **support teams** enable others to do their work, and serve many functions such as quality improvement, strategic planning, and search committees hiring new employees. Note that individuals who serve on work teams may also have a role on support teams. In this situation, they are referred to as **parallel teams**— teams typically composed of people from different work units or jobs who carry out functions not regularly performed in the organization. They usually have limited authority and generally make recommendations to individuals higher up in the hierarchy. Parallel teams include quality improvement teams, employee involvement groups, and task forces. In the health care system, parallel teams may be involved in such activities as continuous quality improvement (CQI) and process improvement, community health needs assessments, and staff search committees. By their nature, they are often multidisciplinary. As suggested by the diversity of teams falling into this category, these teams may be temporary or permanent features of the organization.

**Project teams** are usually time limited, producing one-time outputs such as a new product or service or a new information system. In health care, such teams may exist for purposes of planning a new hospital, developing a new Alzheimer's drug, writing a new employee handbook, or developing a hospital disaster preparedness plan.

Finally, **management teams** coordinate and provide direction to the subunits under their jurisdiction. Management teams may exist at multiple levels, such as board, senior management, or departmental levels. Management teams may also include members from multiple levels of the hierarchy.

Members of management teams, by definition, have defined line responsibilities, although management teams may at times include individuals who are in non-line staff positions. Such individuals may play roles that are different from those of managers. For instance, they may serve the team in an advisory capacity with limited **decisional authority**.

Note that team purposes described in this section may overlap; therefore, teams often include elements of different team types. For example, a support team can be established to complete a particular project, and a treatment team might also function in a quality improvement capacity.

## Decisional Authority

Perhaps one of the most misunderstood aspects of teams is the element we call decisional authority. Decisional authority refers to a continuum of roles that teams may play in decision making. At one end of the continuum, teams may have the authority to make decisions. The hospital board of trustees fits into this category. A self-managed work team comes close to having full decisional authority, although even these teams ultimately report to a higher authority, which may veto or otherwise alter a decision.

At the other extreme are teams with no decisional authority. These types of teams are frequently established to make recommendations, or to generate options for decision making. For example, an organization seeking to install a new information system may assign a team composed of administrative support personnel and IT professionals to provide input on their information technology needs. Alternatively, such a team may be asked to look into different vendors for a new information system and to evaluate the benefits and drawbacks of each vendor. They may or may not be asked to make a recommendation. In any event, final decision-making authority rests with senior management or a specific person or team higher in the hierarchy.

The misunderstanding about a team's decisional authority usually results from a team having misinformation about its decisional role. Often, the decision-making authority of the team is not made clear, and teams may assume more authority than they actually have. The lesson for managers is apparent: the role of a team should be absolutely clear, particularly the role that it plays in decision making. However, even when decisional authority is made clear, team members may become disillusioned if they perceive that their recommendations or input have been ignored by the decision maker. In a team-focused organization, it is critical that managers respect the work and time of teams and team members. Where a decision is made that contradicts a team's recommendation, communication with team members is critical to avoid the frustration that may result from such situations. When unmanaged, disillusionment may inhibit future efforts to engage teams in similar work.

Related to team decisional authority is the decisional authority of individual team members. In some situations, the team leader has decisional authority, and team members simply provide input to the team leader. This is discussed more fully later in the chapter.

## Temporal Nature

The third team dimension is **temporal nature**, or the permanence of a team. As noted earlier, teams can be relatively permanent and ongoing, or time-limited and focused on a particular project or task. The use of time-limited teams is becoming more common in large part because of the rapidity of change and the need to respond quickly. In the area of new product development, for example, changes in technology, shorter product life cycles, and globalization require quick and efficient development of new products (Edmondson and Nembhard, 2009). The health care industry faces similar changes brought on by technological and other environmental changes. A new strain of influenza, for example, may impact multiple segments of a hospital. It is logical to involve a multidisciplinary team approach to devising appropriate responses by the organization. Similarly, teams may be used to identify how changes in laws and regulations will affect the organization.

Whether a team is temporary or not has no bearing on its importance to the organization. What is important, however, is that **team processes** accommodate the speed that is sometimes required of temporary teams. Group process and leadership issues may need to be resolved more efficiently than in more traditional teams. Group process concerns are discussed more fully later in this chapter.

## Time and Space

The vast quantity of research and literature on teams is predicated on teams that exist and function in a particular time and place. Advice offered on managing team meetings is based on the idea that meetings have set starting and ending times; some of this literature prescribes physical details of team management, such as optimal seating arrangements, mechanisms for ensuring full participation, and methods of dealing with people who arrive late and leave early.

With advances in communication and the ease with which **communication technology** can be used, rules of time and space often do not hold. Teams can communicate and work efficiently over any distance. As in an Internet-based chess game, teams need not meet at a specified time, but "meetings" can extend over several days if necessary, feasible, and appropriate to the team task. Team members can take hours or days to respond to a question from another team member, and one's response can be made at any time during the day or night.

The use of the term "virtual teams" implies that much or all communication among team members takes place outside of traditional face-to-face meetings through such mechanisms as e-mail, fax, and video teleconferencing. An additional potential benefit of virtual teams is the potential to store and make accessible to team members relevant data from medical records and other sources.

Of course, not all teams are amenable to the idea of ignoring time and space constraints. A hospital treatment team generally must find times to meet in one place at a physical location. However, technology affords the opportunity for even physically constrained teams to have extended communication outside of the formal team setting. With advances in telemedicine, teams can also obtain specialized advice from experts at any distance. Thus, a radiologist in Mumbai can be a virtual member of a treatment team in rural Oklahoma. Recent studies have shown the potential for virtual teams in health care, including providing care to chronically ill patients (Wiecha and Pollard, 2007). A recent study found that a virtual health care team reduced emergency room visits by high-risk diabetes patients. Carried out at Rush University Medical Center under the auspices of the "Virtual Integrated Practice" (VIP) model, teams consisting of pharmacists, social workers, and dieticians communicated via multiple technologies, such as phone, fax, and e-mail, to help coordinate care for these patients (Rush University Medical Center, 2008). Communication technology provides many new opportunities for enhanced teamwork, including the active inclusion of patients on virtual teams.

While there is potential for growth in virtual teams, it is important to note that virtual teams require additional rules and guidance. Virtual teams enhance the ability for teams to more fluidly shift team membership according to particular needs. This may involve the inclusion of people from outside the organization, including patients. These dynamics present additional challenges for managers. New or modified processes for team management must be designed, tested, and refined. These dynamics may also have implications for traditional reporting relationships, accountability, and reward systems in the organization. Modified measurement and control systems need to be put in place to ensure that performance is effectively monitored. Finally, since technology plays a central role in virtual teams, it is necessary for team members to be comfortable with the multiple communication technologies used by a virtual team. This is not a trivial point, particularly since virtual team members may come from different organizations (or no organization at all) and backgrounds.

## Diversity

**Diversity** provides both opportunities and challenges for teamwork. The advantages include the opportunity to obtain multiple perspectives and expertise that are necessary for effective decision making. A major challenge resulting from diversity is managing these multiple viewpoints and worldviews and the conflicts that may result from interactions among diverse team members.

Diversity itself is multidimensional, and depending upon the team and its needs, diversity will be defined differently. In society at large, we tend to think of diversity in terms of ethnic and racial diversity, and in health care, diversity in professional backgrounds is often used when discussing teams. Among the challenges faced with multidisciplinary teams are differences in social status between professions, different worldviews, and differences in language and professional terminology and jargon. However, diversity extends into other relevant domains, including:

- *Diversity based on age and generation.* This has particular relevance in organizations as they work to accommodate the work styles of baby boomers, Gen Xers, millennials, retired persons, and others.

- *Gender diversity.* This type of diversity requires an understanding of how gender may affect one's worldview and perceptions of problems and solutions. In health care, gender is often correlated with social status in the organization—specifically, the fact that nurses are predominantly female and physicians are now split about equally between male and female.

- *Diversity in hierarchical level.* This is particularly relevant in health care teams, where **team composition** may

specifically require people from different levels in the organization, as well as different departments.

- *Consumer and professional diversity.* Many teams include consumers as team members. It is not uncommon for consumers to feel intimidated on health care teams because of their lack of familiarity with the norms of behavior and professional language used on professionally dominated teams. Consumers may also come from different socioeconomic backgrounds than professionals on a team, adding yet another diversity domain.

- *Demographic and cultural diversity.* Our health care organizations mirror the heterogeneous nature of society. As society in general struggles towards greater inclusiveness, organizations and teams confront the tensions, misunderstandings, and prejudices that sometimes result from a multicultural environment. Because many teams require close collaboration among its members, cultural differences may become magnified in a team setting.

## Accountabilities

Just as teams have different levels of decisional authority, they also vary in the types of accountability required of them. Teams may be internally accountable, externally accountable, or both. A manager may assign a team the responsibility to complete a task; therefore, the team is externally accountable to that manager. On a project team, team members are accountable to the project team leader, but the project leader, representing the team, may be externally accountable to a manager outside of the team. Similarly, team members on a project team may also be accountable to their functional managers, a situation known as a program or matrix structure.

In well-functioning teams, team members perceive that they are accountable to *each other* for their individual contributions. Team communication, coordination, team outcomes, and discipline become the responsibility of team members, largely eliminating the need for external team management. In fact, in certain circumstances, an effective team leader should strive for a team that is self-managing, or has self-managing characteristics.

## Membership Fluidity and Boundary Permeability

This final dimension deals with the nature of membership and team boundaries. It was noted earlier that teams may be temporary or permanent. Membership may also be relatively stable over time, or fluid. In a medical school residents advisory committee, team membership will change quite frequently as residents leave and new ones arrive. There are liabilities to **membership fluidity**, including lack of cohesiveness among team members. Teams with fluid membership may have to continuously reorient team members, and new team members often take some time before they are able to make significant contributions to the work of the team. On the other hand, fluid membership may bring a continuous influx of new ideas that may benefit team performance and keep the team from becoming so inwardly focused that it loses touch with changes in the external environment. Of course, long-standing team members may resent "young Turks" who may be perceived as seeking to change the way things are done.

Related to membership fluidity is team **boundary permeability**. Some teams have a specific core membership that is sustained over time. The board of trustees of a hospital has a relatively stable set of team members, perhaps with a few members beginning and ending their terms each year. A team that is planning a new hospital wing will likely have a core membership that is relatively stable, but will call upon additional team members as the need arises in the course of the building project. Some members of this team may enter and exit the team several times according to the team's needs. Consider as well the team of professionals in a hospital emergency department. Team membership changes quite frequently during the course of a 24-hour day, just as the flight crew of a passenger jet changes its composition with every flight. How do these teams function with such rapid turnover? Certainly, a hockey team that changes its membership every eight hours will likely not be as effective as a team with more stable membership. The difference is that the work in an emergency department or passenger jet is highly standardized, and the professionals who work in these settings are highly trained in the roles they play in those settings. Even in a setting as unpredictable as an emergency department, employees are trained to respond in a planned way to the unexpected. Therefore, while teams may have permeable boundaries and membership, they may still exhibit high levels of performance.

In sum, teams vary along multiple dimensions. As discussed throughout this chapter, where teams find themselves on these dimensions has important implications for team performance and team management. Teams strive for high levels of performance, and the following section addresses team performance.

# UNDERSTANDING TEAM PERFORMANCE

We described earlier how teams represent the building blocks of organizational life and that the performance of a single employee is often determined by how well the team performs. Some may argue that too much importance is placed on how individual performance is affected by team performance. This may be true in certain types of work settings where an individual can outperform team performance. This would have its highest likelihood in a situation where there is a relative lack of interdependence between employees. For example, one could make the case (although it would contain many holes!) that an excellent elementary schoolteacher is unaffected by the overall quality of teaching in the school. We do have occasions in which excellent teachers teach in "bad" schools. It is difficult to come up with a similar situation in health care because the work of health care employees is so dependent upon the quality of others' work.

Moving beyond individual and team levels—to the organizational level—what is the impact of team performance on the overall performance of the organization? Here, the answer is much less ambiguous than the previous discussion about the impact of teams on individual performance. Everyone in a health care organization is a member of a team, and in most cases, employees are members of multiple teams, some of which may overlap in membership. Thus, teams are the entity that makes any kind of productivity possible. It is highly likely that a health care organization with poorly functioning teams will have lower productivity (or other indicator of effectiveness) than an organization whose teams are well constituted and well managed. Given a choice, a surgical patient needing three days of postoperative care would certainly prefer a nursing unit where nurses communicate with each other accurately and often, where physicians and nurses respect each other's views, and where all team members feel a sense of cohesion and share a stake in the quality of care provided in the unit. In a word, an informed patient would prefer a nursing unit that has the attributes of a strong team.

Some years ago, health care entered the era of accountability. Health care organizations have always had "reputations" for high or low quality, but the idea of actually measuring performance according to agreed-upon measures is relatively new. Private organizations and the U.S. government publicize quality ratings and rankings for healthcare organizations (see, for example, http://www.hospitalcompare.hhs.gov for measures of hospital performance, and http://www.medicare.gov/NHCompare for measures of nursing home quality). While measurement and reporting is still incomplete and in need of further development, measurement of organizational performance in health care will be a constant feature of the healthcare environment, with teams playing a major role.

Consider some of the most important measures used by the Department of Health and Human Services to assess hospital quality (USDHHS, 2010).

- Percentage of pneumonia patients assessed and given pneumococcal vaccination

- Percentage of surgery patients given an antibiotic at the right time (within one hour before surgery) to help prevent infection

- Percentage of patients at each hospital who reported "yes," they were given information about what to do during their recovery at home

- Percentage of children and their caregivers receiving a home management plan of care document while hospitalized for asthma

Each of these measures is based on professionally developed guidelines. Implementation of these procedures requires that the appropriate people in the hospital have an understanding of the guidelines and the evidence that informs them. However, knowing the guidelines and the supporting evidence is very different from taking the correct action based on those guidelines. For these procedures and others, it is not difficult to uncover the role that teams play in their implementation.

With hospitals eager to earn good ratings on such quality measures, it is somewhat surprising that they do not pay more attention to those "building blocks" of quality—teams. Much attention is given to assessing the quality of clinicians through review of credentials and past work experience. This provides necessary information about hospital staff members' technical competence, but it is inadequate to ensure that appropriate evidence-based procedures are implemented. Should hospitals have the same type of "credentialing" of teams? Given the importance of teams in implementing evidence-based practices and organizational performance, it seems advisable—at a minimum—for healthcare organizations to engage in periodic team audits that would address such questions as:

- What is the level of communication among team members in our organization? What are the strengths and weaknesses of communication on our teams?

- How satisfied are team members with how members communicate and how teams are managed? To what extent do team members feel as if they have input into decision making?

- What mechanisms do teams have in place to promote **team learning** and improvement in team processes and outcomes?

- To what extent do team members feel that it is safe to express themselves to other team members?

- What are the dominant leadership styles in our teams, and given what is known about team leadership, are these styles appropriate to the work of the team?

- Are we training team members and team leaders, and is there evidence that this training has resulted in improved team functioning and outcomes?

- What is the level of communication and coordination among teams? What are the specific areas that require improvement in inter-team relationships? Do our teams have specific measures to assess their effectiveness in producing desired outcomes? Are team members aware of these measures, and are they reviewed periodically by team members?

Unfortunately, such a systematic ongoing review of team processes and performance is not common in health care organizations. If hospitals and other health care organizations are interested in improving their rankings, it is important to determine the effectiveness of teams—those organizational building blocks whose output in large measure determines the rankings.

Whether we are dealing with sports teams, surgical teams, or public health surveillance teams, it is common knowledge that not all teams are equal. Some are better than others. We have all been members of teams, therefore having the opportunity to observe them in action. From these observations, it is apparent that teams vary in their effectiveness and efficiency. Why is there such variation in the performance of teams? Some variation may be due to differences in the skills of individual members, an explanation that may be salient in teams with little interdependence among its members. However, there are many situations where individual team members may be highly talented, but the team produces poor decisions that may lead to suboptimal outcomes. Later in this chapter, for example, we discuss the concept of **groupthink**, in which disastrously poor advice may be generated and acted upon by a team of highly talented and skilled individuals.

In the following section, we present a model of team effectiveness. Using this model, we incorporate existing evidence on the major factors that make certain teams more effective than others.

# A MODEL OF TEAM EFFECTIVENESS

What makes some teams more effective than others? We know that teams are not naturally effective by simply bringing people together who are highly skilled at their assigned tasks. Basic team member competence is important and necessary, but insufficient to predict effective team performance. There is obviously not a single action that team leaders can take to ensure that their team will function at peak levels of performance. Nevertheless, there are actions and decisions that leaders can take to improve the probability that a team will perform at a high level. Furthermore, there are processes that leaders can put in place to maximize the probability that a team's performance will improve over time. We adopt in this section a model of team effectiveness that includes a range of these actions, decisions, and processes. Some of these are interdependent, where implementation of one strategy is dependent upon another necessary strategy.

Notwithstanding the usefulness of this model, we also need to accept—as all managers must—that certain factors are outside of the control of the organization or manager. For example, we know that **team cohesiveness** is generally a positive attribute for teams, but a manager cannot always control events that may reduce team cohesion, such as turnover among team members. It is absolutely vital, however, that managers and team leaders understand and anticipate how uncontrollable factors may affect team performance. If such uncontrollable factors can be planned for, then negative impacts may be minimized. Of course, there are situations where uncontrollable factors may have a positive impact on team processes and outcomes. For instance, employee turnover tends to decrease during a recession, which in turn may lead to lower turnover among team members and sustained levels of team cohesion. An individual manager is unlikely to have much control over global macroeconomic events! However, a manager can take advantage of such "silver linings" by using the opportunity to strengthen teams and improve working conditions.

Figure 5.1 provides an overview of the multiple factors associated with team effectiveness. In the interests of simplicity, the multiple interrelationships among these factors are not included in the model, although they are addressed in the text. Moving from left to right, the model sets out three sets of factors, referred to as Team Characteristics, Nature of the Work, and the Environmental Context within which the team is situated. For each item listed, note that most are at least partially controllable by the manager, the noted exceptions being Organizational Culture and External Environment.

Moving to the right is a set of Team Process factors, many of which may be modified or controlled by the manager. Finally, Team Effectiveness factors are indicated. These include both performance outputs, such as patient outcomes, as well as team process measures, such as team member satisfaction and the capacity for team effectiveness to be sustained over time. As noted above, not illustrated in the model are potential interrelationships among these outcomes, such as the potential impact of team member satisfaction on patient outcomes.

## Team Characteristics

### Team Size, Composition, and Diversity

Team size has been a subject of research for many years. In general, **team size** has an inverted U-shaped relationship to effectiveness so that too few or too many members may reduce performance (Cohen and Bailey, 1997). As teams grow in size, communication and coordination problems tend to increase, and a climate of cohesiveness may decrease (Colquitt, Noe, and Jackson, 2002; Liberman et al., 2001). However, a team must be sufficiently large to accomplish its work. A useful rule of thumb is that teams should be staffed to the smallest number to accomplish the work (Hackman, 1987).

The U-shaped relationship between size and effectiveness is not precise. In treatment teams, performance has been found to be negatively affected by size (Alexander, Jinnett, D'Aunno, and Ullman, 1996; Vinokur-Kaplan, 1995b); in quality improvement teams, the effect was curvilinear (Shortell, 2004). Most likely, this is due to smaller teams being less cumbersome and having fewer social distractions. Smaller teams also have lower incidences of **social loafing**, a phenomenon in which a team member benefits from the work of the team without

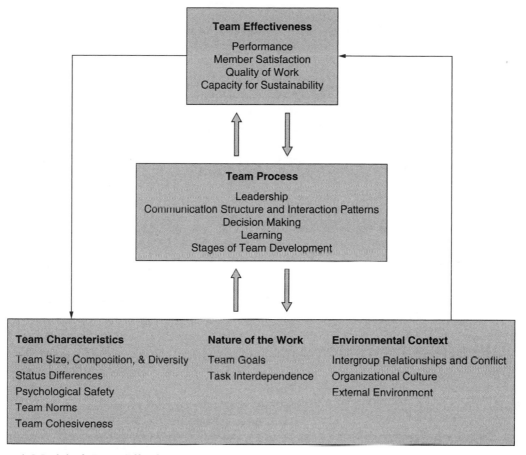

**Figure 5.1** A Model of Team Effectiveness.
SOURCE: Delmar, Cengage Learning.

making a commensurate contribution to the work of the team (Liden et al., 2004). A member's lack of work is more visible on a small team, while individuals in larger teams may be able to maintain anonymity and gain from the work of the group without making a suitable contribution.

However, team size is often out of the control of the manager, particularly when democratic representational norms pervade an organization. In these situations, constituencies may demand to be represented, and the leader may need to design strategies to make the group more manageable (e.g., forming subcommittees). Otherwise, teams may be *overstaffed*. Overstaffed teams may perform work in a perfunctory, lackadaisical manner. Overstaffed teams may also lead to competition and jealousy among team members, with

individuals guarding their particular domain. Alternatively, members of large teams may distance themselves from the team's efforts and lack commitment to the team. On the other hand, breaking a team into subgroups or subcommittees has its own set of problems. When large teams are divided into smaller ones, subgroups may become cliquish and, while cohesive within themselves, may become isolated from the rest of the team.

As noted above, the impact of team size on performance is dependent upon a number of factors. Although the empirical evidence on the relationship between team size and performance is less than definitive, it is useful for managers to keep in mind the potential problems and benefits that may emerge as a result of team size.

Team composition and diversity are important determinants of team performance as well. For certain types of teams, it is easier to control the membership of the group than in others. The CEO of a hospital can select from a wide variety of employees to sit on a strategic planning task force, while the director of nursing may be highly constrained in the nurses chosen for a self-managed nursing team in a pediatric oncology unit. In the latter situation, the director of nursing is limited by the pool of nurses in the unit or trained in such a specialty area. However, an awareness of likely problems related to membership helps, at least, to identify potential problems and to develop strategies to manage them. In our examination of team composition, we consider the following diagnostic questions (Hackman, 1990b):

- Is the team appropriately staffed? Is the diversity of members appropriate?

- Do members have the expertise required to perform team tasks well?

- Are the members so similar that there is little for them to learn from one another? Or, are they so heterogeneous that they risk having difficulty communicating and coordinating with one another?

- Is the team composed of members who have worked together before, and if not, how will team members learn about each other and their work styles?

Team composition may vary along a number of dimensions, such as age, occupation, gender, tenure, abilities, personality, and experience. Diversity, or the distribution of personal attributes among team members, is likely to affect the way individuals perceive each other and how well they work together (Jackson, Joshi, and Erhardt, 2003). These, in turn, may affect team performance. Most research on group composition concludes that diversity in a team is particularly desirable when the work is complex and has a limited time span (Campion, Medsker, and Higgs, 1993). Thus, diversity in team members' abilities and experiences is particularly important (Athanasaw, 2003; Mitchell, Parker, Giles, and White, 2010). However, one study found that a balance between different levels of managerial experience was needed in entrepreneurial teams in the medical and surgical instruments industry (Kor, 2003). That is, the more effective teams were composed of members who had a balance between industry and team experience; too much of either created conflict and decreased the ability of the team to seize new growth opportunities.

Diversity has become a very important concern in health care organizations. Diversity can help to promote quality and competitive advantage by including staff who can best understand diverse cultures. Diversity can also generate a broader perspective on a problem, which may lead to superior problem analysis and suitable solutions. From a legal perspective, diversity is a concern in relation to equal employment opportunity law. Thus, it has become so important that the Joint Commission has instituted requirements for staff diversity and cultural competence (Joint Commission, 2005). Although diversity brings many advantages, it also comes with problems, such as the potential for increased conflict and a loss of cohesiveness. Researchers, finding a negative relationship between diversity and performance in new product development teams, suggest that group heterogeneity might reduce social integration and cohesion (Ancona and Caldwell, 1992b). As a result, conflict begins in the initial stages of group formation and affects performance throughout the team's existence. In multidisciplinary health care teams, this is especially prevalent due to the differences between disciplines in basic philosophy and values, treatment modality, and terminology.

**Tenure diversity**, or the length of time members have been on the team, is also an important consideration in teams. For instance, new members coming into an already functioning team must be socialized to **team norms** (standards shared by team members that regulate team members' behavior) and procedures, which takes valuable time away from the work of the team. Although continuity of staffing is important, boundaries of some groups are, by necessity, more permeable than others. For example, hospital teams often include different physicians and nurses corresponding to the needs of the patients at certain points in their treatment and recovery. It should be noted that having a clear mission and set of task priorities will decrease many problems associated with tenure diversity, while the use of core and peripheral members and full-time and alternate members will increase team continuity and stabilize the process (Ancona and Caldwell, 1998; Topping, Norton, and Scafidi, 2003). The diversity "liability" can also be alleviated if members have previous experience working in teams or have been given training in team-building techniques (Athanasaw, 2003; Topping, Norton, and Scafidi, 2003). Katzenbach and Smith (1993) note that successful teams do not just happen; they become effective when members have certain skills that permit them to function positively in a group situation. Training and previous group experience—especially if members have worked together before—can provide these skills and reduce the potential for conflict.

## Status Differences

Status is a measure of worth conferred on an individual by a group. **Status differences** are seen throughout organizations and occur in all teams. It may have the effect of motivating people and providing them with a means of identification; it may be a force for stability in the organization (Scott, 1967). Status differences can also be a negative force and a source of conflict and tension. These differences exist in all teams and can have a profound effect on team functioning and individual behavior on teams. Status differences cannot be eliminated, but if well managed, can mitigate negative impacts. In this section, we discuss some of the ways that status differences affect teams and suggest strategies for managing status differences.

Status differences in health care are common and well entrenched (Lemieux-Charles and McGuire, 2006; Nembhard and Edmondson, 2006; Topping, Norton, and Scafidi, 2003). Multidisciplinary teams benefit from operating as a company of equals, yet the reality may make this very difficult. For example, in a study of end-stage renal disease teams in which the equal participation ideology was accepted by most team participants, it was clear that the physicians, who had higher professional status than other groups, had greater involvement than others in decision making (Deber and Leatt, 1986). The mismatch between expectations and reality made many team members, particularly staff nurses, feel a sense of role deprivation. That is, they were inhibited in their ability to fulfill completely their role as health professionals. This in turn led to a decrease in morale and job satisfaction. Status issues may be exacerbated in teams characterized by gender diversity, particularly when men comprise the higher status group. High-status members tend to initiate communication more often, are provided more opportunities to participate, and have more influence over the decision-making process. Thus, a lower-status team member may feel intimidated or ignored by higher-status team members. The group, as a result, may not benefit from this person's expertise.

Status differences can profoundly affect team effectiveness. They may impede someone with less authority or status from challenging someone with more authority. Similarly, status differences may inhibit someone of higher status from hearing input from those with lower status. The term authority

*gradient* has been used to describe differences in status and authority. Authority gradients have been identified in the airline industry as one of the causes of aviation accidents. That is, coordination and communication within the cockpit may be inhibited by differences in authority and status. In health care, authority gradients have been discussed among physicians, between residents and attending physicians, and between physicians and nurses, pharmacists, and social workers. Cosby (2009) notes as well the authority gradients between physicians in different specialties.

Status differences may affect patient outcomes. From the well-regarded IOM report, *Keeping Patients Safe: Transforming the Work Environment of Nurses*, "counterproductive hierarchical communication patterns that derive from status differences" are partly responsible for many medical errors (Institute of Medicine, 2003). Further, a review of medical malpractice cases from across the country found that physicians (higher-status team members) often ignored important information communicated by nurses, who had lower status on the team. Nurses in turn withheld relevant information for diagnosis and treatment from physicians (Schmitt, 1990). In a status consciousness environment such as health care, opportunities for learning and improvement can be missed because of unwillingness to engage in communication necessary for improvement.

Some teams have developed positive norms of equality, which can certainly help to minimize the negative impact of status differences. However, norms of equality may run counter to the formal or informal status of individual group members in the larger organization. For example, within a hospital, a physician may possess and exercise his or her power. Within a CQI team, that same physician may be expected to serve as an equal in analyzing problems and recommending solutions. Is it possible for such an individual to adjust his or her attitudes and behaviors according to the norms of the particular social milieu? As discussed later in the section on Environmental Context, this is an example of the larger environment (the hospital) potentially affecting the behavior of individuals on a particular team. This discrepancy between the status one has in the external environment and within the team may pose team management challenges.

CQI teams often use training early in the team development process to cope with problems brought about by status differences. In well-managed multidisciplinary teams, lower-status individuals should feel elevated by being part of such high-profile, effective teams. If status inequality exists, it is advisable for leaders to build a trusting environment in which members can disagree with the leader and others on the team without repercussions. In other words, the team leader should strive to achieve a climate of psychological safety for its members. In one study, NICU medical directors who were more attentive to other professions' ideas and concerns mitigated perceptions of status differences, increased unit psychological safety, and had success implementing quality improvement projects in the units (Nembhard and Edmondson, 2006).

## Psychological Safety

**Psychological safety** describes individuals' perceptions about the consequences of interpersonal risks in their work environment—largely taken-for-granted beliefs about how others will respond when one puts oneself on the line, such as by asking a question, seeking feedback, reporting a mistake, or proposing a new idea in the team context. In psychologically safe teams, people believe that if they make a mistake, other team members will not penalize or think less of them for it. This belief fosters the confidence to experiment, discuss mistakes and problems, and ask others for help. Psychological safety is created by mutual respect and trust among team members, and leader behavior is a powerful influence on the level of psychological safety in teams (Edmondson, 1999, 2003).

Management research on psychological safety started with studies of organizational change, when Schein and Bennis (1965) discussed the need to create psychological safety for individuals if they are to feel secure and capable of changing. Psychological safety helps people overcome the defensiveness, or "learning anxiety," that occurs when people are presented with data that disconfirm their expectations or hopes, which can thwart productive learning behavior (Schein, 1985). However, the need for a team climate conducive to learning does not imply a cozy environment in which people are close friends, nor does it suggest an absence of pressure or problems. Team psychological safety is distinct from group cohesiveness; team cohesiveness can reduce willingness to disagree and challenge others' views, creating groupthink (Janis, 1982). This represents a *lack* of interpersonal risk taking. Psychological safety describes instead a climate in which the focus is productive discussion that enables early prevention of problems and the accomplishment of shared goals, because people feel less of a need to focus on self-protection.

Although few people are without concern about others' impressions, our immediate social context can mitigate—or exacerbate—the reluctance to relax our guard. Research in hospitals and other organizations has found differences across teams in people's willingness to engage in behavior for which the outcomes are uncertain and potentially harmful to their image. When psychological safety is high, teams are much more likely to engage in learning, which in turn promotes team performance (Edmondson, 1999). Just as compelling goals are necessary to motivate learning, psychological safety enhances the power of such goals by facilitating less self-conscious interpersonal interactions. Without a goal, there is no clear direction to drive toward and no motivation to exert the effort; without psychological safety, the risks of engaging wholeheartedly in learning behaviors and other key team processes in front of other people are simply too great. In one recent study, unit psychological safety was associated with implementation success of quality improvement projects; when unit members were able to raise questions and concerns, they were better able to understand the rationale behind proposed changes and more able and willing to implement them quickly (Tucker, Nembhard, and Edmondson, 2007).

## Team Norms

A team norm is defined as a standard that is shared by team members and regulates member behavior. **Behavior norms** are rules that standardize how people act at work on a day-to-day basis, while **performance norms** are rules that standardize employee output. Behavioral norms in teams are far reaching and may vary substantially from one group to another in the same organization. Norms may govern how much each individual participates in the team's work, how humor is used, the use of formal group procedures (e.g., Robert's Rules of Order), and responses to absence and lateness. In their study of operating room nurses, Denison and Sutton (1990) describe their surprise at the behavioral norms present in the operating room:

> At first we were surprised by the norms of emotional expression in the operating rooms. The first time we entered the room where a coronary bypass operation was being done, for example, we were surprised by the loud rock music blaring from the speakers, the smiles on the faces of the surgical team, and the constant joking. Denison observed one surgeon who joked and told a series of funny stories as he performed the complicated task of cutting the veins out of a patient's leg—veins

that would be used to bypass clogged coronary arteries. Similarly, one reason that Sutton almost passed out during a tonsillectomy was that he became very upset when the surgeon laughed, joked, and talked about "what was on the tube last night" while blood from an unconscious child splattered about.

Norms are powerful influences in organizations and teams, and the existence of norms is necessary for effective group functioning. In Hackman's (1976) classic *Work Redesign*, he suggests that norms have the following characteristics:

1. Norms summarize and simplify team influence processes. They denote the processes by which teams regulate member behavior.

2. Norms apply only to behavior, not to private thoughts and feelings. Private acceptance of norms is not necessary, only public compliance is required.

3. Norms are generally developed only for behaviors that are viewed as important by most team members.

4. Norms usually develop gradually, but members can quicken the process. Norms usually are developed by team members when the occasion arises, such as when a situation occurs that requires new ground rules for members in order to protect team integrity.

5. All norms do not apply to all team members. Some norms apply only to newer members, while others may be applied to individuals based on seniority, sex, race, economic status, or profession.

Because of the significance of norms in effective group functioning, it is important to clarify norms publicly so members will know what is expected. This is especially the case for multidisciplinary teams in hospitals and other health care settings (Deeter-Schmelz and Ramsey, 2003). If acceptable norms are established as part of the group process in a multidisciplinary team, there is less chance of the team being dominated by one discipline (Vinokur-Kaplan, 1995a).

## Team Cohesiveness

There are a variety of definitions for team cohesiveness, many of which focus on the degree to which members of a group are *attracted* to other members and, thereby, are motivated to stay in the group. Another, more narrow definition that better fits the purpose of this chapter is used by Goodman, Ravlin, and Schminke (1987): "cohesiveness is the extent that members are committed to the group task." In this definition, the focus is on the decision to produce, and it acknowledges that members can be committed to a common task but not necessarily be attracted to each other. This is a pragmatic view of cohesiveness that is particularly important for focusing on the management of teams in which members, such as nurses, physicians, psychologists, and social workers, are already highly committed to professional standards.

Cohesion is an important component in understanding group process and effectiveness. Highly cohesive teams may exhibit higher levels of performance, greater member satisfaction, and lower levels of turnover (Gully, Devine, and Whitney, 1995; Hoegl and Gemuenden, 2001; Yang and Tang, 2004). The relationship between cohesion and effectiveness is particularly strong when the work of the team is complex, requiring high levels of coordination, communication, and mutual performance. Specifically, research focusing on treatment teams in psychiatric hospitals, engaged in highly interdependent work, found that cohesive teams had higher performance levels than less cohesive ones (Vinokur-Kaplan, 1995a). Similar findings resulted from a study examining the effectiveness of geriatric rehabilitation teams (Wells et al., 2003).

Cohesion among team members is a key determinant of team effectiveness. Cohesiveness can also promote better enforcement of group norms and general control over group members; however, taken to extremes, this can lead to situations of undue or dysfunctional conformity. For instance, there are circumstances under which high levels of cohesiveness can lead to *lower* levels of productivity. That is, if a group's norms favor low productivity, then having a highly cohesive group will likely lead to high levels of conformity to this norm and, hence, lower productivity. Similarly, a highly cohesive team may work against a manager's efforts to involve new team members, or to encourage interaction with other teams. Cohesiveness, therefore, should be viewed in context. In most situations, it is a positive force, while in others, it can lead to conformity and counterproductive norms and practices.

What are the sources of cohesiveness? A central tenet of social psychological theory is that individuals are attracted to others who are similar to them; therefore, homogeneous groups should be more cohesive than heterogeneous ones. All-female groups, for instance, tend to be more cohesive than all-male and mixed sex groups (Bettenhausen, 1991).

The lack of conflict, team training, a positive predisposition for teamwork, and the presence of trust among members also lead to increased cohesiveness (Deeter-Schmelz and Ramsey, 2003). To complicate matters, some research suggests that conflict may be beneficial to group performance, particularly when a group is dealing with complex problem-solving tasks (Cosier, 1981; Janis, 1972; Schwenk, 1983). In this sense, multidisciplinary teams and cultural diverse teams, while potentially exhibiting higher levels of conflict and less cohesiveness, may also be more creative and innovative in their approach to problem solving (Mitchell et al., 2010).

The cohesiveness of a team is also influenced by the goal orientation or reward structure of the team. Let us consider two conditions. First is the situation of goal interdependence in which members are evaluated and rewarded as a team (i.e., equal reward structure). Here, progress to each member's professional/personal goals is identical to progress to **team goals**. The second condition is one in which group members are judged and rewarded as individuals (i.e., unequal reward structure). In essence, one member may reach his or her goal at the expense of another team member. In general, the findings support the first or cooperative condition (Parker, McAdams, and Zielinski, 2000; Yang and Tang, 2004). Team members in the second situation are more likely to be highly competitive, leading to lower cohesiveness due to:

- Less inter-member influence and acceptance of other's ideas

- Greater difficulty in communication and understanding

- Less coordination effort, less division of labor, and less productivity

Following from this, cohesive groups tend to have levels of interaction that are greater and more positive, which is strengthened by conditions of high interdependence. That is, groups that have equivalent reward structures not only perform more efficiently, but also develop cooperative strategies such as teamwork and pooling of information that facilitate achievement of jointly shared goals.

## Nature of the Work

Organizational research has for many years adopted the principle of contingency; specifically, that organizational structures and processes must be aligned with a number of factors. That is, there is no *one best way* to organize; optimal organizational mechanisms depend upon environmental factors, the technology used, and the nature of the work done by the organization. Among the underlying themes in research on teams is that team tasks can be classified according to their critical demands; that is, critical features of a task dictate particular team behaviors essential to successful performance. These specific behaviors include not only individual effort, but also cooperative and interdependent endeavors. This means that effective performance is a function of matching team process to task demands. In this section, we identify key aspects of the tasks confronting teams and the manner in which teams adapt to different task characteristics. In addition, we consider two aspects of the work of a team: goals, and the level and type of task interdependence.

### Team Goals

Team goals and their accompanying tasks can be categorized according to goal clarity, complexity, and diversity. Each of these dimensions has implications for the manner in which a team is organized and managed. For example, some teams work toward goals that are repeated over time. In these situations, communication and coordination mechanisms among team members can be routinized. Although they face variations and some uncertainty, obstetrical teams face a defined set of goals, namely the safe delivery of newborns and the health and well-being of mother and child. The goals and accompanying tasks for such teams and for individual team members are well structured and understood by team members. Where goals and tasks are relatively predictable, and where team members understand exactly what is to be done, the work of a team can become highly routine.

Contrast this situation with teams facing ambiguous, ill-structured goals. A disaster preparedness team is perhaps the epitome of this type of uncertainty. In such a situation, communication is of paramount importance. Team members must be prepared to adapt to new circumstances, and adjust their work according to the situation. Ongoing coordination and mutual adjustment among team members are essential, since routinization may be possible only up to a point.

Goal and task clarity were significant variables in determining the performance of hospital treatment teams, allowing them to meet the hospital's standards of quality, quantity, and timeliness (Shaw, 1990; Vinokur-Kaplan, 1995a). Task complexity is related to team interaction; the more complex the task, the greater the need for interaction, so that it is important that managers plan for enhanced communication among the team members under conditions of complexity. Others have found that an increase in task diversity, as defined by the number of different conditions treated within ICUs, challenges caregivers since their expertise and knowledge can be applied across a wider range of conditions, and leads to better outcomes (Shortell et al., 1994).

## Task Interdependence

Another form of task diversity focuses on interdependence, which is generally the reason why teams form in the first place. **Task interdependence** refers to the interconnections between tasks, or more specifically, the degree to which team members must rely on one another to perform work effectively. A useful way of classifying task interdependence is the hierarchy of task interdependence based on exchange of information or resources (Thompson, 1967; Van de Ven, Delbecq, and Koenig, 1976):

- **Pooled interdependence** is a situation in which each member makes a contribution to the group output without the need of interaction among members. Since each group member completes the whole task, team performance is the sum of the individual efforts. Standardized rules and procedures are needed to enhance coordination of team outputs.

- **Sequential interdependence** is a situation in which one group member must act before another one can. Group members have different roles and perform different tasks in some prescribed order, with the work flowing in only one direction. There is always an element of potential contingency since readjustment is necessary if any member fails to meet expectations. Coordination using schedules and plans is needed to keep the team on track.

- **Reciprocal interdependence** is a situation in which the outputs of each member become inputs for the others, such that each member poses a contingency for the other. Group members often are specialists with different areas of expertise and have structured roles; therefore, they perform different parts of the task in a flexible, "back-and-forth" order. Leaders must provide for open communication between members and scheduled meetings as necessary.

- **Team interdependence** is a situation in which team members must actively coordinate to diagnose and solve problems, or otherwise carry out work or work-related activities. The workflow is simultaneous and multidirectional.

Coordination requires mutual interactions with group autonomy to decide the sequencing of inputs and outputs among members. Leaders should plan frequent meetings, while also encouraging unscheduled ones.

The higher the level of interdependence, the greater the uncertainty faced by a team and its members. Therefore, as the degree of interdependence among team members increases, so does the need for information exchange and processing, coordination, communication, and cooperation. Implicit in this is the need for matching the information exchange and processing needs requirements with appropriate interaction and coordination patterns that facilitate information exchange. If team members perceive low interdependence when high interdependence actually exists, then too little effort will go toward coordination. On the contrary, when interdependence is perceived as higher than it really is, too much effort may be expended in coordination behavior at the expense of performance. For this reason, interdependence and the level and type of coordination must be appropriately matched. Some researchers go so far as to suggest that successful teams are the ones that match interdependence in terms of task, goal, and feedback. That is, a successful team is one in which reciprocal work is matched with group goals and group feedback. Group goals and feedback mean that rewards would be based on the group goal and feedback given on the group's performance as a whole. Conversely, pooled interdependence should be matched with a situation of individual goals and feedback.

Regardless of the task characteristic, the important point for managers is the need to match team tasks with process and structure. One study demonstrating this matching described the reengineering effort in a large urban hospital system that used teams for overcoming care delivery problems, particularly fragmentation and discontinuities in delivery (Schweikhart and Smith-Daniels, 1996). Focused teams, or relatively autonomous operating units, were formed by merging multidisciplinary clinicians into patient care units, so that pharmacists, respiratory therapists, nurses, and other caregivers were integrated through shared governance and cross-training. The teams were given high levels of autonomy and accountability, while sharing responsibility for both care production work—execution of the patient's care plan—and care management work—planning and coordinating the care. In this case, high levels of task complexity and interdependence were matched with a team structure that allowed increased levels of communication and interaction.

In virtual teams, team members may be separated not only by geography and time, but also by culture and language. In this situation, managers are faced with the dual challenges of coordinating work among individuals from different disciplines and from different cultures (Barczak and McDonough, 2003). In health care, this type of team is most common in product development (for example, pharmaceuticals and medical equipment) and in clinical research.

# Environmental Context

Teams do not exist and function in a vacuum, but operate within a broader **environmental context**. They are affected by pressures and events from outside of the immediate team. In this section, we examine several critical external factors that may affect team performance: intergroup relationships and conflict; organizational culture; and the larger external environment.

## *Intergroup Relationships and Conflict*

An important part of a team's external environment is the presence of other teams. In many situations, effective team performance is dependent upon a team's ability to form **intergroup relationships** with other teams in a positive and productive manner. In complex organizations, one of the most challenging tasks of many teams is to interact with other teams whose work is related to theirs (Edmonson, 2002). For example, consider the myriad intergroup interactions among teams that must occur in the merging of two hospitals (see Sidorov, 2003; Dooley and Zimmerman, 2003; Yang and Tang, 2004). Teams assembled to deal with staffing issues, technology, finances, architectural concerns, and countless other factors must work with other teams in both their own group and the merging organization. One could only imagine the confusion if each team chose to work without the advice and input of other teams.

What happens when teams must coordinate their efforts? What are the factors responsible for effective and ineffective intergroup relationships in this context? Intergroup relationships are often lateral, or peer, relationships, rather than hierarchical ones. As health care organizations have moved away from rigid hierarchical structures to manage work, and as they have become more specialized, the need for new coordination mechanisms has increased such as cross-team training, virtual team updates, and joint meetings for planning and coordination.

In the process of working out intergroup challenges and coordination issues, intergroup conflict is perhaps inevitable.

Given the uncertainty and heterogeneity of inputs in health care, it is virtually impossible to design all work processes in advance in such ways as to ensure that the work of all groups mesh perfectly with the work of other groups. When conflicts or disagreements occur among groups, it is important that team members possess a repertoire of conflict resolution strategies. In some cases, the interfaces among teams require only fine tuning; in the worst situations, work processes may need to be overhauled to achieve functional intergroup relationships.

Some intergroup conflict results from interpersonal differences or animosities. However, most intergroup conflict emerges because of factors related to the interdependent multiple teams. This is especially true for health care organizations, which are known for high levels of interaction and, therefore, present more opportunities for the emergence of conflict. Conflict between groups cannot usually be addressed at an individual level; one member of a group can rarely resolve an intergroup conflict in a unilateral manner. If intergroup conflict is viewed as resulting from problems in the *interface* between groups, then the analysis of the causes and sources of conflict should examine the nature of relationships.

First, intergroup conflict is more likely to occur when there is ambiguity about the team's respective task responsibilities and roles. This situation largely explains conflicts that occur between professional groups with overlapping practice domains, such as between psychologists and psychiatrists (Brown and Keyes, 2000; Weist et al., 2001). Task and role ambiguity may also be common in organizations undergoing rapid growth or change, where different groups may have divergent understandings of the nature and implications of change. Consider the conflict that may occur when an organization is in the midst of a merger (Dooley and Zimmerman, 2003). This type of conflict points to the need to articulate team roles clearly and distinguish precisely the responsibilities of similar groups.

Conflict may also arise from intergroup differences in work orientation. Every team develops its own set of norms regarding the manner in which work is accomplished. In many organizations, teams have different perspectives on *time*. This difference in time orientation was identified and managed when strategic planning was attempted with a group of family physicians (Fried and Nelson, 1987):

> By its nature, the activity of planning is at odds with the role orientation of most physicians. Planning is a long-term process in which the results of strategic decisions appear over time. The outcomes of planning

are often intangible in the short term. By contrast, physicians are trained to be action oriented.

It was discovered early in the planning process that physician attendance at meetings decreased when the pace of work lagged. Therefore, whenever possible, the pace of work was increased to a level more acceptable to physicians. A work plan with specific deadlines was followed.

Related to differences in work orientation is the problem of goal incompatibility among teams. Teams whose goals are in conflict (or perceived to be in conflict) must sometimes work together. A common conflict in health care is between teams whose orientation is primarily cost containment and teams whose orientation is focused more on quality concerns. At other times, differences in group culture may cause conflict between teams. Each group develops its own unique norms, communication network, and values, which collectively is referred to as a team culture. When these vary between teams, conflict often occurs. Lastly, intergroup conflict may occur when there is competition for resources. Teams may have much in common and be oriented toward the same goals, yet experience conflict because they are competing for the same limited financial, human, or physical resources. In hospitals, the change to product or program management would tend to increase the likelihood of intergroup conflict as product-line teams develop internal competitive thrusts.

Perhaps of greatest importance for the organization as a whole, as conflict emerges between groups, cooperative relationships may be replaced by a win-or-lose mentality. In this case, victory becomes more important than solving the problem that may have caused the conflict in the first place. Because of this, it is important to develop strategies that can be used in managing and reducing intergroup conflict.

### Organizational Culture

Among the most important environmental factors affecting team performance is the **organizational culture** of the larger organization. For teams to function to their maximum potential, it is extremely important that a suitable culture exists—one that values and emphasizes teamwork and participation (Zarrage and Bonache, 2003). Among the most common complaints about teams in organizations is that they do not receive adequate support from the larger organization. While many organizations claim a commitment to a team-based organization, they often lack effective culture and strategies for accomplishing this transition.

How does senior management of an organization adopt a team-based culture? First, it is important for senior management to internalize the concept of a team culture, and to understand fully how a team culture is consistent with and supportive of its overall strategy. Furthermore, this needs to be communicated throughout the organization. Senior management also needs (1) to believe that employees want to be responsible for their work; (2) to be able to demonstrate the team philosophy; (3) to articulate a coherent vision of the team environment; and (4) to have the creativity and authority to overcome obstacles as they surface (Moorhead and Griffin, 1998; Orsburn, Moran, Musselwhite, and Zenger, 1990).

As with other aspects of organizational life, teams require strong support from senior management to be effective (Liberman et al., 2001). By support, we refer to philosophical backing and resource support. Resource support includes money, human resources, training, and time. Once senior management has made a commitment to teams, it may be necessary to develop a detailed implementation plan. This plan might include a clarification of the organization mission to focus on such things as continuous improvement, employee involvement, and customer satisfaction; selecting sites for teams; preparing a design team to assist with team staffing and operation; planning the transfer of authority from management to teams; and drafting a preliminary plan for implementation. To be successful, teams need an internal champion who can provide motivation, encouragement, and work to acquire the resources and support required (Cohen and Bailey, 1997; Shortell et al., 2004).

Training constitutes a key part of implementing and supporting teams, and to be effective, the organizational culture must support its use (Liberman, 2000). No one would ever consider the possibility of a soccer team being successful without substantial training or practice. Based on the experience of countless non-sports teams, the need for training—in fact, continuous training—is very apparent. There is a vast literature on selecting and training individuals to work in teams, and the knowledge, skills, and abilities necessary for effective teamwork. Such training may include cognitive content, including the rationale or raison d'être of having a team-based organization. Affective content should also be addressed, including the roles and responsibilities of team members and team norms as well as logistical issues dealing with meeting management and the reward system (Moorhead and Griffin, 1998). Other examples include team interaction training that can lead to shared mental models (Marks, Zaccaro, and Mathieu, 2000); problem-solving and decision-making training, which can enhance interdisciplinary team interactions (Doran et al., 2002); and newcomer training, which can speed the socialization process (Chen and Klimoski, 2003). Overall, for team training to be comprehensive, it optimally should include requisite technical, administrative, and interpersonal skills.

The reward system of the organization should optimally reflect the organizational culture. Thus, a particular dilemma facing managers in team-oriented organizations is the question of type of reward system. To what extent should the organization bestow team, as opposed to (or in addition to) individual, rewards? The organization also needs to address one of the unanswered questions in organizational research: do team-based rewards improve team and/or individual performance? Despite the equivocal nature of the literature in this area, there seems to be a natural tendency for team-oriented organizations to at least consider the idea of **team-based rewards**. In a team-based environment, a variety of mechanisms may be employed to reward team and team member performance. Team members may be rewarded for mastering a range of skills needed to meet team performance goals. Compensation or other rewards may also be given for team achievements and performance. **Skill-based pay** may reward employees for acquiring specific skills needed by an employee's team. Team members may increase their compensation by acquiring value-added skill sets. Team bonus plans reward particular teams based on the performance of the team. Finally, gain-sharing plans (usually considered an organization-wide incentive system) typically reward all team members from all teams based on the performance of the organization as a whole.

It should be stressed that while there are many options for rewarding team performance, the number of organizations that actually use team-based incentives is relatively small. A survey of 2,500 corporations found that the number of companies with group incentives grew from 16 percent in 1995 to 19 percent in 1996 (Pascarella, 1997). While this growth is notable, the majority of organizations have not implemented team-based incentive systems. Part of the reason for this is the complexity of such schemes and the lack of agreement on the link between incentives and performance. While there is an intuitive appeal to performance-based compensation, there exists substantial dissent regarding the whole premise of pay-for-performance. Many managers and scholars believe that

such schemes are highly destructive to individual, team, and organizational performance. In addition, there are a number of critical questions that need to be resolved to ensure that a team payment system does not yield unintended negative consequences, including (Pascarella, 1997):

- Does the team as a whole receive rewards, or do individuals on the team receive rewards for outstanding team performance?
- If rewards are not uniformly distributed among team members, how does management assess the relative contributions of different team members?
- Should team members be compensated for results, behaviors, or both?
- How should people be rewarded when they have membership on multiple teams?

These are critical questions, the answers to which depend upon the particular manner in which teams are used in the organization as well as the culture of the organization (Beersma et al., 2003). However, several hybrid compensation structures have been successful in simultaneously motivating low-performing team members to improve while encouraging high-performing members to help in this process (Katz, 2001). An example of a hybrid plan involves a team threshold; once the team as a whole reaches this level, pay increases are based on individual performance. This is especially successful when there are enough highly skilled workers on the team to teach their less-skilled or less-knowledgeable colleagues.

## External Environment

Besides the organizational environment, teams are affected constantly by influences from the external environment as well. This makes it important to understand how external factors influence team process and effectiveness (Ancona, 1990; Arrow et al., 2000). Most research has involved organizational factors that affect teams (e.g., support from senior levels of the organization), so there is little known about the effect of external environment (Lacey and Gruenfeld, 1999). For many groups, the greater external environment may exert influence equal to or greater than the internal organizational environment (Hackman, 2003; Salas, Burke, and Cannon-Bowers, 2000). This is particularly true for multidisciplinary, interagency groups that interact with and depend on not only member organizations but also the community environment and local service network for critical resources and support.

These teams often are used in resource-deficient rural areas to extend services, making it critical to understand how these conditions affect teams and how to develop strategies to override the effects.

In several studies (Fried et al., 1998; Topping and Calloway, 2000), the findings indicated that resource scarcity was an important issue in the development of mental health delivery systems in rural environments. In areas with high levels of resource scarcity, only a few core providers took a central or gatekeeper role, thereby implying that organizations in that system act more autonomously than a system with more resources. This, in turn, will affect the collaborative behavior or **social capital** existing in the provider network, in specific, and community, as a whole. Social capital can be best defined as the web of cooperative relationships between providers in a service system that involve interpersonal trust, norms of reciprocity, and mutual aid (Veenstra, 2000). In situations of scarce resources where social capital may be low since organizations tend to interact less, there will be little impetus to use teams to solve interorganizational problems. For instance, teams including acute care hospital nurses and community providers are used to provide care to older people discharged from the hospital (Robinson and Street, 2004). In these situations, collaboration among team members would be much more difficult.

Another contextual factor influencing collaboration between team members is the collaborative history of the provider network or community. Interagency teams, whose members have a long history of service coordination, tend to report a remarkably easy process of forming and becoming a cohesive, effective team (Topping, Norton, and Scafidi, 2003). There are also rural and urban differences. Many rural areas report that, "everyone knows each other and have worked together before." Thus, a sense of "teamness" is there from the beginning. In addition, urban communities tend to include a larger number of service organizations, so that interagency teams usually are composed of many professionals, while rural areas have to depend on nontraditional groups such as the YMCA, churches, and Boys and Girls Clubs, for members. This, of course, increases diversity, which may also increase team conflict (Jackson, 1992; Kor, 2003).

## Team Processes

Up until this point, we have discussed basic team characteristics such as composition and norms, the type of work done, the environment within which teams operate, and

interrelationships among these factors. In this section, we focus on *how* teams do their work—how they are led, the manner in which communication is handled, how they make decisions, and other processes and procedures. Team process thus refers to the methods of interacting and performing work by team members alone and in interaction with each other. Processes addressed in this section are leadership, communications, decision making, learning, and how the work of the team is affected by its stage of development.

### Leadership

Leadership in teams refers to the ability of individuals to influence other members toward the achievement of the team's goals. This definition permits us to include formal and informal leadership. By **formal leadership**, we refer to legitimate authority given to a team member. In some cases, an external individual in a position of authority can assign leadership, or in other instances, leaders may be designated by team members through voting or other forms of consensus. By **informal leadership**, we refer to individuals who assume leadership roles based on some personal characteristic. A number of factors can give rise to informal leaders, including expertise, experience, or personal charisma.

Related to but distinct from leadership is power. Some team members may acquire and exert power in a team through their relationships with individuals outside of the team. For example, in an academic medical center, a team member whose spouse is a vice president may be in a position to wield considerable power. A team member may also obtain power because they are perceived to be non-substitutable, or difficult to replace, in the organization. Some people may also achieve power because they have the ability to cope with uncertainties faced by the organization. An IT staff member may achieve an inordinate amount of power because her skills and knowledge are scarce, *and* because of her ability to cope with a major uncertainty— the risk that the information system will fail, causing potentially widespread disruption to the work of the organization.

Some teams have multiple leaders. For instance, there may be a formal leader as well as several informal ones. Informal leaders can be supportive of the formal leader, or can undercut the authority of the formal leader. Examples of formal leaders are head nurses, department managers, and project committee chairs. As noted before, formal leaders have legitimate authority over the team. That is, the organization has granted these individuals power along with some ability to use formal rewards and sanctions to support that authority. However, the formal leader may not be the most *influential* person on the team. The extent to which team members accept the formal leader's wishes is, in large part, determined by the reaction of the informal leader(s) to those wishes.

Note that there is a difference between ad hoc groups, such as parallel and project teams, and formal work teams. In a parallel or project team, an informal leader may be selected as the group's formal leader. This is the rationale for appointing high-profile individuals to chair significant CQI teams or to serve as "honorary chairs" of important search committees. In work teams, however, there is no opportunity for choice. It may be that the formal leader is not the person on whom the team depends, but it is the "informal leader who embodies the values of the group, aids it in accomplishing objectives, facilitates group maintenance, and usually serves as team spokesperson" (Hunsaker and Cook, 1986).

Leadership in teams has been studied extensively and has included both formal and informal leadership. That is, the important distinction is often not between formal and informal leadership, but between effective and ineffective leadership. In one study, leadership in intensive care units (ICUs) was positively related to efficiency of operation, satisfaction, and lower turnover of nurses (Shortell et al., 1994). Successful leaders adopted a supportive formal or informal leadership style, emphasizing standards of excellence, encouraging interaction, communicating clear goals and expectations, responding to changing needs, and providing support resources when possible. In another study, surgeon leadership was critical to the successful implementation of a new technology (Edmondson, 2003). Successful leaders communicated a compelling rationale for the change, motivating others to exert the necessary effort, and also minimized the status difference between themselves and other members of the operating room team, to facilitate others' ability to speak up with questions, observations, and concerns.

Team leaders vary in the style of leadership they adopt, and different circumstances call for different styles of leadership. In deciding upon a leadership style, therefore, group leaders need to consider in realistic terms their formal and informal authority within the group. Use of a coercive or forceful style may backfire when the individual does not have the power to back up decisions. Such a leader may find that the informal leader is able to veto, modify, or sabotage demands. Webster et al. (1998), using case management teams, found

that "powerless leaders" were faced with the formation of cliques and competition from more influential members. It is best, therefore, for the formal leader not only to consider the views of informal leaders, but also to collaborate with them if possible. It is therefore wise for a formal team leader to know the identity of the informal leader(s) and positively engage him in the work of the team.

## Communication Network and Interaction Patterns

A team cannot function effectively unless members can exchange information. Team leaders are usually best positioned to help manage communications within a team and between the team and external teams and other entities (Hackman, 1982). Consider the case of a nurse in a neonatal intensive care unit, who has just met with a patient's physician and must pass on vital information to the nurse on the next shift as well as to the parents who will visit during the next shift. How does information get conveyed? Without workable communication structures, important information may be lost or inaccurately communicated. In fact, the evaluation and design of communication processes are important components of many quality improvement projects (Tucker et al., 2007).

Communication speed and accuracy in a team are influenced by the nature of the team's communication network and by the complexity of its task. When a task is simple and **communication networks** are centralized (e.g., a wheel-and-spoke structure), speed and accuracy are enhanced in a team. However, when tasks are relatively complex, centralized communication networks lower both speed and accuracy because people serving as network hubs (i.e., information disseminators) may suffer from information overload. In this situation, communication networks are best decentralized (e.g., a star-shaped structure), relieving a manager of the need to filter (and possibly distort) information before it is passed on. In the example of the neonatal intensive care unit, it would be inefficient and risk error to have a nurse on the earlier shift communicate needed information to a head nurse first, who would then pass it on to the next shift's nurse. Timeliness and accuracy are both served by direct communication between the two nurses on the front lines of care. The team should thus use a communication structure that encourages direct interaction between nurses on sequential shifts.

The team communication network can be best described in terms of process behavior and interaction strategies

(Coopman, 2001; Stewart and Barrick, 2000). This involves the type of interaction that occurs between members (Stewart and Barrick, 2000). Most measurement of this behavior is based on the classic work of Bales (1950), who separated group process into either maintenance behaviors or task behaviors. The maintenance category includes interpersonal activities that lead to open communication, supportiveness, and reduction of interpersonal conflict. Task behaviors are those that relate directly to the team's work on its task. Using such a classification system, it should be possible to determine how team interaction develops and to assess the effectiveness of the process (Hackman, 1987). In a study of multidisciplinary, interagency teams coordinating services to youth with serious emotional disturbances, it was found that new teams engaged in more maintenance behavior than older, more experienced teams (Topping, Breland, and Fowler, 2004). Moreover, the focus on maintenance interactions occurred throughout team meetings indicating that teams in the forming stage do interact differently. As a result, the new teams had less task-oriented interaction; therefore, they reviewed fewer cases and engaged in less task-oriented behavior.

Although most of the focus in teams is on internal communications, teams also rely on external relationships to perform well (Gladstein, 1984). Boundary-spanning activities help teams coordinate with other teams in the organization and ensure that team activities serve the needs of the organization as a whole. New product or new technology teams, for example, use a diverse array of members, including researchers from the marketing department, physicians from the medical staff, and senior managers. All members take on **boundary-spanning roles**, because all members are responsible for representing and communicating with their external function while also working interdependently with other members of the team. Ancona and Caldwell (1992a) use the following classification to describe the range of boundary spanning activities observed in their research:

- **Ambassador activities**: Members carrying out these activities communicate frequently with those above them in the hierarchy. This set of activities is used to protect the team from outside pressures, to persuade others to support the team, and to lobby for resources.

- **Task coordinator activities**: Members carrying out these activities communicate frequently with other groups and persons at lateral levels in the organization. These activities include discussing problems with others, obtaining feedback, and coordinating and negotiating with outsiders.

- **Scout activities**: Members carrying out these activities are involved in general scanning for ideas and information about the external environment. These differ from the other two in that these activities relate to general scanning instead of specific coordination issues.

Generally, effective teams engage in high levels of ambassadorial and task coordinator activities and low levels of prolonged scouting activities. They found that other, "isolationist" teams neglected external activity altogether and thus tended to do quite poorly, probably due to being out of touch with the environment in which they work. In addition, some groups such as R&D teams use boundary spanning as an effective means of communication, but have found that stakeholder (customer) ratings were highest when the project leader—not the team—was the source of information (Hirst and Mann, 2004).

In sum, the increasing reliance on teams in health care organizations and the expanding responsibilities placed on them require strong communication structures both within the team and between the team and other groups outside the boundaries.

### Decision Making

Most teams are involved in making decisions at some point. This does not mean that all team members are involved in making all decisions, or even that the team itself makes decisions. To illustrate, a hospital president may ask for a recommendation on a decision from his or her senior management team, but retain the right to make the final decision. Similarly, a physician may obtain input from a variety of professionals but make the final determination on treatment. Managers and team leaders can decrease the chance of misunderstandings by clarifying the role of the team and the role of each member in a particular decision. Team members can deal with limitations on their influence as long as the boundaries of their influence are clear.

In contrast, decision making in a multidisciplinary research team—set up to produce high-quality research by leveraging a diversity of inputs—calls for a highly participative approach, with considerable dialogue and discussion prior to coming to a decision. Decisions in this setting may be based on consensus and compromise (Edmondson, Watkins, and Roberto, 2003).

A third scenario is a situation in which a decision is needed quickly. Under these circumstances, it may not be possible to obtain extensive participation for a particular decision. For example, decision making in an emergency triage team may be made without full consultation because time is critical and decisions must be made quickly and often by a single individual. Clearly, we would not want to use an elaborate team decision-making process (such as one that might be used by the multidisciplinary research team described above) in an emergency department! Conversely, given the ambiguities faced in research and the need for multiple perspectives (and few urgent time constraints), we would not want one individual making unilateral decisions in that context.

Leaders may also find the need to clarify the difference between problem solving and decision making. Some groups, such as some process improvement teams, are established to solve problems or seek methods for improving a particular organizational process. However, they may not be given authority to actually implement their solutions, particularly when substantial resources are required.

The process by which information is exchanged and decisions made is of central importance. Teams naturally attempt to make correct decisions, applying all available information to the issue at hand. One common problem that prevents complete sharing of information among members of a team is that of the **free rider**. The term "free rider" (referred to also as "social loafing") refers to a member of a team who obtains the benefits of group membership but does not accept a proportional share of the costs of membership (Albanese and Van Fleet, 1985). The free rider is seen as someone who promotes self-interest (the personal acquisition of benefits) over the public interest (the need to contribute to the activity that produces those benefits). It is often observed that the larger the group, the greater the free rider effect (Roberts and Hunt, 1991).

What can managers do to minimize free riding? Through effective use of power, design of organizations (including the size of the organizational units), and control of the incentive system, managers can influence team member behavior (Albanese and Van Fleet, 1985). At a routine level, this influence may be achieved by offering financial incentives or special forms of recognition to particular group members. In the longer term, it is important for managers to deal with the free rider problem by attempting to broaden the individual's concept of self-interest by creating, communicating, and maintaining a group culture that views effort expended on team processes as contributing to a shared goal that is meaningful to each team member.

Information may be available in a team, but effective use of that information for decision making does not always occur.

First, unique information (known by only one member) may not surface in group discussions (Stasser, 1999). Experimental studies have demonstrated that groups tend to dwell on common information (that held by all members), such that privately held information fails to surface; further, when it does surface, its impact is often muted (Larson et al., 1996).

Second, teams can become polarized on an issue in ways that do not reflect the full range of information and opinion in the group. As team members compare their positions on an issue with those of others on the team, pressures emerge to accept one position or the other as the *team* position. Furthermore, when one position is more forcefully argued than another, it gains support, despite initial discussion that revealed no clearly favored argument (Cartwright and Zander, 1968).

A manifestation of the poor use of information is the groupthink phenomenon, which can lead to premature convergence on a poor decision (Janis, 1972). The concept emerged from Janis's studies of high-level policy decisions by government leaders, including decisions about Vietnam, the Bay of Pigs, and the Korean War. Groupthink can occur at all levels of decision making, from the level of a family to high-profile policy decisions. Essentially, groupthink occurs when the desire for harmony and consensus overrides members' rational efforts to appraise the situation. In other words, groupthink occurs when maintaining the pleasant atmosphere of the team implicitly becomes more important to members than reaching a good decision. Some or all of the following symptoms may indicate the presence of groupthink (Janis, 1972):

1. *The illusion of invulnerability.* Team members may reassure themselves about obvious dangers and become overly optimistic and willing to take extraordinary risks.

2. *Collective rationalization.* Teams may overlook blind spots in their plans. When confronted with conflicting information, the team may spend considerable time and energy refuting the information and rationalizing a decision.

3. *Belief in the inherent morality of the team.* Highly cohesive teams may develop a sense of self-righteousness about their role, making them insensitive to the consequences of decisions.

4. *Stereotyping others.* Victims of groupthink hold biased, highly negative views of competing teams. They assume that they are unable to negotiate with other teams, and rule out compromise. This refusal to compromise is also related

to their belief in the inherent morality and "rightness" of the team, as described above.

5. *Pressures to conform.* Group members face severe *pressures* to conform to team norms and to team decisions. Dissent is considered abnormal and may lead to formal or informal censure or punishment.

6. *The use of mindguards.* Mindguards are members who withhold or discount dissonant information that interferes with the team's current view of a problem and its solution.

7. *Self-censorship.* Teams subject to groupthink pressure members to remain silent about possible misgivings and to minimize self-doubts about a decision. This and other symptoms are particularly prevalent when a team has a member with a great deal of power and influence.

8. *Illusion of unanimity.* A sense of unanimity emerges when members assume that silence and lack of protest signify agreement and consensus. Lack of disagreement does not necessarily mean there is not serious disagreement.

The consequences of groupthink are that teams may limit themselves, often prematurely, to one possible solution and fail to conduct a comprehensive analysis of a problem. When groupthink is well entrenched, members may fail to *review* their decisions in light of new information or changing events. Teams may also fail to consult adequately with experts within or outside the organization, and fail to develop contingency plans in the event that the decision turns out to be wrong.

Team leaders can help avoid groupthink. First, leaders can encourage members to critically evaluate proposals and solutions. Where a leader is particularly powerful and influential (yet still wants to get unbiased views from team members), the leader may refrain from stating his or her position until later in the decision-making process. Another strategy is to assign the same problem to two separate work teams. Most importantly, groupthink can be avoided by proactively engaging in a process of *critical appraisal* of ideas and solutions, and by understanding the warning signs of groupthink. Managers might also consider alternative systematic methods of decision making that emphasize member participation. **Nominal group technique** and **Delphi technique** elicit group members' opinions prior to judgments about those opinions. These and other approaches help generate ideas, and facilitate objective debate (Delbeq et al., 1975; Edmondson, et al., 2003).

## Team Learning

In a changing and uncertain world, a team's ability to learn is essential to its ongoing effectiveness (Edmondson, 1999). In the organizational literature, some discuss learning as an outcome, others as a process (see Edmondson, 1999). This chapter joins the latter tradition in treating team learning as a process, and we describe the behaviors and activities through which teams learn. Team learning is defined as an iterative process of reflection and action through which teams may discover and correct problems and errors in their work processes.

Learning processes consist of activities carried out by team members through which a team obtains and processes data that allow it to adapt and improve. Examples include seeking feedback on how well the team's outputs meet its customers' needs, talking about errors, and experimenting. It is through these activities that teams detect changes in the environment, better understand customer requirements, develop members' collective understanding of the situation, or discover unexpected consequences of previous team actions.

A study of cardiac surgery operating room teams learning to use a new technology for minimally invasive surgery found that the teams that were successful did a great deal more reflecting aloud on what they were learning, on how the process was going, and what changes might be made going forward than other teams (Edmondson, 2003). The learning for these teams involved acquiring knowledge and skill related to technical aspects of the new technology. It also involved practicing new interpersonal behaviors, such as speaking up in the operating room in new ways.

The behaviors through which teams learn involve interpersonal risk for individuals. For instance, other team members may think less of an individual for raising a concern, admitting an error, or asking a question for which the answer seems obvious to some. For this reason, learning in teams is greatly enabled by a climate of psychological safety, in which people believe that others will not think less of them for well-intentioned risks. This is an element of team climate, and is described further later in this chapter.

In health care, team learning is particularly important for two reasons. First, medical knowledge is constantly developing; individual providers must keep up with new care protocols, medications, and technologies. Physicians keep up with new developments in biology and medical technology by scanning the medical literature, attending conferences, and consulting with trusted colleagues. In fact, developments in science and medicine have always required continuing education for physicians and nurses. At the same time, however, the organizational context of health care delivery has changed in ways that increase the interdependence of the care delivery process, so that groups must learn how to better coordinate their activities to reflect changes in care protocols and to adjust to the unexpected. One recent study of teams, mentioned above for its findings related to psychological safety, also found that quality improvement teams had greater success implementing new practices when they had found support in the medical literature for the efficacy of the proposed changes (Tucker et al., 2007).

Another vital element of team learning in health care is the detection and correction of error. One way this learning occurs is through Morbidity and Mortality (M&M) rounds; however, physicians are often uncomfortable openly discussing errors with their colleagues, such that much learning about error remains private and individual. The current medico-legal environment, which holds the individual accountable for medical outcomes, together with the ethic of professional conscientiousness, serves to reinforce a model of learning focused on private learning by individual practitioners (Bohmer and Edmondson, 2001). Yet, team learning, where new insights are rapidly shared among providers, is a critical part of the new environment of health care, and increasingly, health care organizations are learning how to learn from their own failures. For example, Children's Hospital and Clinics of Minneapolis instituted "blame-free reporting" and safety action teams to encourage the reporting of mistakes and near misses to learn how to prevent them. Intermountain Health Care in Utah uses an integrated system that blends information technology and behavioral norms to allow the hospitals to learn from error and continuously improve the quality of care (Bohmer and Edmondson, 2002; Edmondson, 2004). Recently, Cincinnati Children's Hospital has embarked upon a similar and highly successful change effort, in which errors and sentinel events are thoroughly analyzed and publicly discussed for the lessons they contain (Tucker and Edmondson, 2009). In these cases, managers have worked hard to help people overcome the stigma of error, for the purpose of continuous, collective learning.

### Stages of Team Development

The effectiveness of a team is affected to varying degrees by its maturity, or **stage of team development**. Teams go through predictable stages of development, although the speed with which they mature varies. The familiar model presented below suggests that teams progress through five stages (Tuckman, 1965; Whetten and Cameron, 1998). Every team may not follow this precise pattern, but maturity and the age of a team need to be taken into consideration as a team leader plans and works. The following sequence of team development is summarized below:

1. *Forming.* During the first stage, members become acquainted with each other and with the team purpose. Members attempt to discover what behaviors are acceptable and unacceptable, while establishing trust and familiarity. This early stage is characterized by polite interactions and tentative interactions. Establishing a clear direction is critical.

2. *Storming.* At this stage, the team is faced with disagreement, counter-independence, and the need to manage conflict. Members may attempt to influence the development of group norms, roles, and procedures; therefore, the stage has high potential for conflict. Focusing on process improvements, team achievement, and collaborative relationships can help overcome emergent conflicts.

3. *Norming.* During this stage, the team grows more cohesive and aligned in purpose and actions. Agreement on rules and processes of decision making, roles and expectations, and commitment emerges. Emphasizing the team's direction or goals is essential for forward progress.

4. *Performing.* Once team members agree on the purpose and norms of the group, they can move forward to the task of defining separate roles and establishing work plans. The team is faced with the need for continuous improvement, innovation, and speed. Leaders must be ready to sponsor new ideas, orchestrate their implementation, and foster extraordinary performance from members.

5. *Adjourning.* For temporary teams, the adjournment stage is characterized by a sense of task accomplishment, regret, and increased emotionality.

As noted, teams may deviate from this model; not all teams pass through all stages as described. Some teams may begin at a norming or performing stage (e.g., members that have worked together before), while some may never move beyond the storming stage. Moreover, teams may not move in a linear fashion through the stages, but exhibit long, stable periods in which little occurs interspersed with relatively brief periods of dramatic progress—a "punctuated equilibrium" model

(Gersick, 1989). Finally, some teams may revert to earlier stages of development, sometimes resulting from new tasks or responsibilities given the team, a change in formal or informal leadership, the addition of a new member, or the loss of a valuable member. Managers should consider the stage of team development in establishing team expectations. For example, research has shown that managers of virtual teams need to know the challenges associated with each stage of the life cycle and time appropriate intervention strategies accordingly (Furst et al., 2004). An example of such a strategy is the active involvement of a senior sponsor in clarifying team mission and goals during the early stages of team development.

### Team Processes as Intermediary

Team processes are thus the intermediary between team structures and the outcome of team effectiveness. Through ineffective processes, teams composed of highly talented individuals can be dysfunctional. Conversely, effective processes allow the team to achieve its potential. Team processes are important because unlike relatively unchangeable inputs, such as the team's composition and task, team processes can be altered and improved upon by team members and leaders. Teams can learn how to better communicate, leaders can improve their ability to manage meetings and coach other team members, team members can experiment with different types of decision making, and teams can learn and improve. The extent to which these and other processes are appropriately used can have a profound impact on team outcomes.

Finally, what constitutes effective team processes is contingent on the context. As noted above, saving lives in an emergency department requires extraordinary and rapid communication, and a unilateral decision-making style, while a medical research team can benefit from a participative consensus-seeking approach. In sum, no single set of team processes meets every team's needs; team processes are dependent upon structural aspects of the team, including team size, the nature of team tasks, and the larger context within which the team operates.

## DEBATE TIME: The Individual versus The Team?

Managers often preach the importance of teams, yet our workforce management systems continue to be oriented largely on the individual. If teams are that important, shouldn't we reengineer our workforce management practices around teams rather than individuals? Consider the following aspects of management:

- Individual employees are given a job description, and this job description is often supported by a comprehensive job analysis. Teams, on the other hand, often have vague goals and unclear work processes.

- Individual employees are provided with an orientation to their job and ongoing training to improve their performance. How often are teams provided with a similar orientation to their work and training to improve team performance?

- Complex systems have been established to select job applicants for work in an organization. With some exceptions, technical qualifications are deemed to be of paramount importance in the selection process. Systematic evaluative techniques are used to assess technical qualifications. If organizations are truly interested in improving team performance, should we not employ similar methods to determine the "team-worthiness" of job applicants?

- Organizations orient their motivational and reward systems around individual employee performance. Given the importance of teams and team performance, should we not spend energy developing effective ways of motivating and improving team performance?

- Performance management systems are designed to provide feedback, coaching, and goal setting for individuals. How often are teams provided with feedback on their performance, along with strategies for improving team performance?

The question is not whether we should ignore the individual and individual reward systems. The larger question is how do we design the workforce management process in our health care organizations to truly do justice to the prominent role of teams, now and in the future? Can our culture change from one that views the individual as the sole unit of value to one where the work team is recognized as having similar value? Is it possible for our bureaucratic organizational systems—such as personnel systems—to recognize and accommodate the value of teams? Are the obstacles insurmountable: is it worth the effort?

# CONCLUSIONS

One of the most important managerial tasks in health services organizations is the development and management of teams. It is now common wisdom that organizations as a whole, as well as individuals, are dependent upon well-functioning teams. As noted, however, teams do not naturally perform optimally. Teams must be set up and led, if they are to succeed. Nor do teams naturally develop and improve. In fact, their level of performance may even erode and become dysfunctional over time without deliberate and continuous supportive efforts. Effective managers understand that improving a team's performance is a complex endeavor and that improvement strategies need to emphasize both design—structure and process—and understanding of the challenges and contributions of individual members of the team (see Debate Time). Finally, while we can make general theoretical statements about teams, each team develops in a distinct way, at its own pace, making its own mark in the organization. Thus, there is both science and art to managing and working with teams.

# SUMMARY AND MANAGERIAL GUIDELINES

Effective team management requires understanding of fundamental team principles and theories as well as an ability to translate those concepts into management action and behavior. The following managerial guidelines provide specific applications of theory with the goal of improving team effectiveness:

1. Team members are both individuals and team members. To ensure a sustained level of motivation, reward systems should be constructed so that individual and team contributions are recognized.

2. Ongoing teams usually have a set of group norms, some of which are functional and others dysfunctional. Team leaders need to be aware of both positive and negative norms, and develop strategies to reinforce positive norms and eliminate norms that limit team effectiveness.

3. Conflict is common in teams, and managers must be able to accurately diagnose the causes of conflict. To resolve team conflict, managers should also be comfortable with a range of conflict resolution strategies.

4. Team leadership is complex, partly because teams often have both a formal leader as well as one or more informal leaders. Managers should be aware of these often unspoken dynamics because they can have a profound impact on team processes and effectiveness.

5. Managers should clarify to team members the role of a team. In particular, team members need to understand clearly the team's role in decision making. Some teams provide input to decision makers, while other teams have the authority to make decisions. Team leaders should clearly understand the decisional authority of the team, and communicate this accurately to team members.

6. Managers should understand the applicability of a variety of approaches to building team consensus and decision making. They should avoid prematurely moving to arbitrary approaches to decision making, such as imposing a decision or voting. Full airing of perspectives, and the identification and discussion of team members' interests (rather than positions) may help to identify areas of agreement among team members.

7. Managers should be aware of status differences among team members and how these differences may affect the fullness of discussion and the airing of differences.

8. Managers should employ specific techniques for managing meetings, including:

   **a.** Team leaders should prepare an agenda, with time limits for each item, and the placement of the most critical agenda items early on the agenda. Some managers include an indication of the purpose of each item, whether it is for information, discussion, decision making, or other purpose.

   **b.** If a specific team member is expected to address an issue at a meeting, the manager should brief those individuals prior to the meeting to be sure there is agreement on the agenda item and the role of the team member during the meeting.

   **c.** Team leaders should review the progress made to date and establish the purpose of the meeting. When appropriate, ask subcommittee representatives to review the progress of their work to date.

   **d.** Team members should be provided with needed materials prior to meetings.

   **e.** Manage team discussions to ensure full participation. For example, it is advisable to ask more junior team members for their input prior to asking for the views of more senior team members.

   **f.** Keep a record of team deliberations, in particular decisions that were made and the discussion that supported each decision.

   **g.** Team leaders should utilize delegation for complex decisions and information-gathering tasks. Managers should maintain an awareness of the flow of discussion and close off discussion when it becomes apparent that further progress requires more information and/or more extensive analysis.

   **h.** Close the meeting by summarizing what has been accomplished and reviewing assignments for the next meeting.

# DISCUSSION QUESTIONS

1. To foster teamwork and a culture of quality improvement, a new director of an ambulatory care center in a hospital has begun holding twice-monthly management team meetings, consisting of several physicians, nurses, physician assistants, financial managers, and others. Attendance at these meetings has been erratic, and enforcing attendance is difficult because many of these people report to their discipline chiefs rather than to the director of the center. What advice would you give to this person to promote more consistent participation?

2. A community task force has been formed to improve the coordination of care for the frail elderly. Given the large number of people and agencies involved in providing services to this population, how would you balance the need for representation with the need to keep the task force size to a manageable level?

3. You are a member of a hospital project team assigned to develop a new pediatric oncology service line. Your team is expected to develop a business plan for presentation to the senior management team and the hospital board. A specific timetable has been established for producing a set of deliverables. The team leader is a well-known oncologist with a very strong clinical background and reputation. However, his team leadership skills leave something to be desired. Among other problems, meetings are cancelled at the last minute, delegation of tasks is ambiguous, and the focus and direction of the project changes scope at virtually every meeting. As a team member, what alternatives do you have to improve team management? Which alternative would you select as having the best chance of success?

4. Along with other hospital business managers, you have been a member of a management team. Recently, you have been promoted, and your former business manager team members now report to you. As the new leader of the management team, what challenges will you face in managing the team? How would you approach these challenges?

5. As described in this chapter, teams go through stages of development. As a team leader, what is the practical value to understanding these stages? How could this knowledge improve your effectiveness as a team leader?

# CASE: Using Teams to Achieve Millennium Development Goals

Childhood mortality continues to be a major health problem in developing countries. A child born in a developing country is over 13 times more likely to die within the first five years of life than a child born in an industrialized country. Sub-Saharan African countries account for about half the deaths of children under five in the developing world. Between 1990 and 2006, about 27 countries—the large majority in sub-Saharan Africa—made no progress in reducing childhood deaths.

The country of Ghana has set a goal of decreasing childhood mortality from 110 per 1,000 live births to 20 per 1,000 live births by 2015. The most common causes of death among children under age 5 in Ghana are malaria and neonatal diseases, primarily asphyxia, sepsis, and prematurity. Tragically, most of these deaths are preventable. Among other initiatives, Project Fives-Alive! was established to reduce childhood mortality in Ghana. The approach being taken by this nationwide project is the Institute for Health Improvement (IHI) Breakthrough Series Improvement Collaborative Network. Through this multiyear project, teams of frontline health providers and their managers meet periodically in learning sessions where they acquire quality improvement knowledge and skills. Teams test system improvement changes, and learn from each other. This is one of the first applications of IHI improvement initiatives in Africa. When the project is fully scaled up, over 1,000 teams will have participated in this improvement effort.

Among the most important factors associated with under-five mortality is underutilization of health services. For example, many women do not receive antenatal care, preventive measures (such as neonatal tetanus protection and folate/iron supplements) are inconsistently provided, and many women lack knowledge about oral rehydration therapy and other life-saving procedures.

Why the focus on teams? The answer is that frontline providers are often in the best position to understand the obstacles that women face in accessing services—and to suggest and test potential solutions. As with quality improvement initiatives elsewhere, teams need training, knowledge, and skills, as well as a framework for applying quality improvement methods. Throughout the country, teams are being trained in quality improvement methods: setting measurable goals, implementing tests of change, identifying best practices, and—perhaps of greatest significance from a country development perspective—sharing their experiences with other teams and disseminating this knowledge to the larger global health community.

Results are encouraging. Teams are enthusiastically sharing their knowledge through collaborative meetings, and evidence is emerging of improvements in the processes of care, and hopefully, in health outcomes. Even more encouraging is evidence that teams are learning how to function as teams, and to apply a systems improvement perspective to other health system problems. Development of well-functioning and highly trained teams could be a key part of achieving important global health goals.

## Questions

1. One feature of the teams in this case is frequent turnover among team members. How might turnover among team members affect team performance? What approaches can team leaders take to minimize potential negative impacts of turnover and gain advantages, if any?

2. Consumers or patients are sometimes involved in quality improvement teams, but in this role, they may feel that their voices are unimportant, or that their participation is symbolic rather than substantive. Do you think that consumers should be involved in the improvement teams in this case? Why or why not? If consumers are involved, how can team leaders and members most effectively utilize their knowledge and insights?

3. Even when team improvement efforts achieve change, the sustainability of change remains a pervasive challenge. In fact, sustainability of the teams themselves may be problematic. What are the particular obstacles to sustaining the improvements achieved by teams in this case? Similarly, what factors might lead to the dissolution of the improvement teams over time? As a team leader, what strategies might be used to sustain change and to uphold the vitality of the team over time?

# REFERENCES

Albanese, R., & Van Fleet, D. D. (1985). Rational behavior in groups: The free riding tendency. *Academy of Management Review, 10*, 244–255.

Alderfer, C. P. (1987). An intergroup perspective on organizational behavior. In J. W. Lorsch (Ed.), *Handbook of organizational behavior*. Englewood Cliffs, NJ, Prentice-Hall.

Alexander, J. A., Jinnett, K., D'Aunno, T. A., & Ullman, E. (1996). The effects of treatment team diversity and size on assessments of team functioning. *Hospital & Health Services Administration, 41*, 37–53.

Ancona, D. G. (1990). Outward bound: Strategies for team survival in an organization. *Academy of Management Journal, 2*, 334–365.

Ancona, D. G., & Caldwell, D. F. (1992a). Bridging the boundary: External activity and performance in organizational teams. *Administrative Science Quarterly, 37*, 634–665.

Ancona, D. G., & Caldwell, D. F. (1992b). Demography and design: Predictors of a new product team performance. *Organization Science, 3*, 321–341.

Ancona, D. G., & Caldwell, D. F. (1998). Rethinking team composition from the outside in. In D. H. Gruenfeld (Ed.), *Research on managing groups and teams* (pp. 21–37). Stamford, CT: MAI Press.

Arnold, H. J., & Feldman, D. C. (1986). *Organizational behavior*. New York: McGraw-Hill.

Arrow, H., McGrath, J. E., & Berdahl, J. L. (2000). *Small Groups as Complex Systems*. Thousand Oaks, CA: Sage Publications.

Ashforth, B. E., & Mael, F. (1989). Social identity theory and the organization. *Academy of Management Journal, 32*, 20–39.

Athanasaw, Y. (2003). Team characteristics and team member knowledge, skills, and ability relationships to the effectiveness of cross-functional teams in the public sector. *International Journal of Public Administration, 26*, 1165–1204.

Barczak, G., & McDonough, E. F. (2003, November–December). Leading global product development teams. *Research Technology Management, 46*(6), 14.

Batalden, P. B., Nelson, E. C., Edwards, W. H., Godfrey, M. M., & Mohr, J. J. (2003). Microsystems in health care: Part 9. Developing small clinical units to attain peak performance. *Joint Commission Journal on Quality Improvement, 29*(11): 575–585.

Beckhard, R. (1967). The confrontation meeting. *Harvard Business Review, 43*, 159–165.

Beersma, B., Hollenbeck, J. R., Humphrey, S. E., Moon, H., Conlon, D. E., & Ilgen, D. R. (2003). Cooperation, competition, and team performance: Toward a contingency approach. *Academy of Management Journal, 46*, 572–591.

Benne, K., & Sheats, P. (1948). Functional roles of group members. *Journal of Social Issues, 2*, 42–47.

Berwick, D. M. (1995). The toxicity of pay for performance. *Quality Management in Health Care, 4*(1), 27–33.

Bettenhausen, K. L. (1991). Five years of group research: What we have learned and what needs to be addressed. *Journal of Management, 17*, 345–381.

Blake, R. R., & Mouton, J. S. (1978). *The new managerial grid*. Houston, TX: Gulf.

Blake, R. R., & Mouton, J. S. (1984). *Solving costly organizational conflicts*. San Francisco: Jossey-Bass.

Bohmer, R., & Edmondson, A. (2001, March–April). Organizational learning in health care, *Health Forum Journal*, 32–35.

Bohmer R., & Edmondson, A. (2002) Intermountain health care. Harvard Business School Case #9-602-145. Boston: HBS Press.

Brodbeck, F. (1996). Work group performance and effectiveness: Conceptual and measurement issues. In M. A. West (Ed.), *Handbook of work group psychology* (pp. 285–315). Chichester: Wiley.

Brown, B., & Keyes, M. (2000). Blurred roles and permeable boundaries: The experience of multidisciplinary working in community mental health. *Health and Social Care in the Community, 8*(6), 425–435.

Burchard, J. D., Burchard, S. N., Sewell, R., & VanDenBerg, J. (1993). *One kid at a time.* Juneau, AK: State of Alaska Division of Mental Health and Mental Retardation.

Campion, M. A., Medsker, G. J., & Higgs, A. C. (1993). Relations between work group characteristics and effectiveness: Implications for designing effective work groups. *Personnel Psychology, 46,* 823–850.

Cannon-Bowers, J. A., Oser, R., & Flanagan, D. L. (1992). Work teams in industry: A selected review and proposed framework. In R. W. Swezey, & E. Salas (Eds.), *Teams: Their training and performance.* Norwood, NJ: Ablex Publishing.

Capelli, P., & Rogovsky, N. (1994). New work systems and skills requirements. *International Labour Review, 133*(2), 205–220.

Cartwright, D., & Zander, A. (1968). Group *dynamics: Research and theory* (3rd ed.). New York: Harper & Row.

Cassard, S. D., Weisman, C. S., Gordon, D. L., & Wong, R. (1994). The impact of unit-based selfmanagement by nurses on patient outcomes. *Health Services Research, 29,* 415–433.

Chen, G., & Klimoski, R. J. (2003). The impact of expectations on newcomer performance in teams as mediated by work characteristics, social exchanges, and empowerment. *Academy of Management Journal, 46,* 591–607.

Cheser, R. (1999). When teams go to war—against each other! *Quality Progress, 32,* 25–29.

Cohen, S. G., & Bailey, D. E. (1997). What makes teams work: Group effectiveness research from the shop floor to the executive suite. *Journal of Management, 23,* 239–290.

Colquitt, J. A., Noe, R. A., & Jackson, C. L. (2002). Justice in teams: Antecedents and consequences of procedural justice climate. *Personnel Psychology, 55,* 83–100.

Coopman, S. J. (2001). Democracy, performance, and outcomes in interdisciplinary health care teams. *The Journal of Business Communication, 38*(3), 261–281.

Cosby K. S. (2009). Authority gradients and communication. In P. Croskerry, K. S. Cosby, S. M. Schenkel, & R. L. Wears, *Patient Safety in Emergency Medicine* (chap. 28). Philadelphia: Wolters Kluwer/Lippincott Williams & Wilkins.

Cosier, R. A. (1981). Dialectical inquiry in strategic planning: A case of premature acceptance? *Academy of Management Review, 6,* 643–648.

Cummings, T. (1978). Self-regulating work groups: A socio-technical synthesis. *Academy of Management Review, 3,* 625–634.

Dailey, R., Young, A., & Barr, C. (1991). Empowering middle managers in hospitals with team-based problem solving. *Health Care Management Review, 16,* 55–63.

Deber, R. B., & Leatt, P (1986). The multidisciplinary renal team: Who makes the decisions? *Health Matrix, 4*(3), 3–9.

Deeter-Schmelz, D. R., & Ramsey, D. R. (2003). An investigation of team information processing in service teams: Exploring the link between teams and customers. *Journal of the Academy of Marketing Science, 31*(4), 409–425.

Delbecq, A., Van de Ven, A., & Gustafson, D. (1975). *Group techniques for program planning.* Glenview, IL: Scott, Foresman.

Denison, D. R., & Sutton, R. I. (1990). Operating room nurses. In J. R. Hackman (Ed.), *Groups that work (and those that don't): Creating conditions for effective teamwork.* San Francisco: Jossey-Bass.

Deutsch, M. (1949). An experimental study of the effects of co-operation and competition upon group process. *Human Relations, 2,* 199–232.

Dooley, K. J., & Zimmerman, B. J. 2003. Merger as marriage: Communication issues in postmerger integration. *Health Care Management Review, 28,* 55–68.

Doran, D., Baker, R., Murray, M., Bohnen, J., Zahn, C., Sidani, S., & Carryer, J. (2002). Achieving clinical improvement: An interdisciplinary intervention. *Health Care Management Review, 27,* 42–57.

Dyer, J. L. (1984). Team research and team training: A state-of-the-art review. In F. A. Muckler (Ed.), *Human factors review: 1984* (pp. 285–323). Santa Monica, CA: Human Factors Society.

Edmondson, A. (1996). Learning from mistakes is easier said than done: Group and organizational influences on the detection and correction of human error. *Journal of Applied Behavioral Science, 32*(1), 5–28.

Edmondson, A. (1999). Psychological safety and learning behavior in work teams. *Administrative Science Quarterly, 44*, 350–383.

Edmondson, A. C. (2002). The local and variegated nature of learning in organizations. *Organization Science, 13*(2), 128–146.

Edmondson, A. C. (2003). Speaking up in the operating room: How team leaders promote learning in interdisciplinary action teams. *Journal of Management Studies, 40*(6), 1419–1452.

Edmondson, A. C. (2004). Learning from failure in health care: Frequent opportunities, pervasive barriers. *Quality and Safety in Health Care, 13*, 3–9.

Edmondson, A. C., Bohmer, R. M., and Pisano, G. P. (2001). Disrupted routines: Team learning and new technology implementation in hospitals. *Administrative Science Quarterly, 46*, 685–716.

Edmondson, A. C., & Nembhard, I. M. (2009). Product development and learning in project teams: The challenges are the benefits. *Journal of Product Innovation Management, 26*, 123–138.

Edmondson, A. C., Roberto, M., and Watkins, M. (2003) A dynamic model of top management team effectiveness: Managing unstructured task streams. *Leadership Quarterly, 219*, 1–29.

Erickson, J. (1997). Turmoil in Tuscon. *American Medical News, 40*(34), 1, 23.

Etzioni, A. (1961). *A comparative analysis of complex organizations.* New York: Free Press.

Fargason, C. A., & Haddock, C. C. (1992). Crossfunctional, integrative team decision making: Essential for effective QI in health care. *Quality Review Bulletin, 7*, 157–163.

French, W. L., & Bell, C. H. (1990). *Organizational development.* Englewood Cliffs, NJ: PrenticeHall.

Fried, B., & Nelson, W. (1987). Strategic planning with family physicians. *Canadian Family Physician, 33*, 1309–1312.

Fried, B. J., Johnsen, M. C., Starrett, B. E., Calloway, M. O., & Morrissey, J. P. (1998). An empirical assessment of rural community support networks for individuals with severe mental disorders. *Community Mental Health Journal, 34*(1), 39–56.

Furst, S. A., Reeves, M. Rosen, B., & Blackburn, R. S. (2004). Managing the life cycle of virtual teams. *Academy of Managament Executive, 18*, 6–20.

George, J. F., & Jones, G. R. (1999). *Understanding and managing organizational behavior* (2nd ed.). Reading, MA: Addison-Wesley.

George, J. M. (1992). Extrinsic and intrinsic origins of perceived social loafing in organizations. *Academy of Management Journal, 35*, 191–202.

Gersick, C. J. G. (1989). Marking time: Predictable transitions in task groups. *Academy of Management, 32*, 274–309.

Gist, M. E., Locke, E. A., & Taylor, M. S. (1987). Organizational behavior: Group structure, process, and effectiveness. *Journal of Management, 13*, 237–257.

Gladstein, D. (1984). Groups in context: A model of task group effectiveness. *Administrative Science Quarterly, 29*, 499–517.

Goodman, P. S., Ravlin, E., & Schminke, M. (1987). Understanding groups in organizations. *Research in Organizational Behavior, 9*, 121–173.

Gordon, J. (1992, October). Work teams: How far have they come? *Training,* 59–65.

Gordon, J. R. (1999). *Organizational behavior: A diagnostic approach.* Upper Saddle River, NJ: Prentice-Hall.

Gully, S. M., Devine, D. J., & Whitney D. J. (1995). A meta-analysis of cohesion and performance. *Small Group Research, 26,* 497–520.

Guzzo, R. A. (1990). Group decision making and group effectiveness in organizations. In P. S. Goodman (Ed.), *Designing effective work groups.* San Francisco: Jossey-Bass.

Hackman, J. R. (1976). Work design. In J. R. Hackman, & J. L. Suttle (Eds.), *Improving life at work.* Santa Monica, CA: Goodyear.

Hackman, J. R. (1982). *A set of methods for research on work teams* (Technical Report No. 1). School of Organization and Management. New Haven, CT: Yale University.

Hackman, J. R. (1987). The design of work teams. In J. Lorsch (Ed.), *Handbook of organizational behavior.* New York: Prentice-Hall.

Hackman, J. R. (1990a). *Groups that work (and those that don't).* San Francisco: Jossey-Bass.

Hackman, J. R. (1990b). Introduction. Work teams in organizations: An orienting framework. In J. R. Hackman (Ed.), *Groups that work (and those that don't): Creating conditions for effectiveness teamwork.* San Francisco: Jossey-Bass.

Hackman, J. R. (2003). Learning more by crossing levels: Evidence from airplanes, hospitals, and orchestras. *Journal of Organizational Behavior, 24*(8), 905–1013.

Hackman, J. R., & Oldham, G. R. (1980). *Work redesign.* Reading, MA: Addison-Wesley.

Hasenfeld, Y. (1983). *Human service organizations.* Englewood Cliffs, NJ: Prentice-Hall.

Hirst, G., & Mann, L. (2004). A model of R&D leadership and team communication: The relationship with project performance. *R & D Management, 34,* 147–161.

Hoegl, M., & Gemuenden, H. G. (2001). Teamwork quality and the success of innovative projects: A theoretical concept and empirical evidence. *Organization Science, 12,* 435–449.

Horak, B. J., Guarino, J. H., Knight, C. C., & Kweder, S. L. (1991). Building a team on a medical floor. *Health Care Management Review, 16,* 65–71.

Huber, G. (1980). *Managerial decision making.* Glenview, IL: Scott, Foresman.

Hunsaker, P. L., & Cook, C. W. (1986). *Managing organizational behavior.* Reading, MA: Addison-Wesley.

Jackson, S. E. (1992). Team composition in organizational settings: Issues in managing an increasingly diverse work force. In S. Worchel, W. Wood, & J. A. Simpson (Eds.), *Group process and productivity.* Newbury Park, CA: Sage.

Jackson, S. E., Joshi, A., & Erhardt, N. L. (2003). Recent research on team and organizational diversity: SWOT analysis and implications. *Journal of Management, 29*(6), 801–830.

Janis, L. L. (1972). *Victims of groupthink.* Boston: Houghton-Mifflin.

Joint Commission on Accreditation of Healthcare Oganizations. (2005). *2005 comprehensive accreditation manual for hospitals: The official handbook (CAMH).* Oakbrook Terrace, IL: JCAHO.

Katz, N. (2001). Getting the most out of your team. *Harvard Business Review, 79,* 22.

Katzenbach, J. R., & Smith, D. K. (1993). The discipline of teams. *Harvard Business Review, 71,* 111–120.

Kirkman, B. L., & Rosen, B. (1997). A model of work team empowerment. In R. Woodman & W. Pasmore (Eds.), *Research in organizational change and development* (pp. 131–167). Greenwich, CT: Jai Press.

Kolodny, H., & Kiggundu, M. (1980). Towards the development of a sociotechnical systems model in woodlands mechanical harvesting. *Human Relations, 33,* 623–645.

Kor, Y. (2003). Experience-based top management team competence and sustained growth. *Organization Science, 14*(6), 707–720.

Lacey, R., & Gruenfeld, D. (1999). Unwrapping the work group: How extra-organizational context affects group behavior. *Research on Managing Groups and Teams, 2,* 157–177.

LaPenta, C., & Jacobs, G. M. (1996). Application of group process model to performance appraisal development in a CQI environment. *Health Care Management Review, 21,* 45–60.

Larson, J., Christensen, C., Abbott, A. & Franz, T. (1996). Diagnosing groups: charting the flow of information in medical decision making teams. *Journal of Personality and Social Psychology, 71,* 315–330.

Latane, B., Williams, K. D., & Harkins, S. (1979). Many hands make light the work: The causes and consequences of social loafing. *Journal of Personality and Social Psychology, 37,* 822–832.

Liberman, R. P., Hilty, D. M., Drake, R. E., & Tsang, H. (2001). Requirements for multidisciplinary teamwork in psychiatric rehabilitation. *Psychiatric Services, 52*(10), 1331–1342.

Liden, R. C., Wayne, S. J., Jaworski, R. A., & Bennett, N. (2004). Social loafing: A field investigation. *Journal of Management, 30,* 285–305.

Lubit, R. H. (2003). *Coping with toxic managers, subordinates ... and other difficult people: Using emotional intelligence to survive and prosper.* Financial Times/Prentice Hall.

Marks, M. A., Zaccaro, S. J., & Mathieu, J. E. (2000). Performance implications of leader briefings and team-interaction training for team adaptation to novel environments. *Journal of Applied Psychology, 85,* 971–987.

McGrath, J. E. (1984). *Groups: Interaction and performance.* Englewood Cliffs, NJ: Prentice-Hall.

McGregor, D. (1960). *The human side of enterprise.* New York: McGraw-Hill.

Mechanic, D. (1962). Sources of power of lower participants in complex organizations. *Administrative Science Quarterly, 7*(4), 349–364.

Moorhead, G., & Griffin, R. W. (1998). *Organizational behavior: Managing people and organizations.* Boston: Houghton Mifflin.

Moreland, R. L., & Levine, J. M. (1988). Group dynamics over time: Development and socialization in small groups. In J. E. McGrath (Ed.), *The social psychology of groups* (pp.151–181). Beverly Hills, CA: Sage.

Mullen, B., & Baumeister, R. F. (1987). Group effects on self-attention and performance: Social loafing, social facilitation, and social impairment. In C. Hendrick (Ed.), *Review of personality and social psychology.* Beverly Hills, CA: Sage.

Nadler, D. A., & Tushman, M. L. (1988). *Strategic organization design: Concepts, tools, and processes.* Glenview, IL: Scott, Foresman.

Nelson, R. E. (1989). The strength of strong ties: Social networks and intergroup conflict in organizations. *Academy of Management Journal, 32,* 377–401.

Nelson E. C., Batalden P. B., Huber T. P., Mohr, J. J., Godfrey, M. M., Headrick, L. A., & Wasson, J. H. (2002). Microsystems in health care: Part 1. Learning from high-performing front-line clinical units. *Joint Commission Journal on Quality Improvement, 28*(9): 472–493.

Nembhard, I. M., & Edmondson, A.C. (2006). Making it safe: The effects of leader inclusiveness and professional status on psychological safety and improvement efforts in health care teams. *Journal of Organizational Behavior, 27*(7): 941–966.

Orsburn, J. D., Moran, L., Musselwhite, E., & Zenger, J. (1990). *Self-directed work teams: The new American challenge.* Homewood, IL: Business One Irwin.

Owens, D. A., Mannic, E. A., & Neale, M. A. (1998). Strategic formation of groups: Issues in task performancer and team member selection. In D. H. Gruenfeld (Ed.), *Research on managing groups and teams* (pp. 149–165). Stamford, CT: MAI Press.

Parker, G., McAdams, J., & Zielinski, D. (2000). *Rewarding teams: Lessons from the trenches*. San Francisco, Jossey-Bass Publishers.

Pascarella, P. (1997, February). Compensating teams. *Across the Board* (pp. 16–22).

Pinto, M. B., & Pinton, J. K. (1990). Project team communication and cross-functional cooperation in new program development. *Journal of Product Innovation Management, 7*, 200–212.

Roberts, K. H., & Hunt, D. M. (1991). *Organizational behavior*. Boston: PWS-Kent Publishing Co.

Robinson, A., & Street, A. (2004). Care of older people: Improving networks between acute care nurses and an aged care assessment team. *Journal of Clinical Nursing, 13*(4), 486–497.

Roethlisberger, F. J., & Dickson, W. J. (1939). *Management and the worker*. Cambridge, MA: Harvard University Press.

Rundall, T. G., Starkweather, D. B., & Norrish, B. A. (1998). *After restructuring: Empowerment strategies at work in America's hospitals*. San Francisco: Jossey-Bass.

Rush University Medical Center. (2008, May 26). Reduced emergency room visits for elderly patients attributed to virtual health care team approach. *Diabetes Week* (p. 222).

Salas, E., Burke, C. S., & Cannon-Bowers, J. A. (2000). Teamwork: Emerging principles. *International Journal of Management Reviews, 2*(4), 339–356.

Salvedra, R., Earley, P C., & Van Dyne, L. (1993). Complex interdependence in taskperforming groups. *Journal of Applied Psychology, 78*, 61–72.

Schein, E. H. (1985). *Organizational culture and leadership*. San Francisco, Jossey-Bass Publishers.

Schein, E. H. and W. Bennis (1965). *Personal and organizational change through group methods*. New York, Wiley.

Schweikhart, S. B., & Smith-Daniels, V (1996). Reengineering the work of caregivers: Role redefinition, team structures, and organizational redesign. *Health Care Management Review, 41*, 19–36.

Schwenk, C. R. (1983). Laboratory research on illstructured decision aids: The case of dialectical inquiry. *Decision Sciences, 14*, 140–144.

Scott, W. G. (1967). *Organization theory*. Homewood, IL: Irwin.

Seashore, S. (1954). *Group cohesiveness in the industrial work group*. Ann Arbor: Institute for Social Research, University of Michigan.

Shaw, M. E. (1976). *Group dynamics: The psychology of small group behavior*. New York: McGraw-Hill.

Shaw, R. B. (1990). Mental health treatment teams. In J. R. Hackman (Ed.), *Groups that work (and those that don't)* (pp. 320–348). San Francisco: Jossey-Bass.

Sherif, M., & Sherif, C. W. (1953). *Groups in harmony and tension*. New York: Harper.

Shortell, S. M., Marsteller, J. A., Lin, M., Pearson, M. L., Wu, S., Mendel, P., ...Rosen, M. (2004, November). The role of perceived team effectiveness in improving chronic illness care. *Medical Care, 42*(11).

Shortell, S. M., Zimmerman, J. E., Rousseau, D. M., Gillies, R. R., Wagner, D. P, Draper, E. A., ...Duffy, J. (1994). The performance of intensive care units: Does good management make a difference? *Medical Care, 32*, 508–525.

Sidorov, J. (2003). Case study of a failed merger of hospital systems. *Managed Care, 12*(11): 56–60.

Stewart, G. L., & Barrick, M. R. (2000). Team structure and performance: Assessing the mediating role of intrateam process and the moderating role of task type. *Academy of Management Journal, 43*(20), 135–148.

Stasser, G. (1999). The uncertain role of unshared information in collective choice. In L. Thompson, J. Levine, & D. Messick (Eds.), *Shared cognition in organizations* (pp. 49–69). Mahwah, NJ: Lawrence Erlbaum Associates.

Stigler, G. J. (1974). Free riders and collective action: An appendix to theories of economic regulation. *Bell Journal of Economics and Management Science, 5*, 359–365.

Stoner, C. R., & Hartman, R. I. (1993). Team building: Answering the tough questions. *Business Horizons, 36*, 70–78.

Sundstrom, E., DeMeuse, K. P., & Futrell, D. (1990). Work teams: Applications and effectiveness. *American Psychologist, 45*(2), 120–133.

Thompson, J. D. (1967). *Organizations in action*. New York: McGraw-Hill.

Thyen, M. N., Theis, R., & Tebbitt, B. V. (1993). Organizational empowerment through self-governed teams. *Journal of Nursing Administration, 23*, 24–26.

Topping, S., Breland, J., & Fowler, A. (2004). Inter-agency teams: The nature of collaboration, interaction, and effectiveness in serving children and youth with SED. Working Paper.

Topping, S., & Calloway, M. (2000). Does resource scarcity create interorganizational coordination and formal service linkages? A case study of a rural mental health system. *Advances in Health Care Management, 1*, 393–419.

Topping, S., Norton, T., & Scafidi, B. (2003). Coordination of services: The use of multidisciplinary, interagency teams. In S. Dopson and A. L. Mark (Eds.), *Leading health care organizations* (pp. 100–112). New York: Palgrave Macmillan.

Tucker, A. L., Nembhard, I. M., & Edmondson, A. C. (2007). Implementing new practices: An empirical study of organizational learning in hospital intensive care units. *Management Science, 53*(6), 894–907.

Tucker, A., and Edmondson, A. (2009). Cincinnati Children's Hospital Medical Center. Boston: HBS Publishing Case # 9-609-109.

Tuckman, B. W. (1965). Developmental sequences in small groups. *Psychological Bulletin, 63*, 384–399.

U.S. Department of Health and Human Services. *Hospital compare*. Retrieved May 2010 from http://www.hospitalcompare.hhs.gov

Van de Ven, A. H., Delbecq, A. L., & Koenig, R. (1976). Determinants of coordination modes within organizations. *American Sociological Review, 41*, 377–338.

Veenstra, G. (2000). Social capital, SES and health: An individual-level analysis. *Social Science & Medicine, 50*, 619–629.

Vinokur-Kaplan, D. (1995a). Enhancing the effectiveness of interdisciplinary mental health treatment teams. *Administration and Policy in Mental Health, 22*(5), 521–530.

Vinokur-Kaplan, D. (1995b). Treatment teams that work (and those that don't): An application of Hackman's group effectiveness model to interdisciplinary teams in psychiatric hospitals. *Journal of Applied Behavioral Science, 31*, 303–327.

Wagner, J. A. (1994). Participation's effects on performance and satisfaction: A reconsideration of research evidence. *Academy of Management Review, 19*, 312–330.

Walsh, J., & Hewitt, H. (1996). Facilitating an effective process in treatment groups with persons having serious mental illness. *Social Work with Groups, 19*, 5–18.

Webster, C. M., Grusky, O., Young, A., & Podus, D. (1998). Leadership structures in case management teams: An application of social network analysis. *Research in Community and Mental Health, 9*, 11–28.

Weist, M. D., Lowie, J. A., Flaherty, L. T., & Pruitt, D. (2001). Collaboration among the education, mental health, and public health systems to promote youth mental health. *Psychiatric Services, 52*(10), 1348–1351.

Wells, J. L., Seabrook, J. A., Stolee, P., et al. (2003). State of the art in geriatric rehabilitation. Part I: Review of frailty and comprehensive geriatric assessment. *Archives of Physical Medical and Rehabilitation, 84*(6), 890–897.

Whetten, D. A., & Cameron, K. S. (1998). *Developing management skills* (4th ed.). Reading, MA: Addison-Wesley.

Wiecha J., & Pollard T. (2004, September). The interdisciplinary eHealth team: Chronic care for the future. *Journal of Medical Internet Research Electronic Resource, 6*(3): e22, Sept. 2004.

Yang, H., & Tang, J. (2004). Team structure and team performance in IS development: A social network perspective. *Information & Management, 41*, 335–350.

Zarraga, C., & Bonache, J. (2003). Assessing the team environment for knowledge sharing: An empirical analysis. *International Journal of Human Resource Management, 14*(7), 1227–1246.

# Chapter 6

# Communication

Mario Moussa

## CHAPTER OUTLINE

- Who Says What to Whom?
- Barriers to Communication
- Stakeholders
- Tools for Managing Organizational Communication
- Social Networks and Social Media
- Communication Networks
- Organizational Politics
- Communication as a Leadership Art

## LEARNING OBJECTIVES

After completing this chapter, the reader should be able to:

1. Understand the classical sender-receiver communication model and later elaborations of it
2. Identify stakeholders and choose the means for effectively communicating with them
3. Describe the most recent research on social networks and apply it in their work settings
4. Appreciate the importance of organizational politics
5. Recognize the importance of effective communication in leading health care organizations

# KEY TERMS

| | |
|---|---|
| **Barriers to Communication** | **Organizational Politics** |
| **Communication Networks** | **Patient-Centered Communication** |
| **Curse of Knowledge** | **Receiver** |
| **Distortion** | **Sender** |
| **Ethos, Pathos, Logos** | **Social Media** |
| **Feedback** | **Social Networks** |
| **Leadership** | **Speaker-Listener Model** |
| **Message** | **Stakeholder** |
| **Organizational Learning** | **Stakeholder Analysis** |

---

## IN PRACTICE: The Debate over Health Care Reform

At a meeting of the American Medical Association (AMA), in June 2009, President Barack Obama addressed a group of the most influential doctors in the country about health care reform (Text: Obama's Speech on Health Care Reform. June 15, 2009). Many people in the audience were skeptical about his plans. Seeking to win them over, the president emphasized a few key points:

- The health care system needs better record keeping. The government should therefore continue investing in electronic medical records. Better records, he claimed, will lead to "lower administrative costs" and "reduce medical errors."

- Americans need to take more responsibility for their own health. They need to quit smoking, go for a run, and encourage their kids to turn off their video games and spend more time playing outside.

- Everybody needs to eat better and swear off the fatty foods that cause obesity. To show he was following his own advice, the president told the doctors he had planted a vegetable garden on the White House lawn.

- Employers should adopt incentive programs like Safeway's. Safeway has a program called "Healthy Measures" that offers rewards, in the form of reduced premiums, for lowering cholesterol levels and blood pressure.

The payoff of these reasonable proposals, claimed the president, is that consumers can reduce the dollars they spend on medical care, make fewer unnecessary visits to their doctors and the hospital, and be healthier. President Obama made it clear that even the doctors in the audience would benefit, too. Research-based treatment guidelines will make their practices more effective, and the cost burden of the entire health care system will become more sustainable.

Sounds like a win-win. Who could object?

But people did—lots of them. Most notably, Sarah Palin, the Republican vice presidential candidate in the 2008 national election, almost singlehandedly derailed President Obama's arguments for reform by raising the specter of "death panels." Two months after the President's AMA speech, Palin famously declared: "The America I know and love is not one in which my parents or my baby with Down syndrome will have to stand in front of Obama's 'death panel' so his bureaucrats can decide, based on a subjective judgment of their 'level of productivity in society,' whether they are worthy of health care. Such a system is downright evil" (Palin doubles down on death panels, 2009). Somehow, the president's suggestions about invigorating jogs and home-grown vegetables were getting lost in the debate over reform.

Even though leading bipartisan policy analysts made it clear that the notion of death panels was fiction rather than fact, the image of somber dark-suited government officials making life-and-death decisions that affect powerless citizens was too gripping to be forgotten. By the end of August, most news outlets were treating the "death panel" question as one of the central issues in the reform debate.

# CHAPTER PURPOSE

Disregard, for the moment, the political jockeying that went on in the public debate over death panels. The debate serves to highlight an essential characteristic of health care information: for technical as well as political reasons, it is astoundingly complex. The complexity is a problem for any professional in communicating about issues related to clinical delivery, financing, outcomes, safety, professional expertise, and patient choice. Whether you are a politician advocating a policy, an administrator managing a hospital, or a physician treating a patient, it is likely that at least some part of your message—the information or feeling you seek to communicate—will be misunderstood.

The purpose of this chapter is to review the communication concepts and frameworks you can employ as an executive or health care provider to avoid this unfortunate outcome. By applying the key concepts described in this chapter, you will increase the chances that you actually get your point across. You will learn:

1. How to think about the act of communication.

2. The theory and practice of managing stakeholders—the people and groups who have an interest in your ideas.

3. The science of relationships and its practical value in health care settings.

4. The importance of organizational politics and how to lead in complex political environments.

# WHO SAYS WHAT TO WHOM?

One of the dominant figures in communication theory is the ancient Greek philosopher Aristotle (2006). His model of communication, which he called "rhetoric," has influenced the way theorists have thought about the topic for over 2,000 years. Aristotle described communication as a mostly linear process involving a speaker and a listener—the speaker-listener model. Figure 6.1 shows a simplified version of this process. Effective speakers "package" their **message** using one or more of the three persuasive means of conveying a message: **ethos** (character), **pathos** (emotion), and **logos** (logic).

Aristotle's means of persuasion are still relevant today. Consider, for example, the enduring importance of character—or "credibility," in modern terms. People tend to believe facts stated by someone whom they see as trustworthy or

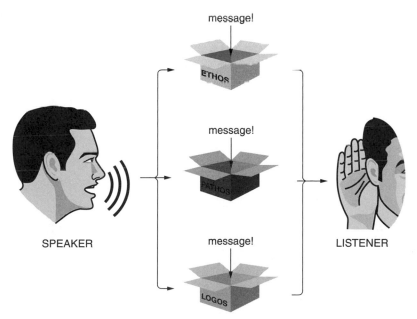

**Figure 6.1** Aristotle's Means of Persuasion.
SOURCE: Delmar, Cengage Learning.

knowledgeable and discount information coming from those whom they mistrust. Indeed, character often trumps logic, as you can see in most political debates. Whether or not you worried about death panels probably had a lot to do with your political leanings: Palin supporters were more likely than others to be suspicious, simply because it was she who had raised a concern about government bureaucrats making life-and-death decisions. Similarly, since people have especially strong reactions to emotion, it is an especially powerful way of making a point—often more powerful than logic alone. Just consider the recent examples of Ronald Reagan or Bill Clinton, who are considered masters of using stories and emotional appeals to win support for complicated policies. But emotion is not always enough. Logic matters most when someone is really paying attention to your ideas. Psychologists have identified a principle called "the power of because," which refers to the fact that arguments backed by logic or reasons tend to be more persuasive than those for which the speaker offers no supporting evidence (Langer, 1989).

The well-known management theorist Nitin Nohria captured the importance of rhetoric and persuasion for modern leaders in a widely cited quote: "Communication is the real work of **leadership**" (Blagg and Young, 2001; Eccles, Nohria, and Berkely, 1994; Nohria and Harrington, 1993). The most effective leaders, Nohria says, know how and when to use each of Aristotle's means of persuasion. Most important, they listen and observe carefully before they communicate, paying attention to social clues that reveal the underlying interests and values of a particular audience: middle managers, front-line staff, external groups, and others. Effective leaders recognize that communication is more than "just words." As the philosopher and linguist C. W. Morris said, language is the "subtlest and most powerful tool" for controlling behavior (Morris, 1949). Modern corporate leaders such as General Electric's former CEO Jack Welch and Apple's CEO Steve Jobs have a deep appreciation for this point, crafting and rehearsing their public statements with the utmost care.

Recent communication theorists have built on Aristotle's **speaker-listener model**, adding an element that Aristotle only implied: **distortion**. The sociologist Harold Laswell, in summarizing his perspective on communication, famously asked: "Who says what in which channel to whom?" (Laswell, 1948). Laswell recognized that many factors affected how listeners understood a message: the **sender** of the message, the content of the message, the medium (face-to-face, written,

or electronic communication), and the listeners themselves. All of these factors influence "impact," which might be completely different from the literal or intended content of a message (Croft, 2004). Later scholars went further and incorporated this possibility of misunderstanding into their theories, leading to the more complex "**feedback**" model illustrated in Figure 6.2 (Longest and Young, 2006).

The feedback model takes account of psychological, cognitive, and contextual factors in communication. From a practical perspective, it shows that you need to pay attention not only to your intended meaning, but also to the entire context in which communication takes place and which ultimately determines how your meaning is construed.

The philosopher of language Ludwig Wittgenstein underscored the centrality of context and the likelihood of misunderstanding in a brief, provocative quote that has stimulated decades of discussion: "If a lion could speak, we could not understand him" (Wittgenstein, 1973). Basically, Wittgenstein's insight is that to communicate effectively, you have to understand the other's situation: their history, social context, values, and psychology. There is no way a human can understand a being so utterly different as a lion. By extension, if another person's values and experience differ dramatically from yours, you will have a hard time communicating with them. The practical implication, for managers and leaders, is that they need to understand the context in which others hear

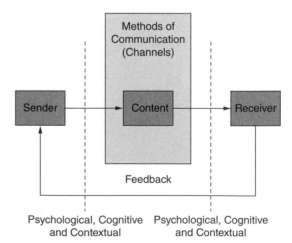

**Figure 6.2** Sender, Receiver, and Feedback Model.
SOURCE: Delmar, Cengage Learning.

| Purpose | Audience | Method |
|---------|----------|--------|
| Manage Public Relations | Employees, Media, Analysts | Press releases, Interviews |
| Build Internal Support for Initiatives | Employees | Town Hall Meetings, Memos, Newsletters |
| Marketing | Physicians, Consumers, Payors | Sales calls, Advertising, Promotions |
| Government Relations | Regulators | Lobbying, one-on-one meetings |

**Figure 6.3** Organizing a Communication Strategy.
SOURCE: Delmar, Cengage Learning.

their words and construct and adjust their communication strategies accordingly.

For organizations large and small, it takes work to construct a communication strategy. The key to an effective strategy is to identify specific audiences within and around your organization, analyze their contexts in terms of values and interests, and choose a means of engaging in two-way interaction with them. Figure 6.3 shows how to organize such a strategy (Argenti, Howell, and Beck, 2005).

This framework makes it clear that a "one-size-fits-all" communication strategy is doomed to fail. In any organization, there are multiple audiences, each of which has its own set of values, interests, and assumptions that require highly customized methods. A standard set of questions helps organize a communication strategy: What is the goal? What is the message? Who is the audience? What is the right "channel"? What are the feedback mechanisms? (Norton and Coffey, 2007).

The consensus among contemporary scholars is that today's leaders need to engage in robust, targeted two-way communication. The era of autocratic, top-down communication is over. Markets and consumer preferences change so fast that organizations must be constantly learning and adapting to internal and external environments. Leading management theorists use the term **organizational learning** to describe the range of communication methods designed to engage people in a collective process of problem solving, planning, and implementation (Senge, 2006).

Each audience is a **stakeholder**—a person or group of people who are affected by your ideas and will have a reaction to them. The full context in which they live and work encompasses their psychological and cognitive biases,

their social networks, and the **organizational politics** that represent their interests. Skillful executives know that they must actively manage stakeholders, tailoring messages to their context and cultivating their support for policies and programs. Otherwise, even the best plans will encounter resistance that slows down or derails execution.

# BARRIERS TO COMMUNICATION

Even when you, the sender, know exactly what you want to say, the distortion within the **receiver** often blocks your message. As George Bernard Shaw quipped, "The single biggest problem in communication is the illusion that it has taken place."

A game created at Stanford University shows why it is that communication so often goes awry. A researcher assigned people two roles: "tappers" and "listeners." Each tapper was asked to tap out a well-known song to a listener. Before this exercise, the tappers were asked to estimate the odds that the listener would recognize the song. The average reply was 50 percent. In actuality, only 1 in 40 listeners recognized the song. The explanation is that the tappers have trouble imagining what the listeners are hearing. The songs seem obvious to the tappers, but to the listeners, they are anything but. The tappers suffer from the **Curse of Knowledge**—the problem of imagining another person's state of mind when you have a piece of knowledge that they lack (Heath and Heath, 2007).

The Curse of Knowledge is evident every day at work, in presentations that hospital CEOs give to staff, in meetings that professionals conduct with colleagues from other disciplines, and in conversations that physicians have with patients.

When a CEO announces that his or her hospital generated $200 million in annual profit, many of his or her listeners, no matter how educated or sophisticated they might be, imagine that the sum is tidily stored in a bank account somewhere. Some will complain that if the hospital "made" so much money, they should get some of it. Only those who have experience working with income statements or have an MBA degree really understand that profit is actually an accounting concept and not a pile of dollars waiting to be spent. Physicians, nurses, and technical specialists are trained in clinical settings, so their frame of reference makes it difficult to understand the practical import of the CEO's message about operational performance. A similar problem occurs in clinical encounters, where misunderstandings are surprisingly common. There is evidence that patients misunderstand up to 80 percent of the information conveyed by their physicians (Britten et al., 2000). Uncertainty, anxiety, and lack of clinical training all get in the way.

Extensive research has revealed that one typically encounters a small number of barriers in communicating a message (Shell and Moussa, 2007). As an organizational leader, to increase the likelihood that important stakeholders will pay attention to you and your idea, you need to assess each situation, decide which barriers are relevant, and employ strategies to turn them into assets. There are five barriers: negative or ambiguous relationships, poor credibility, conflicting belief systems, conflicting interests, and communication mismatches. By systematically planning to turn the barriers into assets, you help yourself imagine what it is like to view a situation from a stakeholder's perspective and how to communicate your message to them. This is the best way to overcome the Curse of Knowledge.

## Relationships

Developing relationships is a fundamental skill in managing and leading health care organizations and in delivering clinical treatments. Relationships give people a level of trust and confidence in each other, facilitating communication and making it easier to cooperate. People respond well to others who take an interest in them, especially when there is no obvious benefit that flows from it.

Even in today's wired world, where you can communicate using e-mail, Twitter, Facebook, and many other **social media**, face time matters in building relationships. In a 1987 experiment, R. F. Bornstein and two other psychologists showed that, in the most literal terms, a face makes all the difference (Bornstein, Leone, and Donna, 1987). They flashed photographs of several people on a screen so quickly that subjects were not even aware of having seen them. Then the subjects had conversations with the people whose photographs had been displayed. Consistently, subjects found those people "likeable" and, even more striking, persuasive. In staged disagreements, subjects sided with them more often than with others they had never seen before.

Similarly, in clinical settings, many patients who value relationships need to feel the connection that comes with a face-to-face encounter. As one patient put it, "I think that if I meet a new doctor and we don't have that face-to-face contact, I would not feel comfortable telling him all my ills" (Armstrong-Cohen, 2009). The following true story about an elderly patient vividly illustrates this preference. One morning, he was touching up the paint on his sailboat. Nearby, another boat owner, who happened to be an emergency medical technician, noticed the man was struggling to breathe and that his lips had turned purple. A trip to the local community hospital led to a barrage of high-tech tests and procedures, a diagnosis of emphysema, later complications with cerebral hematomas, and hospitalizations and re-hospitalizations that brought him into contact with a neurologist, a neurosurgeon, a cardiologist, and a pulmonologist. Throughout this medical ordeal, the team of specialists stayed in touch with each other and the primary care physician via various electronic media. But one person remained out of the loop—the patient. One day, six months into the experience, the primary care physician phoned his wife to check on his patient. The patient recalls thinking, "Why was he calling *her*?" The physician was communicating, but he was emotionally disconnected. He was not paying enough attention to the relationship. Feeling intense frustration, the patient was likely to ignore some or all of the physician's prescriptions, even if he understood them in the first place.

Because of the importance of relationships, you should take the time to get to know what is important to the people you work with. Successful stakeholder management depends upon your ability to establish, maintain, and deepen your connections with people.

## Credibility

As Aristotle first noted, credibility ensures that people take you and your ideas seriously. Most modern experts agree that credibility is based on others' perceptions of three characteristics: competence, expertise, and trustworthiness. Thus, your credibility resides in a subjective experience that others have of your character rather than your objective qualities. Moreover, credibility is highly fragile. You can lose your credibility in a single moment of poor judgment, miscalculation, or misconduct.

You establish competence by reliably making good on your commitments. When you promise that a department chair will receive another assistant professor position, you should be sure you can actually follow through on the pledge. In health care organizations, agreements big and small hinge on reliability. Once you gain a reputation for it, your words carry tremendous weight.

When it comes to expertise, you must choose your sources carefully. You may consider your experience as an administrator to be an important source of authoritative knowledge, but the surgeon you want to influence may consider administration to be simply applied "common sense." In this case, you must find some other way of establishing your credibility. In beginning a conversation, you may need to acknowledge that the *surgeon's* expertise is extremely valuable to the success of the hospital. This shows that at least you know enough to value his or her efforts. As Dale Carnegie pointed in his classic *How to Win Friends and Influence People*, the need to feel important is one of the most powerful desires that everyone has.

Management expert Stephen Covey says that trust is "the one thing that changes everything" (Covey and Merril, 2008). With it, almost any stakeholder can be won over. Without it, you have a hard time getting anything done. In a study of 15 top business leaders of the past 20 years, researchers discovered that the most important skill they had was the ability to convey to others that organization interests always came before personal agendas, including their own (Harrison and Clough, 2006).

## Beliefs

Whenever you can, you should couch your messages in terms that resonate with the core beliefs and values of your stakeholders. These deeply held principles exert a strong influence on their opinions and actions. Psychologists have a variety of explanations for why appeals to core beliefs work: belief bias (the tendency of people to accept any and all conclusions that fit within their systems of belief), the consistency principle (the need for people to behave in ways that are consistent with previously declared values and norms),

and the pull of "power" or "God" terms (the tendency of people to respond to appeals invoking ultimate values such as safety, connection, community, or truth). These explanations all point to the same conclusion: if an idea promises to reinforce one of your stakeholder's core beliefs or the values related to them, the idea gains traction (Gardner, 2006).

Surprisingly, this phenomenon affects researchers as well as dogmatic ideologues. For example, in the historic effort to map the human genome, virtually everyone in the scientific community believed that a painstaking, gene-by-gene mapping process, destined to take decades, was the only way to assure a complete, accurate map. When geneticist James Weber and computational biologist Eugene Myers made a landmark presentation at a 1996 conference in Bermuda outlining a "shotgun sequencing" method for speeding up the process, leading scientists refused to take it seriously. "Flawed and unworkable," said the experts. But one man—a little known researcher and former surfer named Craig Venter—was not so sure. He called Myers, and together they made history, turning the human genome mapping effort into a high-profile race that they won a short four years later in 2000.

The inventor of the theory of evolution, Charles Darwin, once remarked that it was so difficult for him to overcome his own beliefs when he was gathering data that he made a conscious effort to seek out contrary examples. The temptation to skip over evidence that contradicted his beliefs was so strong that Darwin made a habit of immediately writing all such evidence down. Otherwise, he reported, he was sure to forget it.

If even committed scientists have trouble overcoming the biases caused by their own beliefs, imagine the problems such beliefs cause in ordinary organizational life. Under such circumstances, it will not matter how much formal authority you may have as an executive or department administrator. Ideas that violate basic beliefs will simply be rejected. Because belief bias is so powerful, you should frame your ideas using key phrases that honor your stakeholders' core values. In the health care setting, such phrases include "quality care," "patient satisfaction," "scientific rigor," and "outcomes." Hot-button phrases likely to stimulate resistance are "bottom line performance," "market-based competition," and "efficiency."

When you advocate an idea that seems contrary to some core belief, you should break your proposal into small bites that reduce the amount of dramatic change required from your stakeholders. Psychologists have discovered that people sometimes have what they call "anchor positions" on various beliefs and opinions, and their willingness to be flexible on these positions can depend on how much they are asked to change. The less you ask of your stakeholders, the more willing they are to move in your direction.

Another example from the research world illustrates this point. In the early 1980s, it was hard for anyone in the IBM research department to get a hearing for ideas that took personal computers seriously. Senior leaders believed that there were no competitive markets left to conquer. IBM was so dominant that the only measure of real success left to them was promotion within the company. Low-level internal task forces had forecast that the industry was about to change, but the people at the top, blinded by their beliefs, refused to take these warnings seriously. Nevertheless, an IBM senior manager named Bill Lowe succeeded in obtaining development funds for an experimental PC project that set the stage for IBM's entry into that market. He did it by keeping the project so small nobody could be bothered to oppose it. When it became clear that Lowe's little program would take no resources away from the focus on the company's corporate customers, the IBM Management Committee let it pass as one of the dozen or so things it approved in a given week. The PC initiative, in short, flew in under the radar screen of IBM's core beliefs.

## Interests

At the very center of stakeholder management, like the bull's eye in the middle of a target, are their self-interests, problems, and needs. If you can show your stakeholders that your idea furthers their interests, you will usually have a much easier time gaining their support.

Academic studies in psychology confirm two important findings about the role of self-interest in communication. First, people pay much closer attention to messages they see as having important personal consequences for them than ones that do not. Even a glance at nonfiction bestseller lists in publishing, which is perennially littered with titles such as *You on a Diet*, *Why We Want You to Be Rich*, and *Younger You*, confirms this basic truth. Second, self-interest biases the way people think about proposals. Naturally enough, people tend to favor ideas that benefit them and oppose those that will force them to shoulder significant costs. But research has also shown that audiences see arguments as *more persuasive* when they stand to gain from an idea and less persuasive

when they stand to lose. In short, people's interests serve as windows through which they see your ideas. When you can find and address their interests, they open their window to let your ideas in; if they see your idea as running against their needs, the windows close.

To think about your stakeholders' interests in a systematic way, you should ask three important questions:

1. Why might it be in the other party's interests to support my idea?

2. What do other parties want that I can give them to gain their support?

3. Why might they say no?

Your answers to these questions will help you frame your idea so that it appeals to others' underlying interests and gets their attention.

For example, a medical center faced a serious crisis when a change in government regulations forced the hospital CEO to take away a major insurance benefit enjoyed by a low-paid but important group of workers: hospital residents (doctors in training). As the CEO prepared his formal announcement to make this change, rumors spread that the residents were organizing a job action to demand compensation to make up for the loss. The hospital, meanwhile, was in no position to give this group a raise without also raising the pay of many other workers, something it could not afford to do.

Finding himself between a rock and hard place, the CEO asked the residents' leaders to join a committee to explore their overall situation at the hospital. His charge to the administrator leading this committee was simple: find out as much as possible about what the residents' real interests were. His hope was that something would turn up that he could take action on. After a week of meetings, his administrator reported back that the residents would be willing to accept their reduced insurance benefit if the hospital would agree to one very important demand: they wanted to wear the same, somewhat longer white coats that full-fledged physicians wore so patients would treat them with the same respect. The CEO ordered the new coats without delay.

## Communication Styles

Jim Collins wrote in his best-seller *Good to Great* that one of the best practices of the best organizations is a willingness to gather data, analyze it, and "confront the brutal facts"

(Collins, 2001). It sounds easy, but this advice is much easier to give than to follow. You must constantly remind yourself that your audience's point of view is much more important than your own. And you need to return to the questions about your own credibility: How do stakeholders see you, and do you have credibility?

When it comes to communicating the substance of your message, the most important thing you can do is define it simply. Charles Kettering, the great engineer and inventor, stated: "A problem well stated is a problem half solved." And according to noted communications expert David Zarefsky, "definition is the key to persuasion." By providing a crisp answer to the question, "What is the problem?" you establish the context in which your ideas will be evaluated. Cognitive psychologists call this the act of *framing*, and it powerfully affects people's perceptions, the standards they will call to mind, the evidence they will consider relevant, the emotions they will feel and the decisions they will ultimately make. As the American journalist and commentator Walter Lippman once said, "For the most part, we do not first see, and then define. We define first and then see." How you state the problem defines what your audience will see in their mind's eye.

At the World Economic Forum in Davos, Switzerland, in 2005, social activist Bono used framing to influence the AIDS debate. Bono sat on a stage with British prime minister Tony Blair, Former U.S. president Bill Clinton, Presidents Olusegun Obasanjo of Nigeria and Thabo Mbeki of South Africa, and Microsoft CEO Bill Gates. Bono listened as the others detailed all of the difficulties Africa faced in overcoming AIDS, poverty, and political corruption. Then the moderator asked Bono what he would like to see changed. Instead of continuing with the panel discussion, Bono decided to reframe the issue. What he wanted changed, he said, was "The tone of the debate." He continued:

> Here we are, reasonable men talking about a reasonable situation. I walk down the street and people say: "I love what you're doing. Love your cause, Bon." [But] I don't think 6,000 Africans a day dying from AIDS is a cause; it's an emergency. And 3,000 children dying every day of malaria isn't a cause; it's an emergency.

Bono's message got through. The audience of corporate executives, government ministers, and cultural luminaries burst into loud applause. Poverty and AIDS in Africa were not business-as-usual issues for public officials. They were global "emergencies." Emergencies require action, not analysis. They affect everyone, not just specialists.

To return to the earlier example of health care reform in the United States: the biggest mistake that the Obama administration may have made in managing communications on this issue is over-complication. As one critic put it, "the White House has taken an issue more intimate and immediate than perhaps any other in a voter's life and transformed it into an abstract, technical argument about long-term actuarial projections. It's a peculiar kind of reverse political alchemy, transforming gold into lead" (Pinkerton, 2010). Palin knew what she was doing when she adopted a different communication strategy. When asked about her "death panels" remark, she said: "[It's] a lot like when President Reagan used to refer to the Soviet Union as the 'evil empire.' He got his point across. He got people thinking and researching what he was talking about. It was quite effective. Same thing with the death panels." A follow-up comment reveals that she made a conscious choice in emphasizing the phrase: "The term I used to describe the panel making these decisions should not be taken literally" (Davis, 2009).

After simplicity, the second most important quality of your message is vividness. Consider, for example, the strategy used in communicating the importance of hand washing at Cedars-Sinai Medical Center in Los Angeles (Dubner and Leavitt, 2006). Bacterial infections are a serious problem in hospitals, with thousands of people dying each year from germs carried from one patient to another on the hands of doctors and nurses. But getting hospital staff—especially physicians—to wash their hands after each examination is surprisingly difficult, even though everyone knows it is the right thing to do. Hospital hygiene poses, in short, a classic problem of organizational communication: getting people to adopt a new "best practice" when old habits are deeply ingrained.

At Cedars-Sinai, there were several causes for lax hand washing: physicians said they were too busy, the sinks were not always conveniently located, and, even more perversely, the doctors actually believed they *were* washing their hands. Each physician was convinced that "someone else" was the source of the bacteria problem. This presented administrators with a delicate issue of organizational politics: how could they sell doctors on the idea of washing their hands without insulting or alienating them? Administrators tried data-based, inspirational appeals using e-mails, faxes, and posters, but hospital staff assigned to spy on the doctors reported no change in behavioral habits. The hospital then switched to the self-interest persuasion channel and offered doctors $10 gift certificates at the local coffee shop when they were seen washing up by hand-washing "spies." This program had a moderately positive effect, but compliance still fell far short of what the hospital needed to protect its patients.

Finally, the hospital decided to try a vivid, visual way to deliver the hand-washing message. At a formal luncheon for the senior medical staff, the administrator in charge of the hand-washing initiative surprised everyone by bringing out a set of lab trays and asking the doctors to press their hands into these trays to record the bacterial cultures residing on their hands at that moment. The hospital used these hand prints to create full-color, graphic images of the bacterial colonies residing there. They made sure these pictures were as disgusting as possible.

Their final step was to transform these images into screen savers and load them on every computer in the hospital. Thus, no matter where physicians were, these images stalked them. Compliance with the hand-washing rule immediately shot up to nearly 100 percent and stayed there. The pictures of the actual bacteria on the doctors' own hands, as Dubner and Levitt put it, "was worth 1,000 statistical tables."

---

## IN PRACTICE: Patient-Centered Communication

In a study sponsored by the National Cancer Institute, Ronald M. Epstein and Richard L. Street emphasize that communicating clinical health care information is much more than a matter of imparting objective information. Their model, illustrated in Figure 6.4, captures the distinctive factors that make communicating in this setting so challenging.

Notice that exchanging information is just one among six functions that clinicians need to manage in communicating with patients. Two of the others—responding to emotions and managing uncertainty—involve feelings both negative and positive: anxiety, fear, hope, and happiness. Another two aim at empowering patients to manage their own care and make appropriate decisions. The last one is about promoting health-inducing relationships between the clinician and patient and among family members and friends.

This model goes far beyond the linear sender-listener model that Aristotle created. Epstein and Street's framework encompasses the full complexity of information, feelings, relationships, and high-stakes decisions that form the context of health care communication (Epstein and Street, 2007).

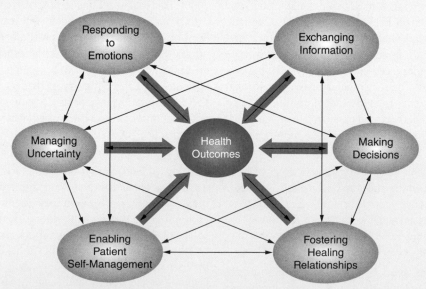

**Figure 6.4** Factors Affecting Communication in Clinical Care.
SOURCE: Delmar, Cengage Learning.

This story is an extreme example of a more general truth about human perception: people respond to ideas that are easy to visualize because they can be recalled from memory more readily. Psychologists call this the "availability" phenomenon. The more "available" an idea is, the more people believe it to be true. The beauty of the Cedars-Sinai screen savers was that the bacteria displayed actually had been found on the physicians' hands.

# STAKEHOLDERS

The "stakeholder" is one of the most important concepts in health care. Effective leaders know their stakeholders, paying close attention to the barriers that distort communication.

The concept of a stakeholder goes back to management research done in the 1960s about the environment in which corporate executives do strategic planning. Building on the

idea of a "stockholder," stakeholder theorists recognized that owners—the stockholders—were just one group among many that influenced a corporation's decisions and actions. There were others who had legitimate or at least de facto "claims" on the corporation: customers, employees, citizens, legislators, and activists, to name a few. Each of these groups has an interest in a corporation's investments, projects, environmental policies, and other commitments because they all have consequences that extend far beyond the narrow circle of profit-and-loss statements (Freeman and McVea, 2001).

Health care organizations are located in especially complex stakeholder environments. Take, for example, a large academic hospital. It can easily have more than two dozen stakeholders, as illustrated by Figure 6.5. Each stakeholder group has interests that predispose it to support or contest the hospital's initiatives.

To understand stakeholder management in action, consider the quality initiatives that hospitals across the country have

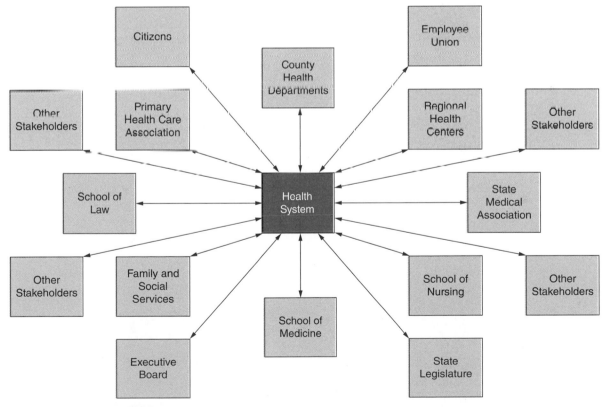

**Figure 6.5** Stakeholder Map for a Large Academic Hospital.
SOURCE: Delmar, Cengage Learning.

recently undertaken. A centerpiece of many endeavors is unit-based clinical teams, composed of a physician, a nurse manager, and a quality specialist. These teams have produced stunning results, decreasing average length of stay, improving the effectiveness of care in a broad range of clinical areas, and reducing patient wait times for scheduled appointments. In the abstract, no one would claim that these are undesirable outcomes. Yet there may be reasons that certain groups might be lukewarm supporters, if not outright opponents, of quality efforts in specific situations. Physicians might feel, for example, that working in a team-based environment rather than the more traditional hierarchical structure in which they were trained compromises their professional status. Or unit staff might resist the introduction of new quality guidelines because they entail learning whole new ways of doing their jobs, with little or no

benefit to be gained in compensation or job satisfaction. Other groups may have other reasons for opposing the initiative that, on the face of it, seem unassailable. As a hospital administrator championing the quality initiative, you would need to assess just who has a stake in it, whether they support or oppose it, and whether they have enough power to make a difference.

This is the essence of **stakeholder analysis**, which is the first step in stakeholder management. A useful tool to guide the analysis is a Power/Interest matrix, such as the one in Figure 6.6 (Block, 1991). By systematically mapping the stakeholders, you can begin to articulate communication strategies for each group.

This matrix reveals that you need to pay a lot of attention to those three people who are powerful and have a strong interest in

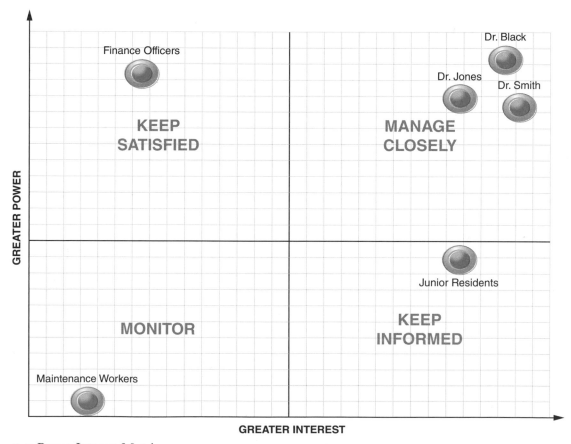

**Figure 6.6** Power-Interest Matrix.
SOURCE: Delmar, Cengage Learning.

the initiative. Assume that two of them (Dr. Jones and Dr. Smith) are top-producing physicians—if they become unhappy, you had better respond quickly with some well-crafted message points. If there is one particular physician among them who wields influence with physicians across the hospital (Dr. Black), you should make a special effort to sit down with him or her and understand how you can address his or her concerns. You can adopt more of a maintenance strategy for those powerful stakeholders who have little interest in the quality initiative. The finance officers in departments that are not directly involved in the initiative fall into this category. Because of their position, they are generally powerful players, but they have no immediate reason to get involved. For the time being, you want to keep it that way, so you should make sure nothing happens to disrupt their peace of mind. As for those stakeholders who have an interest but wield little power, such as junior residents, you can communicate with them on a "need to know" basis. Finally, you can safely expend the minimum effort on communicating with stakeholders who have neither interest nor power in this situation. As valuable as they might be to the hospital's operations, maintenance workers, who fall into this category, should not be at the top of your mind in leading this particular initiative. But you would need to pay a lot of attention to them in a different setting—for example, in a process-improvement project aimed at optimizing the facilities management function.

This kind of analysis, if you are not used to doing it, might seem overly calculating. But your ultimate goal is a practical one—managerial effectiveness. By understanding exactly with whom you need to communicate and how, you can maximize the impact of your ideas. There are two important reasons why broad involvement of many different stakeholders is crucial to your success as a communicator. First, stakeholders can offer their knowledge, expertise, attitudes, and suggestions about your ideas. By organizing this collective intelligence, you sharpen your own thinking. Second, stakeholders will be more committed and knowledgeable through being involved. And the more committed stakeholders are, the more willing they will be to support your ideas.

# TOOLS FOR MANAGING ORGANIZATIONAL COMMUNICATION

After identifying stakeholders, assessing their interests, and developing strategies for overcoming potential communication barriers, the next step is to select methods for consulting with them. Table 6.1 describes various tools for engaging stakeholders in an organizational communication process. You should choose methods on the basis of your goals. "Nominal Group Technique," for instance, helps draw out ideas from a small group of stakeholders, while questionnaires are more successful at representing the opinions held by a larger population. The issue of broad representation generally becomes more important as an organizational initiative moves into the implementation phase.

The methods can be divided between those most appropriate for small- and large-group communication—with the methods listed farther down in the table generally being more appropriate for larger, less personal settings. The methods or mix of methods that work best vary according to the situation. But your managerial focus should always be on tailoring communication as much as possible to fit the profile of a particular person, group, or organizational culture.

# SOCIAL NETWORKS AND SOCIAL MEDIA

The most recent research on communication has highlighted the importance of **social networks**—the connections among a group of people and the broader environment in which they live and work. In settings of all kinds, people get things done and spread information through these informal channels (Burt, 2007; Christatkis and Fowler, 2009; Powell, 1998). The extent of your network constitutes your "social capital" and is one of your most important assets as a communicator. An invaluable addition to stakeholder analysis, a social network map is like an X-ray that reveals the inner workings of your organization and its environment.

In a recent study of treatment guidelines for hypertension, a group of researchers compared two primary-care practices (Scott et al., 2005). Figure 6.7 shows the pattern of relationships for each one. The one on the left has much greater "density"—a measure of the number of connections per person. Other measures reveal that the physicians in this practice spend more time working together collaboratively and engaging in two-way communication. As the researchers predicted, this practice was much more successful at implementing treatment guidelines among its physicians.

Two concepts explain the differences between the practices in adhering to the treatment guidelines: connection and contagion. "Connection" refers to the pattern of relationships that a group of people have. Some networks have mainly

## TABLE 6.1

| Consulting Modes | Time Required | Objectives | Description | Representative | Strengths | Weaknesses |
|---|---|---|---|---|---|---|
| Open-ended interviews | 30 minutes–1 hour | To obtain responses to relatively complex issues and alternatives | Interviewer poses questions to respondent | No | Complicated questions may be entertained; may suggest other questions to be explored in more structured formats | Dependent on the interviewing skills of the interviewer, time consuming, expensive |
| Structured interviews | 15 minutes–1 hour | To obtain responses to relatively complex issues and alternatives | Interviewer poses questions to respondent | Yes, with appropriate sampling | Complicated questions may be entertained. Valuable for generating questions for more standardized formats | Dependent on the interviewing skills of the interviewer, time-consuming, expensive |
| Nominal Group Technique | 1/2 hour–2 hours | To increase and balance participation among meeting participants | Individual generation of ideas in writing, followed by group discussion and ranking of ideas | No | Easy to learn, easy to use, produces broad participation | No interaction among ideas and issues |
| Interview design | 1–2 hours | To stimulate interaction among large groups (16–200) and reveal similarities and differences among their ideas | Several rounds of one-on-one interviewing by group members, followed by summaries of interviews | No | Active involvement of group members, rapid generation of ideas | Not appropriate for exploring a particular idea or proposal in depth |
| Focus group | 2–3 hours | To generate hypotheses about the way members and customers think | Open discussions among 6–12 people, facilitated by a trained moderator | No | Flexibility, open to unexpected responses, good for exploring unfamiliar terrain | Dependent on facilitator's ability, peer pressure can silence some participants, interpretation can be difficult |
| One-minute essays | 1–3 minutes | To provide a brief opportunity for reflection on a discussion | Brief writing exercise or key takeaways from a discussion | No | Quick, easy to do, offers a chance to digest information | Not appropriate for sorting out complex proposals |

**TABLE 6.1** (*Continued*)

| Consulting Modes | Time Required | Objectives | Description | Representative | Strengths | Weaknesses |
|---|---|---|---|---|---|---|
| Short questionnaire | 15–30 minutes | To solicit information about specific topics | Prepared questions with limited range of responses | Yes, with appropriate sampling | Respondents have opportunity to reflect on responses, no chance of interviewer influencing | Low response rate, no opportunity for interviewer to clarify questions, small amount of information gathered, takes time to develop effective questions |
| Long questionnaire | 1/2 hour– 1 hour | To solicit information about specific topics | Prepared questions with limited range of responses | Yes, with appropriate sampling | More information gathered with brief questionnaires | Same disadvantages as brief questionnaires, except length further reduces response rate |
| Mini Delphi | 15–30 minutes (for each round) | To produce a consensus ratio-scaled evaluation of alternatives | Respondents prioritize alternatives, then repeat exercise after seeing the average rankings from previous rounds | No | Gives geographically dispersed respondents the chance to interact with each other; anonymity prevents bias | Assumes the desirability of the average response |
| Workshop designs | 1/2 day– 1 1/2 days | To provide a structured setting where participants collectively explore issues in depth | Events where small and large groups engage in facilitated discussions and exercises | No | Participants have time to focus on a set of topics, collaborative efforts can produce richer ideas and proposals | Time-consuming, requires careful design work, difficult to meet participants' heightened expectations |
| Exploring strategic options | 1/2 –1 day | To develop a strategic agenda | Derives key alternatives from open-ended interviews, then sets data on current state, desired future state and relative importance | No | Helps build common strategic agenda, identifies quickly areas of disagreement | Time consuming, depends on skill in extracting key choices from interviews |

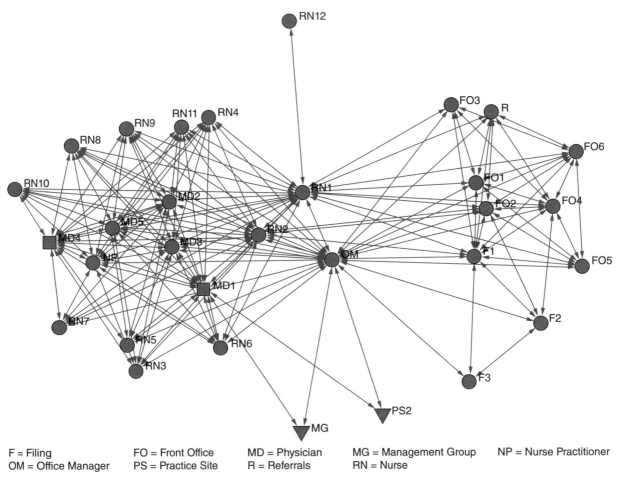

F = Filing            FO = Front Office      MD = Physician        MG = Management Group      NP = Nurse Practitioner
OM = Office Manager   PS = Practice Site     R = Referrals         RN = Nurse

**Figure 6.7** Density of Connections per Physician.
SOURCE: Delmar, Cengage Learning.

a hub-and-spoke configuration, where one person resides at the center of several relationships. There may be several hubs and a few connections between the hubs. Another configuration is mainly hierarchical, where a few people sit "atop" others and send information "down" through a network. And then there are networks like the first primary-care practice, characterized by lots of interconnections between people. These patterns influence whether and how information spreads through a network.

"Contagion" explains how the information spreads. Biologically, people have evolved to mimic others' behavior. In mimicking behavior, they also pick up corresponding emotions. As the authors of *Connected* note, there is a lot of truth in the saying, "When you smile, the world smiles with you." In one of the strangest epidemics ever recorded, in 1962, an outbreak of uncontrollable

laughter spread in Tanzania from one person to another until it "infected" over 1,000 people. Four schools were forced to close, and villages were paralyzed. Just like this "illness of laughing," new treatment guidelines spread among professionals who work closely with each other. You are much more likely to "catch" them than someone who spends most of their time working in isolation.

The practical value of a social network map is that it shows how you should manage the flow of information in your organization and its environment. If you know that it has a hub-and-spoke structure, then you should target the "hubs." You can bring them together for a meeting, using one or more of the consultation methods described earlier. Once the "hubs" have bought into your proposal, you can rely on them to spread it through the surrounding "spokes." Or, if you work in a more hierarchical environment, you should focus on

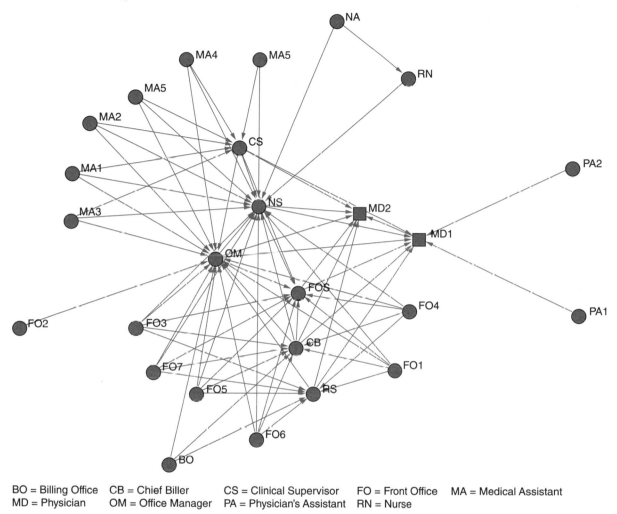

**Figure 6.7** Density of Connections per Physician. (*continued*)

SOURCE: Delmar, Cengage Learning.

BO = Billing Office    CB = Chief Biller    CS = Clinical Supervisor    FO = Front Office    MA = Medical Assistant
MD = Physician    OM = Office Manager    PA = Physician's Assistant    RN = Nurse

reaching out to those at the "top." They will facilitate the flow of information "down" through the rest of the organization.

A recent study of health care outreach organizations is a good example of using a social network map in this way (Michigan Department of Community Health, 2009). Researchers assessed the effectiveness of several Diabetes Outreach Networks (DONs), organizations dedicated to promoting diabetes prevention, detection, and treatment. Their findings reveal that, as illustrated in Figure 6.8, the most successful DONs had a central, "hub" position in their social networks.

From a policy perspective, one of the most important implications is that the DONs play an invaluable role in spreading clinical information and should continue to be funded. The data also suggest a particular set of management practices will maximize the DONs' impact as "hubs": establishing regional advisory councils, offering professional development courses, and disseminating information resources online.

The point about online information-sharing raises an important issue related to social networks: social networking. Web 2.0 technology offers a dizzying array of options for using social media for building social networks: e-mail, blogs, tweets, IMs, wikis, and other electronic communication tools that continue to appear with amazing speed. As a manager and health care provider, which channels should you choose? Research

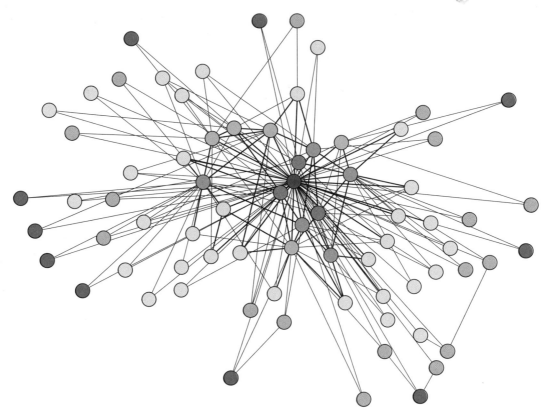

**Figure 6.8** A Social Network Map.
SOURCE: Delmar, Cengage Learning.

into communication has shown that people have different preferences for how they like to give and receive information, online and off-line. One size does not fit all. What counts as "connection," therefore, differs from person to person, depending on their psychological and technological preferences.

You need to be sensitive to these differences in building relationships and disseminating information. Every situation is different, so you need to exercise judgment in choosing the appropriate communication strategy. But in every case, it pays to ask a key question: What is the right balance of psychological and informational needs? When the need for psychological contact is high, you should lean toward "high-touch" encounters. If informational needs are strongest, you should rely more on social media tools.

Consider, for example, patient communication. Since patients do better when they are knowledgeable and actively involved in their care, health care providers must give them

the information they need to make the best decisions. Today, this often requires striking the right balance between virtual and face-to-face communication for each patient. The researchers Ben Gerber and Arnold Eiser found that, as decision makers, patients fall into two broad categories: the "knowledge acquirer" and the "informed decision-maker" (Gerber and Eiser, 2001). The knowledge acquirer is the more passive one—more comfortable with the physician as the ultimate authority. But this patient may still want to learn about his or her condition. In this case, you can "prescribe" a Web site that provides background on healthy diets or home care. These patients are more likely to comply with behavioral advice if a health provider has "primed" them before they review online material that supplements other information sources. The informed decision maker wants to participate more fully in making decisions. You can make face-to-face meetings with these patients more productive by directing them to sites where they can use credible information to educate themselves.

Patients who are comfortable working online can handle routine informational issues using social media tools. At Patientsite.org, at Boston's Beth Israel Deaconess Medical Center, patients read and send e-mail, make appointments, see personal test results, and refill prescriptions. They also access information about wellness services, medication management programs, and decision-making tools. In this setting, social media are useful in "broadcasting" information to a whole population of patients.

In managing organizational communication, you should design a system that includes both face-to-face and virtual channels. Stakeholder preferences should guide your choices about which ones to use and with whom. The benefit for you as a manager will be a social network—an "invisible" but powerful organization existing "inside" the formal hierarchy—that amplifies the impact of your programs and initiatives.

# COMMUNICATION NETWORKS

Another way to view your communication strategy is through the concept of "**communication networks**" (Longest and Young, 2006). You can create these networks to achieve various objectives. Figure 6.9 illustrates five basic patterns that scholars have identified. Each pattern is appropriate to different managerial situations.

The following examples illustrate the practical uses to which you can put the concept of a communication network:

- *Chain*: Simple hierarchical communication is most like a chain. Messages flow downwards and upwards from one level to another. Basic factual information, like work schedules or requests for vacation days, can be communicated in this way.

- *Y*: In a Y pattern, people report up to a superior, who in turn has a dual reporting relationship to two separate superiors. As a chief operating officer, for instance, you might recommend that a senior nurse in a large clinical department report directly to the department chair and to the chief nursing officer, each of whom has a "stake" in his or her performance at the departmental level. This ensures that both departmental and enterprise-wide "interests" are represented in the reporting relationship.

- *Wheel*: A wheel is suitable when you have to communicate with several people who have no need to communicate directly with each other. When you keep important stakeholders from different parts of an organization "in the loop"—department chairs, administrators, and staff—you are following this pattern.

- *Circle*: Peers, such as division chiefs, often communicate in a "circle" between regularly meetings and events. Anyone can communicate with anyone else, but no one is formally managing or controlling the communication. As a senior administrator, you might encourage this kind of self-managing information flow as a conscious strategy.

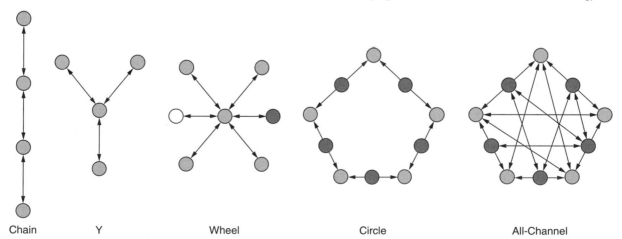

| Chain | Y | Wheel | Circle | All-Channel |

**Figure 6.9** Social Network Typology.
SOURCE: Delmar, Cengage Learning.

- *All-Channel:* Real-time team meetings are venues where "all-channel" communication takes place. Information flows freely as team members speak directly to each other.

Like social networks, communication networks are conceptual tools for managing the flow of information across large and complex organizations. They help organize your thinking about communication strategies.

# ORGANIZATIONAL POLITICS

Even if you are a master of stakeholder management, know how to manage the flow of information through social and communication networks, and are comfortable with social media tools, you cannot avoid organizational politics. There is plenty of evidence showing that politics is a reality in most workplaces. Studies have found that some political activity takes place in nearly all organizations. And in nearly half, it takes place to a "very great" or "fair" extent. If you consider yourself "above" politics, you condemn yourself to being dominated by those who are willing to get into the trenches and fight. As the ancient philosopher Plato said: "Those who are too smart to engage in politics are condemned to being governed by those who are dumber." As a leader, therefore, you must be prepared to get involved in this often rough-and-tumble activity.

A good example of the skillful combination of communication finesse and political savvy is Richard Shannon, a physician who led an effort at Allegheny General Hospital to reduce the incidence of lethal infections in the ICU (Institute for Healthcare Improvement, 2005). He started small, realizing that there would be too much resistance among many stakeholder groups to making large-scale procedural changes all at once. With seed money for a small pilot project, Shannon implemented a zero-defect problem-solving process inspired by Toyota's lean production techniques. The results were stunning: catheter-related bloodstream infections (CRBLIs) and ventilator-associated pneumonias (VAPs) were reduced by 87 percent and 83 percent, respectively. Then Shannon focused on getting traction with two key stakeholder groups: the nurses and residents. "We estimate that our efforts probably saved 47 lives," he said. "Once the staff saw we could have that kind of impact, they were immediately on board."

Next, Shannon turned his attention to getting support from senior management. He adjusted his communication strategy accordingly. He noted that this group of stakeholders had a distinctive perspective: "Their job is to look at costs, but they don't get to see the consequences of poor quality care case by case. They see aggregated data, which blunts the financial impact." Shannon thus highlighted the financial impact of a case involving a single patient who suffered from multiple complications caused by a catheter infection. "The hospital had to absorb more than $41,000 on that one case," Shannon noted. In addition, he discovered, "30 to 70 percent of the total went for treating the infection or the complications it caused." In total, the hospital could save millions by controlling infections—specifically, $2.2 million. This figure got the attention of senior management as well as the hospital's largest insurer, who ponied up a $2.1 million bonus to keep the work going.

Paul Levy, who was featured in Chapter 2, was similarly skilled in responding to the bare-knuckles politicking at Beth Israel Deaconess Medical Center. Soon after he took over as CEO, he laid out his communication ground rules (Grey, 2006). Anybody could criticize his plans, as long as they did so openly and offered constructive alternatives. Following a meeting with department chiefs, Levy received a rude challenge to this principle. One of the chiefs had sat silently through a discussion of operational problems. Afterwards, he sent a harshly critical e-mail to Levy lambasting his plans and copied all of the other chiefs and the chairman of the hospital's board. Rather than address the chief's criticisms in private, as earlier administrators might have done, Levy openly confronted the chief in a bluntly worded e-mail. Levy made it clear he was not going to be bullied. The other chiefs, who were tired of endless sniping and wanted action, became even stronger allies of Levy. But Levy knew when to respond with softer gestures, too. When one group of nurses rebelled over work rules, leading to scores of resignations, Levy established a group of task forces to look into the issue. Once the nurses had an opportunity to work collaboratively on solving their own problems, turnover dropped from 15 percent to 4 percent.

The stories of Richard Shannon and Paul Levy show that effective communication requires that you think carefully about the political interests of key stakeholder groups. For Shannon, the key group was the senior administrators, who had the power to expand the small-scale initiative into an enterprise-wide initiative. Shannon tailored his communication to speak directly to their financial perspective. Levy made an attention-getting point about his leadership in standing up publicly to a disrespectful department chief. But Levy also knew when to back off and let an important stakeholder group—the nurses—find its own solution to a dispute over work rules. Organizational communication is like basketball—skill, timing, judgment, and even luck are all part of the game.

# COMMUNICATION AS A LEADERSHIP ART

Most health care organizations are complex, high-pressure work settings that include multiple disciplines and professional belief systems. To communicate successfully in this environment, you must learn to adapt to the "local culture" and speak many different "languages."

The need to adapt to stakeholders raises an important leadership issue: authenticity. Will you lose credibility and self-respect if you become a shape-shifter, changing yourself for each new audience? As actress Judy Garland once said, "Always be a first-rate version of yourself instead of a second-rate version of somebody else."

The English philosopher and politician Francis Bacon, who rose to become one of the most powerful men in England in the late 1500s under Queen Elizabeth I, tried to manage virtually every impression he made with people at the royal court. He filled his journals with observations and advice to himself on how he should appear to others in pivotal encounters and drew lessons from each success and failure to take to his next meeting. For example, he once wrote that he needed to "suppress at once my speaking with panting and labor of breath and voice" in conversing with one of the queen's closest advisors. Bacon's goal was to create a separate and distinct "public self" as an instrument of persuasion.

Behavioral experts Rob Goffe and Gareth Jones have wrestled with the apparent paradox that impression management presents (Goffe and Jones, 2005). Your personal credibility, which has its roots in perceived consistency and trustworthiness, provides the foundation for influence. Yet effective communicators are, as these authors say, "like chameleons, capable of adapting to the demands of the situations they face."

Is it really possible to be a "credible chameleon"? Yes, in the following sense: You play many roles in your life—spouse, parent, professional, employee, boss, sports fan, customer, community leader, student, and teacher. In each of these roles, you naturally display different aspects of yourself. Your child's third-grade teacher sees a different side of you than does your boss, and your brother or sister probably sees a different person than does your child. Nevertheless, it is always just "you."

Thus, the authenticity paradox diminishes somewhat when you see that you cannot help being a somewhat "different person" depending on who you are communicating with. And your awareness of these various roles gives you a range of "authentic selves" to draw from in each encounter. The art of communicating as a leader involves knowing which "self" to be: sympathetic listener, master of ceremonies, social networker, or harsh taskmaster.

## DEBATE TIME: Is Strategic Communication Really Just Manipulation?

There are many examples in this chapter of leaders who adapted their messages and communication styles to fit a particular situation. Take the case of Dr. Richard Shannon. While he used the language of finance when he was communicating the benefits of lean production techniques to senior administrators at Allegheny General Hospital, he emphasized clinical outcomes when he sought the buy-in of medical staff. In another show of adaptability, Paul Levy at Beth Israel Deaconess Medical Center used strong-arm tactics in dealing with a disruptive surgeon, but he used a much gentler approach with nurses who were upset over work rules. When does "adaptability" become "inauthenticity"?

The very concept of a "stakeholder analysis" might raise a similar question. In using a "Power-Interest Matrix" to categorize stakeholders, you are assigning different levels of importance to people and groups. In executing a communication strategy based on such an analysis, you will pay more attention to some groups than to others. Is this fair?

Finally, management experts Rob Goffe and Gareth Jones propose that leaders should work to become "credible chameleons," adapting themselves to each situation so that they increase the likelihood of being understood. This advice may make some people uneasy. Shakespeare said, "To thine own self be true." Shouldn't you follow this principle rather than trying to be all things to all people?

From the perspective of an organizational leader, weigh the pros and cons of "being yourself" versus being a politically savvy "credible chameleon." In what kinds of situations might it be advisable to show flexibility, and when, if ever, should you simply speak your mind without carefully crafting a communication strategy?

# SUMMARY AND MANAGERIAL GUIDELINES

1. In any managerial situation, pay attention not only to the substance of your intended message but also to the ways your message can be distorted.

2. Map the stakeholders of an organization, creating communication strategies appropriate to each stakeholder group.

3. In designing a communication strategy for an entire organization, use different channels for each purpose and audience: town hall meetings, one-on-one briefings, written memos, e-mails, etc.

4. Use multiple communication styles in disseminating organizational policies and strategy: data-oriented, emotional, and visionary.

5. Maximize "organizational learning" by engaging in robust, two-way communication with staff and external stakeholders.

6. Always work to enhance your credibility as a leader, building your reputation for trustworthiness, competence, and expertise.

7. Analyze and actively manage social networks to influence the flow of information within and around your organization.

8. Be willing, when necessary, to engage in "organizational politics" even if you have implemented a highly structured communication strategy.

9. Work hard to be a "credible chameleon" by getting in touch with your multiple "authentic selves" that enable you to make contact with many different kinds of people.

# DISCUSSION QUESTIONS

1. Describe Aristotle's model of communication.

2. How did recent communication theorists build on Aristotle's model?

3. What are the Five Barriers to communication, and how do you remove them?

4. Identify three different methods for consulting with stakeholders in a complex communication process. Explain the objective as well as the strengths and weaknesses of each method.

5. How is the National Cancer Institute's "Patient Centered Communication Model" different from the simple sender-receiver model?

6. How does the concept of "contagion" help explain how information spreads in social networks?

7. Why do leaders need to take account of organizational politics?

# CASE: The Case of Jesica Santillon

It is extraordinarily difficult to manage communications in health care settings. Few cases offer a better illustration of that difficulty than Jesica Santillon's. She was a 17-year old girl who died in 2003 after undergoing a heart and lung transplant in which, at one of the nation's top medical centers, she received organs with the wrong blood type.

Her tragic story shows how social, technical, and organizational complexity combines to create daunting communication barriers for health providers and administrators. Consider the complicating factors in this situation, and the related leadership questions they raise:

• The Family. Jesica's parents smuggled her into the country from Mexico, hoping to find a cure for a heart and lung disorder that doctors in her home country could not treat. The family settled in North Carolina, settling down in a trailer. They soon came to the attention of a local builder, who started a charity that eventually raised enough money for her to receive a transplant at Duke Medical Center. The procedure went terribly wrong, leading to severe and irreversible brain damage. When the doctors informed Jesica's mother they planned to stop treatment, she announced at a press conference, through a translator, "They are taking her off of the medicine little by little in order to kill her. They want to rid themselves of this problem."

## Questions

1. **Leadership question:** What social and cultural barriers may have made it difficult for the doctors to communicate with Jesica's family? What might have the doctors done to increase the chances that Jesica's family understood the true nature of the problems in this terrible circumstance?

   - *The Procedure.* A heart and lung transplant is obviously a challenging procedure. Though Dr. James Jaggers, the chief of pediatric surgery at Duke University, was a highly skilled and well-regarded physician, he was just one among many professionals involved in a multistep process that began with the location of suitable organs somewhere in North America and continued through transferring the patient to the intensive care unit (ICU). The many handoffs required in this process meant there was a risk of important information being lost or garbled at key transition points, as in the "whisper down the lane" game. This is in fact what happened. Jesica's Santillon's blood type was O, while the organs' was A. Carolina Donor Services located the organs and, they claimed, informed Dr. Jaggers of the organs' blood type. Dr. Jaggers does not remember the conversation about it. Another physician was sent to pick up the organs in Boston. He was informed three times of the blood type, but since he did not know Jesica's blood type, he was not aware there was a mismatch.

2. **Leadership question:** How would you organize the complex set of steps required in this transplant process to ensure that misunderstandings do not occur in handoffs between professionals?

   - *The Stakeholders.* Following the string of errors leading to the mistaken transplant, the Duke Medical Center had to manage a whole set of stakeholders: the Santillon family, the family's lawyers, the community, the press, and the health provider community. Each stakeholder group had its own interests, influenced by their cultural, social, and professional backgrounds.

3. **Leadership question:** If you were the Duke Medical Center CEO, what general communication strategy would you put in place to manage the stakeholders in this case? In particular, how would your messages to each group differ from the others?

Adapted from a CBS News story. Original text retrieved from http://www.saynotocaps.org/trailoftears/jesica_santillan.htm

# REFERENCES

Argenti, P., Howell, R. A., & Beck, H. A. (2005). The strategic communication imperative. *MIT Sloan Management Review, 46*(3), 83–89.

Aristotle. (2006). *On rhetoric: A theory of civic discourse.* New York: Oxford University Press.

Armstrong-Coben, A. (2009, March 5). The computer will see you now. *The New York Times.*

Blagg, D., & Young, S. (2001). What makes a good leader? *Harvard Business School Working Knowledge.*

Block, P. (1991). *The empowered manager.* San Francisco: Jossey-Bass.

Bornstein, R., Leone, D., & Donna, J. (1987). The generalizability of subliminal mere exposure effects. *Journal of Personality and Social Psychology, 53*(6): 1070–1079.

Britten, N., Stevenson, F., Barry, C., Barber, N., & Bradley, C. (2000). Misunderstandings in prescribing decisions in general practice: qualitative study. Retrieved August 12, 2010, from http://www.ncbi.nlm.nih.gov/pmc/articles/PMC27293/?tool=pubmed

Burt, R. (2007). *Brokerage and closure: an introduction to social capital.* Oxford University Press.

Collins, J. (2001). *Good to great: why some companies make the leap … and others don't.* Harper Business.

Covey, S. & Merril, R. (2008). *The speed of trust: The one thing that changes everything. Free Press.*

Croft, R. (2004). Communication theory. Retrieved August 12, 2010, from http://www2.eou.edu/~rcroft/MM350/CommModels.pdf

Christakis, N., & Fowler, J. (2009). *Connected: the surprising power of our social networks and how they shape our lives.* New York: Little Brown.

Davis, S. (2009). Palin's "death panels" charge named "Lie of the Year." Retrieved August 12, 2010, from http://blogs.wsj.com/washwire/2009/12/22/palins-death-panels-charge-named-lie-of-the-year/tab/article/

Dubner, S. and Levitt, S. (2006, September 24). "Selling soap." *The New York Times.* Retrieved August 12, 2010, from http://www.nytimes.com/2006/09/24/magazine/24wwln_freak.html

Eccles, R. G., Nohria, N., and Berkely, J. D. (1994). *Beyond the hype: Rediscovering the Essence of Management.* Boston: Harvard Business School Press.

Epstein, R., & Street, R. (2007). *Patient-centered communication in cancer care: Promoting healing and reducing suffering.* National Cancer Institute, NIH Publication No. 07-6225. Bethesda, MD.

Freeman, R. E., & McVea, J. (2001). A stakeholder approach to strategic management. Working Paper 01-02, Daren Graduate School of Business Administration.

Gardner, H. (2006). *Changing minds: The art and science of changing our own and other people's minds (leadership for the common good).* Boston: Harvard Business School Press.

Gerber, B. S., & Eiser, R. A. (2001). The patient-physician relationship in the internet age: future prospects and the research agenda. *Journal of Medical Internet Research, 3*(2), e15.

Goffe, R., & Jones, G. (2005). Managing authenticity. *Harvard Business Review, 83*(12), 86–94.

Grey, P. B. (2006). Rx for merger trauma. CFO.com. Retrieved August 12, 2010, from http://www.cfo.com/printable/article.cfm/5598469?f=optionss

Harrison, J. K., & Clough, M. W. (2006). Characteristics of "state of the art" leader: productive narcissism versus emotional intelligence and level 5 capabilities. *The Social Science Journal, 43*, 287–292.

Heath, C., & Heath, D. (2007). *Made to stick.* Random House, 2007.

Institute for Healthcare Improvement. (2005). Doing better, spending less. Retrieved on August 12, 2010 from http://www.ihi.org/IHI/Topics/CriticalCare/IntensiveCare/ImprovementStories/DoingBetterSpendingLess.htm

Langer, E. (1989). *Mindfulness.* Reading, MA: Da Capo.

Laswell, H. (1948). The structure and function of communication in society. In L. Bryson (Ed.), *The communication of ideas.* New York: Harper.

Longest, B. B., Jr., & Young, G. (2006). Coordination and communication. In *Health Care Management: Organization Design and Behavior* (5th ed.). Delmar Cengage Learning.

Michigan Department of Community Health. (2009). *An interorganizational social network analysis of the Michigan Diabetes Outreach Networks.* Written by L. Corteville & M. Sun. Retrieved August 12, 2010, from http://www.diabetesinmichigan.org/PDF/SNA%2009.pdf

Morris, C. W. (1949). Signs, language and behavior. New York: Prentice Hall.

Nohria, N. and Harrington, B. (1993). Six principles of successful persuasion. Boston: Harvard Business School Note: 9-494-037.

Norton, D. P., & Coffey, J. (2007). Building an organized process for strategy communication. *Harvard Business Review.* Vol 9(3): 1–5.

Palin doubles down on "death panels." (2009). Yahoo! News. Retrieved on August 12, 2010 from http://news.yahoo.com/s/politico/20090813/pl_politico/26078

Pinkerton, J. (2010). Why Obama-care is doomed: The Hollywood version. Retrieved on August 12, 2010 from http://www.foxnews.com/opinion/2010/01/26/james-p-pinkerton-extraordinary-measures-obamacare-review/

Powell, W. W. (1998). Learning from collaboration: knowledge and networks in the biotechnology and pharmaceutical industries. *California Management Review, 40*(3), 228–240.

Senge, P. (2006). *The fifth discipline: the art and practice of the learning organization.* USA: Broadway Business.

Shell, G. R., & Moussa, M. (2007). *The art of woo: Using strategic persuasion to sell your ideas.* Penguin. (8). Portions of this chapter were adapted from the book, with the publisher's permission.

Scott, J., Tallia, A., Crosson, J. C., Orzano, A. J., Stroebel, C., Dicco-Bloom, B., O'Malley, D., Shaw, E., Crabtree, B. (2005). Social network analysis as an analytic tool for interaction patterns in primary care practices. *Annals of Family Medicine, 3*(5), 443–448.

Text: Obama's speech on health care reform. (2009). *The New York Times.* Retrieved on August 12, 2010 from http://www.nytimes.com/2009/06/15/health/policy/15obama.text.html?pagewanted=1&_r=1&sq=obama%20on%20health%20care&st=cse&scp=21

Wittgenstein, L. (1973). *Philosophical investigations.* New York: Prentice Hall.

# Chapter 7

# Power, Politics, and Conflict Management

## Timothy Hoff and Kevin W. Rockmann

## CHAPTER OUTLINE

- **The Uses of Power in Organizations**
- **Key Power Relationships in Health Care Organizations**
- **The Political Nature of Power**
- **The Abuse of Power in Health Care Organizations**
- **Power as a Key Source of Conflict**
- **Types of Conflict**
- **Common Mistakes in Thinking about Conflict**
- **Key Conflict Management Strategies**
- **Conclusion**

## LEARNING OBJECTIVES

**After completing this chapter, the reader should be able to:**

1. Recognize what power is and how it is used within health care organizations
2. Describe and compare the major sources of power within health care organizations
3. Recognize the differences between managerial and professional sources of power within health care organizations
4. Summarize the interrelationship between power and politics within organizational settings
5. Describe the demographic and contextual factors that affect how power is distributed within health care organizations
6. Classify the various conditions that give rise to power abuses in health care organizations
7. Compare the different roles played by trust, fairness, and transparency in preventing power abuse in health care organizations
8. Distinguish between the different types of conflict and how they might be present in various health care organizations

9.  Understand how emotions affect individuals attempting to manage conflict

10. Describe the various mistakes relating to how individuals think about negotiation and how they think about relationships

11. Identify the difference between interests and positions and describe why understanding that difference is critical in negotiation

12. Compare the benefits of compromise, competition, and collaboration as three distinct strategies for negotiation

13. Describe the tactics to find a better solution, the tactics to acquire information, and the tactics to influence others

# KEY TERMS

| | |
|---|---|
| **Anchoring Bias** | **Network Centrality** |
| **BATNA** | **Nonspecific Compensation** |
| **Coalitions** | **Organizational Politics** |
| **Coercion** | **Power** |
| **Cognitively active** | **Power Abuse** |
| **Collaborating** | **Power Stratification** |
| **Competing** | **Reciprocity** |
| **Compromising** | **Relationship Conflict** |
| **Confirming Evidence Bias** | **Self-Fulfilling Prophecy** |
| **Culturally Derived Power** | **Structurally Derived Power** |
| **Emotional Contagion** | **Study of Conflict Management** |
| **Fractioning** | **Task Conflict** |
| **Functional Fixedness** | **Threat Rigidity Effect** |
| **Inert Knowledge Problem** | **Value in Negotiation** |
| **Knowledge-Based Sources of Power** | **Winner's Curse** |
| **Logrolling** | |

---

**IN PRACTICE: Pay-for-Performance and Power: Influencing and Negotiating the Murky Measurement Waters of Value-Based Purchasing**

The concept of "value-based purchasing" (VBP) has gained traction as a potential means to better link health care outcomes to payment. Numerous national demonstration projects are underway, and the concept's flagship philosophy, "pay-for-performance" (P4P), has been integrated into the majority of physician practices and many hospitals across the United States. VBP rests on a fundamental principle—that practitioners and institutions that produce the best outcomes, from both an efficiency perspective and a quality-of-care perspective, should be rewarded financially, while those who underperform should be subject to earning less. This approach is innovative because traditionally everyone in health care gets paid the same, regardless of their performance excellence, for the services they provide.

**IN PRACTICE:** **Pay-for-Performance and Power: Influencing and Negotiating the Murky Measurement Waters of Value-Based Purchasing** *(Continued)*

However, the VBP approach unleashes the potential for many power dynamics within the health care setting, and for conflict among different stakeholders. For example, the issues of how to measure cost-effectiveness and quality become front and center to making VBP work. Because there can be substantial disagreement as to the "right" ways to measure these outcomes, the use of power can become an integral component of making decisions in this regard. When one stakeholder uses their power to try to influence the kinds of measures used, conflict may erupt. This conflict can undermine the success of pay-for-performance programs by promoting an adversarial relationship among the parties involved. Insurance companies, employers, and government—all of whom pay for health care services—may seek to exhibit greater influence over the measurement debate because of the dependence by providers such as physicians and hospitals on that payment for their economic survival. This may cause consternation and resistance among providers such as physicians and hospitals, especially if they have differing opinions on the measurement issue.

On the other hand, physicians may use their own advantages of control over clinical knowledge and the public's trust in them to counteract the influence of payers in deciding which measurements will form the basis for paying on the basis of quality and value. Hospitals, because they possess the infrastructure that everyone in the system relies upon to deliver complex care, can exert their own influence to shape measures in a way favorable to their interests and constituencies. Moreover, patients may have little ability to influence the measurement debate, simply because they do not have a source of power upon which to draw in getting the other stakeholders to comply with their preferences. In fact, these overall power dynamics have been seen in the current value-based purchasing movement, where many major decisions around how to measure become drawn-out exercises in power use and influence tactics.

The conflict that arises around identifying the best way to measure outcomes in a pay-for-performance incentive program is often managed through a political process in which different stakeholders attempt to use their power in shaping how the debate is conducted. For example, health care payers may push for the establishment of public reporting of clinical outcomes through devices like "report cards," in part as a means to get consumers on their side and to put physicians and hospitals on the defensive. The use of tactics like report cards may be promoted overtly as a rational means to achieve performance transparency. However, these tactics may also be used covertly to exert and enhance the payers' control over how "value" and "quality" should be defined and measured in the eyes of the general public. Alternatively, health care providers may put forth a message of "we know best because we deliver the care" to patients and advocacy groups to try to convince them that they should be allowed to exert greater influence over which measures are used.

This is where conflict management and, more specifically, the process of negotiation can play a role in moving the use of power and politics to a productive end. By treating the discussion around measurement within a VBP approach as one in which multiple stakeholders can simultaneously "win," there is a higher probability that the outcome will have something favorable in it for everyone (including patients) and, as a result, will be more easily accepted by all the relevant parties in the negotiation. In this way, negotiations around how to measure "cost effectiveness" or "quality" that consider multiple viewpoints, provide voice to a diverse group of stakeholders for input, and seek to achieve a level of acceptance and satisfaction among all constituencies are likely to create a more favorable climate for implementing pay-for-performance programs, and to enhance the chances for their long-term success. The use of power and politics goes hand in hand with the use of negotiation, simply because power and politics create the potential for conflict among stakeholders, and this conflict is best managed through a more rational approach that seeks to find the most optimum outcome that can be accepted by all.

# CHAPTER PURPOSE

As the first In Practice example illustrates, perhaps nothing is as potent a force in organizational life as **power**. Power is the ability to exert influence or control over others. It dictates a significant degree of what goes on in organizations, from decision making to performance outcomes. Power involves two key dynamics—influence and dependence—and when these dynamics are present in large quantities, power may be wielded by individuals, groups, and organizations in ways that allow them to achieve their preferred vision and goals.

The purpose of this chapter is to provide students with a clearer understanding of what power is, how and where to look for it, and how it plays out in health care organizations. In addition, emphasis is placed on how power relates to the political aspects of organizational action in settings such as hospitals and physician practices, and the conditions and circumstances that give rise to power abuse are featured as important factors for managers to keep in mind at all times. A key focus in the second half of the chapter is on the role of conflict management in managing the role of both power and politics. A practical guide is offered for how to use the process of negotiation to achieve mutually satisfactory outcomes among organizational stakeholders.

Power and politics can be implemented in dysfunctional, self-interested ways by a variety of organizational stakeholders. This chapter touches upon this issue. But it also stresses the important and necessary functions played by power and politics in getting organizations and workers to perform effectively. In either case, the use of power and politics heightens the level of conflict that may occur in organizations, and such conflict is best managed, this chapter argues, through a more strategic perspective that focuses on an ethical, rational, and results-oriented process of conflict management and negotiation.

# THE USES OF POWER IN ORGANIZATIONS

Power can be used for different purposes within organizational settings. Perhaps the most ubiquitous use of power in organizations involves determining the key choices made at an organizational level to guide overall company strategy (Finkelstein, 1992). The types of choices in this regard most amenable to the use of power include those that involve higher levels of uncertainty and innovativeness (Mintzberg, Raisinghani, and Theoret, 1976). The use of power by chief executive officers, boards of directors, and other top leadership to guide the direction in which the organization moves, how it chooses to compete, which products or services to offer, and the type of business model employed for pursuing profit has existed as long as the concept of the corporation. Leaders can and do use power effectively to make strategic decisions in efficient ways.

Power may also be used to influence the actions of others, be they workers, professionals, other organizations, or the customers that use the organization's products. In this way, power is thought of as a highly coercive mechanism alongside other influence-wielding tactics such as trust, cooptation, and conformity (Hart and Saunders, 1997). Power in this regard is simply another in a toolbox of tactics individuals in organizations employ to get other people to behave in desired ways. While it is worth noting that the use of power in this regard may be no more effective than other "softer" tactics such as gaining people's trust to believe that what is being asked of them is the correct thing to do (McEvily, Perrone, and Zaheer, 2003), nonetheless, it is often viewed as a quick, reliable form of control that can be employed across a diverse array of organizational situations (Pfeffer, 1981).

**IN PRACTICE:** **The Quality Improvement Department, Accreditation, and Power**

Organizations in the health care industry gain a great deal of their legitimacy from accreditation. Many different types of accrediting processes exist, from the Joint Commission for hospitals and other health providers, to the National Committee for Quality Assurance (NCQA) for insurance plans, and to more specialized accreditation for niche providers like laboratories and radiology facilities.

---

**IN PRACTICE:** **The Quality Improvement Department, Accreditation, and Power** *(Continued)*

Nothing shifts the power structure more in a health care organization, at least temporarily, than the process of gearing up for one of these many accreditations. Much of the time, the power shift moves favorably in the direction of quality improvement (QI) staff and units within the organization. These staff and units are often the nerve centers of data collection, analysis, and reporting for the kinds of things accrediting organizations request and verify when they visit. Thus, accreditation offers them an opportunity to gain greater control over scarce resources, influence strategic decision making, shape organizational culture, and change the manner in which the organization's workforce does their jobs.

For example, there may be a particular area or work output of the organization where quality measures lag and a problem regarding quality is thought to exist. While a QI department may be involved over time in addressing the issue, if the issue impacts accreditation, greater resources may be made available to QI staff, and greater freedom provided to them by top management, to try to correct the issue in a timely manner. The resources given to QI may be taken away from some other part of the organization, lessening the influence of other stakeholders in the process.

The QI function may be emboldened by the organization to reshape how work is performed in the particular area, how workers do and think about their jobs, what performance data should be collected, and how that data must be evaluated. In this way, QI staff come to be relied upon by top management and the organization as a whole to help ensure that not only are quality problems identified and fixed, but that the all-important external accreditation is not jeopardized in any substantive way. This may also represent an opportunity for the QI function to solidify its influence within the organization, acquire greater resources for itself, and gain greater control over others competing for the same resources. Thus, even a short-term shift in power and influence within an organization can have long-term consequences.

---

Power can control, allocate, and redistribute resources of all types within organizations (Pfeffer and Salancik, 1978). These resources include human capital such as clinical staff, financial resources such as budget allocations to hospital departments, and knowledge resources like innovations that enable a production process to be done better. For example, power can be used to decide which part of a health care system should have a fully integrated electronic medical record to use first in its everyday work. By being the first to use such a system, favorable benefits may accrue to that part of the system earlier and in greater quantity than later adopters. Resource control and allocation is perhaps the most widely used application of power within organizations. As the sociologist Charles Perrow asserts, this use of power deals with "the size of the pie" within organizations and how it is sliced—i.e., who wins and who loses in getting more of something that they want, while at the same time preventing others from doing the same thing (Perrow, 1989).

Power may also be wielded for purposes of shaping or transforming organizational or work cultures in ways top management desires, or to move the organization toward being more competitive and effective in the marketplace. For example, leaders of both General Electric and IBM used their positions and authority, along with that of their top managers, to help transform these companies during the 1980s and 1990s into global, innovative firms (Gerstner, 2002; Slater, 1999). They did this in large part through a focus on shifting the meaning systems among employees within each of the organizations toward beliefs and values that could support a new way of doing business, one that would enable the companies to meet the challenges of a changing marketplace. However, using power to change organizational culture carries risks, because culture is difficult to change (Martin, 1992).

## What Is Power, and Where Does It Come From?

Power has been defined in a variety of different ways. However, common to all definitions is the notion of one stakeholder's ability to exert influence over others in ways that, among other things, influence them to do things they normally would not do (Pfeffer, 1981). In short, power is defined by the control one group has over another's behavior (Hickson et al., 1971). Central to this definition of power is the idea of influence—i.e., that an individual, group, subunit, or organization has both the ability and opportunity to control how another acts either directly or indirectly (Dahl, 1957). In this way, power by definition involves **coercion**. Coercion is the use of subtle influence dynamics to achieve desired goals, which means that all power brings with it the potential for heightened tension and conflict within the organizational setting. This is one of the reasons why the use of power is often filtered through a political process within organizations that is described later in the chapter. It is also a key reason why negotiation and conflict management, a primary focus of this chapter, are at the center of a more pragmatic view of how to think about, use, and regulate power within organizations.

If influence is at the core of defining power, then this implies that all power is also relational in the sense that its existence, magnitude, and use rely upon an ongoing social exchange between two parties (Dahl, 1957). Thus, power requires two or more parties interacting with each other on an ongoing basis to be fully realized. While it may be understood that one group or unit has power over another, for example, in a hospital or insurance company, by this definition, power would exist in its fullest form only when the powerful group or unit interacts with others in a way specifically designed to control or alter their behavior. In this way, a group of self-employed surgeons working collectively in the same practice may be presumed to have the ability to influence Hospital A's behavior towards them, such as better reimbursement rates or preferred operating room (OR) times, because there is an equivalent Hospital B in the same geographic area where these surgeons can take their business. But as a relational dynamic, power would be evident most during moments when the surgical group, through direct communication or posturing during contract negotiations with Hospital A, actually convinces Hospital A to give them higher reimbursement or better OR times, and Hospital A complies in this regard (see the "In Practice" case study "Pay-for-Performance and Power").

Power comes from several different sources. Three major sources of power within an organization are structural, cultural, and knowledge-based. **Structural sources of power** are sources that derive from the formal or bureaucratic aspects of an organization (Wilson, 1982). Examples of these aspects include the organizational chart, written policies and procedures, job titles and descriptions, and budgets. The potential for power is built into every organization through the existence of a formal structure that orders social relations and provides a guide for behaving to organizational actors. In examining how structure gives rise to power, one need only examine how one or more of these bureaucratic components instill in specific people and groups the ability to exert influence over others.

For example, a simple job title and job description provides insight into the power and influence associated with that position. A job title that includes the word "manager" or "supervisor" means that the person filling the position will have formal authority over one or more persons in the organization. This authority may be implied in the job title (e.g., medical director, chief executive officer, vice president in charge of compliance) and articulated in more detail in the description itself (e.g., "hires, supervises, and evaluates all physicians working in the medical group"). From the title and job description, an individual gains the legitimacy to direct others' actions, evaluate their performance, and serve as the conduit for information between higher levels of the organization and the workers under their direct supervision.

**Structurally derived power** gains its stability and legitimacy by creating resource dependencies that place some individuals or groups in positions to influence others (Pfeffer and Salancik, 1978). This is seen clearly in the situation in which one department or unit in an organization is relied upon to help produce the work of other departments. In health care, such situations abound. For example, all hospital work from emergency medicine to surgery relies heavily for its effective completion upon departments like radiology and laboratory services. The need to test and monitor patient blood levels, screen for infection and disease, and examine bones and organs in detail for proper assessment give both the radiology and laboratory departments the ability to influence how other work in the hospital is performed, and how other actors request and get services from these departments. Without the timely, high-quality assistance of these latter units, both surgical and emergency services can take longer to do, be of lower quality, and cost more. This creates a dependency situation in which radiology and laboratory services, because they are vital to all other work in the hospital, gain additional ability to determine their own work patterns and resource needs. In this instance, the "resource" depended upon is the knowledge and technology associated with radiology and lab work. In other situations, the resources may be financial.

Power also is derived culturally within organizations. Culture is defined as the shared meaning systems that arise out of ongoing interaction between two or more entities (Schein, 1992). Whereas structure represents the formal aspects of organization, culture is associated with the informal aspects, i.e., norms, values, beliefs, and assumptions. **Culturally derived power** is power that derives from these informal aspects, and is less visible but no less potent than structurally derived power. In some situations, power deriving from existing norms or beliefs may become more influential than structural power, in part because it seeks to influence organizational behavior in ways that are more hidden from public view.

Cultural sources of power cannot easily be identified through formal artifacts such as organizational charts or budgets. Instead, they are discerned from an implicit understanding and appreciation for "how things work" in the organization. An example of culturally derived power might be seen in a group of surgeons, where one surgeon in particular who is widely understood to be "the best cutter" or "have the best hands" is deferred to by other surgical colleagues across a variety of work situations, in large part due to the collective belief that such a surgeon must know and be good at a variety of things if they are perceived as the best in the core skill all surgeons value. In this instance, this surgeon gains power and influence due to a shared meaning system within the group that may or may not mirror reality. Similarly, physicians who believe a particular nurse working with them has great sway with other nurses may defer more to that nurse across different work situations, giving the nurse more power to influence not only those physicians, but also her fellow nursing colleagues.

There are also **knowledge-based sources of power** within organizations. Knowledge-based power derives from a group's control over the expertise needed to make key decisions and organize production. This power source is especially potent in industries such as health care, in which much of the work contains higher degrees of uncertainty in terms of both processes and outcomes. Some health care work can be standardized and routinized, but much of it cannot, providing ample opportunity for those with a knowledge advantage to assert control. Knowledge power in the health care industry currently plays out in two major ways. Traditionally, the medical profession has been the primary source of knowledge power. Physicians have been able to define how clinical work should be performed, how patients should be treated, and what success and failure mean in different types of delivery situations (Freidson, 1970). Physicians still remain the most powerful group of health care workers in large part because they retain heavy control over the most important forms of clinical and scientific knowledge available, and others defer to them in setting the terms under which that knowledge is applied on an everyday basis.

More recently, however, knowledge-based power through bureaucratic outlets has proliferated. This is an example of the commodification of knowledge power by standardizing and making it transparent throughout the organization. In one sense, the modern-day quality movement represents an attempt to garner knowledge-based power for the organization and its administrators, either taking it away from or sharing it with physicians. For example, a clinical care guideline that is developed to treat a diabetic or hypertensive patient, where specifics of the diagnostic process, preferred means of treatment, and identification of risk factors are all included in it, can transfer knowledge previously within the exclusive domain of the physician to the organization, reducing the physician's power in the process.

---

**IN PRACTICE:  The Pursuit of Power among Managers and Physicians**

Managers and physicians working in the same health care organization might draw upon different sources for establishing and maintaining their power. Managers work in positions typically associated with the formal organization—i.e., the bureaucratic chain of command that exists to help coordinate work in standard and routine ways. If one examines an organizational chart for a department or the entire organization, it may be clear that persons occupying management or supervisory positions possess specific degrees of influence over different organizational functions, budgets, or staff. Physicians, especially those not occupying formal administrative positions, derive their power mainly from knowledge-based and cultural sources. These sources are not specific to any single organization, as might be the case for management power,

---

**IN PRACTICE:** **The Pursuit of Power among Managers and Physicians** *(Continued)*

which relies upon formal policies or organizational charts. Rather, physician power derives similarly across all organizations from the wider societal belief that doctors "should be in charge," possess the most valuable knowledge for effective health care delivery, and are more likely to represent the views of the customer, i.e., patients and their families.

Within the hospital setting, for example, a "dual hierarchy" exists that recognizes the power of both managers and physicians to direct staff, control work, and make decisions for the organization. One part of the hierarchy recognizes the role played by management personnel in these areas, while the other bestows that same recognition on physicians. It is this dual hierarchy and its everyday implementation that gives rise to ongoing tension between the two groups within settings such as a hospital. With each having power and influence, and each seen as legitimate by key stakeholders within the organization, the imperative becomes one of advancing the positive contributions of each group to organizational functioning while minimizing the conflict and confusion potentially arising from both groups asserting their power in the same situations.

And assert power they do. Managers may use formal devices to both assert and pursue power, such as: the creation of new organizational policies; reorganization; the collection, analysis, and reporting of data around clinical work; and establishment of new domains of authority such as quality assurance or accreditation. They may not be viewed as "knowing what physicians know," but they can seek to offset some of this knowledge advantage by gaining access to the knowledge, standardizing it, and making it transparent throughout the organization. Physicians may counter in their pursuit and assertion of power by making more overt their knowledge advantage in specific work situations, moving to make portions of their work more complex, or look more complex, so it is less subject to management cooptation, and getting others like patients and nurses to believe that they are the most legitimate group to direct care and make decisions. In each case, different sources are drawn upon to promote the group's power and influence. This reality makes health care settings particularly fluid in terms of how such a dual hierarchy works, how power is distributed between the two groups, and which group accomplishes its preferred goals for the organization and themselves at a given period in time.

---

Finally, it is important to note that none of these three power sources often acts alone to generate power in an organization. Sources of power can and do interact with each other, as in the case above where knowledge-based power is embedded formally in the organizational structure through guidelines, policies, and "best practices." The concept of **network centrality** is another illustration of interaction occurring between knowledge-based and structural sources of power. Network centrality refers to a situation within an organization in which one work group or unit lays at the intersection of many other work groups or units, as a result becoming a repository of knowledge and understanding about how the entire organization works (Ibarra and Andrews, 1993). This makes them indispensible sources of information for other parts of the organization, and provides them with a greater ability to influence the actions of others.

The quality improvement (QI) department of a hospital, insurance plan, or medical group is the clearest example of

this in health care. By collecting and analyzing information on each work process in the organization—e.g., what works in one area of the hospital or practice and could be transferred for use to another part—this type of department gains legitimacy and power. Departments and personnel that require knowledge or understanding held by other parts of the organization will come to depend on such a "network-central" entity like the QI department to help improve their own production processes.

# KEY POWER RELATIONSHIPS IN HEALTH CARE ORGANIZATIONS

Health care is a service industry. This means that the key production inputs are the individuals who provide the services—physicians, nurses, and a variety of clinical and nonclinical support staff. Since all power is relational, understanding power within a service industry like health care requires examination of the major stakeholders and their interactions with each other. There are three key power relationships in health care organizations: physician-patient, physician-nurse, and physician-administrator.

The most important relationship in health care involves that of physician and patient. All health care service delivery is built around this relationship, because patients are the ultimate consumers of all health care services. Traditionally, physicians have held great authority over patients. The main reason for this has been the significant asymmetries in knowledge, information, and access. For instance, physicians possess the clinical knowledge and skills patients seek when accessing care. Traditionally, such knowledge and skills were not available for access in any manner other than seeing the physician (Starr, 1982). Society has also granted to physicians exclusive or near-exclusive rights to prescribe medications, order medical services such as MRIs and physical therapy, bill insurance for services rendered to patients, and serve as the final arbiter for which types of services are appropriate and reimbursable. These rights bestow on doctors control over medical decision making. This gives them a significant power advantage over the patients they serve.

For a long time, physician power over patients manifested itself in a paternalistic approach that emphasized the caring doctor to whom the patient must listen and comply. This approach limited conflict and tension in the relationship, as patients were expected to obey the physician's orders and question less. However, this type of relationship and the one-sided nature of the power and influence implied in it have been increasingly criticized as unnecessary and a source of lower health care quality and patient satisfaction (Wachter and Shojana, 2004).

Although the physician continues to maintain a clear and significant knowledge advantage over patients, some believe that information and knowledge asymmetries between doctor and patient are lessening with the advent of new information technologies, such as the Internet, which give patients the ability to access and absorb quick, easy-to-understand medical information (Pew Internet and American Life Project, 2002). Another reason for a potential redress in the balance of power between doctor and patient may stem from increasing distrust of health care institutions, reflected in lower confidence in our health care system, a growing health care consumer movement, and sustained emphasis on consumer-driven issues such as patient safety (Armstrong et al., 2006).

The physician-nurse relationship is also fraught with the use of power and influence. Physicians depend greatly on nursing staff to perform their work effectively. However, this dependence does not translate into equal power for nurses vis-à-vis physicians since the medical profession retains control over key cultural and knowledge-based power sources. This control allows them to maintain legal privileges and exert direct influence over nursing work, pay, and employment status. For example, registered nurses (RN) and licensed practical nurses (LPN) are neither allowed to prescribe their own medications for patients nor diagnose and treat patients. Training for these occupational groups is limited largely to preparing them for work roles where they assist physicians in their clinical work. The pay and prestige of nursing as a field also lags behind physicians' salaries and prestige.

---

## IN PRACTICE:  Patient Empowerment in the Internet Age

Some argue that the advent of the Internet and advanced forms of health information technology such as the electronic medical record (EMR) afford patients an opportunity to rebalance the power inequities in their relationship with physicians. There is no doubt patients have become more consumer-oriented in their health care interactions. For example, a recent survey showed that three-quarters of individuals access the Internet and try to find relevant health-related information first before visiting a doctor for an ailment or complaint (Pew Internet and American Life Project, 2002). Anecdotes abound about the manner in which patients may now come to a physician's office armed with reams of printouts describing some disease the patient feels they have, and the ensuing confusion that can result from the physician trying to explain to the patient why such information is not relevant to the patient's clinical situation. In a key sense, though, these anecdotes miss the main point: that the ability of patients to investigate and consume medical information prior to their interactions with the health care system inevitably creates a more proactive, inquisitive, engaged, and thus powerful health care consumer; a consumer that has to be more respected and addressed in a different, less paternalistic manner.

---

**IN PRACTICE:  Patient Empowerment in the Internet Age  *(Continued)***

---

There are a variety of report cards, rating systems, and performance measures now available online for specific physicians, hospitals, insurance companies, and others doing the business of health care. If one requires cardiac surgery in New York State, for example, there is an easily accessed comparison of morbidity and mortality for all the cardiac surgery programs operating in New York State that helps in deciding which programs are of the highest quality. In turn, these report cards mean that cardiac surgery programs must openly compete on the basis of providing the highest-quality outcome to patients, giving patients more power to help determine the direction such programs take in the way of clinical process improvements, resource investment, marketing, and customer relations.

Whether the types of patient empowerment created by the Internet and health information technology generally give patients more power in their interactions with health professionals, or merely create the perception of additional power, the fact remains that much health care performance is now more transparent and available for consumers to use in comparison shopping. This "information marketplace" levels the playing field, if only in a small way, between health care consumers and producers, aiding in the transformation of an entire industry long built on "knowing what is best for the patient." However, as medical science grows increasingly complex, it may be far-fetched to presume that the availability of more information for consumers empowers as opposed to confuses them. This confusion, along with the information overload that accompanies a fully transparent health care delivery endeavor, may provide physicians and hospitals additional future opportunities to gain back any power loss from the consumer-oriented movement occurring in health care over the past decade.

---

As a result of this relationship, which is based on mutual dependence but asymmetrical power, the physician-nurse relationship has been characterized historically by high degrees of tension. More recently, however, because of workforce shortages in medical fields such as primary care, the nursing profession has advanced a new occupational subgroup, nurse practitioners (NP), which puts them more on a par with certain groups of physicians such as family doctors and pediatricians. In some states, nurse practitioners have independent prescribing power, and can diagnose and treat patients without physician oversight. Recent studies show that NPs may provide care on a similar quality level as their physician counterparts (Horrocks, Anderson, and Salisbury, 2002). Over time, if a subgroup such as NPs can demonstrate equality in work performance in areas traditionally the purview of physicians, they will provide nursing with an opportunity to acquire new sources of power for themselves that allow them greater self-determination as an occupational group.

The physician-administrator relationship is also one characterized by the acquisition and use of power. As noted in the "In Practice: The Pursuit of Power among Managers and Physicians" discussion, physicians and management tend to derive their power and influence from different sources, setting up an ongoing competition for power acquisition that may fester and go unnoticed for some time within the organization. In addition, the presence of dual hierarchies in places like hospitals creates tension between these groups because it legitimizes the claim to power for both simultaneously, while being less specific about where and when one group should have more authority than the other. Finally, physicians and administrators often have performance-related interests that differ, giving rise to sustained attempts by each to use power across a variety of situations to gain a specific preferred outcome.

For example, physicians may remain largely concerned with their individual patients, how they as clinicians or their immediate departments deliver care, and thus they maintain less concern about the overall performance of their peers or that of the organization as a whole. On the other hand, administrators (even physicians who become administrators) are hired directly by the organization to help ensure effective performance at a macro level, whether that is defined by work unit, department, function, or the entire organization. It is a manager's job not to overemphasize individual performance assessment, but instead examine performance from an aggregate or group level. It should be noted that these differences in perspective do not imply that one is bad and the other good. Rather, the important point is that difference in responsibility itself sets up differences in how appropriate performance should be viewed, and this may lead to conflict and the use of power and negotiation in attempts to reconcile.

The modern-day quality movement in health care and the increased emphasis on high-cost, high-tech specialty care are two recent examples of trends that have exacerbated power battles between physicians and administrators. For example, different from a decade ago, these two groups now come into contact frequently in a health care system that seeks greater and more formalized performance variety, transparency, and measurement. This has led health plans, hospitals, and practices to build formal administrative systems, using managers to run them, that provide the resources and authority not only to evaluate how clinicians perform, but to make that information available for patients and the rest of the organization to view. Examples of these systems include elaborate pay-for-performance programs that provide incentives for clinicians to perform higher-quality care, standardized "bundles" of care delivery for specific conditions that require things done in the same manner all the time, and profiling systems that assess provider performance relative to one another. The shift from performance "as defined by the individual physician" to performance based on global, transparent standards has been profound. It may threaten physicians' source of power because it involves transferring knowledge traditionally controlled and disseminated by the medical profession to the health care organization as a whole, and also to patients.

# THE POLITICAL NATURE OF POWER

Power in organizations is often created, maintained, and transferred through a political process. **Organizational politics** has been defined as an ongoing process of "managing influence" (Mayes and Allen, 1977), in which different coalitions of interests or influence vie for the opportunity to achieve their desired goals. This process of managing influence often involves the use of non-legitimate strategies and tactics, one of which is the exertion of power (Mayes and Allen, 1977). This definition is consistent with others that see politics as a process of using dynamics like power to gain desired ends (Eisenhart and Bourgeois, 1988). These definitions point to organizational politics as a key crucible in which power use is amplified and gains greater momentum. For example, the presence of a highly political work atmosphere both denotes and encourages the use of power, because it gives stakeholders greater freedom to assert their rights to control work, each other, and decisions.

The use of politics is characterized by its hidden nature; i.e., it involves strategies and tactics that are not transparent to everyone (Eisenhart and Bourgeois, 1988). This also facilitates power use, especially in situations that are high stakes, are high risk, or involve activities not immediately sanctioned by the organization and its workers. An example of one of these situations is when a company in financial crisis decides they must lay off workers to help reverse its fortunes. While the layoff decision may be known at all levels of the organization, different departments and units will likely engage in a political process designed to minimize the layoff impact on their own workers. This process may include making veiled or overt threats to management about the negative outcomes for the organization of being included too heavily in the layoff decision; moving to get key decision makers to support their specific department or unit cause; and undermining the cases made by other departments or units to top management.

This process can be hidden from view, and often involves only the most senior managers within each department and unit, and top management. The process itself will likely involve a wide range of power demonstrations and attempts to control decision making. For instance, the nursing department in a hospital may threaten to walk off the job, especially if they are unionized, if too many layoffs are aimed at them. The quality improvement or information technology departments may allude to the breakdown in hospital functioning that would occur should too many of their workers be fired. Physician staff may appeal directly to "one of their own" such as the hospital medical director or physician members on the board, and craft arguments geared to what they feel would resonate most with another physician. Often, those areas of the organization that top management perceives as most powerfully affecting how the organization conducts its business, combined with the assessment of threats made about how business could be affected, helps determine which parts of the organization get targeted for layoffs.

The notion of organizations as negotiated orders or coalitions of different interests provides a rationale for why politics becomes a dominant mode of interaction for members. Seen in this way, conflict and struggles for control are endemic, almost natural, in every organizational setting, in large part because it is acknowledged by everyone that melding different and often competing stakeholder interests into a single cohesive set of outcomes remains daunting. Through this lens, much organizational activity becomes preoccupied with two things: (1) determining whose interests and perspectives should rule in a given situation; and (2) determining which specific organizational outcomes are preferred and how they should be attained.

Health care organizations are particularly political organizations. This is due mainly to the presence of several different, powerful stakeholder groups working alongside each other. For example, physicians, nurses, and administrators each have the ability to exert influence over their work settings, make key decisions, and gain control over resources. Much of the management imperative within health care settings revolves around trying to limit political activity that aims to exert power in dysfunctional ways—i.e., ways that benefit the group exerting power without clearly adding value for the organization as a whole. The use of politics can be inefficient for the organization in these situations, because it requires individuals and groups to expend valuable time and resources for self-interested ends, which often reduces the overall time and resources available to pursue collective ends related to productivity and quality (Pfeffer, 1981).

On the positive side, politics plays a critical role in organizations by encouraging groups and individuals to share power, and to ally with each other if only temporarily to achieve common goals or outcomes. This reality can be used by the organization to mount collective efforts aimed at mutually agreed-upon goals. For example, while physicians and nurses may spend a certain portion of their collective time in conflict with one another around different issues in the workplace, or become preoccupied with exerting influence in part to gain resources at the expense of the other group, they may come together and use their political power to help the organization fulfill its accreditation requirements or to address a quality deficiency that threatens the reputation of the organization and its workers. In pursuing these imperatives, physicians and nurses in the same setting use similar informal tactics, share information and best practices, and advocate behind the scenes for similar changes. The political activity generated by two such powerful groups working in tandem may be quite influential.

Generally, the political process creates a fluid power structure within organizations, making it more difficult to predict at a given moment which parts of the organization may exert their influence, and whether or not they will be successful. The fluid nature of power within an especially political environment makes it somewhat risky for organizational leaders to attempt to manage the use and acquisition of power. Add to this the dependence of both power and politics on the type of work environment in which they are embedded, and the ability to harness political activity and the power it encapsulates remains one of the foremost management challenges in modern organization.

## How Power Stratifies: Personal and Contextual Influences

Power is never equally distributed within or across organizations. **Power stratification** means that different stakeholders may have unique opportunities to access power based upon their particular characteristics or circumstances. One key source of power stratification derives from the demographic qualities of stakeholder groups. For example, traditionally, males have been afforded greater chances to assume top management roles in a variety of organizations compared to their female colleagues (Ragins, 1993). In U.S. medicine, the most powerful, highest-paying specialties such as surgery have long been dominated by male physicians, despite an increasing number of female physicians over the past two decades. Much academic medicine in the United States also remains populated disproportionately with male physicians, giving this demographic group inordinate power to control the educational and socialization agenda for medical students and young physicians.

Age is another key demographic source of power stratification in health care. For example, professions such as medicine and nursing are built upon the apprenticeship model of training, where experience is the basis for seniority. In this way, individuals who have the most work experience, almost always older practitioners, retain greater influence and authority among their peers. They set the rules for professional behavior as well as impose their preferred cultural meaning systems onto the group as a whole, with sanctions applied for those choosing to deviate from their norms. Residency and fellowship programs that form the basis of professional training in health care implicitly favor age as a determining factor for which professionals deserve the access to greater power and control within their profession.

Employment status also serves as a source of power stratification in health care. For instance, salaried physicians, who work directly for their medical practices or for a health maintenance organization, generally have less individual and collective power than physicians who own their own practices. In the former situation, the physicians rely on the organization to pay them a salary, structure their workloads, and set policies that they must follow. In the latter case, the physicians may negotiate preferred rates of reimbursement with insurers and hospitals, can self-manage their work and hours, and choose the types of patients and services they offer.

Depending on the size and type of organization in which an individual works in health care, different power opportunities may also be afforded. Being an executive in a large insurance plan that controls a majority of the market share in a geographic area provides numerous opportunities to acquire and exert power with physician practices, hospitals, and employer groups—all of whom may depend on the insurance plan heavily for the success of their business. In the same way, physicians in a particular specialty may come together within a geographic area to form a single practice organization that dominates care in that market. This trend has been seen increasingly in the United States, with specialists such as orthopedists, cardiologists, and urologists, among others, splitting their practices off from academic medical centers to form "super-practices" that contain significant numbers of the available specialty physicians in that geographical area.

Finally, controlling financial resources stratifies organizational power. Within any organization, the "power of the purse" means that those individuals maintaining control over the distribution of resources have additional power opportunities than individuals who do not have this control. Traditionally, departmental units such as finance and accounting retain a great deal of power within the organization because they are sanctioned to review or approve the decisions made by other units in areas such as purchasing, capital acquisition, and hiring. Very often, struggles for power within the organizational setting revolve at least in part around one group's desire for greater fiscal independence or authority over others.

# THE ABUSE OF POWER IN HEALTH CARE ORGANIZATIONS

It is important for managers to view the use of power as necessary at times for their organization in helping to achieve its goals in an efficient manner. Managers should however, balance this functional view of power with a more critical perspective that views the use of power as potentially abusive to the organization's employees and external stakeholders (Hardy and Clegg, 1996). **Power abuse** refers to situations where one or more organizational stakeholders uses power in ways that are not generally acceptable, often involve self-interest and not the organization's best interests, and can inflict negative outcomes on workers, customers, and supporters of the organization.

Power abuses occur within organizations for two main reasons. One reason is the advancement of personal ends at the expense of the customer, shareholder, or employee. Examples of power abuses used to pursue personal ends could involve chief executives creating boards of directors consisting solely of friends or business partners, executives directing staff to misrepresent financial and performance data to outside stakeholders, and executives using unauthorized company funds or resources to enhance personal wealth. All these examples have recently been seen in both health care and other industries.

Power can also be abused to advance organizational ends. This form of power abuse is not easy to discern, nor do all groups within the organization necessarily agree that abusing power to achieve organizational ends in a given situation has negative consequences. In fact, such abuse may be sanctioned by numerous stakeholders both within and external to the organization. Examples of power abuses by managers that are used to pursue organizational ends could include laying off employees to send positive signals to board members or shareholders, without attending to the fundamental organizational problems or bad management decisions causing poor performance, and manipulating performance measurements for the sole purpose of misrepresenting the organization vis-à-vis other competitors in the marketplace.

Regardless of the ends pursued, the abuse of power by managers elevates the potential for negative fallout to occur in the organization. Perhaps most important is the crisis of trust that can occur when managers or executives abuse power. This trust crisis is expressed in two primary ways: (1) loss of faith by customers and external stakeholders (e.g., regulators, shareholders, funders) in the organization, and (2) loss of faith by employees in management. Both crises have recently gained center stage in light of corporate scandals in health care and other industries, as well as in the U.S. financial industry crisis that helped to produce a severe economic recession. Loss of faith by customers and other external stakeholders can meaningfully affect organizational performance and survival, in the form of lost business for the organization, reduced financial capital, stricter regulatory scrutiny, and the development of a negative reputation that allows other competitors to gain a long-term edge over the organization (Fukuyama, 1995; Sitkin and Stickel, 1996).

Loss of trust by employees toward managers when power is abused reduces the potential for positive dynamics within the organization to enhance performance. Examples of positive dynamics negatively affected by power abuse include teamwork, cooperative behavior, communication quality, citizenship behavior, and job satisfaction (Axelrod, 1984; Blau, 1964; Hoff, 2003; Whitener et al., 1998). Other negative fallout that may occur includes increased organizational complacency, decreased work effort or "shirking" on the part of employees, slower organizational adaptation to change, and decreased quality of services or products (Burawoy, 1979). While not a certainty, the abuse of power can seriously impact organizational performance, lead to lost business, and, in some cases, facilitate collapse in the form of bankruptcy or dissolution. Examples of these outcomes are found in recent American corporate history.

Several conditions facilitate the abuse of power within organizations. These include high uncertainty regarding how to achieve goals or desired output; an overly centralized decision-making structure; the scarcity of rival coalitions both internal and external to the organization; a lack of reliance by key organizational stakeholders on each other; an existing culture of organizational complacency; and existing pressure to make quick decisions within the organization (Brass, Burkhardt, and Marlene, 1993; Crozier, 1964; Mintzberg, 1983; Perrow, 1989; Weber, 1978). Ironically, many of the conditions that create the potential for power abuse derive in large part from the same general conditions that give rise to power use. This highlights the paradoxical nature of power within organizations, in that the factors that allow power to grow and be used effectively are also those that, when manipulated in certain ways or taken to extremes, provide fertile conditions for power abuse. Given this reality, a key managerial task is to institutionalize a structural framework and culture within the organization that limits the probability that power use conditions are manipulated.

For example, the ability to create dependencies in relationships on the basis of resources like knowledge or funding is a potential source of organizational power within organizations. However, too much of an imbalance in terms of the extent to which a dependency relationship favors one group over another creates the potential for power abuse (Brass, Burkhardt, and Marlene, 1993). This situation is exacerbated when the resources in question are scarce, essential, and non-substitutable.

Control over information through structural advantages such as network centrality is another legitimate source of organizational power that, when taken to extremes, often results in power abuse. As discussed, individuals or groups who position themselves at the center of communication and information networks within the organization are in a position to exercise power. Information is a resource that allows individuals to set decision-making premises within the organization and control uncertainty (Crozier, 1964; Perrow, 1989). However, to the extent that managers or others within the organization gain exclusive control over information—i.e., to the extent that specific individuals or groups can create gaps or ambiguities in understanding within the organization that only they can fill—a foundation for power abuse is created.

The building of coalitions and alliances is a source of organizational power. However, an organizational environment in which there is a single dominant coalition or alliance provides a foundation for power abuse. Any leader-centered coalition that does not adhere to a diversity of viewpoints and perspectives can create an autocratic situation in which the leader's will and preferences become those of the larger group (Mintzberg, 1983). This leads to negative outcomes such as groupthink. The absence of rival coalitions within the organization creates a situation for power abuse, mainly by lessening the capacity for creative tension and ideas to compete with each other on the basis of their informational, logical, and strategic merits. This decreased capacity encourages the dominant coalition to introduce mechanisms by which to minimize deviation from the preferred status quo (Salancik and Pfeffer, 1977). This may hurt the organization in terms of performance and ability to adapt to changing demands in the environment.

## The Role of Trust, Fairness, and Transparency in Preventing Power Abuse

Managers can take several steps to guard against the abuse of power within their organizations. These steps include structuring communication networks to create greater transparency in terms of organizational decision making, implementation, and evaluation; using boards of directors and advisory groups as counterbalances to managerial authority; creating a strong code of ethics within the organization; designing appropriate appraisal systems; and emphasizing personal integrity in the hiring function (Alford, 2001; Hoff, 2003; Thibodeaux and Powell, 1985; Westheafer, 2000).

---

**IN PRACTICE:** Abusing Power at the Top Levels of the Organization

---

There have been instances in business and health care over the years in which top managers, a chief executive officer (CEO), or a board of directors have abused their power through the creation and maintenance of a single dominant coalition within the organization that controls decisions and discourages dissenting viewpoints. For example, if a CEO desires to have more influence over the organization, she or he may create a board of directors that consists of close friends, business partners, or individuals that share a similar strategic viewpoint. In the extreme, these types of boards become "rubber stamps" that may fail to carry out their fiduciary responsibility as counterbalances to executive control within the organization. They also reduce the quality of strategic decision making because they abdicate their role of critiquing management decisions. In the final analysis, this allows executives to make decisions that potentially benefit their own ends at the expense of customer, employee, or shareholder interests.

Imagine a CEO of a hospital who helps place on its board of directors a banker with whom the CEO used to work, a lawyer who frequents the same country club to which the CEO belongs, the head of a local construction company that has helped perform work on the hospital, and an old college friend who still goes on fishing trips with the CEO and is one of the top cardiologists in the community. The prior and existing relationships between the CEO and these individuals, forged through other work and personal circumstances, may taint the ability of the group as a whole to generate the creative tension and independent thought needed for developing hospital strategy and evaluating the CEO's decision making. For instance, one or more of the board members, because they trust the CEO from other walks of life, may come to rely on the CEO's "version of the world" and align their thinking with the CEO's, leading to unquestioning support for the CEO's actions and take on the world. By owing the CEO for their seats on the board, some directors may be remiss to challenge or disagree with the CEO. Other directors may perceive that if they help the CEO "get his way," there is the possibility of additional rewards for themselves. Still others may simply like the CEO, be friends with him, and so be less likely to contradict his desires or decisions.

Having directors that know the CEO from prior walks of life, or who feel indebted to a CEO for their position, increases the chances that the CEO may abuse his own power, especially if he wishes to make certain decisions or impose a particular strategic decision on the organization. Friendship is important in life, but in the case of a CEO and his board, it may foster a singular alliance of interests at the very top of an organization that crowds out alternative viewpoints and critical debate, producing a leadership group that becomes insular, self-interested, and disconnected from true organizational realities. It is these attributes that can then facilitate power abuse within the group.

---

Creating transparency involves making information a "public good" within organizations. This means, for example, allowing access to performance data at all levels of the organization, so that everyone from line employees to the chief executive appreciates the logic by which specific decisions are made. In establishing greater internal transparency, managers end up becoming more accessible to employees. This enhances trust within the organization, and while it does not preclude the use of power as a necessary dynamic, it is likely to identify instances of abuse in a timely manner. External transparency also limits power abuse. Providing key constituents such as shareholders, regulators, and customers with complete, accurate, and timely performance data prevents executives and boards of directors from making decisions that are not rooted in strategic logic but instead derive more from the manipulation of circumstances on the part of individuals or groups in the organization.

Many recent corporate scandals that involved managerial abuse of power could have been prevented through the use of independent oversight mechanisms in the form of boards of directors and external auditors. Many boards are laden with members who are connected to the organization in some manner that makes them reluctant to enact their oversight role (see the "In Practice: Abusing Power at the Top Levels of the Organization" example). Such characteristics make boards less useful for controlling power abuse in organizations.

Organizations that staff boards of directors with individuals who have the time to fulfill the oversight role, and who have no personal stake involved in the results of that oversight, place themselves in the best position to allow the use, but not abuse, of power by managers.

Creating a strong code of ethics and institutionalizing it into the organization's culture also limits power abuse (Hatcher, 2002). Recent examples of power abuses within organizations have been found to result in part from the presence of work environments that tolerated and even promoted unethical (not necessarily illegal) behavior in relation to the use of power. Establishing a code of ethics gives managers and employees formal guidance as to how to act across different situations where power may be exercised. This limits individual discretion in using power. It also conveys a sense that there are risks or potential sanctions to using power in an abusive way (Thibodeaux and Powell, 1985). Key to the success of a code of ethics is the overt dedication of top management to it.

Designing performance appraisal and hiring systems that emphasize and reward ethical behavior also limit the potential for power abuse within organizations. For example, power abuse by managers toward employees through the use of formal position in the hierarchy is minimized when appraisal systems exist that judge employee performance across a range of objective performance dimensions. Considering personal values and ethical behavior as important factors in the hiring and evaluation of managers and employees heightens the probability that the organizational workforce consists of individuals who are less likely to take advantage of any power at their disposal. Over time, it creates an organizational culture in which a negative view towards power abuse becomes a shared norm.

# POWER AS A KEY SOURCE OF CONFLICT

The use of power within organizational settings, along with the political activity that helps manifest it, can give rise to conflict. Conflict associated with power and politics derives from two primary organizational circumstances. First, conflict can occur when two or more parties have different perspectives, ideas, or agendas; they intend to move them forward in the organization; and each party is willing to behave in ways that require some form of resolution to avert a suboptimal or dysfunctional organizational outcome.

Conflict in organizations can also arise when two or more interdependent parties draw upon different sources for their power, or have unequal access to power opportunities in the organization. This second circumstance is most endemic to health care settings, where different groups have their work highly coordinated and must rely meaningfully upon each other to deliver services to patients. In these instances—high mutual dependence among two or more parties that have different power sources—the key conflict-generating dynamic involves parties trying to figure out who (and therefore also which power source) is more influential or controlling in a given situation.

One such instance of this second source of conflict occurs when there is a specific organizational goal that the interdependent parties are expected to pursue jointly. For example, physicians and nurses working in a hospital may be asked to help reduce the incidence of medical errors occurring to patients during their hospital stays. To accomplish this goal, each group may want the same resource—more staff positions, technology, or decision-making autonomy—and the conflict becomes centered on each group attempting to claim that resource for themselves. This is the type of conflict we generally think about.

However, conflict often occurs at a second, deeper level in this circumstance. This conflict involves disagreements about which power source to rely upon in order to solve the first-level conflict of who should claim the desired resources. When multiple sources of power exist in an organization, ideas for how to resolve conflict are not necessarily shared by all parties. For instance, those who possess a knowledge advantage might think knowledge-based power is most relevant, while those who are in supervisory or high positions and who have structurally derived power might think relying on administrative mechanisms like formal policies is most appropriate (Ashforth and Johnson, 2001).

A related issue is the choice of which conflict management technique to use in a given situation. For example, in the physician-nurse relationship or the physician-patient relationship, the physician has culturally derived power from his or her advanced standing in the medical profession. That power gives the physician authority over the nurse or the patient. When conflict arises between the physician and nurse or the physician and patient, that physician has to decide whether or not to employ the use of power. The physician may draw on that culturally derived power to say

## DEBATE TIME

For those who possess some level of professional or organizational power, it can be difficult to know when and how to use that power in situations that might benefit the organization's customers. As the chapter notes, not all power use is bad. In fact, the use of power is necessary and productive in situations where the customer stands to benefit in the form of a higher-quality or more efficient service provided to them. Often, the carefully planned use of power can help overcome organizational inertia regarding the best decision to implement, resolve infighting between internal stakeholders that may hold up appropriate decision making, and produce needed decisions quickly in situations where time is of the essence. However, knowing the precise moment and manner in which to begin using one's power, regardless of the reason for it, is a challenging task for any health care manager or professional.

When would you use power within an organization? Several considerations should likely guide your decision making. First, consider the type of outcome toward which your use of power would contribute. Is it ethical? Does it benefit the organization as a whole? Would it help produce an outcome that improves the efficiency or quality of services provided, or directly benefit the customer in some meaningful way? Can it be done in a manner that does not undermine other important organizational goals or objectives? The answers to these types of questions are critical for establishing the prerequisite rationale for using power, a rationale that, at some point, others in the organization or external stakeholders may need to hear. Once these questions have been answered, the second consideration is to assess the type of actions required for using power and how disruptive such actions might be for the rest of the organization. For example, using power in a strictly covert, highly political manner that masks its true nature as a control or influence mechanism may not be appropriate, regardless of the type of outcome such a use of power is aiming to achieve. In short, this step requires understanding the right ways to exercise one's power. What should be the level of transparency in using power? Should everyone know that the use of power is guiding organizational action in the given situation? Are certain actions "out of bounds" with respect to how power will be used?

A third consideration involves assessing the potential unintended negative consequences the use of power might cause within an organization. Such consequences may result even if power use is determined to be necessary and the actions taken to use power are appropriate. These types of unintended consequences are important. They may include workforce effects like decreased job satisfaction, productivity, morale, and turnover; organizational outcomes like decreased profitability or client dissatisfaction; increased short-term conflict between different organizational stakeholders or constituencies; and cultural shifts within the organization that might undermine worker or management cohesiveness. Predicting which types of negative consequences might occur is not easy. However, it is imperative to at least discuss openly the probability that some of these could happen, and what could be done to limit the damage done to the organization.

Finally, the use of power, even in an appropriate, required circumstance should be short-lived. Clear consideration must be given to the time frame within which power use will occur, when it is no longer appropriate to use power in a given situation, and agreement on the boundaries within which power will be used and when it will no longer be used, regardless of whether or not all the desired outcomes are achieved. This consideration is important precisely because the use of power takes a toll on the organization, especially the longer its use occurs. Therefore, this dynamic must be used sparingly, strategically, and with careful attention paid to whether or not it is working effectively.

With these things in mind, power may be exercised by individuals and groups within organizations, as well as by organizations themselves. This notion moves us beyond the idea that all power is bad, that its use is immoral, and that the organization never benefits from its employment as a tactical device to achieve particular outcomes. That said, it remains a higher-risk, more unpredictable approach to managing, and must always be assessed within that regard.

"I'm the physician, you are the nurse or patient, and I know better" as an influence attempt, or the physician can take a different approach that relies less on formal power use and more on less coercive models of influence. Effective conflict management is based on appreciating the sources of power for each party involved and knowing how and when a particular power source could be used.

The **study of conflict management** concerns how parties approach, deal with, and resolve conflict and which personal, social, and environmental factors affect that process. The focus here is on one conflict management tool—negotiation—which is presented as a direct way to resolve conflict. In this section of the chapter, we refer to those who engage in conflict management as "negotiators" or "parties in the negotiation." They may include the actual parties involved in benefiting or losing from the negotiation itself. Other strategies to resolve conflict could include avoidance, whereby one or more parties refuses to deal with the conflict; or accommodation, where one party simply concedes to the other(s). While avoidance may work in a situation where emotions are high and time is needed to prepare for negotiation, and accommodation may work in a situation where the outcome is of less importance, negotiation is a viable process when there is a vested interest in the outcome and when each party wishes to manage the situation as effectively as possible for themselves and their interests.

# TYPES OF CONFLICT

There are generally thought to be two types of conflict that occur in groups: conflict related to ideas concerning the task at hand, and conflict related to social factors in the team (Jehn, 1997). The first type of conflict, known as **task conflict**, reflects differences amongst the parties in understanding and carrying out tasks. This type of conflict, while detrimental to overall performance or decision making in the team or group, is seen to be the "better" type of conflict in that it is less personal and somewhat easier to accommodate. For instance, in a task conflict situation, a physician and administrator want different things, but they respect each other and may even like each other. This does not necessarily make the task easier to solve, but it does mean that these parties would likely preserve their relationship after the conflict management situation is over.

Where interdependent parties struggle in terms of both performance and satisfaction is when **relationship conflict**,

or conflict regarding some inherent characteristic of the other party, is present. The causes of relationship conflict could be related to interpersonal styles, personality, political preference, and the like (De Dreu and Weingart, 2003). Relationship conflict is particularly difficult to deal with because judgments are being made about the party above and beyond the task at hand. Even when there is a shared understanding regarding how to solve the task, those groups experiencing conflict rooted in the relationship itself possess heightened negative emotions and perceive a dislike of the other party.

If the conflict is primarily task-based, the challenge is in understanding the viewpoints and perspectives of all of those at the table. If the conflict is more relationship-based, the challenge is how to navigate around the heightened emotions and perceptions in the group, which can interfere with the mutual pursuit of a negotiated outcome. Task conflict can also lead to relationship conflict. For example, if we acknowledge that two different parties can have two different sources of power, such as with a physician and an administrator, the knowledge-based power possessed by the physician might create task conflict with the administrator, who has control over resources. In this case, each thinks they know the "best" way to solve the conflict, which represents conflict over the task at hand. However, if they fail to see the conflict from the other side's point of view, that task conflict can escalate into relationship conflict. Once this happens, not only do they hold different views regarding how to solve the task, but they now also judge each other's values, which can lessen mutual trust and respect. This lack of trust means they do not have a solid relational base from which to work, which makes the resolution of conflict more difficult.

## The Negative Side of Emotions

In 1981, Barry Staw and colleagues published a paper on the **threat rigidity effect**, which states that when individuals feel threatened, their thinking becomes rigid or inflexible (Staw, Sandelands, and Dutton, 1981). As conflict can often result in individuals feeling like their resources are threatened, or that they are being attacked by the other party, threat rigidity is a likely outcome. The result of these heightened emotions produces a decreased ability to cognitively process information, ideas, or possible solutions. The brain goes into "protection" mode instead of "exploration" mode, and consequently the negotiators, or the parties involved in the negotiation, become preoccupied with protecting their own viewpoint rather than trying to come to a creative solution with others. In a study related to this in a negotiation context, Carnevale and Probst (1998) found that when participants expected a hostile situation with high conflict, they showed less cognitive flexibility and creative thinking than if expecting a collaborative situation.

Not only do heightened emotions shut down cognitive processing, but emotions can be contagious (Barsade, 2002). The process of **emotional contagion** occurs when emotions are transmitted from one party to another. If one party becomes angry, others in the room can "catch" that anger, and a negative spiral ensues where they then transfer that anger to others. Parties experiencing conflict who travel through this negative emotional spiral may find themselves with very few options that would result in a positive resolution to the conflict at hand. This is why parties experiencing conflict in general, and relationship conflict in particular, need to be aware of the emotional state of the group.

---

**IN PRACTICE:  A Negative Emotional Spiral in Hospital Human Resources**

In the following example of Mary and her boss Ryan, we can see emotional contagion in action. Mary, an HR benefits administrator in the hospital, has been experiencing a bit of frustration with her career progress. While she started out in patient advocacy and later moved into advocacy training, her current job has taken her from patient contact completely. She feels that her boss, Ryan, has taken advantage of her willingness to work "any task" and forced her away from her passion. Ryan, as her boss, has been quite pleased with Mary's performance, and counts her among his top performers. She is conscientious with all assigned tasks, and seems willing to do whatever he asks. This is precisely why he approached her about moving into a benefits position.

Mary has just had lunch with a colleague who was asking about her career, a conversation in which Mary "realizes" that she is not happy about her position. Without thinking through the conflict, she is placing the blame largely on Ryan and has decided to approach Ryan about this conflict:

Mary (already upset):  "Ryan, I'd like to talk with you right now about my position."

Ryan:  "Sure, Mary, what's the problem?"

Mary:  "Why have you put me into this dead-end job?"

Ryan:  "What are you talking about? You are one of my best performers!"

Mary:  "You know exactly what I'm talking about—no one else wanted to do benefits and you knew that I wouldn't say no to you."

Ryan:  "If you think accusing me of something is going to get you what you want, you are sorely mistaken. I've done nothing but try to help you."

Mary:  "I want out of this job and a move back to patient advocacy. If I don't get that, I'm moving to another hospital."

Ryan:  "If that's your attitude, then my answer is no."

In this case, the negative emotions that Mary harbors when resolving this conflict has not only clouded her ability to negotiate effectively, but they have transferred to Ryan. Her anger has become contagious in this discussion. The effect of this is that Ryan, who may have been happy to calmly discuss Mary's issues, is now unwilling to work with Mary. We can detect this here by noticing that they do not talk about Mary's passion—having direct patient contact. If this were discussed, it is possible that Ryan would agree to try to get her back to what she loves, especially considering she is a high performer. Good negotiators realize that the actions and emotions they portray will be mimicked by the other party.

# COMMON MISTAKES IN THINKING ABOUT CONFLICT

Perhaps the most significant error negotiators make when approaching conflict, and one easily seen with Mary in the "In Practice: A Negative Emotional Spiral" example, is failing to plan or think through the conflict before attempting to deal with it. Failing to plan is more likely to result in a haphazard approach to negotiation marked by an overreliance on techniques most familiar to the negotiator, while planning beforehand is more likely to result in a methodical and well-thought-out approach marked by tactics that would be most effective in resolving the conflict. An effective plan for each party to a negotiation will include a description of one's own interests or underlying needs, possible positions or offers that can satisfy those interests, goals regarding specific positions for the negotiation, and possible tactics to use in reaching the goals. If there is uncertainty regarding the interests and positions of the other party, a plan should also include a listing of questions to ask, as questions will help gain understanding about the interests and positions of the other side.

Interests, rather than positions, are important to discuss because they help a negotiator focus on what is most important to them, which opens up possibilities for creative problem solving through the consideration of multiple positions (see Thompson, 2005). The importance of goals is that it drives motivation on the part of the negotiator (Locke and Latham, 1990). When negotiators have clear goals, they are influenced to keep working toward reaching those goals, which can increase persistence and effort toward conflict resolution. Finally, planning before dealing with the conflict will give each party multiple options for how to resolve the conflict. This will help the negotiators avoid coming to an impasse, which is marked by neither side knowing how to resolve the situation.

A negotiation plan also includes a description of all the logistics in the negotiation. Where will the negotiation take place? For how long? Who will be at the table? Who are the influential stakeholders not present at the table? What are the issues to be discussed? The logistics are important for various reasons. First, there must be enough time to resolve the conflict without a sense of urgency, as a sense of urgency usually results in parties using compromising as a strategy, which is not ideal in all situations as will be discussed later in the chapter. Second, the environment can facilitate information sharing if all parties are comfortable and relaxed. Even the ambient level of noise is important, as a quiet environment will decrease the likelihood of miscommunication. Third, as much information as possible about the parties and issues should be known beforehand so that each negotiator, or person in the negotiation, knows what to expect. Finally, meeting in one's own office instead of another's conveys power and comfort. Meeting at a location and time convenient to another may be seen as a gesture of good faith.

When negotiators fail to plan, they can fall victim to **functional fixedness**, which occurs when a negotiator bases his or her strategy on familiar, rather than the most effective, methods. (Adamson and Taylor, 1954). For example, imagine that a particular physician has had a long, contentious relationship with one hospital administrator. Every time they have to negotiate or solve a problem, the interaction becomes emotional, and each party behaves aggressively toward the other side. Needless to say, this creates tension for them and for those around them, and it results in less-than-effective negotiated agreements—neither side is ever happy. Now imagine that the administrator is replaced by someone new. Given his or her past experiences, that physician immediately begins to rely on those same contentious behaviors with the new administrator—he or she is fixated on those types of behaviors as being the way to negotiate with all administrators. Thus, even though the new administrator may be willing to negotiate in a different way, the physician never uncovers that possibility because they revert to those familiar tactics. A negotiation plan, in this case, could reveal that the physician knows very little about the new administrator and should rely on asking probing questions and building a rapport with them before any competitive behaviors are even considered.

Another hindrance to effective negotiation is cognitive biases, or the mental blocks that impede effective information gathering and synthesis. These biases impede effective conflict management as successful negotiations are based on the information-gathering process of the parties. Each party must seek to understand not only what his or her interests are, but also the interests of the other parties involved in the negotiation. One bias particularly relevant to negotiators is the **confirming evidence bias**, which is the tendency for people to seek out and pay attention only to information that confirms prior beliefs (Eagly and Chaiken, 1993). The confirming evidence bias shuts down the learning process as individuals are no longer attending to information that could potentially help them work through multiple possible offers.

Consider a job negotiation, this time focusing on an applicant who has "fallen in love" with the company. This preexisting belief will severely impair the ability of that person to negotiate because they will be unable to evaluate information objectively. A negotiator who falls victim to the confirming evidence bias will not want to ask questions of the other side, will be hesitant to add issues, and will not pay attention to information suggesting the company is not satisfying their interests. While this may be a peaceful negotiation without much conflict, it raises the potential for the **winner's curse**, or the feeling of unhappiness after a reached settlement where one side feels that they should have asked for more.

Another common problem that exists for many negotiators is the **inert knowledge problem**, or the inability for negotiators to draw on information they have to solve novel situations. The root of the inert knowledge problem stems from the inability to transfer "lessons learned" from situation to situation that are not very similar on the surface. For example, a common conflict between a physician and a patient could revolve around the physician trying to understand patient fears about a certain medication. The physician may believe that the best way to convince a patient that a certain medication is good is by showing expertise through the provision of objective statistics that the patient cannot refute. However, this is only one possible way to convince the patient to use that medication. It could be that the patient does not really care about or understand statistics. Perhaps the patient is worried because he or she knows someone else who took this medication and did not have a positive experience. Or perhaps the patient is worried about the short-term and long-term costs. By ignoring the knowledge about patients and their various fears, the physician might be unable to get what he or she wants, and what is clinically indicated, which is to get that patient on the new drug.

## Common Mistakes in Managing Relationships

Another mistake negotiators make is not thinking about the other party. Most negotiators, especially when negotiating early in their careers or negotiating without much experience, tend to focus primarily on their own needs. They ignore the power of **reciprocity**, which is the tendency for others to exchange equal levels of goods and services (Cialdini, 2001). Reciprocity is powerful in situations of uncertainty, as negotiators are looking for cues regarding how to behave towards the other party. If one side gives a small concession, gives up some information, or behaves competitively, usually the other side will do the same (Weingart et al., 2007). Through reciprocity, the parties in the negotiation can build trust with one another. Thus the mistake made in negotiation is when one side ignores the needs of the other party and yet wants something in return.

Along with not realizing the power of reciprocity, another mistake with regard to not thinking about the other party is "adding up" during the negotiation how much has been personally rather than collectively gained. Think of the negotiation between a physician and a staff member regarding working regular overtime. As discussion proceeds, the physician is focused on how many hours he or she has been able to get the staff member to concede. This leads to thoughts such as "I've gotten 45 hours per week, how much more can I get?" However, this view ignores whether the staff member is going to be satisfied with this agreement, or if the staff member has other ideas about how many extra hours they wish to work. Satisfying the needs of the other party means that party has received enough in the negotiation for them to say "yes" and carry out the agreement. This act of being focused on all parties in the negotiation is called being **cognitively active**— constantly and intentionally focusing on all parties instead of only focusing on oneself.

Finally, failing to trust is another mistake that can severely hamper effective conflict resolution. Deepak Malhotra and colleagues, in recent studies, have investigated how much trust toward another party was beneficial in a negotiation (Malhotra, 2004; Weber, Malhotra, and Murnighan, 2005). This is an important topic as most negotiators find it very hard to trust others, even when they know there is no good reason to believe the other side will take advantage of them. Negotiators tend to protect information, and are hesitant to give even the smallest of concessions, because they worry that the other side will use that information against them and that it will be seen by the other as a sign of weakness. What negotiators fail to realize is that the act of withholding information communicates to the other party that there is no trust between them. This then creates a **self-fulfilling prophecy**, which describes the process by which one party's beliefs cause another party to behave in such a way that supports that belief (Merton, 1968). What Bazerman and Gillespie (1999) found was that partial trust in others—or giving some information—was the worst strategy a negotiator could take. The reason is that while full trust induces reciprocity, and no trust protects information and other resources, partial trust sacrifices resources without invoking reciprocity.

---

**IN PRACTICE: ER Nurse Contract Negotiation and Planning to Negotiate**

Joanne is a nurse who just moved to Springfield with her husband and is going in to negotiate her job at County General Hospital. This hospital happens to be her number-one choice due to the departmental opening (the emergency room) and proximity to her new house. She will be negotiating with Chandra, who is in charge of hiring nurses.

Chandra: "Joanne, we are really excited to have you on board at County General, I think you'll be a great addition to the ER department."

Joanne: "Thank you so much."

Chandra: "I know salary conversations can be touchy, and I definitely want to be fair to you as well as to the hospital. So I thought maybe we could start by discussing what you were making at your last job. That will give us a baseline from which to work."

Joanne: "But I want to make more than I was at my last job."

Chandra: "Well, I'd like to pay you fairly based on your experience and thought that your prior salary would be a piece of information we could use to figure out the right number."

Joanne: "I'm not comfortable with that."

Chandra: "Why not? I thought you were excited about joining us? Do you think I'm trying to take advantage of you?"

Joanne has made both the mistake of failing to plan and the mistake of failing to trust. She has no reason to distrust Chandra and yet is unwilling to give up any information. She reciprocates with denial, instead of either giving the information or reframing the discussion. An alternative would be if the final part of the scenario had gone like this:

Chandra: ". . . That will give us a baseline from which to work."

Joanne: "I appreciate that you would like to know that information and I will provide it, but I was hoping we could focus our discussion around my skills and experience in comparison with the other nurses here as a way to figure out my salary. I've actually done quite a bit of thinking and research on this and would like to share that information with you. Is that okay?"

Chandra: "Absolutely."

Joanne: "I'd also like to discuss the shifts I might be working as well as my vacation. Those items are also very important to me as I have a toddler at home."

Chandra: "Of course. We actually have quite a bit of flexibility on hours as there are two open positions and you are the first offer we've made."

Joanne: "Excellent, let's start there . . ."

By talking about her interests instead of getting defensive with Chandra, she preserves the relationship and provides a solid base for not only discussing salary but for discussing any issue. This negotiation has gone from potentially emotional and contentious to being a comfortable problem-solving environment.

# KEY CONFLICT MANAGEMENT STRATEGIES

When a conflict arises that is important enough to the parties to address it, they engage in strategies to solve the conflict. Each of these strategies is marked by a different approach to **value in negotiation**, defined as the combined benefits among all the parties in the negotiated agreement. The three most common strategies when individuals engage another party and seek resolution (i.e., not avoid the situation) are **compromising, competing, and collaborating** (Pruitt and Rubin, 1986).

> *Compromising*: A negotiation strategy where the parties in the negotiation divide value and find a solution that partially satisfies everyone. This is often a "split-the-difference" solution to a problem whereby no one wins, but also no one loses.
> Example: *I'm going to struggle to cover my Thursday shift this week. If I take the first four hours, can you take the second four hours?*

The main benefit of taking a compromising approach is that it is timely and efficient. If a manager knows that half of his staff want the department meeting at 8:00 a.m. and half would like it at 8:30 a.m., a compromise solution would suggest that the meeting be held at 8:15 a.m. There is little need to try to find a different solution. In cases, then, where the importance of the outcome is of low or modest importance to the parties negotiating, compromising is an effective strategy. The danger with compromise solutions is that negotiators often compromise when they should not—when the importance of the problem is high and they are unable to figure out any other way to solve the problem. The downside to compromising in this situation is that this strategy *prevents* the creation of creative alternatives, which could lead to a more beneficial outcome for all parties.

> *Competing*: A negotiation strategy where one party tries to get as much value for themselves as possible with little, if any, concern for the other party.
> Example: *I'm going to struggle to cover my Thursday shift this week. You should cover my shift for me because I have two little kids at home who are sick and am in a really tough rotation right now.*

A competitive strategy is beneficial when either (1) there is no concern for a lasting relationship with the other party,

or (2) there is reason not to trust the other party. In this case, the physician, rather than trying to collaborate with the other party, is trying to change the perspective of the other side—to get them to say yes without giving up very much or anything. We call this claiming value because they are trying to capture as many of the benefits contained in the agreement for themselves.

> *Collaborating*: A negotiation strategy where parties try to help each other get what they want and in the process maximize the value created in the negotiation.
> Example: *I'm going to struggle to cover my Thursday shift this week. I know you need consecutive days off to go visit your parents—if I cover your shift next week, when you need the days off, can you cover my shift this week?*

Collaboration has been shown to be the most effective negotiation strategy, and should be used when there is high concern for both the other party and high concern for the outcome of the negotiation. When adopting a collaborative strategy, negotiators are focused not only on pursuing self-interest, but also on the needs of the other side. This is why this perspective is so powerful—by showing concern for the other party, negotiators can invoke reciprocity. This force of reciprocity leads the other party to show concern as well.

## Tactics to Acquire More Information

There are three main categories of tactics negotiators can use for pursuing various goals: Tactics to acquire more information, tactics to find a better solution, and tactics to influence the other party. The first category focuses on doing research and asking questions both before and during the negotiation. The second category focuses on creating value in negotiation through creative problem solving. The third category, which also tends to be the one most thought of in the context of negotiation, involves changing the perspective of the other side.

### Do Research

Gathering information before negotiation allows an individual to manage power when resolving conflict. While research can come in several forms, the most influential research that can be done is gathering objective data, as objective data facilitates using knowledge-based sources of power to influence. Examples of objective data gathering when negotiating for a job in health care could be: (1) what others in your specialty or

---

## IN PRACTICE:  Nursing Union Negotiation

Many nurses are unionized, and nurses' unions regularly have to negotiate new contracts with their employers, such as hospitals and health care systems. In recent years, two of the more important collective bargaining issues for nurses and their employers have been economic issues like pensions and work-related issues like staffing levels. These issues can often get contentious. For example, nurses' unions may take the position that they are most interested in good patient care and therefore want a required ratio of patients to nurses at all times, while employers like hospitals may advocate for head nurses to be able to set staffing levels depending on patient need at the time, for quality and financial reasons. Regarding the pension issue, employers may seek to decrease or limit the pension contribution in order to make the system more "economically feasible." Both sides may posture by stating that they want the other side to come back to the table and begin negotiating "in good faith."

The difficulty in union negotiations, as highlighted in this brief summary, is that it tends to be largely position-based and not interest-based. This makes both sides entrenched in their positions and inhibits any potential for a creative solution. In instances like these, the union may take a public position on staffing that states that they want "a required ratio," while the hospital may take a public position on staffing that states that they want a system where "the head nurse dictates."

One reason for this type of stance in union negotiations is because those who are negotiating might have different interests than those whom they represent. The negotiators, in addition to satisfying their constituents, want to "look good." So what often happens is that they make public statements reflecting positions (e.g., "I want a required ratio") to fire up and garner support from their members. But we know that in negotiations, using positions is ultimately defeating—when both sides use positions rather than interests to negotiate, there will ultimately be one winner and one loser—or worse, two losers, depending on how things play out.

So what happens? Because positions have been stated publicly, to give in would be to lose face in the negotiation, which is not something that the negotiators on either side wish to do. This is the hallmark of a competitive strategy, with neither side willing to budge. Of course, the potential to create value is largely destroyed, as the sides are not willing to communicate, much less work with each other. The endgame, then, is determined by power. If the company feels that they have more power, they will let the workers (in this case, nurses) strike until the workers cannot financially maintain the strike. If the workers feel they have more power, they will threaten to strike and hope the company gives in. However, what often happens is that you have two groups who, because they are mired in conflict, each become convinced that they have more power to determine the outcome and, in the process, each fails to see how they can reach out to the other side and bring them back to the table in such a way as would allow them to save face. This produces a longer negotiation process, and one which may not make either side satisfied in the end.

---

subspecialty are making, (2) what others in your city or region are making, (3) what others with your experience are making, (4) what others who graduated from your medical or nursing school or who have your same graduate degree are making, (5) what others in your new (or old) hospital, private practice, or company are making, (6) what certifications, degrees, or experience you have relative to what these others are making, and (7) what the cost of living is in your area compared to what you were making in your previous location. These are all objective sources of data because they are based on fact (rather than opinion) and are not easily refuted. This data can

be researched either online, through personal networks, or through print publications.

### Ask Questions

Asking questions of the other side is a specific way to uncover information in a negotiation. As negotiators often go into negotiations with little if any knowledge about what the other side's interests are, asking questions can help accomplish this part of the research-gathering process. Besides acquiring information, asking questions also communicates to the other party that there is concern for their interests. This invokes reciprocity, which, as described previously, is the tendency for individuals to treat others like they are being treated. However, not all questions are created equally. While some questions are designed to acquire information (e.g., "What are your interests?"), other questions can be insulting (e.g., "Why are you acting this way?"), imply threats (e.g., "Are you sure you want to take that position?"), or simply be poorly worded (e.g., "Would you be willing to share your underlying needs? Because right now I can't figure out what you are talking about"). Questions that are likely to lead to the most revealed information are nonthreatening and are perceived by the other side as conveying genuine interest.

### Find Common Ground

One of the main goals when asking questions is to get the other side to be honest about their interests. This is part of a larger tactic called "finding common ground," which is any behavior that helps multiple parties find shared goals or interests. While this could be accomplished through asking questions, it can also be accomplished through sharing similar experiences or talking about what the parties have in common, which has the effect of making negotiations go more smoothly and amicably (Fisher and Ury, 1983). While common ground could reflect mutual interests in the negotiation (e.g., the employer and employee both want the employee to start on the same day), common ground can also reflect common pastimes (e.g., we both like playing golf), common background (e.g., we both graduated from the same university), or common goals for the negotiation (e.g., we both want the process to be fair). When negotiators find common ground with each other, they are more likely to share information with each other (Cramton, 2001).

## Tactics to Find a Better Solution

### Add Issues

Adding issues is one of the simplest tactics negotiators have at their disposal and means exactly what it says—adding issues to the negotiating table. For example, in a job negotiation, if an applicant inquires of his or her new manager about possibly having a new laptop as a part of the job package in addition to salary, they are adding the issue of having a laptop to the discussion to the focal or central issue of salary. When issues are added, it gives both sides the opportunity to state whether or not that issue is important to them, which facilitates logrolling, described later. It also

may help find common ground as discussed above. Adding issues might also create value in the negotiation. Let's assume that the laptop (the added issue) is worth $1,500 in value to the individual as that is what it would cost him or her to go out and buy one. Let's further assume that that the company bought the laptop, because of a bulk discount, at $1,200, and that because the manager splits technology acquisitions evenly with the information technology (IT) department, it is worth only $600 off the manager's bottom line. So when the issue of the laptop is added, it is +$1,500 for the individual and −$600 for the manager = $900 of value has been created in the negotiation.

### Nonspecific Compensation

**Nonspecific compensation** is a negotiation tactic that involves adding issues that are not tied to money or compensation. These issues are important to consider as individuals care about more in the world than just money. For a billing specialist, getting the chance to telecommute one day a week (nonspecific compensation) might be more important than getting a 3 percent raise.

### Fractionl Issues

**Fractioning** is a negotiation tactic that involves separating out the various components of a specific issue. While we use the tactic of adding issues to refer to situations where completely different issues are added to the table, fractioning issues refers to situations where current issues are split into component parts to find better solutions. For instance, in the job negotiation example, "compensation" is typically thought of as salary. However, compensation can be fractioned into the component issues of starting salary and bonus (obvious), but also tuition reimbursement and when the employee will get their next raise (less obvious). All four of these directly impact the amount of money the new employee will take home in his or her paycheck. As with adding issues, fractioning issues helps to identify additional issues for discussion, and it facilitates logrolling.

### Logrolling

**Logrolling** is a negotiation tactic that involves trading off on issues that are of different value to each party. This involves three steps. The first step is to "add issues to the table." The second step is to negotiate these issues at the same time. The third step is to realize that each party prefers one issue more than another. The fourth step is to negotiate a tradeoff, where each party receives his or her preferred position on a specific issue. In order to understand logrolling, we can take, for example, a negotiation between a manager and employee over an upcoming mundane financial reporting task assignment. A non-logrolling solution would be the manager telling the employee to take on the assignment, which would effectively end the conflict. A logrolling solution would be that they would first talk about future task assignments in addition to this pending task assignment (Steps 1 and 2). The employee may state that her most important interest is to work more on compliance issues instead of financial reporting, while the manager states that his most important interest is getting this financial reporting task done (Step 3). They then agree that the employee will complete this task as soon as possible, which satisfies the manager's interest, but that the manager will try to assign to the employee only compliance tasks in the future, satisfying the employee's interest (Step 4).

### Making a Packaged Offer

This tactic involves making an offer with multiple issues. While logrolling is always making a packaged offer, a packaged offer does not necessarily involve logrolling. The importance of making a packaged offer and thus keeping all issues on the table tentative until agreement is that it gives all negotiators a chance to see where the possibilities lie for adding further issues, fractioning issues, and logrolling issues. This helps negotiators avoid impasses, as by keeping everything tentative, the parties can always go back and try a different combination of alternatives on the various issues. This is in contrast to an issue-by-issue negotiation, where issues are dropped from discussion as soon as agreement is reached. This issue-by-issue approach lends itself to compromising on each issue.

### Contingent Contracts

This tactic involves negotiators making a "bet" on the future in order to resolve a potentially difficult issue facing them in the negotiation (Bazerman and Gillespie, 1999). That is, what one side gives to the other side is contingent on some future event. A classic example of this involves hospital department revenue. Let's say the ER department and the hospital cannot agree on the appropriate resource level for the department. The department wants to be able to hire five new personnel, and the hospital wants to allocate only enough funds to hire three. At the heart of this debate is the number of patients that are going to be serviced by the ER department in the future, especially given that another community-based emergency

care facility is about to downsize, increasing demand for the hospital ER in question. Of course, neither side knows for sure what that number is going to be—the ER department believes that they will have 63,000 patient discharges the following year (with 20,000 in the next three months) while the hospital thinks this number will be closer to 50,000 (with 15,000 in the next three months).

To solve this conflict, the hospital might commit to hiring two personnel right away, and then allocate future resources contingent on how many patients actually show up in the following three months. If the number of patients has been fewer than 15,000, no additional personnel are hired; if the number of patients is greater than 20,000, three additional personnel are hired; and if the number is in between, they can hire personnel on a sliding scale. The reason contingent contracts help negotiators find better solutions is that if 20,000 patients show up, the hospital is more amenable to hiring the additional personnel, and if the patients do not show up, the department probably did not really need the extra resources. Further, contingent contracts make each party think that their interests have been satisfied, as each party thinks that his or her estimates are correct regarding the future. This is why performance-based bonuses are so popular—if the individual achieves the benchmark (the contingency), the company is more amenable to paying the employee.

## Tactics to Influence the Other Party
### A Strong Opening Offer

Many negotiations have central or key issues that must be discussed and that take a central role in the negotiation (e.g., salary in a job negotiation). Whether or not to make an opening offer on one of these central issues involves a two-part process of deciding whether to open, and what the opening should be. If the negotiator has objective data on what the opening should be, it has been shown that there is a benefit from making an opening offer (Galinsky, 2004). The reason a strong opening offer is beneficial in negotiations is because of the **anchoring bias**. Anchoring is a psychological effect whereby one piece of information—an initial offer in negotiation—tends to influence subsequent thinking. As with any cognitive bias, this is most influential when there is uncertainty in the thinking of one party. The anchor becomes a key piece of information that frames the negotiation and influences how much one party thinks they can get or what the other party is willing to give (Tversky and Kahneman, 1974). If there is no good information or a solid objective justification for the opening offer, it is best not to make one, as an uninformed opening offer has a chance of being either too low or too high. If it is a seller making an opening offer and they start out very low, they are shortchanging themselves; if it is very high, they anger the buyer, which can cause them to walk away.

## *Using Objective Criteria*

From the Merriam-Webster dictionary, "objective" is defined as: "involving or deriving from sense perception or experience with actual objects, conditions, or phenomena" (2009). Notice the word "actual" in the definition—using objective criteria means using "actual" data when presenting arguments. Actual data could be facts, figures, and statistics, anything that is defendable with non-biased information. This is in contrast to subjective arguments, which reside only within one person's mind and are based on one's perceptions. Objective arguments are more effective than subjective arguments because they are rooted in logic, not perception, and are therefore more difficult to refute. Here are some examples:

> *Subjective: This task is really tough.*
> *Subjective: My work is better than hers.*
> *Subjective: But I'm worth more than that.*
> *Objective: We have the lowest patient cost of any department in the hospital.*
> *Objective: I have been able to clear 90 percent of the accounts due at the practice in the last three weeks.*
> *Objective: I saw 73 patients last week, which is a 20 percent increase over the same week last year.*

## *Forming a Coalition*

**Coalitions** represent a limited-term alliance among individuals or groups that is formed in order to strengthen the power of each and further their respective interests. The power of coalitions was discussed previously in this chapter in reference to using power in situations of mutual interest, to manage organizational politics. Coalitions work when parties, who have compatible interests, align themselves in order to negotiate with another party. They can present a unified front against the authority and are much more likely to influence that party because they will have increased their power. For example, when negotiating individually, each member of the staff of a physician practice may have very little power with respect to the physician in charge. However, if particular staff band together to negotiate the hours of the practice, they immediately have much more power and are able to influence

the physician. In a more severe situation, those staff members could enact their power by refusing to work in order to get the concession they desire.

## *Using BATNA/Power of Walk-Away*

**BATNA** stands for "Best Alternative to a Negotiated Agreement." This represents the best option remaining if the current negotiations fail and an agreement cannot be reached. When using a BATNA, it is communicated to the other side that a better offer exists and that the person using the BATNA has the power of walk-away. BATNAs are often used when one party has resource dependency power over another. For example, given how important nurses and physicians are to hospital functioning, these two groups may have the ability to use the BATNA in negotiation situations with extreme effectiveness. For example, unionized nurses can threaten a strike that might shut down the hospital. If one party controls a valued resource, their BATNA to reaching agreement would be to hold that resource until a better offer comes along. As with coalitions, using a BATNA immediately increases power in the negotiation, which can influence what the other side is willing to concede.

## *Plan Concessions*

Concessions in a negotiation communicate information to the other party and thus can be quite influential, especially when the negotiation is focused around one or two issues. When a concession of $100 is given off an item selling at $200, it tells the other party that the item has little value. Similarly, when a concession of $100 is given off an item selling at $20,000, it suggests the item is valued highly and that the seller is not willing to move very much off the current price. Concessions can be quite influential because as a specific type of behavior, a concession communicates information to the other side independent of verbal arguments. Planning concessions is a nonthreatening way to communicate to the other side that moving from the current price is not really an option.

Examples of poorly planned concessions are when a negotiator makes all concessions the same value (e.g., you continually give $500 with every concession) or makes unilateral concessions (two concessions in a row without a concession from the other side). A good strategy when a negotiator knows that they can go no lower than a certain price is to use a gradual reduction concession strategy. This strategy involves reducing the amount of concessions with each successive one. Consider the example of hiring an hourly worker where the four offers made by the company are $7.00, $7.50, $7.80, and $7.90. Reducing concessions from $.50 to $.30 to $.10 communicates to the potential employee that the company is quickly approaching the price at which they can go no higher.

# CONCLUSION

The major themes of this chapter are: (1) power is an endemic force within organizations that can be managed but also abused; (2) politics is a means by which power is manifested; (3) conflict management through negotiation is one way to sort out power and conflict within organizations; and (4) negotiation is both a formal and informal process that has specific steps which can be learned and mastered. A major point is that all three dynamics—power, politics, and conflict—require taking an active role in understanding context, relationships, and the specific issues at hand. This puts the manager squarely in the center of ensuring that existing power dynamics in the organization are used for beneficial and collective outcomes. It also places responsibility on managers and leaders of organizations to identify where power can and will be used inappropriately, and where the use of organizational politics may mask that inappropriate use.

Power and politics often create conflict within organizations, and that is an unavoidable fact that should not be ignored, but rather addressed through the art and science of conflict management. By learning and mastering the activities associated with effective negotiation, individuals in organizations become empowered to resolve conflict in productive, organizationally beneficial ways. As repositories for a wide array of interactions and relationships, the organization is a breeding ground for the cultivation and use of power and politics. It is in recognition of this reality that we view these two dynamics as within the normal purview of a well-functioning organization, through a strategic approach that emphasizes proactive conflict management tools and techniques.

# SUMMARY AND MANAGERIAL GUIDELINES

1. Understand where power comes from in health care organizations. It is important when attempting to understand or manage the use of power to know its particular sources. This helps not only to understand better the nature of how individuals or groups assert their power in the workplace, but also provides information by which to consider targeted management strategies to offset and limit dysfunctional power use.

2. Creating new structural sources for power is perhaps the most efficient way to change the existing power distribution within the organization. In particular, establishing new resource dependencies for different stakeholders can quickly shift who has greater influence over decision making. In situations where there is a high potential for power abuse from a single stakeholder source, making that source suddenly more dependent on others in the organization for their status or resources that help them function can be an effective way to prevent the abuse from occurring.

3. Always identify and assess organizational situations in which it appears that one or more parties are attempting to exert control over another party in a given situation. By studying different control attempts occurring within a setting, you can gain a better sense of who is attempting to exert their power and influence. This enables quicker development of effective strategies to manage the use of that power.

4. All power is relational. So to truly understand power, one must know the different types of relationships that define the organization and, more importantly, how these relationships manifest themselves. This involves observing the relationships as they play out under normal everyday circumstances.

5. Try to view and manage organizations as places filled with shifting coalitions of individuals and groups that come together or oppose each other based upon the current issues at hand, or issues particularly important to one or more of them. This view makes the management job a highly daunting political challenge in the sense of trying to maintain order among the different interests. But it provides a realistic perspective that can help managers understand the barriers to change, as well as how to cultivate issue-specific coalitions to move issues of importance to the organization forward in productive ways.

6. Never assume everyone is the same in terms of power just because they are in the same occupation. Not all physicians or nurses, for example, have equal access to power development and use. Some physicians and nurses have greater influence than others, and knowing how power stratifies within such occupations provides a more accurate read of work situations where both power and politics may be at work.

7. Power abuse can be avoided proactively by pursuing principles such as transparency, fairness, and trust within organizations. These principles can be translated into specific types of actions and value systems that all employees can learn about, buy into, and use to help create an ethical organizational climate, and one in which the abuse of power remains something rarer and less destructive for the organization as a whole.

8. Do not assume that just because you have a lot of experience negotiating, you are an expert negotiator. Most individuals have a hindsight bias whereby they evaluate past outcomes more favorably than they actually were. Realize that they are multiple ways to solve conflict—not just in the manner or fashion to which you are accustomed.

9. Resist the urge to use authority just because you have it. In the context of conflict management, resist using formal sources of power and a competitive strategy, which may not be the best option or lead to the most effective solution. This is especially problematic for first-time managers.

10. Think about implementation when you are working on an agreement. In other words, how is this agreement going to affect you one week, one month, and one year down the road in your relationship with the other party? If you know that there is no way you or others are going to work to carry out the agreement, solve that problem before you leave the table.

11. If you reach an impasse, take a break and reevaluate. Emotionally laden negotiations can not only hinder creative thinking and problem solving, but they can also damage relationships and hurt your confidence in future negotiations. Be thinking about this as you approach the impasse and ask the other side if it is okay to take a break and think things over.

12. Get advice from others when solving conflict. Usually when one is involved in a conflict, it is difficult to view that situation objectively from all sides. This is because we are biased creatures—we automatically think that we are right, simply because we have a position that we are trying to achieve. Having a third party, whether it is a mentor or friend outside the negotiation or a mediator in the negotiation, can help you work through the negotiation process and come up with creative solutions.

13. Remember that you have to give the other side enough in the negotiation for them to say "yes" to the deal, because getting them to say "yes" will ultimately get you what you want. When you focus only on your interests and possible positions to satisfy those interests, you ignore the interests of the other side, which may inhibit your ability to get them to agree.

## DISCUSSION QUESTIONS

1. How can managers best use the principles of effective negotiation and conflict management to resolve power struggles within health care settings? What types of power struggles in health care settings do you believe are most amenable to using negotiation and conflict management techniques?

2. What are specific ways to limit the potential for power abuse in health care organizations? What specific human resource strategies and transparency mechanisms could be created within hospitals or physician practices, for example, that would help prevent any stakeholder, particularly the top leaders of an organization, from pursuing self-interested goals in suspect ways?

3. What would be situations in which a collaborative or a competitive strategy might be most beneficial when managing conflict in health care organizations? What issues unique to health care organizations would be particularly difficult to negotiate using each of these strategic approaches?

4. In thinking about the power relationships unique to health care organizations (e.g., physician-patient), what might be some of the challenges to effective negotiation? Think about these challenges in the context of the common mistakes made when thinking about conflict and when managing relationships.

# CASE: To Open or Not to Open—That Is the Question

James had eight years experience in health care human resources and wanted to move up into an administrative position. So he decided to go back to school part time for three more years and get a master's of business administration (MBA). As James was approaching the completion of his MBA, his boss, Jayne, knew that he was looking for a new position with a new salary. Before they sat down to talk, neither of them knew exactly what the new salary should be. James was making $63,000 currently and Jayne had no idea what James could make on the open market—3 percent more, 5 percent more, 10 percent more? She wants to be fair, but she also needs to keep her budget under control. James decided to use this uncertainty to his advantage, so he did research and decided to make a strong opening offer.

**James:** "Jayne, I really appreciate you meeting with me."

**Jayne:** "No problem. I'm really proud of you finishing your MBA. Congratulations!"

**James:** "Thank you. I of course do not want there to be any tension between us, so in anticipation for our meeting, I've tried to do quite a bit of research on what a fair salary increase would be. Is it okay if I present you with this information?"

**Jayne:** "Sure."

**James:** "Okay, so the first thing I did was look at the average starting salaries for everyone graduating from my MBA program. This is based on 330 graduates over the last three years and the number was $91,000. Of course not all of those are based in health care, so the next thing I did was look at those in health care with 10–15 years experience and an advanced degree. It's not easy to get this information, but from three people in this company and three others I know, the salaries ranged from $75,000 to $97,000 with an average of $88,000. Finally, I looked at the last person in my position to get an advanced degree, and she received a 20 percent raise, which for me would be $12,600 and take me to $75,600. So in averaging $75,600, $88,000, and $91,000, I came up with about $85,000. I was hoping we could start the discussion around there."

**Jayne:** "That's really impressive research and I respect that. We probably can't go that high but let me see what I can do."

The impetus is now on Jayne to negotiate James off his number, which is $85,000. This creates a much different negotiation than if Jayne opened with a 5 percent raise, which would have anchored the negotiation around $66,000. The impact is that the $85,000, along with the justification, changes the way Jayne is thinking about the negotiation. She might realize that they need to go to $80,000 to keep James now, whereas perhaps before the negotiation, she might have had $75,000 in her mind as the high number.

## Questions

1. Where do you think this negotiation will end up?
2. What would you have done if you were James?
3. When dealing with conflict, do you think about how to begin?
4. What are other types of opening "offers" that have nothing to do with money but that still set the tone for the negotiation?
5. How can you use various types of openings to your advantage?

# REFERENCES

Adamson, R. E., & Taylor, D. W. (1954). Functional fixedness as related to elapsed time and to set. *Journal of Experimental Psychology, 47*(2), 122–126.

Alford, C. F. (2001). *Broken lives and organizational power.* Ithaca, NY: Cornell University Press.

Armstrong, K. A., Rose, A., Peters N., Long, J. A., McMurphy, S., & Shea, J. (2006). Distrust of the health care system and self-reported health in the United States. *Journal of General Internal Medicine, 21*(4), 292–297.

Ashforth, B. E., & Johnson, S. A. (2001). Which hat to wear? The relative salience of multiple identities in organizational contexts. In M. A. Hogg & D. J. Terry (Eds.), *Social identity processes in organizational contexts* (pp. 31–48). Philadelphia, PA: Psychology Press.

Axelrod, R. (1984). *The evolution of cooperation.* New York: Basic Books.

Barsade, S. G. (2002). The ripple effect: Emotional contagion and its influence on group behavior. *Administrative Science Quarterly, 47,* 644–675.

Bazerman, M. H., & Gillespie, J. J. (1999). Betting on the future: The virtues of contingent contracts. *Harvard Business Review, 77,* 155–160.

Blau, P. M. (1964). *Exchange and power in social life.* New York: John Wiley.

Brass, D. J., Burkhardt, M. E., & Marlene, E. (1993). Potential power and power use: An investigation of structure and behavior. *Academy of Management Journal, 36*(3), 441–471.

Burawoy, M. (1979). *Manufacturing consent.* Chicago: University of Chicago Press.

Carnevale, P. J., & Probst, T. M. (1998). Social values and social conflict in creative problem solving and categorization. *Journal of Personality and Social Psychology, 74,* 1300–1309.

Cialdini, R. B. (2001). The science of persuasion. *Scientific American,* 143–148.

Cramton, C. D. (2001). The mutual knowledge problem and its consequences for dispersed collaboration. *Organization Science, 12,* 346–371.

Crozier, M. (1964). *The bureaucratic phenomenon.* Chicago: University of Chicago Press.

Dahl, R. A. (1957). The concept of power. *Behavioral Science, 2,* 201–215.

De Dreu, C. K. W., & Weingart, L. R. (2003). Task versus relationship conflict, team performance, and team member satisfaction: A meta-analysis. *Journal of Applied Psychology, 88,* 741–749.

Eagly, A. H., & Chaiken, S. (1993). *The psychology of attitudes.* Orlando, FL: Harcourt Brace Jovanovich.

Eisenhart, K. M., & Bourgeois, L. J. (1988). Politics of strategic decision making in high-velocity environments: Toward a midrange theory. *Academy of Management Journal, 31*(4), 737–770.

Finkelstein, S. (1992). Power in top management teams: Dimensions, measurement, and validation. *Academy of Management Journal, 35*(3), 505–538.

Fisher, R., & Ury, W. L. (1983). *Getting to yes: Negotiating agreement without giving in.* New York: Penguin Books.

Freidson, E. 1970. *Profession of medicine.* Chicago: University of Chicago Press.

Fukuyama, F. (1995). Trust: The social virtues and the creation of prosperity. New York: Free Press.

Galinsky, A. D. (2004). Should you make your first offer? *Negotiation Journal, 7,* 1–4.

Gerstner, L. (2002). *Who says elephants can't dance?* New York: Harper Business.

Hardy, C., & Clegg, S. R. (1996). Some dare call it power. In S. Clegg, C. Hardy, & W. Nord (Eds.), *Handbook of organizational studies* (pp. 622–640). Thousand Oaks, CA: Sage Publications.

Hart, P., & Saunders, C. (1997). Power and trust: Critical factors in the adoption and use of electronic data interchange. *Organization Science, 8*(1), 23–42.

Hatcher, T. (2002). Ethics and HRD: A new approach to leading responsible organizations. Cambridge, MA: Persuns Publishing.

Hickson, D. J., Hinings, C. R., Lee, C. A., Schneck, R. E., & Pennings, J. M. (1971). A strategic contingencies theory of intraorganizational power. *Administrative Science Quarterly, 16*(2), 216–229.

Hoff, T. J. (2003). The power of frontline workers in transforming government: The Upstate New York Veterans Healthcare Network. Washington, DC: IBM Endowment for the Business of Government.

Horrocks, S., Anderson, E., & Salisbury, C. (2002). Systematic review of whether nurse practitioners working in primary care can provide equivalent care to doctors. *British Medical Journal, 324*(7341), 819–823.

Ibarra, H., & Andrews, S. B. (1993). Power, social influence, and sense making: Effects of network centrality and proximity on employee perceptions. *Administrative Science Quarterly, 38*(2), 277–303.

Jehn, K. (1997). Affective and cognitive conflict in work groups: Increasing performance through value-based intragroup conflict. In C. K. W. De Dreu & E. Van de Vliert (Eds.), Using conflict in organizations (pp. 87–100). London: Sage.

Locke, E. A., & Latham, G. P. (1990). *A theory of goal setting & task performance*. Englewood Cliffs, NJ: Prentice Hall.

Malhotra, D. (2004). Trust and reciprocity decisions: The differing perspectives of trustors and trusted parties. *Organizational Behavior and Human Decision Processes, 91*, 61–73.

Martin, J. (1992). *Cultures in organizations: Three perspectives*. New York: Oxford University Press.

Mayes, B. T., & Allen, R. W. (1977). Toward a definition of organizational politics. *The Academy of Management Review, 2*(4), 672–678.

McEvily, B., Perrone, V., & Zaheer, A. (2003). Trust as an organizing principle. *Organization Science, 14*(1), 91–103.

Merton, R. K. (1968). *Social theory and social structure*. New York: Free Press.

Mintzberg, H. (1983). *Power in and around organizations*. Englewood Cliffs, NJ: Prentice Hall.

Mintzberg, H., Raisinghani, D., & Theoret, A. (1976). The structure of "unstructured" decision processes. *Administrative Science Quarterly, 21*(2), 246–275.

"Objective." (2009). In *Merriam-Webster Online Dictionary*. Retrieved November 15, 2009, from http://www.merriam-webster.com/dictionary/objective.

Perrow, C. (1989). *Complex organizations: A critical essay*. New York: McGraw-Hill.

Pew Internet and American Life Project. (2002). *Counting on the Internet: Most find the information they seek, expect*. Washington, DC.

Pfeffer, J. (1981). *Power in organizations*. Boston, MA: Pitman Publishing.

Pfeffer, J., & Salancik, G. R. (1978). *The external control of organizations: A resource dependence perspective*. New York: Harper and Row.

Pruitt, D. G., & Rubin, J. Z. (1986). *Social conflict: Escalation, stalemate, and settlement*. New York: Random House.

Ragins, B. R. (1993). Gender gap in the executive suite: CEOs and female executives report on breaking the glass ceiling. *The Academy of Management Executive, 12*(1), 28–42.

Salancik, G. R., & Pfeffer, J. (1977). Who gets power—and how they hold on to it: A strategic contingency model of power. *Organizational Dynamics*, 3–21.

Schein, E. H. (1992). Organizational culture and leadership. San Francisco: Jossey-Bass.

Sitkin, S. B., & Stickel, D. (1996). The road to hell: The dynamics of distrust in an era of quality. In R. M. Kramer & T. R. Tyler (Eds.), *Trust in organizations*. Englewood Cliffs, NJ: Prentice Hall.

Slater, R. (1999). *Jack Welch and the GE way*. New York: McGraw-Hill.

Starr, P. (1982). *The social transformation of American medicine*. New York: Basic Books.

Staw, B. M., Sandelands, L. E., & Dutton, J. E. (1981). Threat-rigidity effects in organizational behavior: A multilevel analysis. *Administrative Science Quarterly, 26*, 501–524.

Thibodeaux, M. S., & Powell, J. D. (Spring, 1985). Exploitations: Ethical problems of organizational power. *SAM Advanced Management Journal*, 42–44.

Thompson, L. L. (2005). *The mind and the heart of the negotiator* (3rd ed.). Upper Saddle River, NJ: Prentice Hall.

Tversky, A., & Kahneman, D. (1974). Judgment under uncertainty: Heuristics and biases. *Science, 185*, 1124–1131.

Wachter, R. M., & Shojana, K. G. (2004). *Internal bleeding*. New York: Rugged Land.

Weber, J. M., Malhotra, D., and Murnighan, J. K. (2005). Normal acts of irrational trust, motivated attributions, and the process of trust development. In B. M. Staw and R. M. Kramer (Eds.), *Research in organizational behavior* (Vol. 26, pp. 75–102). New York: Elsevier.

Weber, M. (1978). *Economy and society: An outline of interpretive sociology* (2 vols.) (G. Roth & C. Wittich, Eds.). Berkeley: University of California Press.

Weingart, L. R., Brett, J. M., Olekalns, M., & Smith, P. L. (2007). Conflicting social motives in negotiating groups. *Journal of Personality and Social Psychology, 93*, 994–1010.

Westheafer, C. (2000). Integrating perspectives within a framework: Taming the dark side. *Organizational Development Journal, 18*(3), 63–74.

Whitener, E. M., Brodt, S. E., Korsgaard, M. A., & Werner, J. M. (1998). Managers as initiators of trust: An exchange relationship framework for understanding managerial trustworthy behavior. *Academy of Management Review, 23*(3), 513–530.

Wilson, J. Q. (1989). *Bureaucracy: What government agencies do and why they do it*. New York: Basic Books.

# Chapter 8

# Complexity, Learning, and Innovation

Bryan J. Weiner and Christian D. Helfrich

## CHAPTER OUTLINE

- **Health Care Organizations as Complex Systems**
- **Complexity and Feedback: A Closer Look**
- **Organizational Learning**
- **Innovation and Learning**
- **Managing Complexity, Learning, and Innovation**

## LEARNING OBJECTIVES

**After completing this chapter, the reader should be able to:**

1. Identify the characteristics that make health care organizations complex systems
2. Describe the five disciplines that promote organizational learning
3. Explain why organizational learning often proves difficult in practice
4. Describe how new-to-the-world innovations develop
5. Identify common myths and misconceptions about innovation
6. Discuss strategies for promoting organizational learning and innovation

# KEY TERMS

Adaptive Learning

Balancing Feedback Loops

Complex Systems

Combinatorial Complexity

Detail Complexity

Discovery

Double-Loop Learning

Dynamic Complexity

Emergence

Generative Learning

Innovation

Learning

Learning Organization

Mental Models

Organizational Learning

Personal Mastery

Policy Resistance

Reinforcing Feedback Loops

Shared Vision

Single-Loop Learning

Systems Thinking

Team Learning

Testing

---

**IN PRACTICE:** Learning from Mistakes: Problems Created by an Access Initiative Turn into Solutions in a Patient-Centered Medical Home

In 2002, Group Health Cooperative launched an ambitious plan to improve access and efficiency in primary care. Group Health is a mixed-model health maintenance organization (HMO) headquartered in Seattle, Washington, serving approximately a half-million members in Washington State and northern Idaho. In the late 1990s, the HMO saw its enrollment decline by 16 percent while the proportion of insured citizens remained stable. Facing declining enrollment and revenues (Robert Wood Johnson Foundation, 2008), Group Health responded with the Access Initiative: five major categories of changes based on the Institute of Medicine's principles of patient-centered care, including Web-based secure messaging with providers, redesigning the primary-care teams, instituting a new productivity-based compensation system for physicians, and allowing members direct access to specialists. Group Health realized several expected benefits from Access Initiative: (1) higher overall patient satisfaction; (2) higher patient satisfaction with specific dimensions of access, such as being able to see the doctor when needed and minimizing time spent scheduling an appointment (Ralston et al., 2009); and (3) improved efficiency, both in terms of relative value units per full-time equivalent employee (i.e., a measure of the complexity of care being delivered by the clinical staff) and in terms of per-patient, per-quarter costs (Conrad et al., 2008).

However, the Access Initiative also brought increases in provider workload and troubling decreases in provider satisfaction. Providers reported routinely serving 12- to 15-hour days and feeling acute emotional burnout. Related consequences included not keeping up with the medical literature and putting information into medical records that they deemed clinically unhelpful but administratively required (Tufano, Ralston, and Martin, 2008). Equally serious, Group Health observed declines in quality of care indicators and increases in patient utilization in "downstream" services, such as specialty care, emergency care, and inpatient days (Reid et al., 2009; Robert Wood Johnson Foundation, 2008).

Because of these unexpected, undesired outcomes (i.e., mistakes) Group Health launched a pilot program to elevate some of the ideals of primary care that the Access Initiative had subordinated in the pursuit of access and efficiency (Ralston et al., 2009). Most notably, the pilot program reversed two Access Initiative components: (1) it radically decreased the providers'

---

**IN PRACTICE:  Learning from Mistakes: Problems Created by an Access Initiative Turn into Solutions in a Patient-Centered Medical Home  *(Continued)***

---

panel sizes, and (2) it exempted providers from the performance-based pay incentives. The pilot also made changes in patient outreach (e.g., systematic follow-up after emergency room visits), point-of-care processes (e.g., pairing of a physician with a medical assistant), organizational structure (e.g., collocation of primary team members), and management process (e.g., daily team huddles). This involved a significant up-front investment by the HMO: increases of 15 percent in physician staffing, 17 percent in medical assistants, and 72 percent in clinical pharmacists. They also had to reassign 25 percent of the clinics' patients to new providers to accommodate the smaller panel sizes and increased visit length (Reid et al., 2009).

Results proved encouraging. Compared to control clinics (which are Access Initiative sites), the pilot clinic saw improvements on six of seven patient satisfaction indicators; 10 percent of providers reporting high emotional burnout versus 30 percent in the control clinics; and improvements in quality-of-care indicators. Group Health also saw a decline in emergency department visits of sufficient size to recoup both the cost of staffing increases and the cost of an unexpected increase in specialty visits, so at the end of 12 months the pilot intervention had paid for itself.

The Commonwealth Fund (McCarthy, Mueller, and Tillmann, 2009) and others have touted the pilot program as a possible national model for a patient-centered medical home. But the story does not end here. The pilot program was, after all, only a pilot program. The rollout of the medical home concept in Group Health Cooperative's remaining 19 clinics is ongoing. Experience tells us that the medical home will bring some new problems—for example, the pilot program already observed an unexpected increase in specialty-care visits. The challenge facing Group Health is not to avoid mistakes in the future; it is to look for those new problems as opportunities to learn and further innovate.

# CHAPTER PURPOSE

The experience of Group Health Cooperative with the Access Initiative, and their subsequent pilot of a patient-centered medical home (see "In Practice: Learning from Mistakes"), illustrates three major themes of this chapter: (1) health care organizations are complex systems that respond to stimuli in expected *and* unexpected ways; (2) organizational learning becomes essential to managing complex systems; and (3) mistakes *and* unexpected outcomes can serve as the basis for novelty and innovation—provided that learning occurs.

For managers, one of the most perplexing features of health care organizations is that they frequently exhibit counterintuitive behavior. Health maintenance organizations (HMOs) begin requiring physicians to choose less expensive generic drugs, only to find that pharmaceutical costs rise rather than fall due to unintended changes in physicians' prescribing behavior. Hospitals implement quality management tools and practices that have been proven effective in manufacturing settings, only to find that quality of care worsens rather than improves. A physician group practice introduces electronic medical records and medical errors decrease, but only for a few months, after which they rise to levels even higher than before. A department manager introduces a flexible work schedule to improve job satisfaction and job retention, only to see morale plummet and turnover increase as nurses find themselves working longer hours with less predictability in assignments.

Social systems rarely behave the way we want them to, or even the way that we predict they will. Due to unanticipated consequences, yesterday's solutions become today's problems. Our efforts to introduce change provoke opposition by those who seek to maintain the status quo. We apply solutions that worked well before or work for others, only to find that they do not work again or do not work for us. So, we try harder, applying them with even greater fervor, but the problem only gets worse. Or the solution works, but introduces such deleterious side effects that the cure seems worse than the disease.

To understand and mitigate such counterintuitive dynamics, health care leaders need to rethink their views of how organizations work and how they can be improved and changed. In this chapter, we introduce a perspective of health care organizations as complex systems whose future states are unpredictable. Moreover, we regard innovation and change not as rational, controllable processes, but instead as complex, uncertain, nonlinear sequences of events and activities, often driven by actors' perceptions that are necessarily limited and flawed. Bridging these perspectives and integrating them is the notion of the **learning organization**, where innovation and change (and for that matter, mistakes) are seen as routine and as inputs for further learning (McGill and Slocum, 1993). The chapter concludes with guidelines for managing complexity, learning, and innovation.

# HEALTH CARE ORGANIZATIONS AS COMPLEX SYSTEMS

Management theories reflect the "governing ideas" of their time. At the turn of the last century, management theories embraced a mechanistic view of social systems inspired by Newtonian physics (see Chapter 1). In the 1960s and 1970s, management theories took an organic view of social systems, reflecting developments in biology, ecology, and evolutionary theory. Since the 1990s, new management ideas have appeared as scholars and practitioners absorb the new science of complexity emerging in meteorology, biology, physics, chemistry, and mathematics (Arndt and Bigelow, 2000; Begun, 1994; Burnes, 2005; Lemak and Goodrick, 2003; Plsek and Greenhalgh, 2001; Senge, 2006; Stacey, 1995; Wheatley, 2006). According to this view, organizations are dynamic, nonlinear systems that operate "at the edge of chaos," constantly changing, never quite settling into a predictable pattern, yet displaying complex forms of order within boundary conditions.

What do weather systems, ant colonies, human economies, and health care organizations have in common? They are all **complex systems**: arrangements of interacting, interdependent parts that produce emergent behavior—that is, collective behavior that cannot be predicted based on the behavior of individual parts. Not all systems are complex systems. Complex systems exhibit three defining characteristics. First, complex systems are richly interconnected. That is, system elements are connected in many different ways, and these connections vary in levels of

responsiveness (Marion and Bacon, 2000). Some connections respond rapidly and strongly, some slowly and weakly, and some moderately in terms of timeliness and intensity. Management theories have long recognized that organizations are comprised of numerous, diverse, interdependent parts. Complexity theory suggests that organizations are more than simply open systems; they are "massively entangled" systems (Begun, Zimmerman, and Dooley, 2003).

Second, complex systems are nonlinear (Stacey, 1995). In *linear* systems, output is directly proportional to its input. Small causes have small effects. Big causes have big effects. By contrast, in *nonlinear* systems, output is not directly proportional to its input. Small changes can produce big effects, small effects, or no effects at all, depending on the complex chain of cause-and-effect loops operating in the system. Nonlinearity, combined with dense interconnectedness, makes the behavior of complex systems impossible to reliably predict.

Third, complex systems are dynamic. Not only do systems have the capacity to change, but prior states can influence present events. Management theories are often criticized as discounting the importance of time and history (Pettigrew, 1985). Complexity theory suggests that a system's history cannot be ignored. The set of decisions one faces for any given circumstance is limited by the decisions one has made in the past, even when those past circumstances no longer exist.

These characteristics—interconnectedness, nonlinearity, and dynamism—make complex systems unpredictable and challenging to manage. Managers can be caught off guard when seemingly small, incremental, local changes in one part of the organization rather quickly produce large, undesirable effects in other parts of the organization. Modest changes in the standard operating procedures of the intensive care unit, for example, can quickly cascade into bed shortages in general nursing wards and disruptions in operating room schedules. Likewise, minor "technical" fixes in information systems to address patient registration problems can lead to hundreds of thousands of dollars in lost billing. Contrary to our usual thinking, effects are not always proportional to causes, nor are causes and effects always closely linked in time and space.

Likewise, in complex systems, small differences in initial conditions can send these systems down different developmental pathways. Two community health centers with comparable levels of financial resources, management support, and technical assistance trying to implement the same diabetes registry can follow very different trajectories and experience radically different outcomes due to seemingly small differences in how the physician champion frames the change effort for other providers and staff. Given the sensitivity of complex systems to initial conditions, complexity science warns that programs, processes, or practices that work well in one health care organization may work poorly (or not at all) in another health care organization even when faithfully implemented (Wheatley, 2006).

Finally, complex systems can adjust to a wide variety of environmental conditions. In the language of complexity theory, they are robust, meaning that they resist perturbation or invasion by other systems (Marion and Bacon, 2000). Health care organizations have exhibited a remarkable ability to adjust to policy and market shocks (e.g., prospective payment and managed care) and slower, cumulative changes in operating conditions (Begun and Luke, 2001). While admirable, such resiliency gives rise to **policy resistance**: the tendency for interventions to be delayed, diluted, or defeated by the response of the system to the intervention itself (Sterman, 2000). Much to the consternation of policy makers, managers, clinicians, and patients, health care organizations often respond in ways that confound our understanding and thwart our intentions.

Paradoxically, the same features that make complex systems perplexing and seemingly unmanageable also create endless potential for innovation, creativity, and novelty. Although complex systems behave unpredictably, they do not behave randomly. Rather, they exhibit a complex form of order that Ralph Stacey (1995) calls "bounded instability." In this state, a complex system's behavior follows an inherently unpredictable path, but it does so within limits. While we cannot predict the specific course of the system's behavior over time, we can discern a pattern to its long-term behavior, and we can make somewhat accurate predictions about its short-term behavior. To use a meteorological example, we cannot make accurate predictions of what the weather will be three weeks from now, but we can make reasonably accurate predictions of what the weather will be tomorrow or the day after tomorrow. Moreover, we can see recognizable patterns of temperature, precipitation, and humidity over the long term, even if we cannot predict precisely the weather pattern more than a few days hence.

Complexity-oriented management scholars contend that organizations also exhibit bounded instability (Black, 2000; Fitzgerald, 2002; Hock and VISA International, 1999; Stacey, 1995; Tetenbaum, 1998). That is, organizations never quite settle into a stable equilibrium, but they generally do not fall apart, either. Between order (stability) and chaos (instability), there is an intermediate zone that some scholars poetically call "the edge of chaos" (Hock and VISA International, 1999). When organizations operate at the edge of chaos, new ideas, products, practices, and relationships can spontaneously emerge that are neither predicted nor anticipated by participants or observers. Complexity theorists refer to this phenomenon as **emergence**. The challenge for managers, complexity-oriented management scholars say, is not to give in to the pull of either order (stability) or chaos (anything goes), but rather to sustain organization at the edge of chaos, where continuous innovation and adaptability are possible (Brown and Eisenhardt, 1997; Jenner, 1998; Tetenbaum, 1998).

So, where does complexity science leave the health care manager? How do you manage, let alone lead, a complex system? No new management theory has emerged from complexity science, but scholars and practitioners see two implications for management. First, if we embrace the notion of health care organizations as complex systems, then we need new concepts and new tools to inform our thinking about how innovation, performance, and change occur in health care organizations (Mintzberg, 1994; Senge, 2006; Stacey, 1995). In particular, we need to look closely at our ideas about complexity and feedback and, perhaps, employ systems dynamics and other modeling approaches to simulate the implications of the decisions we make. Second, viewing health care organizations as complex systems entails a fundamental shift in thinking about the role of management (Beeson and Davis, 2000; Rowe and Hogarth, 2005; Sullivan, 1999; Tetenbaum, 1998; Wheatley, 2006). Complexity science draws attention to the limits of managerial control and the ease with which policy resistance occurs because of, not in spite of, our efforts to impose change in complex systems. From a complexity science perspective, managing involves seeing systems as "wholes," looking for leverage points that turn small changes into large effects, and creating conditions for organizational members to learn and improvise in real time (Senge, 2006). In the sections that follow, we explore these two implications of complexity science in the context of innovation and learning.

## DEBATE TIME: How to Manage Complex Systems

Is there still a role in complex systems for the classical management tasks of planning, organizing, deciding, and controlling? Some management scholars and practitioners argue that organizational survival depends on managers giving up their "obsession with control, knowing what is going on, and seeking stability" (Berquist, 1993; McDaniel, 1997; Vaill, 1989; Wheatley, 1992). Others contend that classical management tasks still have a place in complex systems. For instance, Stacey (1995) proposes that, in complex systems, selecting the appropriate management or leadership approaches depends on two factors: the amount of certainty about cause-and-effect linkages ("If we do X, then Y occurs") and the amount of agreement about an issue or decision ("What should we do?"). When high certainty and high agreement exist, then classical management tasks work well. Plsek and Greenhalgh (2001) observe, for instance, that a surgical team doing a routine gallbladder surgery exhibits high certainty about the surgical procedures that lead to successful outcomes and high agreement about how to do the work together. Managing such situations calls for using data from the past to predict the future, planning paths of action to achieve outcomes, and monitoring actual versus expected outcomes in order to reduce variation. When uncertainty is high and disagreement reigns, chaos and anarchy often result. In such situations, few management or leadership approaches work. When only modest levels of certainty and agreement exist, organizations enter the "zone of complexity," or the "edge of chaos," where high levels of creativity and innovation become possible. In this zone, managers cannot hope to understand what a complex system will do or how to optimize it. Hence, traditional management approaches lose their effectiveness. Instead, managers should lead by setting a few simple rules, establishing a "good enough" vision, and creating a wide space for innovation.

## IN PRACTICE: New Concepts for Leading Healthcare Organizations

For James Roberts, MD, senior vice president of VHA, Inc., the concepts of self-organization, co-evolution, and emergence proved useful for understanding and guiding the creation of the VHA's Physician Leadership Network. The concept of co-evolution, for instance, sensitized him to the interdependence that existed within VHA. As the organization developed a comparative database of physician practices, the relationships among the VHA's Dallas headquarters, the regional offices, and the physicians began to change. When relationships are co-evolving rather than being dominated by one partner, ideas for new products, services, and processes emerge that no participant alone could have created or anticipated. "This idea of co-evolving with our customers is one of the most powerful ideas around today. It's really forced me to think about the barriers to us really working together, coevolving. How do we blur the distinctions between providers, customers, and suppliers? After all, we are all in this together" (Zimmerman, 1999).

# COMPLEXITY AND FEEDBACK: A CLOSER LOOK

Like other complex systems, health care organizations exhibit two forms of complexity. **Combinatorial complexity**, or **detail complexity**, arises from the number of constituent elements of a system or the number of interrelationships that might exist among them (Senge, 2006). For instance, the problem of optimally scheduling a suite of operating rooms in a hospital is highly complex. However, the problem's complexity lies in finding the best solution out of an astronomical number of possibilities. For some perspective, imagine that the world operated according to 138 logical, independent propositions, such as, "Consumers will select the lowest price option, all things being equal." These 138 propositions produce so many combinations of potential outcomes that a super-computer operating since the beginning of time would still be evaluating them (Cherniak, 1986).

**Dynamic complexity**, or nonlinearity, arises from the operation of feedback loops (Sterman, 2000). There are two basic types of feedback loops. **Reinforcing feedback loops** amplify or intensify whatever is happening in a system. In everyday language, we refer to reinforcing feedback loops as self-fulfilling prophecies, or the "Pygmalion Effect." For instance, a physician group practice that delivers high-quality care develops a positive reputation, which, through positive word of mouth, generates more referrals. More referrals, in turn, generate more resources that could be invested to further increase quality of care. **Balancing feedback loops** counteract or oppose whatever is happening in a system. For example, when the physicians in a group practice see more patients than they can realistically manage, patient satisfaction and possibly quality of care begin to suffer. Over time, negative word of mouth leads to fewer referrals and lighter schedules. Whereas reinforcing feedback loops drive a system toward disequilibrium and constitute the engines of accelerating growth or accelerating decline, balancing feedback loops drive a system toward equilibrium and constitute the engines of steady states or goal-oriented behavior. It is important to emphasize that reinforcing feedback loops can produce desirable or undesirable consequences. So, too, can balancing feedback loops.

Although combinatorial or "detail" complexity is important, dynamic complexity is critical to understanding the behavior of complex systems. When dynamic complexity exists (that is, when feedback loops operate), the same action can have different effects in the short term and the long term. Likewise, actions can have one consequence locally and a different consequence elsewhere in the system. Policy resistance itself signals the presence of dynamic complexity. What makes dynamic complexity "complex" is that feedback loops often contain delays—or interruptions between actions and consequences—that are poorly understood and often ignored. People have difficulty grasping system dynamics when cause and effect are distant from one another in space or time. In addition, most complex systems possess dozens or even hundreds of interlocking feedback loops. People can sometimes infer correctly the dynamics of systems possessing isolated loops; however, a system possessing multiple, interlocking loops quickly exceeds human perceptual and cognitive limitations (Sterman, 2000).

Systems dynamics can be a useful method for overcoming these limitations and gaining insight into the behavior of complex systems. Systems dynamics is a set of concepts and tools developed at Massachusetts Institute of Technology in the 1950s to help corporate managers improve executive decision making about industrial processes. Systems dynamics applications typically involve the development of computer simulations. Just as airlines use flight simulators to help pilots, managers can use systems dynamics to develop what Sterman (2000) calls "management simulators" that help them understand dynamic complexity, gain insight into sources of policy resistance, and explore implications of managerial decisions. In the field of health policy, systems dynamics models have been used to assess the impact of telecare innovations (Bayer, Barlow, and Curry, 2007), examine the perils and promises of chronic disease management strategies (Homer et al., 2004; Homer, Hirsch, and Milstein, 2007), and explore options for expanding health care system capacity to meet rising demand (Wolstenholme, 2004).

Systems dynamics models, particularly in the form of computer simulations, have several virtues (Sterman, 2000). First, they permit controlled experimentation, enabling managers to test strategies and learn more rapidly than the real world permits. In simulations, time can be compressed in order to reduce delays between cause and effect, acts can be reversed entirely or repeated under different conditions, and action can be stopped to permit reflection and dialogue. Second, simulations relax the performance pressures of the real world, creating a safe environment for managers to explore "what if" scenarios involving high-risk strategies or implausible situations. Finally, simulations can provide managers with "perfect, immediate, undistorted, and complete outcome feedback" (Sterman, 2000). Such high-quality outcome feedback allows managers to see the underlying structure of the complex system that they manage—and, importantly, to examine their own mental representations of it—in ways that the real world rarely, if ever, provides.

Systems dynamics models are not forecasting tools. Their value lies not in the prediction of some future state of the world, but rather in the creation of *low-cost laboratories* for learning in complex systems. Effective systems dynamics models as learning laboratories, however, requires systems thinking and other "disciplines" that support organizational learning.

# ORGANIZATIONAL LEARNING

**Learning** involves the acquisition of knowledge or skills through study, instruction, or experience. Learning is essentially a feedback process. We take action, we gather information about the effects of our action, and then we revise our understanding of our world and ourselves. In its simplest form, learning resembles a balancing feedback loop in which we compare a desired (or anticipated) state of affairs with the actual results of our conduct, and then act in ways that we believe or hope will close the gap (Cyert and March, 1992). Argyris and Schon (1978) refer to this type of learning as **single-loop learning**, a relatively simple error-and-correction process whereby problem solvers look for solutions within an organization's policies, plans, values, and rules. A more complex form of learning, **double-loop learning**, occurs when problem solvers attempt to close the gap between desired and actual states of affairs by questioning and modifying those organization's policies, plans, values, and rules that frame organizational problems and guide organizational action (Argyris and Schon, 1978). Changes in underlying values and assumptions, in turn, prompt changes in action strategies (see Figure 8.1).

Both single-loop and double-loop learning are necessary and useful for health care organizations. Single-loop learning promotes **adaptive learning**, in which problem solvers adjust their behavior and work processes in response to changing events or trends. For instance, a quality improvement team might invoke the Plan-Do-Study-Act (PDSA) cycle (Berwick, 1998)—a form of single-loop learning—in order to test the effectiveness of putting hand sanitizer dispensers in hallways and patient rooms to reduce hospital-acquired infections and thereby shorten lengths of stay. Double-loop learning promotes **generative learning**, in which problem solvers attempt to eliminate problems by changing the underlying structure of the system. This underlying structure includes the "operating policies" of the decision makers and actors in the system (i.e., their values and assumptions). For instance, a quality improvement team seeking to reduce handoffs among clinical professionals and thereby increase quality and safety might begin questioning deeply held assumptions about the value of staff specialization. On the basis of such

questioning, they may redesign the care delivery system to employ multiskilled employees working in small, empowered work teams (Leander, 1996; Wermers et al., 1996).

We often think of learning as an individual process. However, learning is a not solitary activity. Learning is a social enterprise that involves the creation, retention, and transfer of knowledge at individual, group, and organizational levels. In organizations, learning exhibits a circular dynamic where knowledge flows from the individual level to the group level to the organizational level, and back again (Argote, 1999; Chuang, Ginsburg, and Berta, 2007). As Chuang and colleagues (2007) explain:

> When an individual's learning processes are shared with other members of a workgroup, individual learning is recombined with the learning, experience, and interpretation of other group members to share learning at the group level. Through this process, group members may develop mutual understandings of one another's experiences and perspectives, which in turn modify the practices that are collectively perceived to be effective or ineffective. Practices that are deemed to be effective are likely to be retained in the group and transferred to other groups within an organization [Argote, 1999].... Then, what has already been learned feeds back from the organization to the group and individual levels, influencing, if not constraining, how individuals act and think [Crossan, Lane, and White, 1999].

**Organizational learning** is thus a multilevel phenomenon. Moreover, different factors influence knowledge creation, retention, and transfer within and across different levels. Individual learning is influenced, for example, by experience, feedback, and deliberate practice (i.e., focusing on techniques and understanding principles). Group learning is influenced by group member diversity, intergroup linkages, and group norms, such as psychological safety (see Chapter 5). Organizational learning is influenced by organizational leadership, culture, policies, and routines. Although the factors that facilitate or stymie learning at various levels are intertwined, we focus below on five management practices that characterize a learning organization.

## Learning Disciplines

While scholars and theorists have discussed organizational learning for some time, Peter Senge's 1990 book, *The Fifth Discipline*, popularized the term learning organization. In poetic terms, he described learning organizations as places where "people continually expand their capacity to create the

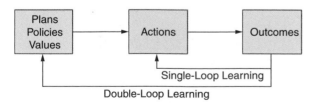

**Figure 8.1** Single-Loop versus Double-Loop Learning.
SOURCE: Delmar, Cengage Learning.

results they truly desire, where new and expansive patterns of thinking are nurtured, where collective aspiration is set free, and where people are continually learning to learn together" (Senge, 1990). Others, in more prosaic language, define a learning organization as "an organization skilled at creating, acquiring, and transferring knowledge, and at modifying its behavior to reflect new knowledge and insights" (Garvin, 1993).

Senge (2006) describes five disciplines that, when combined, produce an organization capable of "expanding its capacity to create its future." He refers to these organizational practices as disciplines because each involves a body of theory and techniques that must be practiced in order for mastery to develop. The disciplines are systems thinking, personal mastery, mental models, shared vision, and team learning.

- **Systems thinking** refers to the discipline of seeing wholes, perceiving the structures that underlie dynamically complex systems, and identifying high-leverage change opportunities. Systems thinking involves not only the recognition of the properties of complex systems, but also the skilled application of "systems archetypes" to illuminate the deeper structures that shape everyday organizational behavior and performance (see the textbox "Using Systems Archetypes to Understand Organizational Behavior"). Through training and practice, organizational members can see "where actions and changes in structures can lead to significant, enduring improvements" (Senge, 1990).

- **Personal mastery** is the discipline of individual learning, without which organizational learning cannot occur. Personal mastery involves continuously clarifying our individual sense of purpose and vision, and continuously learning how to see the world as it is without distortion. The tension created by the gap between vision and reality, if tapped creatively, generates energy for exploration and growth. Organizational members who demonstrate personal mastery are apt to exhibit greater commitment, take more initiative, learn faster, and feel greater responsibility. Fostering personal mastery requires, at a minimum, adopting Theory Y assumptions about human behavior and instituting organizational policies and practices that promote employee growth and development (see Chapter 2).

- **Mental models** refer to the discipline of constantly surfacing, testing, and improving our assumptions about how the world works. Mental models actively shape what we see and, therefore, how we act (see the textbox "Mental Models of Learning"). By training and encouraging organizational members in the dual skills of reflection and inquiry (e.g., recognizing leaps of abstraction and uncovering censored thoughts and feelings), managers can promote organizational learning by loosening the grip of tacit, often faulty mental models (e.g., higher quality always costs more).

- **Shared vision** is the discipline of generating a common answer to the question, "What do we want to create?" Shared vision connects people through common aspiration and derives its motivational power by tapping people's personal visions. From shared vision comes the focus and energy for learning, the willingness to take risks and experiment, the mutual alignment of individual effort, and the commitment to the long-term view. Creating shared vision requires encouraging organizational members to develop and communicate personal visions, inquiring into the deeper vision that unites the diversity of expressed views, and staying the course through difficult times.

- **Team learning** refers to the discipline of creating alignment such that team members think insightfully about complex problems, synergize their knowledge and skills, and produce coordinated action. Team learning requires an organizational climate that promotes trust and respect—where it is safe for individuals to share both strengths and weaknesses. Such an environment diminishes individuals' inclination toward defensiveness as a protection from embarrassment or vulnerability to threat they may perceive in exposing such weaknesses to their colleagues (see Chapter 5). This can be achieved by promoting a mastery of open-minded dialogue where each individual learns from the others, the net result being a collective, organizational search for alternative meanings and new perspectives (Isaacs, 1999).

Senge (2006) emphasizes that all five disciplines matter because each builds upon and reinforces the others. Personal mastery, for instance, facilitates the integration of reason and intuition, which, in turn, enhances one's ability to see interrelationships among seemingly discrete events. Similarly, working with mental models loosens the grip of deeply held, often tacit assumptions that hinder systems thinking, shared vision, and team learning.

## Limits of Organizational Learning

Although the promise of learning organizations is exciting, managers' enthusiasm for learning organizations needs to be tempered not only by the significant challenges involved in

## USING SYSTEMS ARCHETYPES TO UNDERSTAND ORGANIZATIONAL BEHAVIOR

System archetypes—or patterns of structure that occur again and again—represent the key tools of systems thinking. System archetypes enable people to *see* how interlocking reinforcing and balancing feedback loops influence the behavior of social systems; by seeing these structures at play, it becomes possible to identify "high-leverage" actions that can produce lasting change. Senge (2006) describes several system archetypes, including one he calls "Limits to Growth." As illustrated below (Figure 8.2) in Limits to Growth, a reinforcing feedback loop generates a spiral of success, but also triggers a balancing feedback loop that, after a delay, slows down the success.

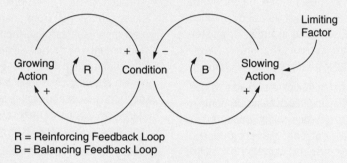

**Figure 8.2** Limits to Growth Archetype: Generic Template.
SOURCE: Delmar, Cengage Learning.

Limits to Growth structures explain that overexpansion can lead to performance decline. For example, a physician group practice that delivers high-quality care develops a positive reputation, which, through positive word of mouth, generates more referrals (Figure 8.3). More referrals, in turn, generate more resources that could be invested in high-quality care. However, if patient volumes increase more rapidly than quality-enhancing investments can be made, patient satisfaction and possible quality of care begin to suffer. Over time, negative word of mouth leads to fewer referrals and lighter schedules.

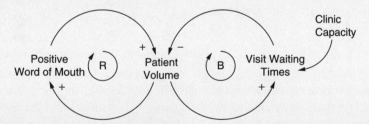

**Figure 8.3** Limits to Growth Archetype: Example.
SOURCE: Delmar, Cengage Learning.

building such organizations, but also the seemingly intractable limits of organizational learning. First, organizational members usually possess only limited information, much of which is ambiguous or inaccurate. As Sterman (2000) observes: "No one knows the current sales rate of their company, the current rate of production, or the true value of the order backlog at any given time. Instead, we receive estimates of these data based on sampled, averaged, and delayed measurements. The act of measurement introduces distortions, delays, biases, errors, and other imperfections, some known, others unknown and unknowable." In addition, expectancy gives rise to selective perception. In other words, we see or hear

# MENTAL MODELS OF LEARNING

Mental models not only shape our actions, but also our capability to learn from our actions. Richard Bohmer and Amy Edmondson contend that health care managers and professionals share a widely held, yet implicit mental model that learning is an individual activity involving a linear process of repetition and error detection and correction (Bohmer and Edmondson, 2001). In this model (see Table 8.1), health professionals gain knowledge and skill through a one-way transfer of knowledge and "best practice" in their initial and continuing professional education. Through repetition, they increase their proficiency ("practice makes perfect"). On-the-job learning occurs primarily through error detection and correction, as in the case of Morbidity and Mortality conferences, or trial-and-error learning, as when a psychiatrist prescribes various antidepressants to find the one that works best for a given patient. According to Bohmer and Edmonson, this mental model of learning is incomplete. They propose an alternative model that, they argue, more fully describes what really happens in health care and that more effectively guides improvement efforts. In this model, learning is a dynamic, cyclical process in which experience gained in routine practice (i.e., knowledge-in-use) is reflected upon, reinterpreted, and refined not just by individuals, but also by groups and organizations. Experience may be the best teacher, but learning from experience is not automatic. Bohmer and Edmonson observed, for example, that surgical teams with the same amount of experience, measured in terms of number of cases, exhibited varying levels of performance improvement. Team and organizational learning, they argue, does not follow inevitably from repetition and experience; rather, team and organizational learning processes must be managed. Moreover, as their research on psychological safety shows (see Chapter 5), effective team and organizational learning involves both single-loop and double-loop learning.

How can managers nurture organizational learning? The first step is to recognize that the prevailing, but largely implicit mental model of learning contains faulty, or at least incomplete, assumptions that limit collective learning capability. By examining this mental model through reflection and dialogue, managers can loosen the grip of these assumptions on their own and others' perceptions, attributions, and actions. Without a change in people's mental models, efforts to increase organizational learning through quality improvement methods, computer simulations, debriefing sessions, and other strategies do not "make sense" and therefore get little support from those who hold an individualistic, linear, single-loop model of learning.

## TABLE 8.1 Mental Models of Learning

| How We Think Learning Happens | How Learning Really Happens |
|---|---|
| Learning is an individual activity | Learning is an individual, group, and organizational activity |
| Learning is a linear process involving a one-way transfer of knowledge and "best practice" | Learning is a cyclical process involving knowledge interpretation, application, feedback, reinterpretation, and refinement |
| Repetition is the path to best practice | Repetition is necessary but not sufficient |
| Learning occurs through error detection and correction (single-loop learning) | Learning occurs through error detection and correction, and through diagnosis of systems and policies (single- and double-loop learning) |

SOURCE: Adapted from Bohmer RM, Edmonson AC. Organizational learning in health care. Health Forum Journal Mar/Apr 2001.

what we expect to see or hear, rather than what actually occurs (Bowditch and Buono, 2001). For instance, our mental models about what is meaningful and important inform what we choose to define, measure, and monitor with our information systems; in turn, our information systems shape the perceptions that we form (Sterman, 2000). In this sense, we "enact" the environment in which we live (Weick, 1979).

Second, even with perfect and complete information, organizational members routinely engage in unscientific reasoning due to judgment errors and biases (Hammond, Keeney, and Raiffa, 1998). The human mind relies upon unconscious routines, called heuristics, to cope with complexity and uncertainty (Kahneman, Slovic, and Tversky, 1982). These heuristics, while efficient, often distort reasoning and judgment. The five learning disciplines can dampen the effects of recall bias, overconfidence, and other judgment errors, but they cannot eliminate them or the poor learning that they produce.

Finally, organizational learning often bumps up against practical problems and competing priorities. For instance, many decisions and programs experience implementation delays or alterations as they encounter technical obstacles, resource constraints, or political resistance. Imperfect implementation hinders learning, especially when long time spans are involved. In addition, as Sterman (2000) observes, "In the real world of irreversible actions and high stakes, the need to maintain performance often overrides the need to learn by suppressing new strategies for fear that they would cause present harm even though they might yield great insight and prevent future harm."

---

## IN PRACTICE: Failing to Learn from Failure

Health care managers and professionals often ask, "Why do we keep solving the same problems time after time?" Organizational learning is frequently inhibited by the system dynamic called "Fixes that Fail." This archetype describes a pattern wherein people act expediently to solve an immediate problem. The quick fix works, but it triggers unintended consequences that makes the problem reappear after some delay, often worse than before.

Anita Tucker and Amy Edmondson's study of nursing care processes illustrates how the "Fixes that Fail" dynamic prevents hospitals from learning from failure (see Figure 8.4) (Tucker and Edmondson, 2003). They observed that nurses often encounter work-flow problems like missing or broken equipment or missing or incorrect information. Nurses overwhelmingly engaged in first-order problem solving (i.e., single-loop learning) to address such problems. That is, they used short-term fixes that allowed them to return quickly to patient care. They did not try to address the underlying causes of the problem through second-order problem solving (i.e., double-loop learning). For example, when an oncology floor nurse working the night shift ran out of clean linens for patients' beds, she went to a unit that had linen in stock and took from that supply. She did not communicate to the person or department responsible for the problem, or bring the problem to managers' attention, or share with others ideas about how to prevent this problem from recurring. She solved the immediate problem, but no organizational learning occurred.

Why do nurses rely so heavily on first-order problem solving? Tucker and Edmonson suggest four reasons. First, industry norms encourage nurses and other health professionals to take personal responsibility to solve problems. Counterintuitively, norms promoting personal responsibility prompt nurses to take decisive, independent action to solve immediate problems without considering the systemic causes of the problem or the systemic consequences of their short-term fixes. Second, nursing units seek to maximize individual unit efficiency through lean staffing. Nurses have little time to resolve the underlying causes of the problems they face in their daily work. Short-term fixes are efficient solutions, even if they are not effective in the long term. Third, for a host of reasons, nurse managers are less involved in the daily work activities of those whom they supervise. This makes it more difficult for overburdened frontline staff to tackle problems that cross organizational boundaries. Finally, Tucker and Edmonson observed that nurses found it personally gratifying to overcome problems on their own; they reported a sense of satisfaction knowing that they did everything they could for their patients.

One of the lessons of systems dynamics is that the cure is often worse than the disease. First-order problem-solving works, but only in the short term. Systemic causes go unaddressed. Things get worse, but only after a delay. For nurses, frustration and exhaustion builds over time as they confront the same problems again and again, ultimately resulting in burnout and the nurse leaving the organization and possibly the profession—representing the loss of a very expensive knowledge asset. Taken to the extreme, first-order problem solving can also actually precipitate catastrophic failure of the system they are meant to support. This is because the consequences of some chronic problems accumulate like a toxin. Paul Levy wrote about the Nut Island sewage treatment plant in Boston Harbor, where employees took pride in first-order problem solving in dealing with facility maintenance (Levy, 2001). They went to heroic lengths to keep the plant operating without bothering their

## IN PRACTICE: Failing to Learn from Failure (*Continued*)

superiors, which resulted in failure to complete critical strategic maintenance and upgrades. Ultimately, the plant experienced catastrophic failures resulting in billions of gallons of raw sewage being dumped in the harbor.

What can managers do to escape the "Fixes that Fail" dynamic like that depicted in this situation? Look for leverage points that promote second-order problem solving. Tucker and Edmondson highlight two such leverage points: (1) increasing managerial support by increasing managers' availability for at least part of all shifts, providing assistance to frontline problem-solving efforts, and acting as a role model for second-order problem solving; and (2) creating an environment where frontline staff feel safe to speak up about work-flow problems without fear of embarrassment or punishment.

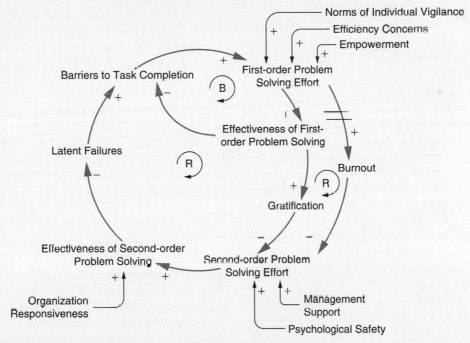

**Figure 8.4** First-Order and Second-Order Problem-Solving Behavior.

SOURCE: Copyright 2003 by The Regents of the University of California. Reprinted from the *California Management Review*. Vol. 45, No. 2. By permission of The Regents.

# INNOVATION AND LEARNING

Learning lies at the heart of innovation. When we innovate, we introduce something new into a setting for the first time, or as if for the first time. Learning—the acquisition of knowledge or skills—occurs throughout the innovation "journey" of discovery, exploration, experimentation, and reflection. Not all learning involves innovation, but all innovation involves learning.

It is important to recognize that innovation is both a noun and a verb. Researchers, consultants, managers, and policy makers often talk past one another because they forget this simple fact. As a noun, **innovation** refers to an "idea, practice, or object that is perceived as new by an individual or other unit adopting it" (Rogers, 2003). Although an innovation can be something that is "new to the world," it does not have to be so for this definition to apply. All that is necessary is that the idea, practice, or object be new, or perceived as new, to the individual, group, organization, community, or other social entity that decides to put that idea, practice, or object into use. For example, we could use the term innovation to refer to a computerized diabetes registry if the federally qualified community health centers that are adopting it have had no prior experience with computerized disease registries, or even paper-based registries (Helfrich et al., 2007). One of the central concerns for those who think about innovation as a noun is: how do new ideas, practices, or objects diffuse through a social system over time? Other concerns include: what factors influence individual or organizational decisions to adopt an innovation, why do some individuals or organizations adopt innovations more quickly than others do, and how can individuals and organizations implement innovations more effectively and sustain innovation use?

As a verb, innovation refers to the act (or process) of introducing something new into an environment or setting. In other words, innovation is something that one does rather than some "thing" that one adopts. In a landmark study, Van de Ven and his colleagues (1999) defined innovation as "a purposeful, concentrated effort to develop and implement a novel idea." They observed that innovation often involves collective effort by many people for a considerable amount of time, frequently under conditions of substantial technical, organizational, and market uncertainty. Moreover, the effort usually requires more resources to complete than those who undertake it possess. One of the central concerns for those who think about innovation as a verb is: how exactly do organizations create something new? Other concerns include: why are some organizations more innovative (i.e., innovation-generating) than others; how can organizations innovate more quickly, efficiently, and effectively; and how can less innovative organizations become more innovative?

Hundreds of studies have examined the adoption, implementation, and diffusion of new ideas, technologies, programs, practices, and services (for a review, see Rogers, 2003, and Greenhalgh et al., 2004). By comparison, few studies have examined the generative process through which new ideas, technologies, programs, practices, and services develop. Instead, much of what we know, or think we know, about the process of innovation comes from the anecdotes, reflections, and reports of current and former executives, management consultants, and popular business publications (Greenhalgh et al., 2004). Although conventional wisdom contains useful insights, it also contains misconceptions,

biases, and myths that do not withstand empirical scrutiny. Here, we mention three.

## "Innovation Is Good"

A strong cultural presumption exists, especially in the United States, that innovations are economically and socially valuable and, further, that innovating is desirable and admirable. Researchers call this presumption the "pro-innovation bias" (Kimberly, 1981; Rogers, 2003). Not all innovations are economically or socially beneficial (e.g., crack cocaine). Some have harmful unanticipated consequences, even when used correctly (e.g., Vioxx). Others have disastrous unintended consequences, especially when overly diffused or improperly used (e.g., financial derivatives). The process of innovation itself is disruptive and fraught with risk for organizations and managers alike. Although some companies innovate themselves into prosperity, others innovate themselves into insolvency (Pfeffer and Sutton, 2006; Rosenzweig, 2007; Van de Ven, 1999); the failure rate of new products (i.e., failure to ever return a profit) appears to be on the order of 30–60 percent, and is higher for new start-ups (Pfeffer and Sutton, 2006). Successful innovation journeys can enhance managers' careers; unsuccessful innovation journeys can lead to stigmatization, demotion, or termination (Van de Ven, 1999).

## "There's a Formula"

Popular management books often promise spectacular results from simple formulae, such as "stick to your knitting" (Peters and Waterman, 1982) or "set audacious goals" (Collins and Porras, 1994). Yet, empirical studies indicate that the innovation journey, even when successful, is a complex, messy affair that cannot be easily summarized, let alone reduced to a dictum (Van de Ven, 1999). Rosenzweig (2007) suggests that the pervasive belief that organizational innovativeness can be attributed to simple formulae arises from a form of observational bias called the *halo effect*: the tendency to infer specific characteristics of a person or organization from our overall impressions or feelings about that person or organization. Much of what we know, or think we know, about innovation comes from studies of successful cases: businesses that have done exceptionally well (Collins, 2001; Collins and Porras, 1994; Peters and Waterman, 1982). Management experts first identify successful companies and then try to reconstruct what these companies did to set themselves apart from their less-accomplished peers. The problem with this sort of retrospective analysis is that management experts interpret what they see in the glow (i.e., the halo) of what they already know about the companies' performance. The halo that surrounds these companies can lead experts to accept uncritically the simple formula or rules of thumb that executives use to describe the secrets of the company's success. Unfortunately, many companies from which management experts derive simple formulae subsequently *underperform* the rest of the market in the years *after* they are profiled (Rosenzweig, 2007).

## "Innovation Is Linear"

The most pervasive misconception of the innovation journey is that it follows a logical, predictable sequence of stages or phases of activity. In the typical stage model, innovation begins with needs assessment or problem identification and proceeds from basic or applied research, to development, and then to commercialization (Rogers, 2003; Van de Ven, 1999). These stages are seen as a linear progression: one stage follows another in a predictable, orderly fashion. Stage models can be useful as heuristics for talking about the innovation journey. But, the simplicity, clarity, and predictability of linear stage models belie the complex, uncertain, and indeterminate nature of the innovation journey revealed by empirical research (Greenhalgh et al., 2004; Van de Ven et al., 1989).

What, then, does the innovation journey look like? Over the course of 17 years, Andrew Van de Ven and a group of management scholars at the University of Minnesota sought to answer this question by studying 14 new-to-the-world innovations, including the development of cochlear implants at 3M, the formation of multihospital systems in the 1980s, and the creation of new programs in schools. The Minnesota Innovation Research Project (MIRP) was conducted prospectively, meaning the researchers began collecting data at the beginning of the innovation journey. MIRP researchers thus avoided the twin problems that Rosenzweig (2007) cites as the main culprits in falling victim to the halo effect: selecting your case studies based on outcomes and collecting data that are not independent from the outcome. To foreshadow the discussion below, MIRP results suggest that the innovation is neither predictable nor random. Instead, the journey reflects the nonlinear dynamics of a complex system. MIRP researchers identified 12 patterns, which they categorized according to three broad phases of activity (Van de Ven et al., 1999). These categories lend these disparate, nonlinear patterns a degree of narrative coherence. But, importantly, in every case, the essential pieces of the

innovation story changed radically over time: the people involved in the effort, the objectives of the effort, even the idea of what the innovation itself was. Finally, MIRP results reveal a more complex picture of organizational learning in the innovation journey than prior innovation and learning research suggested.

### *Innovation Journey*

The MIRP researchers began with assumptions that managers and researchers generally at the time held, and that many still hold today. They assumed that "innovation" involved a single, common idea or technology that retained its identity through the development process. While different stakeholders might hold varying or even opposing views about the innovation, they nonetheless would see the innovation as the same (identifiable) thing. A team of individuals pulled from their other duties would work primarily, if not exclusively, on innovation development; moreover, the team would remain intact through the development process. Likewise, the team's relationships with venders, suppliers, and other external stakeholders would remain stable once established. The team would shepherd the innovation through a linear progression of stages that would culminate in a definitive outcome: success or failure.

What the MIRP researchers found was quite different from what they expected. Innovation involved a proliferation of ideas, frequent reinvention, with multiple entrepreneurs engaging, disengaging and reengaging over time. None of the 14 innovations that they studied developed in a simple, linear sequence of stages. Most produced indeterminate or ambiguous results. MIRP researchers described the complex, messy progression of events that they observed in terms of three broad phases of activity: genesis, development, and termination. Although they parsed the innovation journey into three phases for the purposes of description and reporting, they emphasized that these phases were fuzzy, incomplete, and nonlinear.

### *Genesis*

Innovations do not arise from a single, spur-of-the-moment event. The essence of the idea develops over years, with unpredictable events setting the stage. For example, MIRP researchers studied the development of the cochlear implant, a device implanted within the cochlea (the auditory portion of the inner ear) with an external processor that would allow the profoundly deaf to hear. The 3M Corporation began development of the cochlear implant when researchers at the University of Melbourne contacted one of 3M's Australian subsidiaries about commercializing research they had conducted on a "bionic ear." At the same time, independent of this work, another 3M division was doing similar work based on hearing aids. These research streams evolved independently but converged when university researchers initiated contact.

At some point, some shock or event, often external, triggers concentrated effort to develop the innovation. The innovators submit a plan to those who control the resources needed to initiate intensive innovation development. These sponsors might be senior executives within the company, or external investors such as venture capitalists. This plan marks the beginning of concerted efforts to develop the innovation; but the plan generally serves first and foremost as "sales vehicles" to get sponsors on board. Initial plans often include vague goals, optimistic projections, and downplayed risks. For example, with the cochlear implants, initial projections of the market were based on an assumption that nearly all profoundly deaf adults would be interested in the technology, which put the potential market in excess of $100 million.

## Development

Once intensive work begins, the original idea quickly proliferates into multiple, often divergent ideas and activities. There is no uniform "innovation." There is a nebula of related and evolving ideas, and it is not always clear where one draws the boundaries around this shifting cloud. Though it makes linear narrative nearly impossible, this divergence is logical given how uncertain innovation is. Pursuing multiple development paths is adaptive because innovators and managers do not know which ideas are going to pay off. In the face of such uncertainty, the best bet is to invest limited resources in a number of plausible alternatives simultaneously, in the hope of eventually shifting resources to the most promising option as uncertainty diminishes.

Innovators invariably experience setbacks, often due to unexpected changes in the external environment that alter their original ideas and assumptions. Perhaps a competing technology emerges, a new market opens up, or a financial crisis occurs and capital becomes scarce. In the case of the cochlear implant, the innovators discovered that to the profoundly deaf, "Deaf" (with a capital D) was a whole subculture and community, not a disability they hoped to escape. This throws the original plan into disorder. At first, the innovators successfully petition their sponsors for allowances: more time, additional funds, and a change in the goals. But, typically, problems continue to accumulate. The innovators think of the original plan as an aspirational statement, to be revisited and revised as unexpected problems and opportunities arise. The sponsors, however, think of the original plan as a contract, and, as time passes, seek to hold the innovators accountable to it. For example, as it became clear that the market for the cochlear implant among the profoundly deaf was not sufficient, the 3M innovation managers began exploring options for adapting the technology for hearing aids.

The goals evolve over time. Sponsors and innovators change the criteria by which they judge innovation a success or failure, often diverging and sometimes fighting over these criteria. Likewise, the people themselves—the innovators and their teams—fluctuate over time, becoming involved and subsequently leaving, and in some cases coming back again. These shifting criteria and turnover in staff inhibit learning. It is difficult to understand if planned strategy leads to the desired goals when the goals change repeatedly and unpredictably. Likewise, much of learning that occurs in the innovation journey is tacit: held by individuals and hard to express in words or images. Tacit knowledge is susceptible to loss when individuals leave or get reassigned.

Sponsors (investors and top managers) are frequently involved throughout the process of innovation development, often serving a variety of changing and conflicting roles. Van de Ven and colleagues concluded that no significant innovation problems were solved without the direct involvement of sponsors. Power dynamics between innovators and sponsors change over the course of the innovation development processes (see the textbox "The Role of Management in the Innovation Journey"). Initially, the sponsors hold the essential power as innovators negotiate for support to develop their innovations. After the sponsors have invested significant resources into the innovation, the investment translates into greater influence for the innovators, as sponsors are reluctant to do anything that jeopardizes their investment. Innovators develop relationships with other organizations, and these relationships lock the innovators into certain courses of action, curtailing others, often with consequences they could not foresee. Innovation occurs within an ecosystem of competitors, trade associations, regulators, legislators and others, all of whom contribute to a common infrastructure that supports or inhibits the innovation. So the innovation does not evolve just as a function of what the innovators do, but also as a function of the support and inhibition provided by the broader ecosystem.

### Termination

The innovation continues to evolve as users integrate it and adapt it to local situations. Eventually, the innovation ceases. Either it gets "implemented" and is no longer an innovation, or the innovators exhaust their resources and cease work on the innovation. However, even when work ceases, it could begin again if some new confluence of events triggers interest.

At some point, sponsors draw conclusions about innovation success or failure and assign credit or blame. The greater the consequences of failure, the greater the tendency to attribute failure to the innovation team. In many cases, MIRP researchers found that the attribution of credit or blame is misdirected, but even invalid attributions have important implications for the ultimate fate of the innovation (in cases where the innovation persists) and the innovator's careers. This was particularly striking, because many of the companies that the MIRP researchers studied explicitly or implicitly espoused a culture of risk taking, where employees ostensibly are not punished for taking reasonable risks but failing.

In lieu of a simple stage-model diagram of the innovation journey, the MIRP researchers captured the nonlinear, dynamic nature of the process in a figure they call the "fireworks" diagram (so named for the branching lines, which evoke the shower of sparks as from a Roman candle—though it could equally allude to the drama that marked nearly every case they studied). Overall, the cases studied by Van de Ven and colleagues demonstrated that the process cannot be reduced to stages or phases. Instead, it is a cycle of divergent and convergent activities operating at multiple organizational levels, and it continues for as long as there are resources to sustain it.

## Learning in the Innovation Journey

When we think about innovation, we imagine a process that involves a great deal of trial-and-error learning. Indeed, innovation conjures the popular image of an inventor tinkering in his or her workshop, experimenting with materials and processes to find the right combination that will realize his or her idea. Thomas Edison's comment that "invention is 1 percent inspiration and 99 percent perspiration" reinforces the notion that innovation is essentially an extended process of single loop (or adaptive) learning. The inventor acts, compares the results of his or her actions to some goal, and then acts in ways that he or she believes will close the gap between desired outcomes and actual results. The MIRP researchers observed that the innovation journey did feature single-loop (or adaptive) learning, which they termed **testing**. Through

---

### THE ROLE OF MANAGEMENT IN THE INNOVATION JOURNEY

One of the lessons from the MIRP studies was that multiple managers, at multiple hierarchical levels, played multiple roles in bringing along each and every innovation. They alternately served as sponsor, mentor, critic, and institutional leader, with different managers serving different roles at different times. In doing so, they served as checks and balances to each other. As sponsors, managers advocated for the innovation and the innovation team when investment decisions and other issues were considered. As mentors, managers coached, counseled, and served as role models. As critics, managers played "devil's advocate," taking a "hard-nosed" view of innovation goals, progress, and prospects. As institutional leaders, managers sought to balance these opposing roles by establishing structure and settling disputes. MIRP researchers observed that these management roles were reciprocally related to one another and counterbalanced each other over time through self-correcting cycles (i.e., balancing feedback loops). They also noted the importance of balance and timing in the performance of these roles.

testing, innovators learn about action-outcome relationships; in particular, they learn through successive experimentation which actions reliably produce desired outcomes. However, MIRP researchers also observed that learning by testing did not occur until relatively late in the innovation journey. Learning by testing requires some prior knowledge about the tasks to be performed. In particular, learners must first know what courses of action are possible, what goals or outcomes are preferable, and what rules, resources, and other contextual factors are relevant to the learning process. For the first several months, and in some cases years, of the innovation journey, the conditions necessary for learning by testing did not exist. That did not mean, however, that no learning occurred during the developmental period. Instead, a different kind of learning took place, which MIRP researchers termed **discovery**. Through discovery, innovators learn about possible action alternatives, outcome preferences, and contextual factors. Learning by discovery resembles double-loop (or generative) learning in that it opens up and investigates possibilities. Whereas testing involves a process of error detection and correction, discovery involves a process of exploration. Pathways multiply and diverge rather than winnow and converge.

The MIRP studies further indicate that learning by discovery is a precondition to learning by testing. Innovation typically begins with a high degree of uncertainty. To illustrate, Van de Ven and his colleagues (1999) described the innovation journey of two new-to-the-world biomedical innovations as follows:

> The initial plans contained vague but optimistic proposals to develop and commercialize new technologies that were believed to have the potential to sustain the organizations' businesses in the next generation [Van de Ven et al., 1989]. The plans indicated that the starting conditions were highly ambiguous; they focused on possibilities and opportunities, not specific project goals, objectives, or outcome criteria. The action plans were also highly uncertain; they emphasized exploratory research and discovery, not testing or evaluation, because the innovations represented novel undertakings for the organizations.

Before innovators can test which actions led to which outcomes, they first have to discover what courses of action are possible, what outcome goals and criteria they and others prefer, and in what kind of environmental context they are expected to work. It is during this time of learning by discovery

that the initial idea for the innovation proliferates to many ideas and the actions that innovators take proceed in many different directions at once. While this expansive, divergent period of activity seems random and unproductive, Van de Ven and his colleagues (1999) write, this chaotic process of learning by discovery is necessary before innovators can "converge into the still confusing, but better defined period of trial-and-error learning."

The MIRP studies also shed light on how and when transitions occur from learning by discovery to learning by testing. MIRP researchers noted that innovation efforts must import energy and resources from the organization itself and from outside sources in order to continue. Start-up companies, for example, require a constant flow of venture capital to sustain product development. Similarly, innovation efforts within established organizations require a constant flow of internal "venture capital" in the form of human resources, managerial support, and budgetary allocation. Moreover, innovation efforts occur within a context of institutional rules that shape the timing, pace, content, and process of innovation efforts. Drug development, for example, is strongly affected by U.S. Food and Drug Administration rules, regulations, and procedures. Management directives, institutional rules, and resource flows can trigger transitions from discovery to testing by constraining the freedom of innovation efforts to move along multiple, diverse developmental pathways. For example, managers can impose specific goals for the innovation effort or impose a set of outcome criteria judging the success of the innovation effort. Requiring a tighter linkage between actions and outcomes focuses attention on testing which action alternatives optimally produce a chosen outcome or goal. Likewise, looming deadlines imposed by resource holders and institutional rule makers can shift innovation efforts from exploring action alternatives and possible outcomes to finding the best linear combination of feasible actions and desired outcomes. MIRP researchers contend that learning in the innovation journey does not simply progress in a one-way direction from discovery to testing. While the search for a tighter coupling of actions and outcomes narrows the focus of attention, it also opens new questions and issues that require exploration and resolution. Thus, the innovation journey involves repeatable, but not predictable, cycles of learning by discovery and learning by testing. As noted earlier, the cycles continue until the innovation effort succeeds or runs out of resources.

Finally, the MIRP studies indicate that the innovation journey is characterized by a long delay, sometimes lasting years, between actions and outcomes. "During the developmental period, intensive investments and efforts are required to transform a vague inventive idea into a concrete reality without having any objective information that is useful for narrowing developmental activities toward specific outcomes" (Van de Ven et al., 1999). Indeed, the most definitive information about outcomes does not become available until the innovation is launched into the market or implemented by an adopting organization. This long delay in the feedback loop between action and outcomes explains why adaptive, single-loop, trial-and-error learning often occurs late in the innovation journey. In the absence of concrete goals and timely feedback on outcomes, action persistence appears to be the prevailing and preferred strategy for narrowing the complexity of innovation efforts to manageable proportions. In other words, when faced with ambiguity about goals, means, and performance, the best and perhaps only strategy available is to pick what seems like the best course of action and stick to it. As a prominent organization scientist notes, action persistence is psychologically satisfying. "Commitment marshals forces that destroy the plausibility of alternatives and remove their ability to inhibit action" (Weick, 1993). MIRP researchers agree that there is some value in treating probabilistic information as if it were deterministic information and regarding beliefs that are only relatively true as if they were absolutely true. However, such action persistence underscores a key feature of complex systems: sensitivity to initial conditions. If one persists in certain courses of action in the absence of any feedback that might signal the need for correction, then small differences in starting points can take an innovation journey in very different directions. Persisting in "veering left" at every fork in the road could ultimately lead one to a desired destination, or not. It all depends on the starting point. As MIRP researchers point out, if the innovation journey is successful, action persistence creates heroes. If the journey is not successful, action persistence creates tragedies and scapegoats.

# MANAGING COMPLEXITY, INNOVATION, AND LEARNING

Complexity-oriented management scholars tell us that continuous innovation and learning occur when organizations operate at the "edge of chaos," that intermediate zone between stability and instability where new ideas, products, practices, and relationships spontaneously emerge that are neither predicted nor anticipated. But, keeping organizations poised at the edge of chaos is challenging. It requires constant managerial vigilance to avoid falling into too much structure (order) or too little (chaos). Complexity-oriented management scholars contend that, when it comes to fostering innovation and learning, managers should neither impose order by adopting top-down, command-and-control approaches, nor should they neglect order by adopting freewheeling, "anything goes" approaches. Instead, they should create conditions in which order can emerge in a spontaneous, creative, and self-organizing fashion. One way to accomplish this is to rely on minimum specifications (a few simple rules) rather than detailed planning. As Plsek and Wilson (2001) note, minimum specifications can create a wide space for novel ideas, creative solutions, and new relationships to emerge by establishing four key conditions or parameters: direction, boundaries, permission, and resources. Similarly, managers should keep the whole system in mind when setting goals and allocating resources. Like minimum specifications, global targets and pooled budgets create a context for productive, generative interactions to occur among the various stakeholders in the system. The general idea is to create just enough structure to support innovation and learning, but not enough to stifle it.

## Nurturing Foresight

Organizations that sustain continuous innovation even in the face of rapidly changing, highly competitive environments do so by developing capabilities and processes to "spot developments before they become trends and to grasp the relevant features of social currents that are likely to shape the direction of future events" (Tsoukas and Shepherd, 2004). Consistent with the principles of complexity science, these organizations do not develop comprehensive strategic plans or invest in any one vision of the future. At the same time, they do not leave the future to chance by falling into a reactive mode. Instead, they use a variety of practices to probe the future, explore weak or ambiguous signals, and develop viable options for the future that they in part create. Specific practices for nurturing foresight include: (1) rapid experimentation using prototypes, pilot programs, and computer simulations (Andriopoulos and Gotsi, 2006); (2) knowledge brokering—making connections between ideas from different industries, business units, or projects

(Hargadon and Sutton, 2000); (3) forging alliances with existing and potential customers and other firms in order to learn about unmet needs in current markets and future needs in new markets (Brown and Eisenhardt, 1997); and (4) regular internal meetings to engage in cross-functional dialogue about implausible, unthinkable, and "forbidden" futures (Day and Schoemaker, 2005; Roberto, Bohmer, and Edmondson, 2006). Practices for nurturing foresight allow organizations to avoid the rigidity of planning with as well as the chaos of reactivity. They also promote rapid learning by discovery—that double-loop, generative process whereby innovators gain knowledge of possible action alternatives, outcome preferences, and contextual factors.

## Fostering Improvisation

Organizations that sustain continuous innovation in products and services emphasize improvisation over disciplined problem solving (Brown and Eisenhardt, 1997). Although improvisation involves "making it up as you go along" (Moorman and Miner, 1998), it is not the same as "winging it." In jazz, for example, individual expression and mutual adjustment occur within a few specific rules (e.g., order of soloing, valid chord sequences). In fact, the adherence to a few simple rules makes improvisation possible; if everyone "did their own thing," the result would be cacophony. Consistent with the principles of complexity science, organizations sustain continuous innovation by coupling limited structure with extensive communication (Brown and Eisenhardt, 1997). Specifically, these organizations combine well-defined managerial responsibilities and clear-cut project priorities with loosely specified development processes. They complement these "semi-structures" with frequent formal and informal communication within and across project teams. Improvisation in the form of novelty, creativity, and spontaneity occurs within, and is facilitated by, minimum specification and social interaction. By comparison, organizations that struggle to sustain continuous innovation invoke either too much structure (e.g., highly specified, sequential development processes) or too little (e.g., poorly defined responsibilities, uncertain project priorities). Brown and Eisenhardt's (1997) notion of "semi-structures" seems somewhat at odds with the ambiguous, fluid, and messy process depicted in the MIRP studies. Recall that MIRP researchers found that top managers and other resource holders did not impose explicit goals, priorities, and deadlines until late in the process. Contextual differences might account for the discrepancy: whereas MIRP researchers focused on new-to-the-world innovation, Brown and Eisenhardt (1997) focused on rapid, but nonetheless incremental, product innovations. Alternatively, the discrepancy might relate to differences in success. All of the MIRP innovations failed.

## Maximizing Serendipity

Discoveries occur when we find things we did not know we were looking for, when we see unexpected connections among seemingly unrelated events, objects, or facts. Discovery, by definition, involves an element of surprise. The discovery of penicillin, for example, was a fortunate accident. So too was the discovery of vaccinations, X-rays, anesthesia, coronary catheterization, Viagra, Lithium, Valium, insulin, quinine, antibiotics, antidepressants, and cancer therapies. In almost every case, scientists were looking for, and expecting, one thing but found something completely different and unanticipated. Medicine is not unique. Innovation in other fields is equally dependent on serendipity (e.g., cellophane, Post-it Notes, safety glass, corn flakes, microwave ovens, vulcanized rubber, and even chocolate chip cookies). Louis Pasteur famously remarked, "In fields of observation, chance favors the prepared mind." For managers, the practical question arises: what can organizations do to create, recognize, and act on favorable chance circumstances? Recognizing that old ideas are the main source of new ideas, some innovative companies create situations whereby employees can make connections between ideas from different industries, business units, or projects (Hargadon and Sutton, 2000). Consistent with the principles of complexity science, these firms use knowledge-brokering strategies like cross-product meetings, job rotation, and visits to other industries and new locations as means for promoting generative interaction and making fortuitous connections. Further, psychological science suggests that people can better recognize and act on unexpected opportunities to pursue pending or postponed goals by: (1) thinking about the circumstances required for goal accomplishment, (2) picking a few salient features of such circumstances, and (3) committing the goal and the cues to memory together (Patalano and Seifert, 1997; Seifert and Patalano, 2001). By creating a strong mental association between goals and circumstances, one is more likely to perceive environmental cues indicative of an opportunity to pursue pending goals, even when engaged in other activities.

## Learning from Mistakes

Mistakes and other unintended, undesirable outcomes can create a valuable opportunity for organizational learning. However, learning from mistakes does not happen accidentally. In successful teams, leaders actively manage how their teams learn. For example, Edmondson and colleagues studied cardiac surgical teams implementing a new, minimally invasive surgical technique (Edmondson, Bohmer, and Pisano, 2001). They examined oft-cited factors such as the lead surgeon's status or experience level; the degree of senior management and financial support; and use of team debriefs and audits—none of which appeared to have much, if anything, to do with how rapidly the teams integrated the new procedure. Successful teams did do several things differently, however. First, successful team leaders selected members for their ability to work together and being open to input. Moreover, the team leader did not regard members as interchangeable cogs based on their particular profession and expertise; instead, they emphasized keeping the same team together, which maximized their opportunities to build trust and effective communication. Second, the successful team leaders framed the implementation of the new surgical technique as a fundamentally *organizational* challenge rather than a technical one—i.e., the successful team leaders got their teams thinking about the challenge of the new surgery in terms of how they worked together, rather than in terms of learning new technical competency. Leaders of the slower-learning teams not only framed the challenge as chiefly one of technical skills, but in some cases also downplayed the relatively difficulty of the change. The result was frustrated, unmotivated team members. Third, the most successful teams created a climate of psychological safety, where they felt comfortable suggesting ideas that might not work, identifying potential problems, and admitting mistakes. Psychological safety may have been particularly important because the communication about new ideas and problem solving occurred on the fly, during the surgeries.

Mistakes and other unintended, undesirable outcomes can also be a fertile source of innovation. Peter Drucker, an internationally renowned management scholar, has argued that success in innovation results not from eureka moments of insight, but from systematic pursuit of opportunities that emerge from common dynamics, notably "unexpected occurrences," which are frequently experienced as mistakes. Mistakes provide particularly important opportunities for innovation precisely because most firms treat them as anomalous and undesirable and therefore minimize them instead of exploring their causes (Drucker, 2002). One of the ways that managers and consultants perpetuate this attitude is by treating mistakes or unexpected occurrences as, well, *unexpected*. As Pfeffer and Sutton point out in their manifesto calling for an evidence-based management movement, *every* intervention, program, or idea has a downside (Pfeffer and Sutton, 2006). Even innovations we ultimately find highly desirable, such as a Total Quality Management or lean production, will have some unintended, undesirable consequences. Part of the answer for managers is not to wait to find out *if* unexpected problems emerge from a new program or strategy, but to ask *what* unexpected problems will likely arise. As we observed in our opening vignette on the Group Health patient-centered medical home, unexpected problems create opportunities for better solutions.

What about making a mistake on purpose—that is, deliberately trying a course of action that according to your current thinking will fail? That too can be valuable, argue management consultants Schoemaker and Gunther (2006). The problem, they say, is that our natural tendency is to look exclusively for confirmatory evidence to support previously held assumptions. If we conduct an experiment, we typically select options that we believe will succeed, or at least will not perform any worse than the status quo. That works fine for identifying solutions that do not fail outright, but it is a poor strategy for discovering optimal solutions. This is similar to the problem of single-loop versus double-loop learning; double-loop learning involves examining underlying assumptions, which is precisely what confirmation bias precludes (Schoemaker and Gunther, 2006). For example, if we believe patients will find automated telephone calls intrusive and impersonal, we may decline to explore using interactive-voice response as an option for improving medication adherence. This may even be based on past experience or data. The problem is that assumptions, once made, are rarely revisited, while the conditions that created them may change dramatically. To choose which "mistakes" are likely to lead to significant learning, Schoemaker and Gunther suggest considering several factors, of which we think three are particularly important:

1. *The potential gain to the potential cost:* Obviously to try something you think has a high likelihood of failure, it must entail a reasonably low-cost relative to the potential benefit. It makes no sense to wager the firm's existence on a long-odds bet.

2. *You test core assumptions that drive large numbers of decisions:* If the deliberate mistake tests an assumption that drives large numbers of routine decisions, you can both find out more rapidly if your assumption is incorrect (abandoning your new course of action if your original assumptions were correct), and it is more likely to pay off because the consequential benefits accumulate rapidly.

3. *Conditions have changed:* We develop our assumptions under one set of conditions; those conditions may change.

---

## MOVING BEYOND EXPERIENCE TO DELIBERATE PRACTICE

Common wisdom holds that experience is the best teacher. But, is it really? In his recent bestseller *Outliers*, Malcolm Gladwell (2008) introduces the "10,000-hour rule," the idea that across a range of professions—from music to physics to chess—those who become highly accomplished have amassed 10,000 or more hours at the activity. An extensive body of research in cognitive psychology supports the 10,000-hour rule. However, Gladwell misses half the story: repetition may lead to proficiency, but it does not inevitably lead to excellence. Most performers achieve competence where they are able to complete a task without having to concentrate on it. At that point, their performance plateaus, and they cease to improve. Experts achieving the highest levels of excellence, on the contrary, continue to focus consciously on the task; they engage in *deliberate practice*. As a consequence, they continue to improve (Ericsson, 2006).

The hallmarks of deliberate practice are breaking a task into discrete components that can be learned sequentially; engaging in tasks of increasing difficulty in order to stress existing capacity and ultimately expand it; and having a mechanism for monitoring and correcting performance (Ericsson, 2006).

Though it is often perilous to apply literally lessons from individual behavior to the collective, the hallmarks of deliberate practice have clear parallels for the organization. For example, one of the tenants of systems engineering is to map an organizational process, breaking it into discrete components that can be assessed for opportunities to improve (Anderson and Johnson, 1997). Likewise, managers can use "stretch goals," i.e., setting a goal well beyond current performance such that it cannot reasonably be met by existing processes and that requires teams to find new ways of doing things (Wright et al., 1993).

Perhaps the most important lesson from deliberate practice relates to the third point, the use of feedback mechanisms. While performance measures such as HEDIS and Joint Commission measures abound in health care, these are largely summative; they are reported well after the care processes occur and are frequently linked to incentives. Implicitly, they become more tools of motivation and less tools of information. Managers can use other techniques to provide their teams with monitoring mechanisms that put the emphasis on learning and improving rather than proving that they are performing well. Two underused techniques are team debriefs and huddles. Team debriefs are meetings after a specific event or encounter to walk back through what occurred and identify potential areas for improvement. Team huddles are regular, brief meetings to confer and identify issues as they occur.

The important point to remember with all three of these hallmarks is that the objective is to keep teams from falling into a pattern of operating by rote, without opportunity to consciously evaluate the work and how it is accomplished.

# SUMMARY AND MANAGERIAL GUIDELINES

1. Health care organizations exhibit three characteristics of complex systems: interdependence, nonlinearity, and dynamism. There are no hard and fast rules for managing learning, and innovation in complex systems, though management scholars propose a range of ideas for balancing between too much structure (order) or too little (chaos). These include: (1) relying on a few simple rules rather than detailed planning; and (2) thinking about the effects on the whole system when setting goals and allocating resources.

2. Organizational learning is a feedback-loop process. Single-loop learning (adaptive learning) occurs when problem solvers compare desired states of affairs with actual results and seek to close the gap. Double-loop learning (generative learning) occurs when problem solvers attempt to close the gap between desired and actual states of affairs by questioning and modifying the underlying conditions that contribute to the actual state, such as an organization's policies, plans, values, and the rules that frame organizational problems.

3. Five "disciplines" promote organizational learning: (1) systems thinking, (2) personal mastery, (3) mental models, (4) shared vision, and (5) team learning. A powerful way to spread the discipline of systems thinking is to encourage organizational members to learn and make use of systems archetypes.

4. Organizational learning is constrained by: (1) the availability of limited information, often ambiguous or inaccurate; (2) human errors of judgment and biases, often related to the heuristics we rely on to cope with complexity and uncertainty; and (3) competing priorities, resource constraints, and broader political considerations. Systems dynamics models can help people overcome these "learning disabilities" by helping people grasp the underlying structure of the organization as a complex system, surfacing people's mental models about how the system "works," and allowing managerial strategies to be tested through rapid, low-cost, controlled experimentation.

5. Beware of three common myths or misconceptions about innovation: (1) innovation is good; (2) there is a formula, and (3) innovation is linear.

6. Learning in the innovation journey involves both discovery and testing. Discovery resembles double-loop (generative) learning. Testing resembles single-loop (adaptive) learning. One way to promote discovery is to encourage constant scanning for information about conditions and practices outside the organization's boundaries. Scanning promotes alertness, surfaces discrepant information, and uncovers new ideas. Scanning methods include benchmarking; ongoing contact with purchasers, suppliers, and partners; and soliciting feedback from employees, physicians, and patients.

7. The innovation journey often begins with discovery, but thereafter cycles in non-predictable ways between discovery and testing. It is important to manage expectations about the impacts of innovation. Even highly technical innovations involve major organizational challenges, such as shifting roles, prerogatives, and responsibilities. Acknowledging the challenging nature of the innovation journey upfront will help mitigate frustration and keep lines of communication open.

8. Organizations can promote learning and innovation by nurturing foresight, fostering improvisation, maximizing serendipity, and learning from mistakes. Actively look for mistakes—unanticipated, unwanted consequences—from new programs. Repeatedly let your staff members know that mistakes are bound to occur, and the most essential thing is to understand how they occurred as a result and why. These mistakes may prove the most fertile ground for future innovation.

# DISCUSSION QUESTIONS

1. Complexity theorists advise organizational leaders to abandon command-and-control styles of management and instead set global performance targets and establish a few simple rules. This approach can unleash creativity and innovation, but it can also promote conflict and waste. How can managers "let go of control," yet still ensure that organizational activities are coordinated with each other aligned with organizational goals? What could managers do to mitigate the potentially negative consequences of following complexity theorists' advice?

2. Organizational learning requires a climate of openness, trust, and honesty. What can managers do to establish and maintain such a climate?

3. How can managers hold health professionals and employees accountable for personal and organizational performance, yet still encourage them to try new ideas and take prudent risks to improve quality, safety, and efficiency?

4. If innovation is inherently unknowable, and creates unintended consequences, often far downstream, how can managers effectively evaluate the outcomes of innovation initiatives? Is there ever a point when a manager can reliably draw a conclusion about whether an innovation has been a success?

5. The Minnesota Innovation Research Project found that innovation managers' careers were often unfairly penalized when innovations turned out poorly. Is this an important concern for senior managers? If so, what can they do to mitigate it? What, if anything, should innovation managers do to protect themselves and their teams?

6. Schoemaker and Gunther (2006) recommend making deliberate mistakes as ways of breaking out of ineffective or suboptimal strategy borne of flawed or outdated assumptions. They provide some guidelines for which kinds of mistakes to deliberately make, such as those with a limited cost versus the potential gain. Based on their criteria, can you think of a potential "mistake" you might suggest to your primary-care provider to improve their clinic performance? For example, you might suggest that they eliminate visit co-pays. What are the costs or harms that make this a mistake? What are the assumptions that underpin the practice? What are the potential advantages?

# CASE: Innovating through Quality: Does Developing a New Program Make Sense?

Alliance Health Care is a small hospital chain in the Northwest that has been on the leading edge regionally in adopting an integrated electronic health record (EHR) and was an early participant in one of the first voluntary, public reporting systems for surgical quality. That role, as regional innovator, has served Alliance well, giving it an excellent reputation.

The vice president for quality and safety has been working with researchers at the state's flagship university, who are developing appropriateness criteria for cardiology. They have an idea to integrate appropriateness criteria in the EHR and produce real-time feedback reports to providers. They want to create a pilot program for cardiac surgery.

Appropriateness criteria are essentially very sophisticated practice guidelines. They comprise branching algorithms derived from past cases that give an assessment of whether procedures such as cardiac catheterization, imaging, and medications are right for a specific patient, given their comorbidities, disease severity, life expectancy, and other factors.

The VP has informal discussions with several internal stakeholders, including the chiefs of surgery and radiology at the flagship hospital; the chief information officer; and the chief financial officer. They are cautiously interested, though all bring up major concerns. The chief of surgery worries that no matter how sophisticated, these algorithms can never reflect the complexity of real cases, and that using them will just create another legal vulnerability. The chief of radiology worries that the appropriateness criteria will be used primarily for identifying cases of overuse (when patients get care that is of questionable benefit) and not underuse (when patients fail to receive care they would likely benefit from). The CFO brings up similar concerns and notes that imaging accounts for approximately 10 percent of operating profit; if the new system mainly curtails procedures, it could have a major deleterious effect on your revenues. The CIO really likes the idea, but warns that it could take years to test and fully integrate the algorithms, and the cost will be significant.

In light of these concerns, the VP decides to engage in a generative or double-loop learning cycle.

## Questions
1. What are the underlying assumptions that drive the VP's interest in an appropriateness criteria program?
2. How can she/he explore or test those assumptions?
3. In other words, how can they determine if they are incorrect?
4. What environmental events could change those assumptions?

# REFERENCES

Anderson, V., & Johnson, L. (1997). *Systems thinking basics: From concepts to causal loops.* Cambridge, MA: Pegasus Communication.

Andriopoulos, C., & Gotsi, M. (2006). Probing the future: Mobilising foresight in multiple-product innovation firms. *Futures, 38*(1), 50–66.

Argote, L. (1999). *Organizational learning: Creating, retaining, and transferring knowledge.* Boston: Kluwer Academic.

Argyris, C., & Schon, D. A. (1978). *Organizational learning.* Reading: MA. Addison-Wesley.

Arndt, M., & Bigelow, B. (2000). Commentary: The potential of chaos theory and complexity theory for health services management. *Health Care Management Review, 25*(1), 35–38.

Bayer, S., Barlow, J., & Curry, R. (2007). Assessing the impact of a care innovation: telecare. *System Dynamics Review, 23*(1), 61–80.

Beeson, I., & Davis, C. (2000). Emergence and accomplishment in organizational change. *Journal of Organizational Change Management, 13*(2), 178–189.

Begun, J. W. (1994). Chaos and complexity: Frontiers of organization science. *Journal of Management Inquiry,* 329–335.

Begun, J. W., & Luke, R. D. (2001). Factors underlying organizational change in local health care markets, 1982–1995. *Health Care Management Review, 26*(2): 62–72.

Begun, J. W., Zimmerman, B., & Dooley, K. (2003). Health care organizations as complex adaptive systems. in S. S. Mick and M. F. Wyttenbach (Eds.), *Advances in health care organization theory* (pp. 253–288). San Francisco: Jossey-Bass.

Berquist, W. (1993). *The postmodern organization: Mastering the art of irreversible change.* San Francisco: Jossey-Bass.

Berwick, D. M. (1998). Developing and testing changes in delivery of care. *Annals of Internal Medicine, 128*(8), 651–656.

Black, J. A. (2000). Fermenting change—capitalizing on the inherent change found in dynamic non linear (or complex) systems. *Journal of Organizational Change Management, 13*(6), 520–525.

Bohmer, R. M., & Edmondson, A. C. (2001). Organizational learning in health care. *Health Forum Journal, 44*(2), 32–35.

Bowditch, J. L., & Buono, A. F. (2001). *A primer on organizational behavior* (5th ed.). New York: John Wiley & Sons.

Brown, S. L., & Eisenhardt, K. M. (1997). The art of continuous change: Linking complexity theory and time-paced evolution in relentlessly shifting organizations. *Administrative Science Quarterly, 42*(1), 1–34.

Burnes, B. (2005). Complexity theories and organizational change. *International Journal of Management Reviews, 7*(2), 73–90.

Cherniak, C. (1986). *Minimal rationality: Computational models of cognition and perception.* Cambridge, MA: MIT Press.

Chuang, Y. T., Ginsburg, L., & Berta, W. B. (2007). Learning from preventable adverse events in health care organizations: Development of a multilevel model of learning and propositions. *Health Care Management Review, 32*(4), 330–340.

Collins, J. C. (2001). *Good to great: Why some companies make the leap—and others don't.* New York: HarperBusiness.

Collins, J.C., & Porras, J. I. (1994). *Built to last: Successful habits of visionary companies.* New York: HarperBusiness.

Conrad, D., et al. (2008). Access intervention in an integrated, prepaid group practice: Effects on primary care physician productivity. *Health Services Research, 43*(5), 1888–1905.

Crossan, M. M., Lane, H. W., & White, R. E. (1999). An organizational learning framework: From intuition to institution. *Academy of Management Review, 24*(3), 522–537.

Cyert, R. M. & March, J. G. (1992). *A behavioral theory of the firm* (2nd ed.). Cambridge, MA: Blackwell Business.

Day, G. S., & Schoemaker, P. J. H. (2005). Scanning the periphery. *Harvard Business Review, 83*(11), 135–148.

Drucker, P. F. (2002). The discipline of innovation. *Harvard Business Review, 80*(8), 95–102.

Edmondson, A., Bohmer, R., & Pisano, G. (2001). Speeding up team learning. *Harvard Business Review, 79*(9), 125–132.

Ericsson, K. A. (2006). The influence of experience and deliberate practice on the development of superior expert performance. In K. A. Ericsson (Ed.), *The Cambridge handbook of expertise and expert performance* (pp. 683–703). Cambridge: Cambridge University Press.

Fitzgerald, L. A. (2002). Chaos: The lens that transcends. *Journal of Organizational Change Management, 15*(4), 339–358.

Garvin, D. A. (1993). Building a learning organization. *Harvard Business Review, 74*(1), 78–91.

Gladwell, M. (2008). *Outliers: The story of success.* New York: Little, Brown and Company.

Greenhalgh, T., et al. (2004). Diffusion of innovations in service organizations: systematic review and recommendations. *Milbank Quarterly, 82*(4), 581–629.

Hammond, J. S., Keeney, R. L. & Raiffa, H. (1998). The hidden traps in decision making. *Harvard Business Review, 76*(5), 47–58.

Hargadon, A., & Sutton, R. I. (2000). Building an innovation factory. *Harvard Business Review, 78*(3), 157–166.

Helfrich, C. D., et al. (2007). Adoption and implementation of mandated diabetes registries by community health centers. *American Journal of Preventive Medicine, 33*(1 Suppl.), S50–S58; quiz, S59–S65.

Hock, D., & VISA International (1999). *Birth of the chaordic age.* San Francisco: Berrett-Koehler.

Homer, J., et al. (2004). Models for collaboration: how system dynamics helped a community organize cost-effective care for chronic illness. *System Dynamics Review, 20*(3), 199–222.

Homer, J., Hirsch, G., & Milstein, B. (2007). Chronic illness in a complex health economy: the perils and promises of downstream and upstream reforms. *System Dynamics Review, 23*(2–3), 313–343.

Isaacs, W. (1999). *Dialogue and the art of thinking together.* New York: Random House.

Jenner, R. A. (1998). Dissipative enterprises, chaos, and the principles of lean organizations. *Omega-International Journal of Management Science, 26*(3), 397–407.

Kahneman, D., Slovic, P., & Tversky, A. (Eds.). (1982). *Judgment under uncertainty: Heuristics and biases.* Cambridge: Cambridge University Press.

Kimberly, J. (1981). *Managing innovation.* In P. C. Nystrom and W. H. Starbuck (Eds.), *Handbook of organizational design.* Oxford: Oxford University Press.

Leander, W. J. (1996). *Patients first: Experiences of a patient-focused pioneer.* Chicago: Health Administration Press.

Lemak, C. H., & Goodrick, E. (2003). Strategy as simple rules: Understanding success in a rural clinic. *Health Care Management Review, 28*(2), 179–188.

Levy, P. F. (2001). The Nut Island effect: When good teams go wrong. *Harvard Business Review, 79*(3), 51–59.

Marion, R., & Bacon, J. (2000). "Organizational Extinction and Complex Systems." *Emergence, 1*(4), 71–96.

McCarthy, D., Mueller, K., & Tillmann, I. (2009). *Group Health Cooperative: Reinventing primary care by connecting patients with a medical home.* New York: The Commonwealth Fund.

McDaniel, R. R. (1997). Strategic leadership: A view from quantum and chaos theories. *Health Care Management Review, 22*(1), 21–37.

McGill, M. E., & J.W. Slocum, J. W. (1993). Unlearning the Organization. *Organizational Dynamics, 22,* 67–78.

Mintzberg, H. (1994). *The rise and fall of strategic planning: Reconceiving roles for planning, plans, planners.* New York: Free Press.

Moorman, C., & Miner, A. S. (1998). Organizational improvisation and organizational memory. *Academy of Management Review, 23*(4), 698–723.

Patalano, A. L., & Seifert, C. M. (1997). Opportunistic planning: Being reminded of pending goals. *Cognitive Psychology, 34*(1), 1–36.

Peters, T. J., & Waterman, R. H. (1982). *In search of excellence: Lessons from America's best-run companies.* New York: Harper & Row.

Pettigrew, A. M. (1985). *The awakening giant: Continuity and change in imperial chemical industries.* Oxford: Blackwell.

Pfeffer, J., & Sutton, R. I. (2006). *Hard facts, dangerous half-truths, and total nonsense: profiting from evidence-based management.* Boston: Harvard Business School Press.

Plsek, P. E., & Greenhalgh, T. (2001). Complexity science: The challenge of complexity in health care. *British Medical Journal, 323*(7313), 625–628.

Plsek, P. E., & Wilson, T. (2001, 29 September). "Complexity, leadership, and management in health care organizations." *BMJ, 323,* 746–749.

Ralston, J. D., et al. (2009). Group Health Cooperative's transformation toward patient-centered access. *Medical Care Research and Review, 66*(6), 703–724.

Reid, R. J., et al. (2009). Patient-centered medical home demonstration: A prospective, quasi-experimental, before and after evaluation. *American Journal of Managed Care, 15*(9), E71–E87

Robert Wood Johnson Foundation. (2008). *Improving access to improve quality: evaluation of an organizational innovation.* Washington, DC: AcademyHealth.

Roberto, M. A., Bohmer, R. M. J., & Edmondson, A. C. (2006). *Facing ambiguous threats. Harvard Business Review, 84*(11): p. 106–112.

Rogers, E. M. (2003). *The diffusion of innovations* (5th ed.). New York: Free Press.

Rosenzweig, P. M. (2007). *The halo effect and the eight other business delusions that deceive managers.* New York: Free Press.

Rowe, A., & Hogarth, A. (2005). Use of complex adaptive systems metaphor to achieve professional and organizational change. *Journal of Advanced Nursing, 51*(4), 396–405.

Schoemaker, P. J. H., & Gunther, R. E. (2006). The wisdom of deliberate mistakes. *Harvard Business Review, 84*(6) 108–115.

Seifert, C. M., & A. L. Patalano (2001). Opportunism in memory: Preparing for chance encounters. *Current Directions in Psychological Science, 10*(6), 198–201.

Senge, P. M. (2006). *The fifth discipline: The art and practice of the learning organization* (Rev. and updated ed.) New York: Doubleday/Currency.

Senge, P. M. (1990). *The fifth discipline: The art and practice of the learning organization.* New York: Currency Doubleday.

Stacey, R. D. (1995). *The science of complexity: An alternative perspective for strategic change processes. Strategic Management Journal, 16,* 477–495.

Sterman, J. D. (2000). *Business dynamics: Systems thinking and modeling for a complex world.* Boston: Irwin McGraw-Hill.

Sullivan, T. J. (1999). Leading people in a chaotic world. *Journal of Educational Administration, 37*(5), 408–423.

Tetenbaum, T. J. (1998). Shifting paradigms: From Newton to chaos. *Organizational Dynamics, 26*(4), 21–32.

Tsoukas, H., & Shepherd, J. (2004). Coping with the future: Developing organizational foresightfulness—introduction. *Futures, 36*(2), 137–144.

Tucker, A. L., & Edmondson, A. C. (2003). Why hospitals don't learn from failures: Organizational and psychological dynamics that inhibit system change. *California Management Review, 45*(2), 55–72.

Tufano, J. T., Ralston, J. D., & Martin, D. P. (2008). Providers' experience with an organizational redesign initiative to promote patient-centered access: A qualitative study. *Journal of General Internal Medicine, 23*(11), 1778–1783.

Vaill, P. B. (1989). *Managing as a performing art: New ideas for a world of chaotic change.* San Francisco: Jossey-Bass.

Van de Ven, A. H., Polley, D. E., Garud, R., & Venkataraman, S. (1999). *The innovation journey.* New York: Oxford University Press.

Van de Ven, A. H., et al. (1989). Processes of new business creation in different organizational settings. In A. H. Van de Ven, H. L. Angle, & M. S. Poole (Eds.), *Research on the management of innovation: The Minnesota studies* (pp. 221–298). New York: Ballinger/Harper & Row.

Weick, K. (1979). *The social psychology of organizing.* Reading: MA: Addison-Wesley.

Weick, K. E. (1993). Sensemaking in organizations: Small structures with large consequences. In J. K. Murningham (Ed.), *Social psychology in organizations: Advances in theory and research* (pp. 10–37). Englewood Cliffs, NJ: Prentice Hall.

Wermers, M. A., et al. (1996). Planning and assessing a cross-training initiative with multiskilled employees. *Joint Commission Journal on Quality Improvement, 22*(6), 412–426.

Wheatley, M. J. (2006). *Leadership and the new science: Discovering order in a chaotic world* (3rd ed.). San Francisco: Berrett-Koehler.

Wheatley, M. J. (1992). *Leadership and the new science: Learning about organization from an orderly universe.* San Francisco: Berrett-Koehler.

Wolstenholme, E. (2004). Using generic system archetypes to support thinking and modelling. *System Dynamics Review, 20*(4), 341–356.

Wright, P. M., et al. (1993). Productivity and extra-role behavior—the effects of goals and incentives on spontaneous helping. *Journal of Applied Psychology, 78*(3), 374–381.

Zimmerman, B. J. (1999). Complexity science: A route through hard times and uncertainty. *Health Forum Journal, 42*(2), 42–46.

# Chapter 9

# Improving Quality in Health Care Organizations

**Ann Scheck McAlearney and Jeffrey A. Alexander**

## CHAPTER OUTLINE

- **Quality Improvement in Health Care**
- **Quality Measurement and Quality Improvement**
- **Approaches to Quality Improvement**
- **Getting to Higher Quality and Quality Improvement**
- **Applying Quality Improvement Frameworks**

## LEARNING OBJECTIVES

**After completing this chapter, the reader should be able to:**

1. Explain the importance of quality improvement (QI) in health care
2. Define quality and performance measures for organizations
3. Differentiate the important issues in defining, measuring, and using quality and performance measures
4. Recognize the challenges of undertaking QI and QI implementation in HCOs
5. Distinguish among QI frameworks
6. Describe opportunities to apply QI tactics and strategies to support QI in HCOs
7. Assess conditions for QI change
8. Justify the need to manage for QI in health care
9. Explain the importance of people and focusing on people issues in QI efforts
10. Describe management roles to create high-performance, quality-focused organizations

# KEY TERMS

Benchmarking

Clinical Practice Guidelines

Continuous Quality Improvement

High-Performance Work Practices (HPWPs)

Implementation

Lean

Outcome Measures of Quality

Process Measures of Quality

Quality Improvement (QI)

Quality Improvement (QI) Interventions

Quality Measures

Six Sigma

Structural Measures of Quality

Transactional Leadership

Transformational Leadership

---

## IN PRACTICE: Sharp HealthCare and Their Quality Improvement Journey

Sharp HealthCare is a large, not-for-profit health system based in San Diego, California. With over 14,000 employees and 2,600 physician affiliates, the system is comprised of four acute-care hospitals, three specialty hospitals, and two medical groups, and also includes a wide range of other facilities and services. Given its location in a highly regulated state, Sharp faces particular challenges associated with corporate practice of medicine laws and the laws regulating nurse-staff ratios as they impact Sharp's abilities to employ and deploy health care professionals throughout their organization. Yet despite these challenges, Sharp HealthCare has received increased attention over the past decade as it has received national recognition for Magnet designation for nursing excellence at two of its acute-care hospitals, national designation as a Planetree hospital at another acute-care hospital, and the prestigious 2007 Malcolm Baldrige Award for Quality for the system as a whole.

Sharp's self-described quality improvement "journey" has been multifaceted and has touched the entire health system. In the late 1990s, Sharp had a solid reputation in the San Diego area, and patient satisfaction scores collected by the organization were high, indicating that there was not much to worry about. A change in system leadership, however, created an opportunity to focus on quality and quality improvement in a new way.

Curious about how they were doing, Sharp decided to convene some focus groups to find out how patients felt about their health care experience. Much to the surprise and chagrin of health system leaders, Sharp's patients told them the experience was not all that good, and health care in general left much to be desired from a customer perspective. Instead of confirming their belief that Sharp was well regarded by satisfied patients, these focus groups indicated many opportunities for improvement. The health system began to benchmark data against other health systems and contracted with Press-Ganey for patient satisfaction measurement. Patient satisfaction scores as measured by the new scale were in the lowest quartile.

Sharp's leaders used these data to spark employee interest in quality and performance improvement, and to motivate employees to address needed changes. Over the course of the next decade, Sharp made a substantial investment in **Lean** and **Six Sigma** methods as its selected approach to **performance improvement**, and built a QI focus into the culture of the organization. In addition, as an organizing framework for the QI journey, Sharp designed The Sharp Experience as a performance improvement initiative designed to help Sharp realize its mission-driven goal to be *the best place to work, the best place to practice medicine, and the best place to receive care.* Sharp's receipt of the coveted Baldrige Award for Quality in 2007 provided public recognition of Sharp's success in their QI journey. Now beyond Baldrige, Sharp continues to capitalize on opportunities for QI, and is currently driving improvements in patient safety, including "just culture," transparency, Team Training, standardized communication processes, handoff standardization, and design change to improve quality of care and patient safety throughout the health system.

SOURCE: Nancy G. Pratt, RN, MS, Senior Vice President, Clinical Effectiveness, Sharp HealthCare; Sharp HealthCare Web site (http://www.sharp.com)

# CHAPTER PURPOSE

With the release of the IOM's report, *To Err is Human: Building a Safer Health System* (IOM, 1999), quality and patient safety reemerged as sentinel issues in health care delivery. The Institute's report prompted renewed effort to identify and implement **quality improvement interventions**, interventions designed to decrease medical errors and enhance patient safety. It also rekindled attempts to hold HCOs accountable for quality. Government agencies, accrediting bodies, employer groups, and other organizations have developed an ever-growing number of quality indicators and patient safety goals against which they intend to measure a health care organization's quality performance and improvement. Some states have implemented mandatory quality reporting systems for hospitals (Morrissey, 2002). Thus, health care organization quality is likely to remain under intense scrutiny for some time. This chapter outlines how HCOs can improve quality and patient safety through QI efforts, and describes the challenges and strategies for changing organizational systems to ensure that QI is an accepted part of organizational behavior.

# QUALITY IMPROVEMENT IN HEALTH CARE

Most everyone agrees that high quality is an important characteristic of health care services. However, quality can be a difficult concept to define. Donabedian (2005) observed that although quality can be very broadly defined, it usually reflects the values and goals of the current medical system and of the larger society of which it is a part. According to Donabedian (1988), there are three major elements of quality: structure, process, and outcomes. *Structure* pertains to having the necessary resources to provide adequate health care; *process* focuses on how care is provided, delivered, and managed; and *outcomes* refers to changes in a patient's health status as a result of medical care.

Another definition of quality that is commonly used and widely accepted is contained in the influential report from the Institute of Medicine (IOM), *Crossing the Quality Chasm: A New Health System for the 21st Century*. This report defined quality as "the degree to which health services for individuals and populations increase the likelihood of desired health outcomes and are consistent with current professional knowledge" (IOM, 2001). The report also discussed the six major aims for improvement in health care, built around the need for care to be: *safe, effective, patient-centered, timely, efficient,* and *equitable* (IOM, 2001). Health care organizations (HCOs), then, are challenged to provide care, or support the micro-systems that deliver care, that achieves these aims (Berwick, 2002).

Quality problems in the U.S. health care system are expressed in numerous ways, stem from different sources, and have different consequences for individuals and organizations. With respect to medical errors, for example, it is estimated that preventable medical errors cause between 44,000 and 98,000 deaths in hospitals each year (IOM, 1999). Further, although Americans receive only 55 percent of recommended treatments for preventive care, acute care, and care for chronic conditions (McGlynn et al., 2003), slightly more than 10 percent receive too much care; care that is not recommended or is potentially harmful (McGlynn et al., 2003). Additionally, poor quality can result in increased expenditures; research suggests that 20 to 30 percent of a typical organization's expenses are due to issues such as redundancy of effort, rework, error, inefficiency, persistent problems, and untrained employees (Leebov and Ersoz, 2003).

## Quality Improvement (QI)

**Quality Improvement** (QI) is an organized approach to planning and implementing continuous improvement in performance. QI emphasizes continuous examination and improvement of work processes by teams of organizational members trained in basic statistical techniques and problem-solving tools, and empowered to make decisions based on their analysis of the data. Typically, these QI efforts are strongly rooted in evidence-based procedures and rely extensively on data collected about the processes and outcomes experienced by patients in organizations. Although QI practices were originally developed in the manufacturing sector, quality experts contend that QI methods can be successfully applied to service delivery. Juran (1988), for example, argues that although service outcomes are difficult to measure, due to the intangibility of the product and the interactive nature of service delivery, it remains conceptually feasible to identify customer requirements, to translate these requirements into behavioral routines and standards for personnel, and to monitor these processes. Several HCOs report having measurable success in applying QI practices to clinical care processes (Gregor et al., 1996; Krein et al., 2004; Lynn, West, Hausmann, et al., 2007; Monteleoni and Clark, 2004; Pestotnik et al., 1996; Solberg et al., 2006; Ullman et al., 1996).

Like other systems-based approaches, QI stresses that quality depends foremost on the processes by which services are designed and delivered. The systemic focus of QI complements a growing recognition in the field that the quality of the care delivered by clinicians depends substantially on the performance capability of the organizational systems in which they work. While individual clinician competence remains important, many increasingly see that the capability of organizational systems to prevent errors, to coordinate care among settings and practitioners, and to ensure that relevant, accurate information is available when needed is critical in providing high-quality care. This systems-based perspective on QI emphasizes organization-wide commitment and involvement because most, if not all, vital work processes span many individuals, disciplines, and departments in all clinical settings.

## QI Interventions

**QI interventions** vary widely (Lucas et al., 2007). On the one hand, *externally developed* QI involves looking outside the organization for new or redesigned practices—often evidence-based—to bring into the organization. The emphasis of the intervention is on the desired new practice. Many efforts to bring research into practice, such as guideline implementation, fall into this category. By contrast, in *locally developed* QI, the improvement process begins with a problem, but participants do not know what the improved practices will look like; solutions evolve through analysis and experimentation. In this case, the emphasis is on changing the process by which a service or product is produced. Still other QI initiatives are broadly predefined but allow for considerable flexibility and local tailoring. The chronic care model introduced through the Improving Chronic Illness Care Collaboratives is a good example of such an approach. The Chronic Care Model consists of six interrelated system components: effective team care; planned interactions among providers; self-management support; community resources; integrated decision support;

and patient registries and other information technology (IT). Registries, decision support, provider communication, and information exchange for care coordination are all important QI enablers. Registries, for example, track groups of patients with specific chronic diseases, helping medical teams to make the most of each office visit and to follow evidence-based care guidelines. Although the model provides general guidelines and identifies specific elements that should be included in a care delivery system, the way in which these elements are adapted by primary care practices will vary as a function of available resources, the types of patients treated by the practice, the size of the practice, and experience with similar forms of QI.

In practice, QI interventions can also be described in organizational terms. Interventions can be described (1) by the *levels of organization* at which the intervention is targeted (e.g., individual level, microsystem level such as teams, work units or departments, or at the macrosystem level of the full organization); and (2) by the *scale of the intervention* (e.g., single medical center or clinics, multiple sites, or national rollout). Specifying the level and scale of QI interventions can help organizational members to better understand the nature of the QI goals, as well as the potential reach and impact of the QI intervention.

# QUALITY MEASUREMENT AND QUALITY IMPROVEMENT

In order for organizations to focus on quality and QI in health care, they must understand how quality is measured and monitored. The following sections describe measures and measurement of quality and discuss some of the issues related to the definition and use of different quality and performance measures to drive QI efforts in HCOs.

## Quality Measures and Measurement

Based on Donabedian's (1966) definition of quality in health care, three basic classes of **quality measures** have been specified: structural, process, and outcome measures. First, **structural measures of quality** are defined as based on aspects of an organization or an individual's actions that could impact overall quality or organizational performance. From a business operations standpoint, these structural measures are associated with the capacity of an organization to promote effective work. Examples of structural measures of quality in health care are numerous and include indicators such as the number and type of beds in a given organization, the presence of shared governance structures, and the existence of a computerized provider order entry (CPOE) system with decision support features. Even the presence of certain organizational certifications or accolades can be used as structural measures of performance, including accreditation by the Joint Commission, or receipt of Magnet status in nursing. While structural measures of quality are often under the control of a manager or an organization, they are often seen as quite distal indicators of care quality.

Next, **process measures of quality** refer to indicators of the activities involved in carrying out work in an organization. Activities such as reviewing medical records to ensure completion of patient education, monitoring physician and nurse compliance with organizational standards for cleanliness, or evaluating the use of central lines are all examples of process metrics. Process measures are often favored over structural measures because they are perceived to be more closely linked to clinical care quality, and because they are still within the span of control managers have to influence and improve work processes.

Third, **outcome measures of quality** are metrics based on the results of work performed. In many ways, outcome measures can be considered measures of work process outputs. Examples of outcome measures in health care are numerous and include metrics such as health status, patient satisfaction, and mortality. Often outcome measures are viewed as superior to other classes of quality measures because clinical outcomes are of most concern and relevance to patients and the organizations in which they receive care.

## Using Quality Measures

A key foundation of any QI effort is the ability to accurately measure quality and use those measures to identify problems, monitor progress, and formulate strategies to improve quality of care. Although this seems intuitive, a variety of technical, organizational, and management issues often impede the development and use of quality metrics in HCOs. Perhaps the most fundamental problem is that many managers and boards simply do not know what to do with quality measures even when they have access to them. Whereas measures of financial performance such as ROI (return on investment) and debt-to-asset ratio are immediately recognizable to most managers and board members, many quality measures remain strange and unfathomable to these same individuals. Often this reflects a lack of training in QI, which would enable managers to translate the measures into actionable changes in care processes. Instead, managers often delegate responsibility for quality performance shortfalls to individual clinicians or medical staff who are assumed to be either the source of knowledge about the problem or its cause, rather than linking the measures to failures in the systems that are the underlying root of the problem (Alexander and Young, 2010). For example, because of their lack of proximity to actual care delivery, managers may not understand the clinical processes and support infrastructure that affects quality indicators such as medication error rates or in-hospital mortality due to cardiac arrest.

A second problem that prevents more widespread use of quality measures is the nature of the measures themselves. The validity and attribution of many outcomes-based quality measures are vigorously debated. In the first case, for example, many clinicians place very little credibility in quality metrics derived from insurance claims data, citing a lack of clinical input in such measures and considerable "noise" in the data used to produce the measures. From a managerial perspective, it makes quality measures much more difficult than, say, financial indicators to motivate change in behavior. Similarly, some quality measures are rejected because they are seen to be affected by factors other than the care provided by the organization or its members. For instance, a patient's responsiveness to a particular treatment for heart failure will likely depend upon whether the prescribed treatment actually works (based upon the patient's genetics and biology), what other (comorbid) conditions that patient has, and whether the patient is compliant with the prescribed treatment, among other things. Thus, while the care provided could have been evaluated as successful based on structural or process measures (e.g., the physician was board-certified, the bed was available without delay, the medications were available and prescribed appropriately), the outcome measure might indicate poor quality of care if the patient suffered a heart attack or died while in the hospital.

Attempts to "standardize" for such extraneous factors often take the form of debates around so-called risk adjustment in quality metrics such as hospital mortality rates. In this case, simply counting the number of in-hospital deaths would inaccurately reflect the quality of the institution unless this rate were adjusted for the complexity and severity of cases treated by the hospital, the ages of the patients, and other risk-related factors. Because there is no standard way to adjust for these risk factors, the resulting quality measures may not be accepted by those who are being held accountable for them, and organizational members may be reluctant to assume responsibility for performance over which they feel they have no control.

A third problem centers on the focus of quality measures. As noted above, many outcomes-based measures are exceedingly difficult to assess and are subject to problems of lack of buy-in by key stakeholders. Other quality metrics focus on either process or structure and rest on the key assumption that if such processes or structures are in place, then better quality outcomes will result. Such measures avoid the problems of outcomes-based measures, but carry important assumptions about the link to actual patient outcomes. On the positive side, such measures are rarely subject to risk adjustment controversies, and data on which these measures are based are usually more readily obtainable and accurate. CMS and HEDIS now incorporate a range of process-based quality measures in their Hospital Compare and health plan performance reports.

## Developing Quality Measures

The issues above notwithstanding, health care managers should attempt to follow several basic guidelines in developing quality measures for QI purposes. First, quality measures should be economical. They must be easy to create, and they should not place excessive burdens on the organization or its members for new data systems, time to collect and assemble the data, or time to analyze the measures once they are created. Quality reporting systems that are not economical tend to assume a life of their own and actually become diversions from the initial purpose of the system: a tool to improve quality. Such systems are also likely to collapse under their own weight if users consider them expensive and time-consuming.

Second, the data on which quality measures are based must be timely. This means that the process of data collection/ abstraction, measurement creation, and measurement reporting needs to occur in as close to real time as possible. This makes the measures relevant to those who will act on them because they reflect the current situation. If quality measurement creation and reporting take an excessive period of time, or if the measures are based on data that are several months old, the measures will not be regarded as current, and it is unlikely that such measures will be used to direct changes in care processes.

Finally, and perhaps most important, quality measures must be actionable. Accurate performance measures tell HCOs where they are on quality standards, and to take action if they are not on track or if performance does not meet expectations. That is, the measures must contain clear signals for change. It is important to note that this does not mean that the measure(s) will tell organizations or their members what needs to be changed in specific terms. In fact, a key premise underlying QI is that quality improvements result through a team-based process of analysis and process redesign. However, quality measurement is an important component because actionable measures will provide clear signals about what constitutes acceptable versus unacceptable quality, and will provide clear indications as to whether quality is improving, declining, or maintaining at a steady state level. In practice, this means that the number of measures should be kept to a few key indicators that best reflect quality in order to avoid contradictory signals from too many measures. It also means that standards and operational definitions for the measures must be clearly defined and communicated to those who will use them.

Table 9.1 provides examples of quality measures that an organization might consider. The column showing Organizational Metrics highlights measures that could be derived from data an organization may already collect, thus in keeping with the goals for quality measures to be economical, timely, and actionable. For example, most HCOs collect data on employee satisfaction through an organizational survey, and results from questions on this survey could be compiled to create a quality measure that allows an organization to monitor employees' perceptions of the "quality of work life" in that organization. On the clinical side, the IOM's aims for improvement could be used as a framework around which to develop clinical quality measures. The column showing Clinical Metrics provides examples of how these measures could be developed using commonly available clinical and organizational data.

**TABLE 9.1** **Examples of Quality Measures**

| Organizational Metrics | Clinical Metrics (Institute of Medicine's Aims for Improvement—IOM 2001) |
|---|---|
| *Quality of Work Life*<br>• Perceptions of work-life balance<br>• Often derived from organizational survey | *Safe*<br>• Standardized mortality rate for unit, for organization<br>• Adverse drug events per doses (1,000) administered |
| *Employee Satisfaction with the Organization*<br>• Willingness to refer a friend or relative to the organization<br>• Willingness to seek care within the organization<br>• Employee turnover rates | *Effective*<br>• Lost days of work per employee<br>• Growth in market share for organization<br>• Statistics related to patient safety<br>• Perceptions about quality of care within organizational culture |
| *Financial Metrics*<br>• Margins, etc.<br>• Bed days per 1,000<br>• Market share | *Patient-Centered*<br>• Patient satisfaction with unit, with organization<br>• Drill down into patient education statistics |
| *Patient Satisfaction*<br>• With care, safety, providers<br>• Willingness to refer friend/relative for care | *Timely*<br>• Access to care as measured by waiting times, other process measures<br>• Measurement of delays in care |
| *Achievement of Strategic Goals*<br>• Alignment with balanced scorecard goals<br>• Achievement of national patient safety goals<br>• Participation in Institute for Healthcare Improvement (IHI) campaigns | *Efficient*<br>• Cost per adjusted hospital admission<br>• Operating margin as measured by cash from operations<br>*Equitable*<br>• Disparities in care access<br>• Disparities in utilization<br>• Disparities in referrals made |

# APPROACHES TO QUALITY IMPROVEMENT

All forms of QI share certain principles. QI approaches focus on making improvements that are systematic, guided by data, and efficient (Lynn et al., 2007). Key elements of QI approaches include continuous improvement, customer focus, structured processes, and organization-wide participation (Shortell et al., 1995). These approaches are often based on experiential learning, view improvement as part of the work process, and involve deliberate steps that are expected to improve care (Lynn et al., 2007). Often, an organization employs multiple QI approaches together. Table 9.2 presents a glossary of common terms and programs associated with QI in health care, and includes relevant Internet addresses when available.

## TABLE 9.2  Glossary of Common Terms and Programs Associated with QI in Health Care

*AIDET:*  A communication tool espoused by the Studer Group, designed to help clinicians establish trust with patients in order to improve compliance and clinical outcomes. AIDET is an acronym that stands for Acknowledge, Introduce, Duration, Explanation, and Thank You (http://www.studergroup.com/dotCMS/detailProduct?inode=110454).

*Baldrige Award:*  A prestigious national award to companies in several categories, including health care, that recognizes demonstrated excellence in seven categories: leadership; strategic planning; customer and market focus; measurement, analysis, and knowledge management; workforce focus; process management; and results. Applications are reviewed by an independent Board of Examiners (http://www.baldrige.nist.gov/).

*Benchmarking:*  A key feature of many QI approaches, benchmarking is the process of comparing an organization's performance metrics (e.g., quality, cost, operational efficiency) to those of other "best practice" or peer organizations.

*Business Process Reengineering (BPR):*  Term used to describe efforts to radically review and reorganize existing work processes, or adopt new and innovative work processes, designed to improve customer value, organizational efficiency, and market competitiveness. A key to BPR is the development of organizational and management structures to effectively support the redesign (e.g., information technology) (see Hammer, 1990).

*Clinical Practice Guidelines:*  Typically developed by expert panels, clinical practice guidelines synthesize evidence from the literature and make recommendations regarding treatment for specific clinical conditions (see IOM, 2001). The National Guideline Clearinghouse (http://www.guideline.gov) is a publicly available resource for evidence-based guidelines covering a full range of clinical conditions.

*Continuous Quality Improvement (CQI):*  A participative, systematic approach to planning and implementing a continuous organizational improvement process.

*Crew Resource Management (CRM):*  A technique from the aviation field that addresses errors resulting from communication and decision making in dynamic environments, such as teams, that has been adopted in the health care field to improve patient safety. CRM is among the evidence-based safety practices included in the Agency for Healthcare Research and Quality's document entitled "Making Health Care Safer: A Critical Analysis of Patient Safety Practices Evidence Report/Technology Assessment, No. 43" (**http://www.ncbi.nlm.nih.gov/bookshelf/br.fcgi?book=erta43&part=A64100**).

*Crucial Conversations:*  Refers to concepts and techniques articulated in Patterson et al. (2002).

*Fortune "Best Places to Work:*  *Fortune* magazine's annual ranking of U.S. companies with greater than 1,000 FTEs that have been nominated as a "great place to work." Awards are based on results of employee surveys (in 2009, 81,000 employees surveyed across 353 companies) and a "culture audit" conducted in each company (http://www.greatplacetowork.com/).

*High-Reliability Organizations:*  High-reliability organizations (HROs) are those that have incorporated a culture and processes to "radically reduce system failures and effectively respond when failures occur" (http://www.ahrq.gov/qual/hroadvice/hroadviceexecsum.htm).

*High-Performance Work Practices (HPWPs):*  Workforce or human resource practices that have been shown to improve an organization's capacity to effectively attract, select, hire, develop, and retain high-performing employees.

*Just Culture/Just Safety Culture:*  Term used to describe an organizational culture that encourages open dialogue to facilitate patient safety practices; often described in contrast to a "blame" culture (that focus on individuals, rather than systems, as the source of safety infractions). A just culture gives some "leeway to individuals, but is still premised on . . . accountability and bureaucratic control." More recently, scholars are advocating that just culture focus on organizational learning in the areas of quality and safety (Khatri, Brown, and Hicks 2009).

## TABLE 9.2 Glossary of Common Terms and Programs Associated with QI in Health Care *(Continued)*

*Lean:* A management and operations improvement approach, often described as a "transformation" that focuses on eliminating waste across "value streams" that flow horizontally across technologies, assets, and departments (as opposed to improving within each). The intent of a Lean approach is cost-effectiveness, error reduction, and improved service to customers. The term "Lean" was originally coined by Jim Womack, PhD, to describe innovations in Toyota's manufacturing processes (http://www.lean.org).

*Magnet Status:* A prestigious external designation from the "Magnet" program, this status recognizes hospitals that demonstrate 14 characteristics that comprise an excellent working environment for nurses (e.g., nursing leadership, quality of patient care, level of nursing autonomy, staffing ratios, professional development) (http://www.nursecredentialing.org/Magnet.aspx).

*Pay-for-Performance (P4P):* Reimbursement for health care services that is designed to link payment incentives to quality and performance outcomes. Demonstration programs to test various approaches have been under way through the Centers for Medicare and Medicaid Services (see IOM, 2007).

*Pebble Project:* An initiative through the Center for Health Design, which works with partners to develop facilities that incorporate "evidence-based design" features that have been demonstrated to reduce errors, improve quality and efficiency, and improve work experience (http://www.healthdesign.org/research/pebble/).

*Performance Improvement International:* A consulting company that espouses a system-oriented, engineering-based performance improvement methodology, which uses performance indicators and root-cause analysis to reduce errors and improve performance (http://www.piionline.com/company/index.html).

*Planetree:* The Planetree Institute has developed a model of care that is a "patient-centered, holistic approach to healthcare, promoting mental, emotional, spiritual, social, and physical healing. It empowers patients and families through the exchange of information and encourages healing partnerships with caregivers. It seeks to maximize positive healthcare outcomes by integrating optimal medical therapies and incorporating art and nature into the healing environment." Planetree partners adapt the model to fit their unique circumstances (http://www.planetree.org/).

*Quality Improvement Organization (QIO):* The Centers for Medicare and Medicaid Services contracts with QIOs in each state to monitor, report on, and facilitate improvements in the appropriateness, effectiveness, and quality of care provided to Medicare beneficiaries (http://www.cms.gov/QualityImprovementOrgs/).

*Six Sigma:* A data-driven methodology for eliminating defects in any process by applying a consistent framework of DMAIC (define, measure, analyze, improve, control) to minimize variation and improve processes. Six Sigma was started at Motorola and has been widely adopted at other companies, including General Electric (http://www.isixsigma.com).

*Studer Group:* A health care consulting organization "devoted to teaching evidence-based tools and processes that organizations can immediately use to create and sustain outcomes in service and operational excellence." Additional ideas and methods are available from leader Quint Studer (e.g., Studer, 2003) through Web-based resources, a newsletter, and organizational consulting engagements (http://www.studergroup.com).

*Studer Group "Pillars":* A strategic organizing framework developed by the Studer Group (see above) for communicating strategy and performance improvement efforts, as well as holding employees accountable to organizational goals and standards. According to the Studer Group, these five pillars, tailored for an organization's vision, provide a consistent framework for organizations to set goals and develop metrics for key components of their business (http://www.studergroup.com/dotCMS/knowledgeAssetDetail?inode=109970).

*Total Quality Management (TQM):* A participative, systematic approach to planning and implementing QI in quality.

Two popular approaches to QI are *continuous quality improvement* and *Six Sigma*. **Continuous quality improvement** (CQI) is a QI approach that originated in the mid-1980s (Nichols, 1995). Blumenthal and Kilo (1998) wrote that CQI is a series of methodologies designed to improve quality and promote a vision of leadership. The CQI movement focuses on improving organizational processes, which in turn creates better quality. Through CQI, one applies scientific work processes using effective, straightforward techniques. As opposed to QI approaches such as clinical practice guidelines, CQI focuses on the use of generic analytic techniques that facilitate improvement of both clinical and nonclinical processes. CQI is also characterized by its encouragement of managerial reforms that are designed to bring about organizational change. Such reforms include the need to empower employees to learn and participate in the continuous improvement process.

**Six Sigma** is a QI strategy invented by Motorola in the mid-1980s. "Sigma" is a term used in statistics that measures variation. The premise for this strategy is that if you can measure the number of defects that occur in a process, you can systematically work to eliminate them, getting as close to zero defects as possible. The goal is to reduce variation by employing the DMAIC (define, measure, analyze, improve, control) system to improve processes (Adams et al., 2004). Although this strategy was first applied to manufacturing, it is relevant to the health care field as well. In health care, the number of defects might be the number of diabetes patients who do not receive an annual eye exam, per million diabetes patients. The principles of Six Sigma can be used in health care to ensure that we always provide effective care to those who could benefit, never provide ineffective services, and eliminate all preventable complications of medical care (Chassin, 1998).

CQI and Six Sigma differ in several ways. CQI is known as an "evolutionary" method of QI, which is often used when the problem is relatively minor and localized. CQI attempts to implement smaller, incremental improvements when a major redesign of processes is not thought to be necessary. In contrast, Six Sigma is known as a "revolutionary" QI approach, which is often used when more major improvements are necessary (Benedetto, 2003). Compared to CQI, Six Sigma often uses more advanced data analysis tools, incorporates financial results more explicitly, and is often performed under a tighter time frame (Kwak et al., 2006).

# GETTING TO HIGHER QUALITY AND QUALITY IMPROVEMENT

## The Challenge of Implementation

Although QI holds promise for improving quality of care, HCOs that adopt QI often struggle with its implementation. **Implementation** is the critical gateway between the decision to adopt the QI innovation and the routine use of the QI innovation, or integration of a new idea or practice into the operating system of the organization. For example, implementation occurs when clinical and nonclinical staff apply QI principles and practices routinely to improve clinical care processes. There are three general classes of success or failure in QI implementation: (1) widespread or unit/role-specific avoidance of the QI innovation (nonuse); (2) meager and unenthusiastic use (compliant use); and (3) skilled, enthusiastic, and consistent use (committed use) (Klein and Sorra, 1996). The frequency of the first two categories is disturbingly high. Recent studies estimate implementation rates of evidence-based practices to be less than 50 percent (Burstin et al., 1999; Li et al., 2004; McGlynn, Asch, and Adams, 2003). More importantly, QI programs are unlikely to be effective in improving quality of care unless they are fully implemented and become part of the standard operating routines of organizations.

Why is the level of QI implementation so low? In a general sense, implementation of most new, innovative practices is demanding on both individuals and organizations. It requires

## DEBATE TIME

Health care systems are being challenged to increase value through both improvements in care quality and reductions in service delivery costs. Many different strategies can be deployed to address these issues, such as the process improvement techniques outlined by Six Sigma, Lean, and CQI, among others. For an organization deciding among the various alternatives, what should be considered? How much do you think it matters which QI approach is selected? What other factors could affect the success of a QI strategy?

a complex mix of sustained leadership, extensive training and support, robust measurement and data systems, realigned incentives and human resource practices, and cultural receptivity to change. Further, QI initiatives are often complex interventions that, by definition, evolve over time. Assuming that the intervention will immediately function exactly as planned is both unrealistic and impractical. Finally, the context in which improvement initiatives are implemented (i.e., the structures, processes, and culture of the larger organization and environment) can exert a powerful influence on the success of a QI initiative, independent of the initiative itself.

In addition, QI implementation in HCOs is particularly challenging due to the nature of the work, the workforce, and considerations related to performance measurement and control systems in this industry. These issues and their relationships to QI implementation are discussed further below. Table 9.3 is provided to highlight some of the key

**TABLE 9.3  Health Care Organization Features, Implications, and Principles for QI Implementation Effectiveness**

| Industry Feature | Contribution to Implementation Failure | Key Principle for Implementation Success |
|---|---|---|
| *Nature of work*<br>• High uncertainty<br>• Risk of customer fatality<br>• Hinges on clinician discretion | • Workforce aversion to the experimentation required for successful implementation | • Create opportunities for nonthreatening workforce experimentation and adaptation of innovation |
| *Workforce*<br>• Interprofessional interactions governed by an established hierarchy<br>• Strong professional identification, weak organizational identification | • Workforce aversion to the collaborative learning required for mastering increasingly interdisciplinary innovations<br>• Little workforce interest in participating in organizational improvement efforts | • Frame implementation as a learning challenge<br>• Increase the attractiveness of the perceived organizational identity and construed external image to generate interest in organizational citizenship behavior |
| *Leader-workforce relations*<br>• Transactional exchanges are prevalent<br>• Perceived conflict of goals between leaders and workforce | • Leaders and workforce unable to place collective goal (i.e., innovation implementation) above self-interest | • Incorporate transformational leadership processes for innovation implementation |
| *Performance measurement and control systems*<br>• Underdeveloped<br>• Performance/implementation not rewarded<br>• Founded on calculus-based trust, not relational trust | • Difficult to detect implementation problems and thus make adjustments<br>• Incentives do not favor implementation | • Involve workforce in development of system<br>• Measure and reward implementation efforts |

SOURCE: Adapted from Nembhard et al. (2009).

issues of concern and show how these issues are related to QI implementation success in HCOs.

## The Nature of Work in Health Care

As discussed in other chapters of this textbook, work in health care is often distinct from work in other industries. Three areas of difference are particularly salient when considering the importance of quality and QI in health care: risk; work norms; and clinician discretion.

**Risk (Aversion).** Although many QI innovations are designed to improve quality in the long run, their implementation often increases the risk of failure in the short run while staff become familiar with the new practice. Early implementation efforts often result in failures, including damage to the QI innovation, damage to the organization's reputation, or harm to patients. Individuals' fear of failure limits their willingness to experience failure. However, willingness to experience failure is critical to improvement in many areas of health care delivery. Failures offer valuable insights on what does and does not work. "Controlled" failures are therefore instructive on how to improve existing care processes and avoid implementation failure. Despite health care workers' aversion to risk, it is important to try to create safe environments in which workers can strive to improve quality of care without debilitating fear (Nembhard et al., 2009).

**Work Norms.** The aversion to implementation that health professionals feel stems not only from the fear of failure in general, but also from the specific fear of causing harm to patients. When a behavior is consistent with existing norms, individuals deem it appropriate and are more likely to behave accordingly. Conversely, when behavior seems inconsistent, individuals refrain from participating. Unfortunately, to many health professionals, QI implementation appears inconsistent with occupational norms because it can lead to patient harm. For example, a clinician may resist using a single evidence-based procedure for diagnosing a tumor if she feels that the risk of harming the patient would increase if she does not perform a wider battery of tests. This potential violation is sufficient cause for many health professionals to resist QI implementation. A review of 76 studies identified concerns about harming patients as a primary reason for implementation avoidance (Cabana et al., 1999). Avoidance of a new practice is a natural response when it threatens deeply held norms (e.g., "do no harm").

**Clinician Discretion.** Outside of health care, workers do not have the same liberty to avoid implementation of new practices. By contrast, health care professionals' high level of discretion over implementation is related to their discretion over clinical practice. Because of their monopolistic and protected control over medical knowledge, health professionals are given unparalleled authority over clinical practice. Health care managers' authority pales in comparison because, unlike in other industries, most health care managers do not have the professional credentials of their workers (e.g., MD), and because most professional workers (e.g., physicians) are not bound by employment contracts to abide by manager dictum (Nembhard et al., 2009).

In other industries, managers' authority gives organizations an implementation advantage. Once managers articulate QI implementation as an organizational policy, workers are compelled to comply with implementation efforts. Health care managers do not have such authority because QI implementation often affects the clinical work of health professionals, who frequently decide against innovation implementation for the reasons described. Once professionals decide against an innovation, implementation failure almost inevitably occurs (Nembhard et al., 2009).

## Workforce Characteristics and Implementation Challenges

**Specialization.** Burgeoning medical knowledge and the complexity of health care delivery have resulted in increasing specialization in the health care workforce. For example, physicians specialize in one of 120 disciplines including internal medicine, cardiology, adult cardiothoracic anesthesiology, hand surgery, pediatric endocrinology, and abdominal radiology. Other specialized health care professionals include nurses, therapists, nutritionists, phlebotomists, pharmacists, and so forth.

The high degree of specialization in health care means that each professional brings only partial knowledge needed to care for patients. In practice, the expertise of over 20 health professionals must be integrated to provide care for a single patient in a hospital. There is increasing recognition that these professionals must collaborate to be effective (IOM, 2004). Yet despite the imperative for collaboration, it is often missing from professional interactions, and its absence is a leading cause of quality problems. At a children's hospital in Boston, a five-year-old boy died from a seizure because he received no treatment. An investigation later revealed that his physicians had never communicated with each other about who was in charge of his care. Instead, each assumed another had taken charge, and each therefore removed himself from the boy's care, leaving no one to provide treatment.

**The Physician Culture.** Collaboration problems in the health care workforce result largely from the hierarchical, individualistic culture of medicine, which is deeply rooted in the socialization process for health professionals. Health professionals are socialized before employment through their specialty training programs, which often span a period of 10 or more years—a period longer than is required in most service industries. During training, professionals learn not only how to treat patients, but also how to view themselves and how to interact with others inside and outside of their profession. Physicians, for example, learn to be independent, authoritarian, autonomous, competitive, conservative, reactive, quick, detached actors. They learn to treat others in their discipline with respect and in high regard. They learn to treat individuals in other professions in accordance with the established medical professional hierarchy. In this professional hierarchy, specialists rank higher than primary care physicians, who rank higher than nurses, who rank higher than therapists, and so on. The lower an individual's professional rank, the less consideration given to that individual in clinical decision making. In practice, all individuals are mindful of the hierarchy, and feel a strong sense of professional identification—characteristics that affect not only quality of care, but also efforts to improve quality of care through QI, which depends fundamentally on team-based approaches to change rather than top-down control (Nembhard et al., 2009).

**The Professional Hierarchy.** Health care QI increasingly requires interdisciplinary teamwork, meaning its implementation cannot succeed without professionals from multiple disciplines collaborating both to develop new approaches to care and to learn to use them. Unfortunately, HCOs' hierarchical culture stifles organizational members' willingness to participate in the collaborative learning that is necessary for QI success. Collaborative learning is the iterative process of individuals or groups of individuals *working together* to improve their actions by incorporating new knowledge and understanding. It involves jointly analyzing information, openly discussing concerns, and consciously sharing decision making and coordinating experimentation. In turn, individuals must be willing to challenge others' views, acknowledge their own errors, and openly discuss failed experiments. These behaviors are interpersonally risky because they create the possibility for an individual to appear incompetent or belligerent and thereby potentially diminish that individual's reputation among colleagues (Nembhard et al., 2009).

Individuals take such risks only when they perceive a psychologically safe work climate. Unfortunately, the medical professional hierarchy has undermined the psychological safety of individuals whose professions fall lower in the hierarchy. Nurses frequently report that "it is difficult to speak up" and "nurse input is not well received." Moreover, they report negative consequences (e.g., punishment, rejection, embarrassment) of voicing concerns and suggestions to individuals of higher status and of participating in failed experiments. Hence, they shy away from collaborative learning situations such as QI implementation.

Professionals at the higher end of professional hierarchies shy away as well. A study of employee involvement programs in eight manufacturing plants showed that those in higher-status positions (i.e., supervisors) often resisted the implementation of these programs because they felt that these programs, which were premised on collaborative learning, undermined their control and authority. In some plants, this belief led supervisors to criticize the program, which then discouraged lower-status staff from participating. In the end, the programs failed because neither high- nor low-status staff would participate (Klein, 1984).

**Professional Identification.** Professional identification has effectively limited organizational identification (i.e., individuals' sense of alignment with the organization). This weak organizational identification negatively affects QI implementation in two ways. First, it limits the organization's ability to motivate the collaboration needed for implementation success. Collaboration among individuals who are otherwise pulled in different directions by professional allegiances is a function of group (e.g., organizational) identification. When this identification is weak, it is more difficult to motivate collaborative learning and successful implementation.

Second, weak organizational identification is problematic for HCOs' QI implementation because health professionals historically regard QI implementation as an additional and distinct activity from their core task of patient care delivery. When a workforce holds this view, the organization is dependent on its staff's positive, extra-role behavior—also called organizational citizenship behavior—to accomplish the "additional task." Staff are more likely to engage in this type of behavior when they strongly identify with the organization. For example, studies suggest that physicians who strongly identify with a hospital participated more in the hospital's committees (Dukerich, Golden, and Shortell, 2002). Similarly, physicians are more likely to implement new clinical practices when they feel aligned with the HCO (Nembhard et al., 2009).

## *Performance Measurement and Control Systems*

Performance measurement and control systems collect data and reward specific behaviors and outcomes. Historically, performance measurement and control systems in health care have been underdeveloped. Few HCOs collect data regarding their own processes and performance. Unlike other service or manufacturing organizations, the most common quality data available to physicians come from third-party payers, which suggests a dependence on others for information about their own organizations. Whether received from external sources or self-collected, data often tend to be underutilized to inform organizational behavior (Nembhard et al., 2009).

The lack of well-developed performance measurement and control systems in health care reflects a number of factors. First, HCOs and their members often equate working hard to deliver patient care with delivering the best possible care. As a result, any instances of poor performance are seen as random and not subject to prevention or intervention. Thus, there is little perceived need to invest in performance measurement and control systems. Second, by not investing in these systems, professionals minimize their exposure to information that would challenge the belief that their effort was associated with the best quality care. Avoidance or use of "selective exposure" is a common strategy for minimizing cognitive dissonance (Festinger, 1962). Third, defining and developing valid measures of quality and performance in health care is inherently difficult because of the inherent nature of the work. Much debate remains about what should be measured (e.g., structure, process, or outcomes) and what constitutes a valid measure. Fourth, because HCOs and health professionals have been paid the same amount regardless of whether they provide high- or low-quality care, they have had little incentive to invest in costly measurement systems (Nembhard et al., 2009).

## Implementation Policies and Practices

As described above, QI initiatives are often unsuccessful due to implementation failures. Klein and Sorra's (1996) innovation implementation model describes the determinants of the effectiveness for organizational implementation. They posit that the quality and consistency of the use of an adopted innovation (such as a QI approach) is a function of (1) the organization's climate for the implementation

of the innovation, and (2) the employees' perceptions of the fit of the innovation to their values. The organization's climate refers to the shared summary perceptions of targeted employees concerning the degree to which their use of a particular innovation is rewarded, supported, and expected within the organization. Organizations can encourage innovation implementation by ensuring that employees have the skills necessary to use the innovation, providing incentives for using the innovation and disincentives for not using the innovation, and removing obstacles that prevent use of the innovation.

Implementation policies and practices (IPPs) refer to an array of organizational policies, practices, and characteristics that influence QI use (e.g., training, user support, incentives, recognition, end-user participation, and workload changes) and can be used to support innovation implementation. IPPs facilitate implementation by increasing employees' capabilities, motivations, and opportunities to put the innovation into use. IPPs can be classified into three interdependent categories: organizational infrastructure and support; QI tactics and strategies; and perception management.

## *Organizational Infrastructure and Support*

Implementation policies and practices within this category range from how the organization is structured and financed to how the organization addresses learning. These distinct types of IPPs are each addressed individually below.

**Organizational Structure.** Increasing organization around clinical processes rather than traditional functional (or disciplinary) departments facilitates QI implementation by lowering organizational and professional barriers to clinical QI. Such clinical integration supports QI by creating a cultural mind-set that emphasizes meeting customer needs instead of accommodating professional needs, calling attention to processes of care instead of individual tasks, and promoting the formation of cross-functional, multidisciplinary teams to analyze and improve care delivery processes.

**Financial Support.** Developing robust information systems and reorganizing around clinical processes require significant financial resources (Greenhalgh et al., 2004; Cummings et al., 2007). Allocation of resources to QI efforts represents a key indicator of organizational commitment. The support of QI with hard resources may differentiate those organizations that are serious about QI from those that are simply mimicking the latest trend. Hence, beyond the organization's general financial health, its specific investment in QI may be an important feature of a supportive organizational context. Although financial support is a key aspect of QI infrastructure, other resources such as training, education, physical space, and even time have been positively associated with QI implementation. For example, organizations that have "slack resources" that allow people to "squeeze" time to experiment with a new QI innovation without disrupting existing routines may lead to higher rates of implementation (Damschroder et al., 2009).

**Organizational Culture.** Culture comprises the fundamental values, assumptions, and beliefs held in common by members of an organization. It is often treated as if it is stable, socially constructed, and subconscious. Employees impart the organizational culture to new members, and culture influences in large measure how employees relate to one another and the manner in which they approach their "work." Although nearly all QI change efforts are targeted at "objective" aspects of an organization, such as work tasks, structures, and processes, many of these initiatives fail because there is no corresponding change in organizational culture. In other words, these changes often do not stick because they are inconsistent with prevailing values, understandings, and unspoken "rules" in the organizations. For example, organizational cohesion and adaptability to change are important features found in entrepreneurial-leaning organizations. By contrast, organizations with more formalized cultures may be less prone to adopt QI innovations because of the emphasis on maintaining rules and policies, low acceptance of new ideas, and continuance of the status quo. Cultural change is difficult and time-consuming, but any long-term commitment to sustainable QI needs to address this important aspect of organizational context.

---

## MANAGING THE DISNEY WAY

The importance of quality and QI is not limited to health care. Even though other industries are concerned with different products and services, those in the health care industry can still learn valuable lessons by studying other companies and management techniques.

In his book, *If Disney Ran Your Hospital: 9½ Things You Would Do Differently* (2004), Fred Lee shares insights from his experience working for a short time as a Disney cast member. Lee develops his perspective by examining Disney and the Disney culture based on comparisons with his experiences in the health care industry, and specifically drawing on his perspective as senior vice president at Florida Hospital in Orlando.

Lee ties together his list of things hospitals could do differently by focusing on the importance of culture in organizations. Rather than emphasizing service, he notes, a focus on cultural excellence can tie together an organization and its employees' pursuit of common, valued goals. Disney's four areas of "quality focus" are prioritized: (1) safety; (2) courtesy; (3) show (i.e., the areas of Disney that create a "sensory impression"); and (4) efficiency. By clearly delineating these strategic priorities, employees have an accessible map by which to guide their actions.

The 9½ things Lee highlights as opportunities for hospitals to learn from Disney include the following:

1. Redefining the competition
2. Emphasizing courtesy over efficiency
3. Reducing reliance on patient satisfaction as a metric
4. Focusing on measurement for improvement
5. Decentralizing authority
6. Changing the concept of work
7. Harnessing the power of employees' imaginations to motivate them

## MANAGING THE DISNEY WAY *(Continued)*

8. Creating a climate of dissatisfaction

9. Ending the use of competitive monetary rewards as a means of motivating employees

10. Closing the gap between knowledge and action

Lee acknowledges that being a manager in a hospital is considerably more challenging than being a manager at Disney, where customers want to be and where the lower-risk environment presents situations that can be standardized. Yet despite the obvious differences, Lee's list and accompanying discussion present intriguing opportunities for QI in hospitals that those working in the health care industry may wish to consider.

SOURCE: Lee (2004).

**Leadership and Management Support and Engagement.** Leadership refers to leaders at all levels of an organization who have a direct or indirect influence on QI implementation. In addition to high-level leaders, middle managers are important because of their ability to network and negotiate for resources and because they are often in a position to assign greater (or lesser) priority to QI relative to other organizational demands. Commitment, involvement, and accountability of leaders and managers have a significant influence on the success of QI implementation. Management support in terms of commitment and active interest leads to a stronger implementation climate that is, in turn, related to implementation effectiveness. Managers can be important conduits as they can help persuade stakeholders via interpersonal channels and by modeling norms associated with implementing an intervention. Managerial patience (taking a long-term view rather than a short-term view) allows time for the often-inevitable reduction in productivity that occurs until the intervention takes hold; this patience is also more likely to lead to implementation success. However, if the decision to adopt and implement is made by leaders higher in the hierarchy who mandate change with little user input in the decision to implement an intervention, then implementation is more likely to fail. Middle managers are more likely to support implementation if they believe that doing so will promote their own organizational goals, and if they feel involved in discussions about the implementation.

**Governance Leadership.** Governing boards have an important role to play in overseeing QI efforts and patient safety initiatives because they are the organizational entity legally accountable for quality of care. Beyond fulfilling their oversight responsibilities, boards can potentially play a leadership role by establishing quality and safety as organizational priorities, allocating resources to support QI efforts and patient safety initiatives, revising executive compensation and performance evaluation criteria, and fostering a corporate culture that values quality and safety. In HCOs, the governing board responsibility for quality is clearly delineated in statutory law, regulatory requirements, and accreditation standards.

The board's contemporary role in ensuring quality of care emerged from an expanding legal accountability. Hospital licensure law in all 50 states underscores the board's responsibility for quality and for overseeing the medical staff (Orlikoff and Totten, 1991). In addition, the federal government requires hospitals receiving Medicare reimbursement to comply with the quality-related regulations set forth in the Conditions of Participation in the Medicare Program (Anthony and Singer, 1989). Finally, the Joint Commission sets forth expectations and responsibilities for HCO boards (Joint Commission, 2005).

Although boards have a potentially valuable role to play, several features of board composition, structure, process, and context must be addressed to ensure the board's fulfillment of its responsibility for quality. First, few board members possess health care backgrounds or clinical expertise. Board members are often selected on the basis of their business experience, professional skills (e.g., legal, marketing, finance), community ties, personal values, time availability, or a combination of these factors. Although board members from manufacturing and service industries may be familiar with quality issues in their own organizations, they often report feeling confused about

## IN PRACTICE:  Research on High-Performance Work Practices in Health Care Organizations

Critical in providing high-quality care is the presence of a competent and capable workforce. Outside health care, a breadth of research suggests that innovative human resource (HR) practices (or, **high-performance work practices** [HPWPs]) can be an important element of efforts to improve quality and performance. These HPWPs include activities such as systematic personnel selection, incentive compensation, and the widespread use of teams, and they can help organizations in their efforts to attract and retain highly qualified employees.

Within health care, the question was raised as to whether the use of HPWPs could have a similarly important effect on quality of care and organizational performance. Subsequently, a research team funded by the Agency for Healthcare Research and Quality (AHRQ) designed a project to investigate the use of HPWPs, with particular interest in exploring potential links between the use of HPWPs and factors related to quality of care and patient safety in U.S. HCOs.

The team's first task was to undertake an extensive review and synthesis of the literature available—both academic and "gray" literature, such as reports and publications available outside peer-reviewed journals. Next, the team developed a preliminary model that outlined four key subsystems (or "bundles") of HPWPs, and delineated the relations among these subsystems as well as their potential organizational effects. Then, the team performed five case studies of U.S. HCOs that had been selected based on the HCOs' known success with HPWP implementation. The team conducted site visits in 2009, where they performed 71 interviews with key organizational and clinical informants and collected organizational documents related to the HPWPs that were in use. All the key informant interviews were recorded and transcribed for further analysis.

The team found that all four of the HPWP subsystems they had previously characterized as directly relevant to health care (organizational engagement, staff acquisition/development, frontline empowerment, and leadership alignment/development) were emphasized in the five case study organizations. They found substantial variation in what HPWPs were selected, and also noted innovative applications in the HCOs. The group also found evidence of links between the use of HPWPs and employee outcomes (e.g., turnover, higher satisfaction/engagement). While the team was unable to collect hard data, they noted that the key informants consistently reported believing that HPWPs made important contributions to both care system and organization-level outcomes (e.g., fewer "never events," innovation adoption, lower agency costs, and lower turnover costs), some of which were directly related to quality of care.

The results of this research provide preliminary evidence and examples of ways that HPWPs can be used to improve operations in HCOs. The results also suggest that HPWPs have promise with respect to their ability to impact quality and safety. The team concluded that HPWPs should be considered when addressing the challenges of performance improvement in health care, and suggested the need for further research to investigate which HPWP practices and combinations might have the greatest potential for health care QI.

SOURCE: McAlearney et al. (2010).

their responsibility for quality of care, ill prepared to evaluate quality of care, and uncomfortable taking action to rectify a quality problem (e.g., denying physician reappointment or disciplining an incompetent physician). Boards also face a disjointed quality committee system. In hospitals, for example, both board committees and medical staff committees are charged with improving quality of care and service. This dual committee structure complicates the board's ability to perform effective quality oversight. Third, many boards do not possess adequate *governance information systems*—that is, information systems designed to support governance work. Board members receive either too much information or too little to monitor quality effectively. Moreover, they do not receive information in a format that makes it easy to discern what action they should take to rectify a quality problem or improve quality. Finally, boards spend much of their meeting time focused on financial issues; quality may not even appear as a regular agenda item in every board meeting.

To meet the challenges that have been identified for hospital governance, boards require training to strengthen capabilities around managing the hospital/physician interface and quality of care. Boards need to first engage in careful self-assessment of their own development and orientation relative to their responsibilities. As noted, many board members lack the experience and skills to effectively carry out the activities necessary to strengthen hospital/physician alignment and oversee quality of care. Board members also need to understand the cultural barriers that separate hospital management from physicians, and to determine who can take the steps to help close those barriers through the development and communication of a common vision and related strategies. Rather than the traditional hands-off posture taken by many boards, successful boards need members who are able to reach out to medical staff members and cultivate a culture that supports a quality-driven agenda that does not rely exclusively on structural arrangements to align the board with the organization.

**Learning Climate.** Developing a climate that promotes learning is a "core property" that health care organizations need for ongoing QI. Similar to culture, a positive climate creates a receptive context for change. Specifically, a learning climate is one with a set of interrelated practices and beliefs that support and enable employee and organizational skill development, learning, and growth. In a learning climate, stakeholders are not constrained by failure. A climate of psychological safety is promoted. Key characteristics of a learning climate that promotes QI implementation are that: (1) a compelling and inspiring reason for QI innovation use is clearly articulated; (2) leaders express their own fallibility and need for team members' assistance and input; and (3) leaders communicate to team members that they are essential, valued, and knowledgeable partners in the change process. Having the time and space for reflective thinking and evaluation is another important characteristic because it promotes learning from past successes and failures to inform future QI efforts. It is important to note that learning "climates" often vary across subgroups, and unit- or team-based expressions of these attributes may have a stronger influence than overall organizational learning.

---

## MANAGEMENT LESSONS FROM MAYO CLINIC

Mayo Clinic is known worldwide for excellence in both quality of care and service. Founded in Rochester, Minnesota, over 140 years ago, Mayo Clinic has expanded to include additional hospitals in Rochester and new Mayo Clinic facilities in Jacksonville, Florida, and Scottsdale, Arizona. Leonard Berry and Kent Seltman, in an effort to learn more about the success behind this "100-Year Brand," undertook a study of Mayo Clinic's service culture and systems through interviews and observations of clinician-patient interactions. Their book, *Management Lessons from Mayo Clinic* (2008), describes their findings.

Throughout the book, Berry and Seltman provide multiple examples of the important roles of culture, teamwork, learning, communication, and professional integration in providing excellent care and succeeding with efforts to implement improvement interventions that can ensure quality and service. With respect to quality and QI, for instance, at Mayo Clinic, "quality is defined by clinical outcomes, safety, and service" (p. 229). While Mayo Clinic is consistently listed among the best when ranked by objective metrics assessing quality of care, the Clinic continues to strive for improvement. As explained by one leading Mayo Clinic physician, "No one is better positioned to break away from the rest of the leaders in clinical reliability than an integrated group practice that values teamwork, understands the dividends of a more horizontal, cross-functional team of nurses, technicians, doctors, pharmacists, and administrators, and has a century-long history of patient-centered care facilitated by a large contingent of systems engineers" (p. 229). With an attitude that "we can do better," physicians and administrators at Mayo Clinic work together in a learning environment, united by the Mayo Clinic core value of "the needs of the patient come first" that is embedded in the organization's culture.

SOURCE: Berry and Seltman (2008).

# APPLYING QUALITY IMPROVEMENT FRAMEWORKS

## QI Tactics and Strategies

### Create Opportunities for Staff Experimentation and QI Adaptation

HCOs' members' reluctance to participate in QI implementation may be addressed by creating opportunities for them to experiment with QI innovations in nonthreatening ways. Nonthreatening opportunities (e.g., training, pilot projects, dry runs) create low risk settings where failures have little or no consequence for patients. They enable staff to gain familiarity with the innovation, experience its benefits, and develop user competence. As a result, staff in such settings are less likely to view the innovation as posing high risks, and thus are less likely to resist its implementation.

When staff are not resistant, implementation success is more likely. For example, staff having time to train with a QI innovation is a positive predictor of implementation success. Similarly, units that used activities such as dry runs (with a dummy serving as the patient in clinical procedures) and pilot projects to implement innovative practices experience greater implementation success (Tucker, Nembhard, and Edmondson, 2007). Use of these activities facilitates implementation success not only by reducing risk-derived resistance, but also by fostering "attitudinal commitment," or commitment that generates staffs' active involvement in QI implementation.

### Frame QI as a Learning Challenge

To counter the negative psychological and behavioral effects of the hierarchical culture of medicine with respect to implementation, QI innovations must be appropriately framed. Framing is the process of providing a lens through which to interpret a situation. Challenges can be framed in terms of performance or learning. Individuals or groups that adopt a performance frame view a new task as similar to current practice, while those that adopt a learning frame see the task as different and therefore an opportunity to explore new actions and relationships. Consequently, the behavior that follows from adoption of each frame differs. Teams whose leaders explicitly framed implementation as a learning rather than as a performance challenge were more likely to abandon existing interpersonal routines, including those premised on hierarchical interactions, and were more likely to adopt collaborative learning behaviors (Edmondson, 2003). Moreover, members of these teams (regardless of professional rank) felt psychologically safe and excited about offering their input (Edmondson, 2003).

### Promote Organizational Identification

While professional identification may often conflict with the need for organizational identification associated with successful QI implementation in health care, such conflict is not necessary. There are at least two strategies for fostering the organizational identification needed for implementation success in HCOs: (1) increase the attractiveness of the perceived organizational identity, and (2) increase the attractiveness of the external image

---

**IN PRACTICE: Pursuing Patient Safety through Safety Coach Training**

Hospital Z recognized an opportunity to improve care quality through the empowerment of frontline staff to identify potential safety risks and to address those risks in real time. Using the organization's existing safety-coach structure, the hospital provided training on speaking up using a "crucial conversations" framework. A comparison of pre-post surveys revealed substantial improvements in the percentage of staff indicating that they "speak up and completely express their concerns" across all areas measured. For example, pre-training, survey results showed that 10 percent of staff indicated speaking up about observed use of shortcuts, compared with 36 percent post-training. Other comparisons pre- and post-training showed similar differences (e.g., speaking up about mistakes observed: 43 percent pre-training versus 16 percent post-training; about observation of poor competency: 33 percent versus 10 percent; about observation of poor teamwork: 26 percent versus 8 percent; about observation of disrespect: 21 percent versus 7 percent; and about observation of abuse of authority: 11 percent versus 4 percent).

SOURCE: McHugh, Garman, Song, and McAlearney (2010).

of the organization (i.e., the image held by those outside of the organization) (Dukerich et al., 2002). The former strategy builds on research finding that physicians feel stronger organizational identification when they perceive alignment between their goals and values and those of the organization. The second strategy reflects the finding that physicians' feelings about organizations with which they are affiliated are influenced by how outsiders view those organizations. Thus, the challenge for HCOs is to find ways to highlight the similarities between their goals and their workforce's values. Also, they must showcase their positive attributes (e.g., pro bono work, awards, new facilities) to enhance their external image and their affiliates' perceptions of them.

Applying these principles helped the Royal Devon and Exeter NHS Foundation Trust in England dramatically shift from weak to strong organizational identification (Bate, Mendel, and Robert, 2008). Until the late 1990s, identification with the Trust had been so weak that professionals refused to implement innovations that the Trust desired. Moreover, the Trust had a negative reputation due to high turnover in management and the perception that some physicians were "difficult." The turning point came shortly after a devastating incident in which 82 patients were given incorrect diagnoses, with 11 of them dying. At that point, the CEO decided to make organizational identification a priority and took actions to build identification without tampering with professional identity. For example, she instituted meetings between the executive team and the clinical directors to discuss issues of mutual interest, used quarterly reviews to link individuals across the organization who were working on similar issues, invited the staff to develop its own improvement projects, stressed the importance of interprofessional dialogue, and used "the incident" as a story that exemplified the need to unify as an organization. The Trust now has a positive reputation for organizational identification and QI.

## Use Transformational Leadership Processes

**Transformational leadership** is defined as influencing followers by "broadening and elevating followers' goals and providing them with confidence to perform beyond the expectations specified in the implicit or explicit exchange

---

### IN PRACTICE: The Sharp Experience

A noteworthy part of Sharp's QI journey has been Sharp's conceptualization and launching of "The Sharp Experience" in 2001. This internally branded program is described as "a sweeping performance improvement initiative" and is credited with helping Sharp to improve clinical outcomes, patient safety, and organizational and service metrics. The Sharp Experience is also explained as "what we call our Sharp culture" on the Sharp Web site (http://www.sharp.com), and it provides a central rallying point for employees and patients connected with Sharp.

Overall, the Sharp Experience was designed as an improvement initiative designed to transform the health care experience and make Sharp *the best place to work, the best place to practice medicine, and the best place to receive care*. As described in Sharp's application for the Malcolm Baldrige award, "The Sharp Experience infuses Sharp's Mission by reconnecting the hearts, minds, and attitudes of its almost 14,000 team members, 2,000 volunteers, and 2,600 affiliated physicians to purpose, worthwhile work, and making a difference. Sharp is creating the culture and discipline necessary to provide outstanding care and service."

As part of the Sharp Experience, all employees participate in periodic retreats for which the entire workforce is bused to the San Diego Convention Center for a program featuring internal and external speakers focused on the many dimensions of performance excellence emphasized at Sharp HealthCare. The Sharp Experience is now well entrenched within Sharp HealthCare, providing a platform for consistent organizational communication about organizational goals and achievements, and reportedly giving employees a sense of ownership and pride in Sharp as they are encouraged to continually recommit themselves to the organization and to health care.

SOURCES: Nancy G. Pratt, RN, MS, Senior Vice President, Clinical Effectiveness, Sharp HealthCare; Sharp HealthCare Web site (http://www.sharp.com)

agreement" (Dvir, Eden, Avolio, and Shamir, 2002). Transformational leaders provide vision and a sense of mission, communicate high expectations, promote intelligence, and provide personal attention to employees.

In contrast, **transactional leadership** is based on transactions between managers and employees, such as managers initiating and organizing work and providing recognition and advancement to employees who perform well while penalizing those who do not. Transactional leaders provide rewards for effort and good performance, watch for deviations from rules and standards or intervene only if standards are not met, and avoid making decisions (Bass, 1990).

With respect to QI implementation, transformational leaders use processes that effectively shift the focus of organizational members from their individual goals to collective goals such as QI implementation. By being intellectually stimulating, transformational leaders motivate the workforce to consider how individual goals overlap with collective goals. By being charismatic, they elicit positive feelings in organizational members, which lead members to commit to the leader's and the organization's goals. By modeling collaborative behavior, transformational leaders inspire organizational members to work as a collective. By being individually considerate, they ensure that individuals' developmental needs are fulfilled while working on organizational goals. The workforce often responds to this goodwill by working diligently towards the organizations' goals, including implementation (Gilmartin and D'Aunno, 2007).

The workforce also responds to the support for implementation that transformational leaders provide to them (e.g., allocating needed resources, removing organizational barriers such as existing institutional policies, soliciting and addressing feedback, and championing the work of members). This support greatly facilitates implementation success through legitimation, further motivating organizational members' commitment to implementation. Moreover, it cultivates a climate in which the workforce feels comfortable offering feedback to leaders about how to improve QI implementation. Lastly, leadership support helps maintain the momentum for change in the face of setbacks and performance declines, which are common in implementation efforts.

Given the demonstrated effectiveness of transformational leaders at eliciting targeted organizational members' commitment to organizational change goals such as QI implementation, HCOs are advised to use transformational leadership processes. The inclusion of this behavior does not necessitate the exclusion of transactional behaviors. Indeed, the transactional and transformational leadership styles are complementary, coexist well, and are equally needed to manage the dual challenges of QI implementation and addressing current organizational needs.

There are at least two strategies for increasing transformational leadership in HCOs. One strategy is to hire leaders who innately use transformational processes or who are equally strong users of transformational and transactional processes. Children's Hospitals and Clinics in Minnesota took this approach in hiring Julie Morath, who, during her interviews for the position of chief operating officer, explicitly talked about how she would create a culture of teamwork and safety at Children's (Edmondson, Roberto, and Tucker, 2005). In Morath's case, her reputation preceded her, and the change platform she presented in her job interviews reinforced her reputation as a transformational leader.

A second strategy is to train current leaders in the appropriate use of transformational leadership processes via leadership development programs. Many have debated whether individuals can be trained to be effective leaders and whether leader development programs truly improve the leadership capabilities of individuals. However, management research increasingly affirms the value of such training, especially for HCO leaders, including improvement in leadership style and communication skills in physician leaders. Leaders at all levels within the HCO should learn to use transformational leadership processes adeptly. Use of these skills at the senior level is important because transformational behavior cascades down the organization (see the preceding discussion of governance leadership). Staff tends to adopt the behavior and suggested behaviors of senior leaders with this style. When senior leaders with transformational styles commit to QI implementation, organizational members are likely to commit to this collective purpose as well. However, to enlist organizational members' sustained commitment to implementation, the implementation message must also come from transformational leaders who are closer to them in the hierarchy. These leaders' actions are even more salient and motivating.

---

**IN PRACTICE: The Role of Leadership Development in Quality Improvement**

Expanded use of leadership development programs in HCOs has been relatively recent, particularly in comparison with the use of leadership development programs in other industries (McAlearney, 2006, in press). However, formal leadership development programs are increasingly viewed as a means of helping HCOs to focus on organizational priorities such as quality of care and patient safety (McAlearney, 2010).

Study of leadership development activities in HCOs has highlighted several important opportunities for these programs to improve quality and patient safety in health care (McAlearney, 2008, 2010). First, leadership development programs are typically developed to increase the caliber of the health care workforce. By including education and training in QI techniques, these programs can help ensure that employees can understand and participate in QI activities deployed by the organization. Further, this attention paid to developing leaders who will be able to lead QI activities can help HCOs accelerate the QI process within the organization.

Second, leadership development programs can be used to focus organizational attention on strategic priorities. When quality and QI are included in the organization's strategic priorities, alignment of leadership development goals with organizational objectives can help ensure consistency of communication and clarity of organizational messages about quality as a priority. Through leadership development programs, emerging leaders learn how to emphasize organizational messages about quality in their management and leadership practices.

Finally, leadership development programs can be specifically designed to emphasize and reinforce an organization's culture, particularly cultures that value care quality. Mission, vision, and values are public indicators of what organizations value, and weaving quality into those statements creates an opportunity to focus on quality, since it is embedded in the culture. Leadership development programs can provide specific and focused opportunities to highlight the value of quality as it fits into the HCO's culture. Further, under those circumstances when increasing the amount of attention paid to quality-of-care issues involves a change in organizational culture, leadership development programs can be a particularly important component of the culture change effort.

---

### Involve the Workforce in Performance Measurement and Control System Development

Successful QI implementation depends on the availability and timeliness of information that is used to identify problems and benchmark changes in care processes. Organizations that have developed their information systems and integrated both clinical and financial data have a stronger foundation upon which to build successful QI practices.

However, HCOs must overcome organizational members' distrust of performance measurement and data systems if they are to develop and sustain the systems they need for QI implementation success. To overcome these problems, managers need to increase the perceived fairness of these systems. For example, managers must (1) allow targeted organizational members an ongoing voice (but not necessarily control) in system development, maintenance, and evaluation; (2) share decision-making authority over aspects of the system of particular concern to targeted organizational members (e.g., whether individual performance will be publicly reported); and (3) foster regular communication and information dissemination between organizational leaders and staff (Nembhard et al., 2009).

Perceived fairness facilitates QI implementation in two ways. First, it enhances targeted organizational members' relational trust of and commitment to the organization and its systems. In turn, members cooperate with implementation efforts. Second, perceived fairness derived from involvement in the process causes targeted organizational members to feel personally responsible for implementation results. This feeling makes them more willing partners in implementation efforts, more accepting of comparisons on designated measures, and more willing to be rewarded accordingly.

## Measure and Reward QI Implementation Efforts

HCOs may miss an important avenue for promoting QI implementation when they do not use performance measurement and control systems to appropriately reward implementation efforts. These systems should provide rewards (financial and otherwise) that reflect the nature of the work required for effective innovation. Health care innovations such as QI increasingly amplify the task interdependence among health professionals. In such instances, group-level incentives work best. These incentives result in higher performance for interdependent tasks because they motivate peer monitoring and increased willingness to work together to optimally perform the task. The next best performance is obtained by providing individual incentives for independent components of the task. Misaligned incentive structures (e.g., group incentives for independent work and individual incentives for interdependent work) produce the worst performance because they motivate behavior that contradicts the nature of the task.

Often, the best action for HCOs striving to implement QI innovations that rely on teamwork is to use group-level incentives. For example, Geisinger Medical Center in Pennsylvania provided rewards at the group practice level to encourage staff to abide by the "patient-centered medical home," a QI innovation that aims to improve the quality of care by establishing care coordination processes among patients' care providers (Paulus et al., 2008). Geisinger also provided individual-level rewards. By utilizing this combination of (first- and second-best) approaches at two pilot sites, it experienced a remarkable 20 percent decrease in hospital admissions in its first year of use (Nembhard et al., 2009).

---

## CREATING HIGH-PERFORMANCE HEALTH CARE ORGANIZATIONS

In Jody Hoffer Gittell's book, *High Performance Healthcare: Using the Power of Relationships to Achieve Quality, Efficiency and Resilience* (2009), she synthesizes a decade of her research in the health care industry to emphasize the importance of what she conceptualizes as "relational coordination." Gittell explains, "While coordination is the management of interdependencies between *tasks*, relational coordination is "the management of interdependencies between the *people* who perform those tasks" (p. 15). Further, she notes, "relational coordination is the coordination of work through relationships of shared goals, shared knowledge, and mutual respect" (p. 23).

Gittell's studies of relational coordination and surgical performance, medical performance, and long-term care performance build upon her work investigating relational coordination and airline performance (her 2003 book, *The Southwest Airlines Way*, emphasized these concepts in airlines). Her conclusion across studies is that process improvements in relational coordination can help organizations to improve both quality-of-care and efficiency outcomes.

Acknowledging that there are major challenges in applying these concepts to the health care industry, Gittell recommends focusing improvement efforts on building high-performance work systems. Specifically, Gittell describes 12 work practices that HCOs can adopt or address in order to improve relational coordination:

1. Select for teamwork
2. Measure team performance
3. Reward team performance
4. Resolve conflicts proactively
5. Invest in frontline leadership
6. Design jobs for focus
7. Make job boundaries flexible
8. Create boundary spanners

## CREATING HIGH-PERFORMANCE HEALTH CARE ORGANIZATIONS *(Continued)*

9. Connect through pathways

10. Broaden participation in patient rounds

11. Develop shared information systems

12. Partner with suppliers.

By adopting these work practices, her research results suggest that HCOs will be able to improve relational coordination and thereby improve the important outcomes of quality performance, efficiency performance, and job satisfaction.

As HCOs are known for both high levels of interdependency and less-than-perfect coordination of care and care systems, the opportunity to focus on process improvements that lead to better coordination is clear. Gittell's findings provide compelling preliminary evidence that focusing on people and the relationships among them in delivering care can be an important component of QI efforts.

SOURCE: Gittell (2009).

### Build Evidence for QI

**QI Intervention Source.** Perceptions of key stakeholders about whether the QI innovation is externally or internally developed may influence the success of QI implementation. The QI innovation may enter into the organization through an external source such as through information from a formal research entity; as a market, system, or governmental mandate; or through another external source. Alternatively, a QI innovation may have been internally developed as a good idea, a solution to a problem, or from a grassroots effort. For example, using coated catheters to prevent infections may have been formally studied and reported in the literature, and a nurse may have decided that her organization needs to use these devices to help decrease infection rates. Stakeholders within the organization may regard this QI innovation as external (e.g., the literature for the Centers for Disease Control and Prevention strongly recommends using them), or as an internally developed QI innovation (e.g., the IV nurse team believes these offer the best solution to the problem). However, selection of an externally developed QI innovation coupled with lack of transparency in the decision-making process about implementation of that QI innovation may lead to implementation failure. Though there is empirical evidence of a positive association with an authoritative decision to use the QI innovation, there is also a negative relationship between full implementation or routinization of the QI innovation. On the other hand, key ideas that come from outside the organization and that are then tailored to the particular organization more often result in successful implementation.

**Evidence Strength and Quality.** Strength of evidence includes stakeholders' perceptions of the quality and validity of evidence supporting the belief that the QI innovation will have the desired outcomes. Sources of evidence may include published literature, guidelines, anecdotal stories from colleagues, information from a competitor, patients' experience, results from a local pilot, and more. Though there is no agreed-upon measure of "strong evidence," there is empirical evidence of a positive association with dissemination of the QI innovation if evidence is solid. However, the influence of solid evidence on implementation may be dependent upon the influence of other variables, such as relative advantage, cost, complexity, and congruence with existing practices. External and internal evidence, including experience through piloting, may be combined to build a case for implementing a QI innovation. Credibility of the developers of evidence, transparency of the process used to develop the intervention, and intentionally mapping out the implementation can be used to counterbalance negative perceptions of the QI innovation by potential adopters.

---

**IN PRACTICE:** **Building Evidence Through Practice-Based Health Services Research**

As emphasized in this chapter, increasing evidence suggests that success in achieving QI goals depends on implementation processes and contexts and not only on the nature of the QI intervention. Hence, to advance QI, additional research is needed to study what types of QI activities work, including considerations about where, when, and how they work. Researchers gain this understanding when they learn about the effects of introducing QI interventions in different practice contexts, as well as the effects of using different implementation strategies, thus contributing to the evidence base supporting future QI implementations.

Evidence of this sort typically comes from practice-based research. Federal programs fostering this type of research include the Quality Enhancement Research Initiative (QUERI) of the Veterans Administration (http://www.queri.research.va.gov) as well as the Accelerating Change in Transforming Networks (ACTION, http://www.ahrq.gov/research/ACTION.htm) and the Practice Based Research Networks (PBRNs, http://pbrn.ahrq.gov/portal/server.pt) funded by the Agency for Healthcare Research and Quality. Managers and policymakers alike can use the results of these research projects to inform decisions about QI interventions, helping to maximize the likelihood of QI success.

---

## Keys to Successful QI Change-Perception Management

All QI change occurs in the context of organizational events and histories related to that change, which shape the likelihood that the change will be successfully implemented. These contexts are often socially constructed rather than objective and are perceived though the eyes of the organization members involved in or affected by the change. For example, full participation in a QI initiative requires a positive affective reaction to the QI innovation. Often, subjective opinions obtained from peers based on personal experiences are more accessible and convincing and are key in shaping both individuals' and groups' affective responses (more so than objective evidence requiring cognitive responses).

Perhaps most fundamentally, both the change and the reason for the change have to be understood. Individuals are reluctant to embrace change if they feel its purpose is unclear. This is a cognitive function that relies on knowledge of underlying principles or reasons for adopting the QI innovation. If this knowledge is not obtained prior to trial and individual adoption of a QI innovation, rejection and discontinuance are likely.

A second key principle affecting individual perceptions of a QI change is that almost all forms of change pose potential threats to security—whether job security, financial security,

professional prerogatives, or feelings of self-worth. A proposed QI innovation or change that is perceived as threatening is less likely to be embraced. Change agents should therefore treat these perceived threats as real (rather than unfounded) and take appropriate steps to address them in the change process. This might take the form, for example, of a peer who can champion the QI change in conjunction with repeated assurances by management that such fears are heard (rather than dismissed as unfounded), and that the change will have positive benefits for patients, a goal to which all in the organization can subscribe.

The sequencing of QI can also shape perceptions of those who participate in the change or who are potentially affected by the change. Specifically, managers should attempt to avoid introducing a QI initiative too closely on the heels of another initiative. This may result in perceptions that change for change's sake is the perceived goal, and also does not allow sufficient time for the previous change to be effectively assimilated. Cognitively, individuals will have greater difficulty focusing on the new change because they are still mentally attuned to the previous one. Although too many changes too fast should be avoided, it is also important that managers deliberately connect a QI innovation with a previous change that has been perceived to be successful (or at least not harmful). This can lay a positive foundation for the new change, as perceptions are shaped by prior experience with similar situations. Rather than having to sell the change from the beginning, QI leaders can benefit from the association with a prior experience.

Finally, planning for change should acknowledge the importance of this "perception as reality" perspective and incorporate the following elements. First, plans should fully consider stakeholders' needs and perspectives, with particular attention paid to costs and benefits. How others view the change and its perceived effects on them and the organization is an important basis for the planning process. Second, the complexity of HCOs and the differentiation along professional and occupational lines strongly suggest that organizations need to tailor strategies for appropriate subgroups within the HCO (e.g., delineated by professional, demographic, cultural, and organizational attributes). Third, and for similar reasons, individuals and subgroups will respond to different messages and channels, and some of these will be more or less effective in terms of shaping perceptions of change. Therefore, organizations should deliver information using appropriate style, imagery, and metaphors, and should identify and use appropriate communication channels. Finally, planning for QI change should not rely on faith alone to sustain the change. HCOs need to employ rigorous monitoring and evaluation methods to track progress toward goals and milestones to reinforce and validate the results of the change to organizational members and to provide them with targets/goals.

## DEBATE TIME

When considering QI, some people believe that major opportunities for improvement can be realized by increasing clinicians' skills and competence. However, others believe that more opportunities for improvement can result from changes made to the organization and management of clinical care units. A third group believes that quality of care is tied to technology availability or to participation in teaching activities. What do you think? Where do you think the most emphasis should be put? In considering these questions, what conditions, factors, or variables might influence your decision?

SOURCE: Adapted from Shortell and Kaluzny (2005).

# SUMMARY AND MANAGERIAL GUIDELINES

1. HCOs have strong imperatives to initiate and support efforts to improve quality of care and patient safety. Quality improvement (QI) interventions can be designed and implemented to address many of these issues. Address quality issues proactively by looking for opportunities to improve quality by detecting and preventing potential problems in processes of care delivery. Quality measures must be defined so that organizations striving to improve quality have a basis on which to evaluate improvement or identify problems. The development and deployment of such measures can affect how QI success is defined. Managers must recognize the problems and tradeoffs associated with different definitions of quality measures, and different approaches to quality measurement.

2. Undertaking QI efforts within an HCO can be challenging due to the uncertain nature of work in health care, as well as the professional makeup of the health care workforce. Set high standards by establishing "best practices" in one's own organization as well as using benchmarking to make comparisons with competitors and industry leaders.

3. The selection of performance measurement and control systems can affect how QI efforts proceed, and how achievement of improvements in quality is measured. Select such systems based on accurate and timely data, and develop incentives to improve quality based on work activities under the control of organizational members.

4. Specific implementation policies and procedures will directly affect the use of QI interventions in HCOs. Factors such as organizational structure, financial support, organizational culture, leadership and management support and engagement, governance leadership, and a learning climate are all critical elements of organizational context that will affect the implementation of QI. Focus energy on working smarter, and consider these factors when developing implementation policies and procedures.

5. Seven QI tactics and strategies hold particular promise for QI implementation efforts in HCOs: (1) creating opportunities for staff experimentation; (2) framing QI as a learning challenge; (3) promoting organizational identification; (4) using transformational leadership processes; (5) involving the workforce in performance measurement and control system development; (6) measuring and rewarding QI implementation efforts; and (7) building evidence for QI. Apply these tactics in combination when undertaking QI interventions in HCOs in order to maximize the likelihood of success in QI initiatives.

6. Focusing on the "people" processes associated with QI can help HCOs become high-performance organizations. Strive to develop a participative, team-oriented organizational culture that encourages input from professionals and other workers from all levels of the organization, and seek opportunities to cross-train staff to gain greater flexibility.

7. A crucial element of QI is focusing on organizational change issues and the management of participants' perceptions; if the reasons for QI are understood, if it does not threaten security, if it has involved those affected by it, if it follows a series of successful changes, if it is inaugurated after the previous change has been assimilated, and if it has been planned, there will be a much higher likelihood of successful QI within an HCO. Involve organizational members, particularly professionals, in the development, implementation, and monitoring of QI initiatives.

# DISCUSSION QUESTIONS

1. Take the perspective of the CEO of a large health care system that owns its own managed-care health plan. Describe three major ways that you could improve the quality of health care in your organization. Critique your solutions regarding the extent to which your solution may cause other problems to surface (what kind?), and the extent to which you as the CEO should have the responsibility and power to implement these changes.

2. Using an HCO that you know well, provide three examples each of possible structural, process, and outcome measures of care quality. Would you expect these measures to be highly associated? Why or why not?

3. Consider a community hospital, a major teaching hospital, and a hospital in a large for-profit system. For each, list the major stakeholder groups (both internal and external). Indicate what kinds of quality criteria each group would be most likely to promote.

4. Hospital A and Hospital B both have as their major goal for this year the implementation of a QI program. Hospital A hired a consultant firm and sent its top managers to a program to learn how to change the corporate culture and to set up quality teams to investigate problems. They formed teams to plan strategies for meaningful QI in two specific areas: billing and use of the emergency room. Hospital B, lacking funds, tried to have study groups and use self-teaching but involved everyone from the CEO to the janitor. Which hospital do you think will succeed in implementing QI? Why?

5. Health System Q is located in the same geographic area as Health System P, its main competitor. While Health System Q touts its status as a community-based integrated delivery system, Health System P leverages its role as a research-intensive academic medical center. Both health systems have achieved Magnet designation for nursing, both have been listed among the "Most Wired" by HIMSS, and both have centers of excellence (or service lines) in the areas of cardiology, cancer, and women's health. You have heard that community members seem to favor Health System Q for most conditions, but appreciate having a local academic health system if they have problems that are out of the ordinary. You are considering a job with one of these health systems in the area of QI, and are trying to decide where your expertise will have the most impact. What factors would you consider in trying to evaluate which place might be better positioned to leverage your skills and move forward with QI efforts?

# CASE: Moving Beyond Data Access to QI Action

After a considerable investment of both money and time, executives at Leman Healthcare were delighted that the new incident-reporting system at Leman was now fully operational. The incident reporting system had been deployed across the health care system; frontline and management staff as well as physicians in both inpatient and ambulatory settings had been trained and were able to use the incident-reporting system to access patient information, document adverse events, and report as required to senior management, risk management, and the QI department.

However, even with full system deployment, QI activities across the health system had not changed. The QI department had full access to the data warehouse that housed data collected through the incident-reporting system as well as data from the electronic health record (EHR) and other information systems, yet QI staff members were apparently not using these data. Instead, QI projects continued to follow historical patterns involving laborious efforts to develop queries and reports rather than use the new system's immediate reporting capabilities to supply information for managers and to drive process improvement projects both locally and across the hospital system.

Similarly, the potential for clinicians to use the newly accessible data was not being realized. Physicians were reluctantly compliant with requirements to use the incident-reporting system for documentation and reporting events, but the general consensus seemed to be that the system was just a way to point fingers at the medical staff. Despite efforts from the senior management team to work individually with clinicians to educate and explain the importance of error and near-miss reporting that would provide information to reduce errors, these physicians continued to view the incident-reporting system as a punitive tool, not as an opportunity for them to explore ways to improve their work.

## Questions

1. Given this situation, what are the apparent barriers to using incident reporting systems for QI?

2. How can these barriers be overcome?

3. What steps would you propose to engage both clinicians and QI staff in enhanced QI activities?

# REFERENCES

Adams, R., Warner, P., Hubbard, B., & Goulding, T. (2004). Decreasing turnaround time between general surgery cases: A six sigma initiative. *Journal of Nursing Administration, 34*(3), 140–148.

Alexander, J. A., & Young, G. (2010). Overcoming barriers to improved hospital-physician collaboration and alignment: Governance issues. In J. Crossan & L. Tollen (Eds.), *Partners in health: How physicians and hospitals can be accountable together.* San Francisco: Jossey-Bass.

Anthony, M. F., & Singer, L. E. (1989). The legal basis for the board's quality assurance duties. *Trustee, 42*(1), 2, 19.

Bass, B. M. (1990). From transactional to transformational leadership: Learning to share the vision. *Organizational Dynamics, 18*(3), 19–31.

Bate, P., Mendel, P., & Robert, G. (2008). *Organizing for quality: The improvement journeys of leading hospitals in Europe and the United States.* Oxford: Radcliffe Publishing.

Benedetto, A. R. (2003). Six sigma: not for the faint of heart. *Radiology Management, 25*(2), 40–53.

Berry, L. L., & Seltman, K. D. (2008). *Management lessons from Mayo Clinic: Inside one of the world's most admired service organizations.* New York: McGraw-Hill.

Berwick, D. M. (2002). A user's manual for the IOM's "Quality Chasm" report. *Health Affairs, 21*(3), 80–90.

Blumenthal, D., & Kilo, C. M. (1998). A report card on continuous quality improvement. *Milbank Quarterly, 76*(4), 625–648.

Burstin, H. R., Conn, A., Setnik, G., Rucker, D. W., Cleary, P. D., O'Neil, A. C., ... Brennan, T. A. (1999). Benchmarking and quality improvement: The Harvard Emergency Department quality study. *American Journal of Medicine, 107*(5), 437–449.

Chassin, M. R. (1998). Is health care ready for six sigma quality? *Milbank Quarterly, 76*(4), 565–691.

Cummings, G. G., Estabrooks, C. A., Midodzi, W. K., Wallin, L., & Hayduk, L. (2007). Influence of organizational characteristics and context on research utilization. *Nursing Research, 56*, S24–S39.

Damschroder, L., Aron, D., Keith, R., Kirsch, S., Alexander, J., & Lowry, J. (2009). Fostering implementation of health services research findings into practice: A consolidated framework for advancing implementation science. *Implementation Science, 4*(50): 543–555.

Deming, W. E. (1986). *Out of the crisis.* Cambridge, MA: Massachusetts Institute of Technology.

Donabedian, A. (1966). Evaluating the quality of medical care. *Milbank Memorial Fund Quarterly, 44*(2), 166–206.

Donabedian, A. (1980). *Explorations in quality assessment and monitoring, vol. 1: The definition of quality and approaches to its assessment.* Chicago: Health Administration Press.

Donabedian, A. (1988). The quality of care. How can it be assessed? *Journal of the American Medical Association, 260*(12), 1743–1748.

Donabedian, A. (2005). Evaluating the quality of medical care. *Milbank Quarterly, 83*(4), 691–729.

Dukerich, J. M., Golden, B. R., & Shortell, S. M. (2002). Beauty is in the eye of the beholder: The impact of organizational identification, identity, and image on the cooperative behaviors of physicians. *Administrative Science Quarterly, 47*, 507–533.

Dvir, T., Eden, D., Avolio, B. J., & Shamir, B. (2002). Impact of transformational leadership on follower development and performance: A field experiment. *The Academy of Management Journal, 45*(4), 735–744.

Festinger, L. A. (1962). *A theory of cognitive dissonance.* Palo Alto, CA: Stanford University.

Flood, A. B., Zinn, J. S., & Scott, W. R. (2006). Organizational performance: Managing for efficiency and effectiveness. In: S. M. Shortell & A. D. Kaluzny (Eds.), *Health care management: Organization design and behavior* (5th ed.). Clifton Park, NY: Delmar Cengage Learning.

Gittell, J. H. (2003). *The Southwest Airlines way: Using the power of relationships to achieve high performance.* New York: McGraw-Hill.

Gittell, J. H. (2009). *High performance healthcare: Using the power of relationships to achieve quality, efficiency and resilience.* New York: McGraw-Hill.

Greenhalgh, T., Robert, G., Macfarlane, F., Bate, P., Kyriakidou, O. (2004). Diffusion of innovations in service organizations: systematic review and recommendations. *Milbank Quarterly, 82*, 581–629.

Gregor, C., Pope, S., Werry, D., & Dodek, P. (1996). Reduced length of stay and improved appropriateness of care with a clinical path for total knee or hip arthroplasty. *Joint Commission Journal on Quality Improvement, 22*(9): 617–627.

Hammer, M. (1990). Reengineering Work: Don't Automate, Obliterate. *Harvard Business Review*, July–August.

Helfrich, C. D., Weiner. B. J., McKinney, M. M., & Minasian, L. (2007). Determinants of implementation effectiveness: adapting a framework for complex innovations. *Medical Care Research and Review, 64*, 279–303.

Institute of Medicine. (2000). *To err is human: Building a safer health system.* Washington, DC: National Academy Press.

Institute of Medicine. (2001). *Crossing the quality chasm: A new health system for the 21st century.* Washington, DC: National Academy Press.

Institute of Medicine. (2004). Keeping patients safe: Transforming the work environment of nurses. Washington, DC: National Academy Press.

Institute of Medicine. (2007). *Rewarding provider performance: Aligning incentives in Medicare.* Pathways to Quality Series. Washington, DC: National Academy Press.

Joint Commission on Accreditation of Healthcare Organizations (2005). *Comprehensive accreditation manual for hospitals (CAMH).* Oakbrook Terrace, IL: Joint Commission.

Juran, J. M. (1988). *Juran on planning for quality.* New York: Free Press.

Juran, J. M. (Ed.). (1988). *Juran's quality control handbook* (4th ed.). New York: McGraw-Hill.

Khatri, N., Brown, G. D., & Hicks, L. L. (2009). From a blame culture to a just culture. *Healthcare Management,* October–December, pp. 312–322.

Kimberly, J. R., & Minvielle, E. (2000). *The quality imperative: Measurement and management of quality in health care.* London: Imperial College Press.

Klein, K. J. (1984). Why supervisors resist employee involvement. *Harvard Business Review, 84*(5), 87–95.

Klein, K. J., & Sorra, J. S. (1996). The challenge of innovation implementation. *Academy of Management Review, 21*(4), 1055–1080.

Kohn, L., Corrigan, J., & Donaldson, M. (Eds.). (1999). *To err is human: Building a safer health system.* Washington, DC: National Academy Press.

Krein, S. L., Klamerus, M. L., Vijan, S., Lee, J. L., Fitzgerald, J. T., Pawlow, A., Reeves, P., & Hayward, R. A. (2004). Case management for patients with poorly controlled diabetes: a randomized trial. *American Journal of Medicine, 116,* 732–739.

Kwak, Y. H., & Anbari, F. T. (2006). Benefits, obstacles, and future of six sigma approach. *Technovation, 26,* 708–715.

Lee, F. (2004). *If Disney ran your hospital: 9½ things you would do differently.* Bozeman, MT: Second River Healthcare Press.

Leebov, W., & Ersoz, C. J. (2003). *The health care manager's guide to continuous quality improvement.* Lincoln, NE: Authors Choice Press.

Li, R., Simon, J., Gillies, R. R., Casalino, L., Schmittdiel, J., & Shortell, S. M. (2004). Organizational factors affecting the adoption of diabetes care management processes in physician organizations. *Diabetes Care, 27*(10), 2312–2316.

Lukas, C. V., Holmes, S. K., Cohen, A. B., Restuccia, J., Cramer, I. E., Shwartz, M., & Charns, M. P. (2007). An organizational model of transformational change in healthcare systems. *Health Care Management Review, 32*(4), 309–320.

Lynn, J., Baily, M. A., Bottrell, M., Jennings, B., Levine, R. J., Davidoff, F., et al. (2007). The ethics of using quality improvement methods in health care. *Annals of Internal Medicine, 146*(9), 666–673.

Lynn, J., West, J., Hausmann, S., Gifford, D., Nelson, R., McGann, P., et al. (2007). Collaborative clinical quality improvement for pressure ulcers in nursing homes. *Journal of the American Geriatrics Society, 55*(10), 1663–1669.

McAlearney, A. S. (2006). Leadership development in healthcare organizations: A qualitative study. *Journal of Organizational Behavior, 27*(7), 967–982.

McAlearney, A. S. (2008). Improving patient safety through organizational development: Considering the opportunities. *Advances in Health Care Management, 7,* 213–239.

McAlearney, A. S. (2008, September–October). Using leadership development programs to improve quality and efficiency in healthcare. *Journal of Healthcare Management, 53*(5), 319–332.

McAlearney, A. S. (2010). Executive leadership development in U.S. health systems. *Journal of Healthcare Management, 55*(3), 206–222; discussion 223–224.

McAlearney, A. S., Garman, A., Song, P., McHugh, M., Robbins, J., & Harrison, M. (2010). High-performance work practices in healthcare management: Five case studies of best practices in healthcare organizations. *Best paper proceedings of the 70th annual Academy of Management meeting.*

McGlynn, E. A., Asch, S. M., Adams, J., Keesey, J., Hicks, J., DeCristofaro, A., & Kerr, E. A. (2003). The quality of health care delivered to adults in the United States. *New England Journal of Medicine, 348*(26): 2635–2645.

McHugh, M., Garman, A., Song, P. H., and McAlearney, A. S. (2010). Unpublished data from research study, "Using high-performance work practices to improve quality and safety in healthcare."

McLaughlin, C. P., & Kaluzny, A. D. (2006). *Continuous quality improvement in health care* (3rd ed.). Sudbury, MA: Jones and Bartlett Publishers.

Monteleoni, C., & Clark, E. (2004). Using rapid-cycle quality improvement methodology to reduce feeding tubes in patients with advanced dementia: Before and after study. *British Medical Journal, 329,* 491–494.

Nembhard, I. M., Alexander, J. A, Hoff, T., & Ramanujam, R. (2009). Understanding implementation failure in health care delivery: A role for organizational research and theory. *Academy of Management Perspectives, 23*(1), 1–27.

Nichols, J. O. (1995). *A practitioner's handbook for institutional effectiveness and student outcomes assessment implementation.* Edison, NJ: Agathon Press.

Orlikoff, J. E., & Totten, M. K. (1991). *The board's role in quality.* Chicago, American Hospital Publishing, Inc.

Patterson, K., Grenny, J., McMillan, R., & Switzler, A. (2002). *Crucial conversations: Tools for talking when stakes are high.* New York: McGraw-Hill.

Pestotnik, S. L., Classen, D. C., Evans, R. S., & Burke, J. P. (1996). Implementing antibiotic practice guidelines through computer assisted decision-support: Clinical and financial outcomes. *Annals of Internal Medicine, 124,* 884–890.

Senge, P. (1990). *The fifth discipline: The art and practice of the learning organization.* New York: Free Press.

Shortell, S. M., O'Brien, J. L., Carman, J. M., Foster, R. W., Hughes, E. F., Boerstler, H., et al. (1995). Assessing the impact of continuous quality improvement/total quality management: Concept versus implementation. *Health Services Research, 30*(2), 377–401.

Solberg, L. I., Hroscikoski, M. C., Sperl-Hillen, J. M., Harper, P. G., & Crabtree, B. F. (2006). Transforming medical care: case study of an exemplary, small medical group. *Annals of Family Medicine, 4,* 109–116.

Studer, Q. (2003). *Hardwiring excellence. Purpose, worthwhile work, making a difference.* Gulf Breeze, FL: Fire Starter Publishing.

Thomas, E. J., & Helmreich, R. L. (2002). Will airline safety models work in medicine? In M. M. Rosenthal & K. M. Sutcliffe (Eds.), *Medical error: What do we know? What do we do?* San Francisco: Jossey-Bass.

Tucker, A. L., Nembhard, I. M., & Edmondson, A. C. (2007). Implementing new practices: An empirical study of organizational learning in hospital intensive care units. *Management Science, 53*(6), 894–907.

# PART THREE

# Macro Perspectives

# Chapter 10

# Strategic Thinking and Achieving Competitive Advantage

Stephen L. Walston and Ann F. Chou

## CHAPTER OUTLINE

- **Strategic Management**
- **Values, Mission, and Vision**
- **Strategy and Health Care**
- **Evaluation of Organizational Environment**
- **Internal Resources: A Source of Competitive Advantage**
- **Use of Generic Strategies**
- **Conclusion**

## LEARNING OBJECTIVES

**Upon completion of this chapter, the reader will be able to:**

1. Understand concepts of strategy and strategic management

2. Learn the importance and the formulation of mission, vision, and values in strategy

3. Discern how strategic advantage can be different in health care

4. Perceive how strategy is developed and can evolve in organizations

5. Understand the concept and components of business models

6. Learn how to analyze the internal and external environments and the integration of these analyses into strategic planning

7. Recognize different generic strategic approaches and apply them in the health care setting

8. Acquire skills in strategy evaluation methods

9. Understand how strategy and strategic management applies to health care markets

# KEY TERMS

| | |
|---|---|
| Business Model | Perfect Competition |
| Buyer Power | Porter's Five Forces Framework |
| Competitive Advantage | Portfolio Analysis |
| Barriers to Entry | Product Life Cycle |
| Economies of Scale | Rivalry |
| External Environment | Strategy |
| First Mover Advantage | Strategic Group |
| Generic Strategies | Strategic Management |
| Internal Environment | Supplier Power |
| Market Structure | SWOT Analysis |
| Market Niche Strategy | Switching Costs |
| Mission | Threat of Substitution |
| Monopolistic Competition | Values |
| Monopoly | Vision |
| Oligopoly | |

## IN PRACTICE: How Strategos Evolved

Strategy literally means "the art of the general," from the Greek word "strategos" that signified the planning of a military campaign. This concept of strategy has been discussed for thousands of years. Strategy, along with the concept of organizational structure, was refined and articulated to further military purposes. Military campaigns motivated the training of leaders to obtain competitive advantage on the battlefield. Generals often logged their experiences and wisdom to improve their army's prospects in the next battle. Some of the first recorded history in China from the period between 500 BCE and 700 CE documented significant treatises on warfare, the most familiar of which was Sun Tzu's *The Art of War* (Sawyer, 2007). In the Mediterranean basin, modern military strategy and tactics were developed under such leaders as Philip II (382–336 BC) and Alexander the Great (356–323 BC) of Macedonia and Hannibal (247–183 BC) of Carthage. Philip combined infantry, cavalry, and primitive artillery into a trained, organized, and maneuverable fighting force backed up by engineers and a rudimentary signaling system. His son Alexander became an accomplished strategist and tactician with his concern for planning, keeping open lines of communication and supply, security, relentless pursuit of foes, and the use of surprise. Hannibal was a supreme tactician whose crushing victories taught the Romans that the flexible attack tactics of their legions needed to be supplemented by unity of command and an improved cavalry. The Romans eventually replaced their citizen-soldiers with a paid professional army whose training, equipment, and skill at fortification, road building, and siege warfare became legendary. The Byzantine emperors studied Roman strategy and tactics and wrote some of the first essays on the subject.

The Middle Ages (1000 CE to 1500 CE) saw a decline in the study and application of strategy—with the exception of the great Mongol conqueror Genghis Khan. Medieval tactics began with an emphasis on defensive fortifications, siege craft, and armored cavalry. The introduction, however, of such new developments as the crossbow, longbow, halberd, pike, and, above all, gunpowder, began to revolutionize the conduct of war, changing strategies and tactics.

---

**IN PRACTICE: How Strategos Evolved** *(Continued)*

This notion of strategy applied exclusively to military and warfare until the advent of the Industrial Revolution, when the size of companies grew to a point that warranted more coordination and direction. In the twentieth century, the need for explicit strategy was initially emphasized by executives at large companies, such as Alfred Sloan of General Motors and Chester Barnard of New Jersey Bell (Ghemawat, 2001). During this time, eminent economists also sought to answer questions of the purpose of firms and the relationship between resource allocation and business success (Ghemawat, 2001).

Different perspectives of strategy have developed over time. Strategy has been seen as a deliberate, purposeful behavior that allows a firm to plan decisions that maximize opportunities while minimizing threats. This perspective of strategy allows for conscious action to take advantage of opportunities with a firm's own internal capabilities. Strategies are developed to guide behaviors and achieve organizational goals. Methods and means for achieving success are prescriptive, and often strategists seek to distill how strategy can be executed in the most efficient fashion. For example, Napoleon I had 115 specific principles, and the Confederate general Nathan Bedford Forrest had but one: "Get there first with the most men" (Wills, 1998). Another view of strategy presents an emergent or descriptive perspective. This perspective explains a firm's past actions by examining the patterns of decisions and past choices that reflect environmental changes, organizational learning, and innovations. Both views are necessary for successful strategic management and decision making. Scholars suggest that both deliberate action and nonlinear thought are needed to allow a firm the ability to establish routines and processes, while maintaining the ability to be flexible and adaptive (Burns, 2002; Ghoshal and Bartlett, 1995; Mintzberg et al., 1998).

Today, strategy and strategic management have become widely accepted. Courses about strategy are widespread in business schools, and strategic management is an integral part of leadership training. Yet, given its diverse nature, teaching strategy is a difficult task that involves instructing how to craft future-directed plans, while developing an intuitive insight and the ability to learn, adapt, and change (Burns, 2002). The concept and importance of strategy has proliferated beyond the field of business administration. A search for strategy on Amazon.com in April 2010 produced over 110,000 results. The varied nature of strategy is reflected by the diverse nature of these books, which include strategic maps, marketing, game theory, military, and managerial economics. Overall, the nature of strategy remains very complex, but widely accepted.

---

# CHAPTER PURPOSE

This chapter informs the reader regarding an important aspect of management: strategy and strategic management. Understanding strategy and strategic thinking helps students and health care leaders improve their decision making. This chapter provides a foundation to understand the principles of strategy and strategic management and methods for their application.

# STRATEGIC MANAGEMENT

**Strategic management** involves the creation, implementation, and overall direction for a firm. As such, it requires both internal and external management functions to facilitate the development, implementation, and monitoring of strategy within an organization. Steps in the process of strategic management may include: (1) goal formation; (2) environmental scanning; (3) strategy formulation; (4) strategy evaluation; (5) implementation; and (6) strategic control. Internally, strategic management involves the participation of everyone in the organization, especially the leadership. Organizational leadership and management play key roles in formulating strategies and integrating them into the organization's mission, visions, and goals and leveraging organizational mechanisms, cultures, and resources to support the strategic implementation as well as to conduct analyses and evaluation. Externally, strategic management enhances organizational success by anticipating possible changes in the environment in which the organization operates, and by enabling organizations to change and maintain their **competitive advantage**, the long-term market position and uniqueness that is not easily duplicable by rivals. Both external analyses and internal mechanisms are important in the strategic management processes (Ginter, Swayne, and Duncan, 2002; Luke, Walston, and Plummer, 2004; Mintzberg, Ahlstrand, and Lampel, 1998; Schendel, 1994).

## Environment

No organization is immune to influences that come from its **external environment** (the conditions, entities, and factors surrounding an organization that influence its activities and choices), and strategic management is a process that helps organizations respond appropriately to potential threats and opportunities. Strategic management has become increasingly important in health care. As an industry, health care is particularly sensitive to its environment, which undergoes rapid demographic, societal/cultural, economic, technological, political/legal, and global influences (Fahey, 1999; Walter and Priem, 1999). For the most part, health care organizations cannot directly control these factors in their environment. However, these factors have a direct impact on the competitiveness of these organizations.

One external factor that will have a direct impact on health care strategies is the demographics of our communities. Demographics are represented by population size, age structure, geographic distribution, racial/ethnic mix, and income levels (Fahey and Narayanan, 1986). The demographic

trends in the United States are perhaps the most immutable factor affecting the demand of health care services. The U.S. population is getting older as well as more racially, ethnically, and geographically diverse. The Department of Health and Human Services estimates that more than a quarter of the U.S. population will be older than age 60 by 2050 (Figure 10.1). The population has also become more diverse in its racial/ethnic mix, where racial/ethnic minorities make up about 30 percent of the overall population in the 2000 census (Figure 10.2). In addition, there is no longer a racial or ethnic majority group in the state of California, and the trend is likely to continue in other states. As the 2010 census concludes, racial/ethnic minority groups will assume a larger proportion of the overall population.

The increased diversity will drive greater variations in strategies and force successful health care organizations to be agile and adapt to the cultural and demographic needs of their constituents. Culture, race, ethnicity, and primary language have been shown to be associated with access to care and compliance with prevention and treatment among patients. As our society becomes more diverse, strategies that would lead to culturally sensitive and linguistically appropriate care should be emphasized to ensure equity and quality across patient groups. Professional organizations like the American Hospital Association have encouraged their members to take

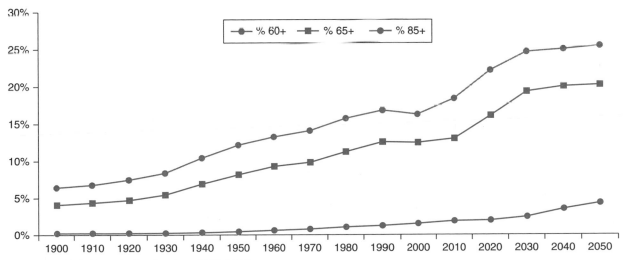

**Older Population by Age: 1900–2050—Percent 60+, Percent 65+, and 85+**

**Figure 10.1** U.S. Population by Age 1900-2050.

SOURCE: Administration on Aging, Department of Health and Human Services. http://www.aoa.gov/AoARoot/Aging_Statistics/future_growth/docs/By_Age_Total_Population.xls

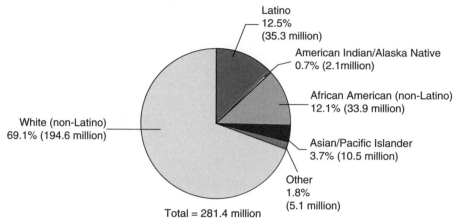

**Figure 10.2** Percent of U.S. Population by Race/Ethnicity.

SOURCE: U.S. Census Bureau, Census 2000 Redistricting Data.

the lead in addressing these diverse needs (AHA, 2010). Health care organizations that evaluate patient satisfaction using instruments such as the Consumer Assessment of Healthcare Providers and Systems are systematically collecting information about possible racial and ethnic disparities in access to and experience with health care.

Moreover, patients have become increasingly more complex as many have multiple comorbidities due to the prevalence of obesity and chronic conditions. At the time when patients have become more difficult to manage, the health care industry also faces a workforce shortage of both clinicians and allied health workers, creating a supply-demand imbalance.

Economically, escalating insurance premiums and health care costs pose threats to the industry as these trends, if they continue, are unsustainable long term. Competition has also broadened to include global players. Due to high prices, patients have turned to other alternatives to meet their health care needs, such as purchasing medications across the border. Medical tourism to South America and Asia has seen a steady growth as Americans are going abroad for surgeries or procedures that they cannot afford in the United States.

Changes in the global health care markets as well as politics are also affecting foreign nationals who come to the United States for health care. For decades, the United States has attracted foreign medical tourists because it offers health

care that has been perceived as cutting edge. In 2008, more than 400,000 non-U.S. residents sought health care services in the United States, which accounted for almost $5 billion and about 2 percent of total services rendered (Deloitte and Touche, 2009). To facilitate access, many large health care systems, such as Stanford Hospital & Clinics and Methodist Hospital in Houston, offer international offices that assist in arranging care. Although foreign visitors make up only a small percentage of the total patient volume, these patients typically pay full prices for their health care services and have therefore been an important source of revenue for many U.S. hospitals. However, the number of foreign patients has fallen steadily and substantially since 2001. This is due in part to the increase in global competition through improved quality of care, lower price, and greater travel restrictions imposed by the United States following the events of September 11, 2001 (Lee and Davis, 2009).

Health care as well is one of the most technologically innovative industries, but the technological advancement has also contributed to the escalating costs. Recently, the health care industry has placed greater emphasis on the adoption and utilization of health information technology (HIT). In particular, the Institute of Medicine has promoted the use of health information technology as a transforming strategy to reduce medical errors and improve quality (IOM, 2001).

In addition, health information technology has a large role in the federal health care reform of 2009, with a mandate for "meaningful use" of HIT among all providers. This also reflects the political environment for health care organizations and for the industry as a whole. Health care is a unique industry that is particularly susceptible to political and legal influences because the government has a complicated relationship with the industry as a provider, regulator, and payer.

In all, the health care industry exists in a very large, dynamic, complex, and challenging environment with many opportunities as well as threats. With an aging and diverse population making up a changing customer base, increased competition, technological innovations, and a changing political landscape, health care organizations must have a good grasp of the relationship between the larger environment and its future. Understanding their industry environment allows the organization to craft strategic actions that will more likely achieve the organization's mission, improve its profitability, and more appropriately establish a strong position in relation to competitors.

## What Is Strategy?

The formation of strategy is often not a rational process. Earlier decisions imprison statesmen within the logic of their choices and finally impose policies and actions that these leaders would have preferred to avoid. (Murray, Knox, and Bernstein, 1994)

Modifying the definition offered by Porter (1980), we identify **strategy** as the development of a broad formula prescribing a way in which a business competes and collaborates, sets goals, and establishes policies to carry out those goals in order to achieve the organizational mission. Strategy occurs at all levels of firms and organizations. It is a concept that has been readily embraced by organizational leadership and defined in many ways. Various other definitions have been suggested, ranging from cognitively directed, documented goals to unintentionally generated patterns of decisions. Strategy has been described as a plan or guide for future action, a pattern of past behaviors, the process of launching products into a particular market, the fundamental way an organization operates, a ploy or feint to outwit a competitor, etc. (Mintzberg, Ahlstrand, and Lampel, 1998). This chapter does not seek to evaluate the many suggested definitions, constructions, and purposes of strategy, which is covered elsewhere in this book. However, herein we focus on the purposeful aspects of strategy that address strategy in a practical sense and provide students and health care leaders with the knowledge and skills to improve their understanding and practice of strategy through intentional and cognitive decisions.

Strategies are important, requiring significant commitment of resources, and are often not easily reversible. Strategy can mean different things, but in general, strategy has these characteristics, where it:

1. Concerns both organizations and the environment
2. Is complex
3. Affects the welfare of the organization
4. Involves issues of content and process
5. Is not purely deliberate
6. Exists on different levels
7. Involves various thought processes
8. Involves the allocation of resources
9. Should be mission based (adapted from Chaffee, 1985)

Strategy ultimately is about making better decisions. Leaders are faced with many critical choices: where to invest, whom to hire, what services to offer, etc. Leaders who embrace strategic thinking and develop strategic skills make better decisions. Strategies assist organizations to choose wisely among the many available options. Strategic planning consists of making decisions that are concerned with positioning a firm relative to its competitors and the allocation of assets for current and future activity. Through strategic analyses and discovery, leaders come to better understand the chain of cause and effect. This directs resource allocation in terms of personnel and physical assets. Strategy does not create a blueprint for future decisions, as the future is full of uncertainties. Strategy must be flexible enough to allow for changing circumstances. However, strategic actions often commit resources that may be difficult to recover. Personnel are often fungible and can frequently and relatively quickly be transferred with minimal cost to new projects, products, and directives. However, most physical assets, such as hospital buildings and medical equipment, are difficult to transfer, requiring a long period of time from conception to implementation. For example, some health care systems are investing in proton therapy units that may cost over $125 million, despite the lack of evidence in the efficacy of the proton treatment (*Forbes*, 2009). Successful strategies consider resource allocation by balancing the need for flexibility and capital asset investment. These choices represent decisions leaders must make after careful consideration of their situation and environment. Strategic planning must be flexible to accommodate the changing environmental conditions, and yet significant enough to sustain competitive advantage. Within these choices, strategy provides a unifying theme that provides coherence and direction to the actions and decisions of the organization.

Strategy has two very important functions. First, good strategies should improve decisions about resource allocation to yield long-term benefits for the organization. A large part of what leaders do is to make decisions of how to allocate finite resources. A good strategist can delegate limited resources to maximize outcomes. Second, developing strategies should challenge existing assumptions and be open to new possibilities. By doing so, leaders and managers can be aware of new realities to manage change effectively.

Often, our assumptions are based on facts and data that may well be outdated or sometimes based upon faulty information. For example, when asked about the location of Lima, Peru, relative to that of Miami, Florida, most people would believe that Lima is west of Miami. In reality, Miami is actually west of Lima (Figure 10.3). In health care, an example was demonstrated in the late 1980s and early 1990s when many assumed that HMOs would be the dominant model for health care delivery. Based on this assumption and early growth of HMO plans, many believed integrated delivery systems would be the type of organizational arrangement that would prevail in health care. This assumption drove the strategic plans of many systems to create systems of insurers, physicians, and hospitals. Some hospitals even redesigned their mission to become an integrated system. Yet, by the late 1990s, it was apparent that HMO's growth had dissipated, and PPOs began to dominate the health care market. Health care systems that did not update this

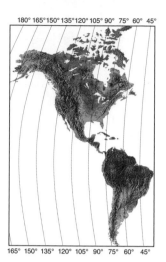

**Figure 10.3** The Americas.
SOURCE: Delmar, Cengage Learning.

assumption could have made significant strategic blunders, and many did.

## The Strategic Process

Successful strategies require direction, resources, and institutionalized processes. Too often, organizations believe that strategy is accomplished when direction is formulated. This, however, is only the first step in taking strategic action. Strategic thinking involves crafting direction that eventually evolves into goals and objectives. Strategies require action, which involves assigning responsibilities, assignments, expected outcomes, and follow-through. Many strategies fail as a result of improper or inattentive implementation. Poor implementation and inadequate follow-up can render the best strategic plan futile. In fact, developing strategies without corresponding implementation planning can create many organizational problems. For example, new strategies can raise expectations

---

## UNDERSTANDING AND DISCOVERING OUR BIASES

When asked which city is farther west, Miami, Florida, or Lima, Peru, almost all would choose Lima. However, on a map or comparing the degrees of longitude, one would find that Miami is actually further west than Lima. Miami has a longitude of −80° 11′ 37″; while Lima's longitude is only −77° 3′ 0″. Why do most individuals have this inaccurate knowledge? Generally, people perceive South America directly below North America, an incorrect fact. South America actually protrudes to the East of North America.

---

**IN PRACTICE:** How Fixed Assumptions Affected the Battle of Gettysburg—July 1863

---

The American Civil War had entered its third year of bloody conflict. During the first two years, the South, under the able direction of General Robert E. Lee, had won many battles, notwithstanding their being outnumbered and outgunned. By the summer of 1863, General Lee was confident that he could invade the North and defeat the Union Army to end the war. In mid-June, General Lee invaded Maryland and Pennsylvania with almost 72,000 troops. The Union Army, led by the newly appointed General George Meade, finally found the Confederate Army at the small town of Gettysburg, Pennsylvania. The Union Army consisted of almost 94,000 troops.

The battle commenced on the morning of July 1, with Lee's armies pushing the Union forces out of the town of Gettysburg and into the surrounding hills. However, darkness halted the South's advance. On the morning of July 2, Lee ordered attacks on both the right and left flanks of the Union forces. The battle swung back and forth, with the Confederates temporarily breaking the Union line but not gaining significant advantage before darkness fell on the second bloody day.

As the third day of battle began, Lee made one of the worst decisions of his career. Against the advice of Lieutenant General James Longstreet, Lee ordered 12,000 men to attack the center of the Union lines. To reach the Union troops, they would have to walk across almost one mile of open field. General Lee's mistake was not so much in tactics or strategies, but in not updating his assumptions and facts. Firearms had been used for about 500 years. However, they had been historically very inaccurate—so inaccurate that strategies called for troops to march until they could see the "whites" of their enemies' eyes, fire their weapon, and then attack with the bayonet, the most important part of the gun. This was because guns traditionally had smoothbores, or smooth insides of the barrels. This caused bullets to rotate randomly, much like a knuckleball baseball pitch. This diminished its accuracy and limited the distance at which it was effective.

Lee was trained in these classical tactics and did not update his strategies, given the advances in weapons. Until the eighteenth century, the standard infantry weapon was a smoothbore musket. However, by 1863, most soldiers had "rifles," such as the U.S. Springfield and the British Enfield that would spin the bullet in the barrel, which increased the range and accuracy from 30 yards to about 300 yards. Marching 12,000 soldiers across open ground enacted a terrible toll on these men, before they were close enough to engage the Union forces. Only about 300 men reached the center of the Union Army, and these were quickly killed or captured. As the battle quieted at the end of July 3, the Confederate Army prepared to retreat. Over 46,000 casualties occurred across the three days of battle. This was the "high-water" mark for the Confederacy, and the beginning of their end. Never again would they significantly challenge the North. Lee later commented that this attack was one of the worst decisions he had made as a commander, and his unchallenged assumptions may have been the reason that the battle and war was lost (Coggins, 1990; Eicher, 2001).

---

that can be dashed with inaction, resulting in employee cynicism and low morale.

Within an organization, strategic priorities should be elaborated, and projects with goals and objectives should be developed, implemented, and monitored for each area. Appropriate individuals should be assigned responsibility and authority for achieving strategic goals, and key performance indicators should be established to measure progress. A regular process of review and feedback should then be set. For instance, one of the strategic priorities of a large international hospital established to provide primarily tertiary services was to improve service capacity. This goal was further defined by measurable and actionable outcomes to: (1) reduce the non-tertiary patient load, (2) increase the efficiency and throughput of patients, (3) expand existing facilities, (4) better coordinate patient care with other institutions, and (5) expand off-site patient care services. Each outcome area was further segmented into specific objectives that had assigned staff with responsibilities, key performance indicators, and reporting timeframes.

Strategic planning processes must involve the right people. Often organizations struggle to involve the right set of people. The top executive should lead the strategic planning and exhibit his/her commitment by the dedication of time, resources, and intellect. Organizational boards, if appropriate, should also be involved in the strategic planning process and its monitoring. In many health care organizations, the board represents the community and has responsibility to assure that management actions and direction align with its mission and vision. This is a critical function of a board. Frequently, the board's direct involvement with strategic planning is coordinated by a strategic planning committee.

It is important to identify all stakeholders who should be involved and clearly define the terms of their involvement and responsibilities. Employees, medical staff, other organizations dependent on the services of the health care organization, and other stakeholders have a vested interest in the firm's strategic planning and may be asked to participate in the planning process. Lack of clarity in responsibilities and tasks can lead to frustration and withdrawal of key stakeholders, which will lead to greater impediments to creating and implementing the strategies.

Figure 10.4 illustrates the strategic management process that we will discuss throughout this chapter. Strategic management begins with a plan to plan, founded on organizational values, followed by mission formulation, strategic modeling, and implementation. The plan should outline steps to be taken, establish the committees and meetings, and the time frames involved should be explicit. It is also important to assess organizational resources such as personnel, facilities/physical assets (e.g., building, work stations, etc.), culture, organizational competencies, and external (political and governmental) support. Processes established can facilitate the implementation process. For example, is the entire process planned and monitored? How does the organizational structure and decision-making hierarchy affect implementation? The processes should also be established to facilitate the establishment or review of the organizational values, mission, and vision, to drive development of strategic analyses and objectives. Finally, clear communication channels to disseminate information and evaluation and feedback loops to continuously improve the implementation process should exist.

As stated above, the most difficult aspect of strategic action is the actual implementation of strategic plans. Organizations often spend an incredible amount of time and resources developing strategic plans. Yet, many of these plans do not get implemented. This waste of resources is caused by an inward focus on the need for the planning process and not understanding that the purpose of strategic thinking should be outcome oriented, where the organization improves its competitive position by achieving its mission and vision.

To facilitate implementation, health care organizations should seek to:

- Establish the competencies, capabilities, and resources needed to achieve strategic action. Firms should embed the organizational skills and allocate the manpower and resources needed to engage in strategic action through specific goals, projects, and programs.

- Identify responsibility and outcomes with definite timelines and key performance indicators. This should include managerial responsibility and related resources necessary to accomplish the targeted strategic objectives.

- Develop and promote policies that facilitate strategic action. Organizations should establish policies that encourage innovation and aid in change.

- Appropriately use information and operating systems to drive the strategies. Health care organizations generally have far too much data, but lack good information to drive strategic decisions. Strategic thinking requires accurate, timely information delivered to the decision maker.

- Tie rewards to the achievement of strategic action. Successful strategic-oriented firms are results oriented and motivate and celebrate achievement of strategic outcomes. Rewards and incentives should be tied to the strategic outcomes.

- Tie budgets to strategies. Too often strategic plans are divorced from organizational budgets. Strategies need to be integrated into annual budgets and be used to drive strategic action.

- Establish a monitoring and evaluation process that will communicate the progress and challenges implementing the strategies.

- Incorporate strategic action into annual evaluations. Annual employee evaluations should be tied into the organizational strategies. Especially, organizational values should be directly reflected in each evaluation. Employees and managers should determine how closely the employees are living the values in their work.

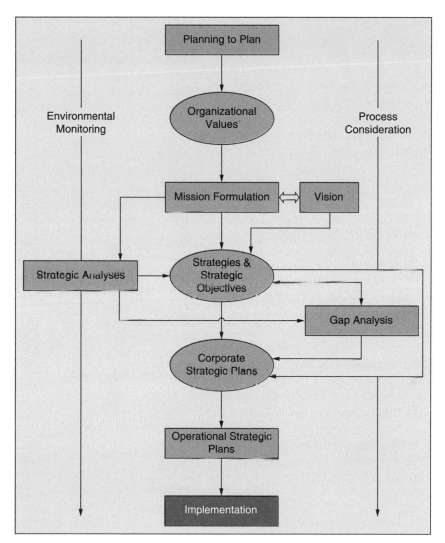

**Figure 10.4** The Strategic Process.
SOURCE: Delmar, Cengage Learning.

# VALUES, MISSION, AND VISION

Organizations can be effective with radically different strategies. Even similar organizations in geographic proximity may have different strategies that each produces spectacular results. How could this be possible? Frankly, as we will discuss, there is not a one right, optimal, or "one-size-fits-all" strategy, but effective strategies are created by matching internal abilities

and resources to the external environment to meet the purpose for the firm's existence. Since organizations exist for many reasons, an effective and successful outcome may be different for different organizations. For example, a for-profit hospital may seek high financial returns, while a church clinic might define success by the greater number of patients they serve.

The definition of success should be based upon the important values and purposes of an organization. Each organization may have different values and stakeholders who will influence their objectives and how they should define their success. Different organizational models may also be associated with different statements of values, mission, and vision as well as with differences in their approaches to strategy. This is especially the case in the health care sector, where strategies often differ significantly across for-profit versus not-for-profit organizations, academic medical centers versus community hospitals, rural versus urban facilities, multi-market systems versus single-market hospitals, and so on.

The basis of all successful strategies should originate with the organization's mission, vision, and values (Luke, Walston, and Plummer, 2004). These should be the foundation of organizational strategies. Too often, however, they end up as a written document sitting on a shelf or a plaque hanging on the wall and are disconnected from the strategic formulation and implementation. Strategy experts have observed that few organizational participants, including executives, demonstrate knowledge of elements of the organizational strategic plans (Collis and Rukstad, 2008). When this disconnect occurs, organizations frequently find themselves in trouble with their stakeholders. For example, HealthSouth, HCA, and Tenet, among many others, experienced indictments, huge fines, lower stock prices, and tarnished public images as a result of their actions in contrast to the stated mission, vision, and values. HCA paid almost $1.7 billion in criminal fines, civil restitution, and penalties in 2000 and 2003 to resolve fraudulent actions that violated their very visible mission and values statements that had been displayed ubiquitously in their hospitals (http://www.usdoj.gov/opa/pr/2003/June/03_civ_386.htm).

## Values

What are values and why are they important? **Values** are the expression of the ethics that guide employees' actions. They should constrain how the mission and vision is accomplished. Certain behaviors, no matter how they accomplish the organizational mission, are unacceptable, and even if the mission is accomplished, if the values have been violated, the organization has failed.

In many organizations, one or more employees may have asked: "Is there any value in articulating our values?" In general, employees may be in the best position to observe whether or not an organization's expressed values have been incorporated into its culture. Employees might perceive that an organization's value statements are mere gestures, that they lack real purpose. The more observant might even fail to see a connection between the expressed values and an organization's intended strategy.

Formalized, written organizational values are important for a number of reasons. For one, they serve as an ethical compass, the absence of which could leave an organization without a viable rudder to direct its strategies. During times of stress, especially, an organization lacking such a compass might feel pressure to deviate from standards and take decisions contrary to normal ethical practices. Pressure to achieve goals may also generate personality conflicts that could motivate individuals and groups to act in inappropriate and unethical ways. Written values serve as visible reminders of the organization's commitment to basic beliefs.

Failure to embed values also subjects an organization to the risk of contingent ethics—values that shift with the circumstances. Written values assist in grounding organizational ethics over time. They keep those values from fluctuating based on the situation. Put another way, values and ethics should endure and not fluctuate based on current encounters or challenges. Strategies will (and should) change over time. However, values should not.

Thomas Watson Jr., former chairman of IBM, expressed the need for common beliefs upon which a business should be founded: "I believe that any organization, in order to survive and achieve success, must have a sound set of beliefs on which it premises all of its policies and actions" (Watson, 1963).

In theory, organizational values represent the sum total of individual values held by each person affiliated with an organization—the stakeholders. In practice, however, the values of top executives almost always exert the greatest influence on an organization's prevailing tone and practices. More generally, it is the role of the CEO, other top executives, and the board of directors to formulate an organization's values and to assure that they are lived throughout the organization. As a consultant once said, "Values should not be just written on a wall, but to be effective they must be written on the hearts of employees." Organizational leaders are responsible to move the values from the wall and into the hearts of their employees.

Expressed values can also be the means by which an organization shapes the attitudes of its members toward selected categories of stakeholders. This is especially important in health care, given the diversity and importance of different stakeholders. A good example of this can be found in the value statements offered by All Saints Healthcare System, a hospital system based in Racine, Wisconsin. All Saints is a member of the Wheaton Franciscan System, a Catholic multi-hospital system. Four of their expressed values (retrieved August 14, 2010, from http://www.mywheaton.org/about/mission_vision_values.asp) are:

*Respect:* We value each person as sacred, created in the image and likeness of God, which gives worth and meaning to each person's life.

*Integrity:* We value honesty, words and actions that build trust.

*Development:* We value personal and professional growth that combines the physical, emotional, spiritual and relational aspects of life and work.

*Excellence:* We value superior performance in our work and service.

*Stewardship:* We value our responsibility to use human, financial, and natural resources entrusted to us for the common good, with special concern for those who are poor.

Note how these values craft expected behaviors toward patients and the poor. Assuming that these values are inculcated within the system's culture, one should expect the provision of excellent care and that the poor are treated with dignity by this system. Furthermore, the location of their facilities and financial policies should reflect these values. One might expect their hospitals to be located near lower socio-economic areas to provide generous discounts from billed charges to the poor.

### How Should Values Be Established and Evaluated?

Values should be established and evaluated based on the values and expectations of key shareholders.

- *Obtain key stakeholders' expectations for the organization.* In some organizations, the owners might be the only group truly deemed to be important. For others, multiple groups including owners, customers, employees, and suppliers might be influential enough to be included in a search for values. One way to identify key stakeholders is to identify those groups that would suffer the most if the organization ceased to exist. The organization can conduct surveys and interviews to see what values are believed to be important. They should seek to answer questions such as (1) For what do they want the organization to be known? (2) What

makes them proud to be affiliated with the organization? And (3) Who are the heroes of the company and why?

- *Identify common values among stakeholders.* Commonly expressed values should be identified and related values merged to express the ethical base of the organization's purpose. A firm should seek to identify those values that set them apart and make them distinctive.

- *Values should be visible and tangible to employees.* Organizational values must be visible and tied to performance. The values should be clearly incorporated into employees' (including the CEO's) evaluations, and the employees should be appraised as to how well they are living the values. The firm should also link the values to measurable strategic outcomes, as reflected in satisfaction scores, error rates, availability of mental health care for the homeless, and other such indicators.

- *Values should be memorable.* Values should be in terms that stakeholders will understand and can remember. As a rule of thumb, there should be no more than 5 to 7 values.

## Mission

A **mission** should be the foundation of strategic direction. The existence and enactment of a company mission should be critical to a firm's success. A mission keeps management focused on what their primary purpose is. Authors have suggested that a mission should address the reason for being and why you do what you do (Ginter, Swayne, and Duncan, 2005; Luke, Walston, and Plummer, 2004). It is a key indicator of how the organization views its stakeholders. As such, it should be a direct outgrowth of its values. A mission provides the reason for the company's existence and forms the basis for strategy. It should guide the firm to focus its energies and frame its choices of strategy and commitments of resources. A mission should be the solid base upon which strategic direction is established that drives resource allocation.

What should be included in a mission? Most successful statements have measurable, definable, and actionable content. They contain as well an emotional appeal that stakeholders can recognize and act upon. Key components should include the definition of product or service, the standards employed, and the population or segment served by the organization. A mission should describe what the organization does or its scope. What does it do? What are the boundaries beyond which it will not venture? They should also reflect the organization's values through expressed standards and objectives. In health care,

## IN PRACTICE: How Values Dictate Actions and Outcomes: The Mongol and Arab Conquests

The values an organization holds can directly influence their behavior and outcomes. Two different peoples conquered huge swaths of the known world across different centuries with different outcomes, demonstrating how values can readily dictate actions and outcomes. The Arab or Muslim armies emerged in 632 CE, as the Arab Peninsula was unified. By 732 CE, the Muslims controlled land from Spain to India. The Muslims were skilled warriors, but held deeply rooted values that dictated how war was to be conducted. Muslims felt a deep need to share Islam with others. Historically, Muslim travelers and traders have peacefully spread the religion to Africa, China, Malaysia, and Indonesia. The sharing of Islam was a primary objective of the Arab armies even during conflict, which was reflected by the army's values and actions.

War was strongly discouraged (see Al-Baqarah 2:190 in the Quran), but necessary against oppressive nations and for self-defense. Muslims, when engaged in war, were never to fight against noncombatants, especially women and children. Trees were not to be harmed. Justice was to be highly valued, as during peace. Medical assistance was to be available to all, regardless of religion or creed, even enemies. Captives were to be shown mercy, fed, and allowed to gain their freedom through ransom, labor, or on their word. When a people were conquered, they were still allowed religious freedom and, generally, had more freedoms and opportunities. As a result, most of the conquered converted to Islam, over time, achieving their primary mission (DeWeese, 1994).

In contrast to the Muslim expansion, the Mongol Empire arose during the thirteenth and fourteenth centuries. At its height, it covered lands from China, Russia, India, and the Middle East. The Mongols lacked a religious motive, but were a warlike people who enjoyed hunting and conquest. The original Mongol leader, Genghis Khan, is reputed to once have asked and then answered, what was the greatest joy in life. He stated that "The greatest joy a man can know is to conquer his enemies and drive them before him. To ride their horses and take away their possessions. To see the faces who were dear to them bedewed with tears, and to clasp their wives and daughters in his arms." (Prawdin and Chaliand, 2005)

Yet, the Mongols had a strict sense of honor and loyalty. The Mongol "mission" was conquest and win. They were very intelligent and used superb tactics and strategies. They gained accurate knowledge of their enemies prior to attacking, used superior technology and tactics, and were highly mobile. The Mongols were extremely ruthless in battle, but also displayed extraordinary military discipline. Resistance was met by ruthless annihilation. Captured enemies might be killed, enslaved, or used as a human shield in subsequent battles. Cooperative territories received relatively benevolent rule that included religious tolerance. When a Mongol army first approached a city, the city's residents were often given an opportunity to surrender and pay tribute. If rejected, the city would be ransacked and destroyed. Everyone and everything was likely to be attacked, including armies, animals, women, and children. For instance, Baghdad, the capital of the then-existing Muslim empire, was destroyed in 1257 CE. As many as a million people were estimated to have been killed (Frazier, 2005). Total destruction occurred to many cities, including Kiev and Moscow among others. The Mongols expanded their empire to the gates of Vienna, Austria, but the empire began to unravel in less than two centuries. Ironically, most of the Mongol controlled areas eventually converted to Islam.

these standards often include wording such as "providing world-class services" or "setting the community's quality standards." The mission should represent the essence of the organization's competitive advantage. What will the organization do differently, or how can it perform better than others? The mission statement may also target a specific customer base. Organizations may state in their missions that they serve a special demographic segment, like women or children, or a nation or region.

Missions are expressed in many ways. Some are short and others lengthy. Mission statements should be long enough to be distinctive and guide an organization's strategies, but short enough that employees can comprehend and apply them. If a mission statement is too long, it may not be readily communicated to organizational participants or used effectively to drive strategies. Collis and Rukstad (2008) suggest that a mission statement should contain no more than 35 words.

Business also should avoid using nondescript, generic statements like "providing the highest quality of care for the lowest possible cost," or "maximizing shareholder wealth by exceeding customer expectations," which in some derivation often appear in many mission statements. A hospital stating that its mission is "is to provide the highest possible quality" expresses a virtually meaningless declaration. Another example of an ambiguous mission is one expressed by a large health care system that claimed that its mission was to "remain at the forefront of health care delivery." What does this mean—the forefront in clinical technology, in market share, in quality, in innovation?

Missions should also be crafted to express the core function and purpose of the organization's existence. One large, sophisticated health care organization had the following as its mission:

> [The] Center provides medical services of a highly specialized nature and promotes medical research and education programs, including postgraduate education training, as well as contributes to the prevention of disease.

After extensive discussion, the leadership agreed that the purpose and reason for the medical center's existence was to provide highly specialized health care and education and research existed to support the delivery of specialized care. As a result, they altered their mission to this:

> [The] Center provides the highest quality specialized health care in an integrated education and research setting [for the nation of ...].

Although the differences may seem subtle, they are important. The hospital's primary purpose and the reason for its existence were to provide tertiary and quaternary care to its service population. In the context of their strategic development, education and research were to be instituted chiefly to support the primary mission and not to be developed in an isolated, self-supporting manner that had occurred before.

A mission should also not be too restrictive. During the early 1900s, the railroads in the United States fell on hard times because they had narrowly defined their mission as providing rail service, rather than being in the transportation business. The railroad companies remained committed to transportation on two rails, while much transportation shifted to roads and air. Likewise, hospitals that narrowly define their mission to be in the acute-care business might encounter competitive difficulties in markets in which more integrated services are demanded. However, organizations establish many different kinds of missions. For example, HealthTrust, Inc., a company formed in 1987 from Hospital Corporation of America, used a narrow, succinct mission that they were the "Hospital Company" that focused exclusively on hospital care. If strictly followed, the company would not have been able to expand into rapidly growing outpatient and non-hospital care.

In contrast to the railroads and HealthTrust, Xerox has more broadly defined itself as "The Document Company," and its mission as "to help people find better ways to do great work—by constantly leading in document technologies, products and services that improve our customers' work processes and business results." Note that Xerox does not portray itself as a copier company, but expands and widens its purpose to be a "document company." As such, they can provide both electronic and hard-copy documents that serve to improve their customers' business.

In summary, a mission must "call employees to action." A mission should direct the organization to focus its energies in certain products, standards, and market/geographic segments. The mission statement should express why the organization exists and motivate employees to action. The organizational mission should both constrain and guide strategies and tactical actions.

## Vision

A **vision** is a statement about what the organization wants to become. It focuses on the future. The vision should resonate with members of the organization and help them feel proud, excited, and part of something much bigger than themselves. A vision should challenge and stretch the organization's capabilities and image of itself. It gives shape and direction to the organization's future. Better vision statements describe

## DEBATE TIME: Missions

Missions can be written in many different ways. Which of the following could you as an employee understand and use in your work? What could be done to improve each? What is the value of a long versus a short mission? The first is an academic medical center, the second and third are hospitals owned by a religious order, and the last is a major pharmaceutical firm.

1. At [Name], our mission is leading health care.

2. Through our exceptional health care services, we reveal the healing presence of God.

3. As a Christian health center, our mission is to improve the health of the people in the communities we serve.

4. We, the management and employees, are striving for entrepreneurial success. Entrepreneurial success starts with people. Our goal is to operate a worldwide business that produces meaningful benefits for consumers, our market partners and our community. Through efficient research and development, production and marketing of pharmaceutical and chemical specialties, we want to extend opportunities to our customers. To achieve this, we focus our endeavors on business areas where we can achieve a competitive advantage through the excellent quality of our products, systems and services. Our objective is to establish permanent business relationships and not merely short term success.

   On the basis of these principles, we operate as an independent and profit oriented enterprise. We expect a high level of performance from each other, and reward this accordingly. We wish to secure an acceptable return on capital for our investors.

   We respect the cultural distinctions and national interests of all countries in which we operate. We strive to achieve positive recognition for our company within the community. [Company] attaches particular importance to its responsibility for safety. We have an obligation to respect the environment.

   We will deal honestly and constructively with one another. We regard open communication, both internal and external, as a fundamental prerequisite for reaching an understanding of our common goals and for giving meaning to what we do. We shall not be constrained by borders between business areas or countries. All employees, male or female, have equal opportunities to develop their careers. All of us make a personal contribution to the company's entrepreneurial success through our mutual initiative, creativity and sense of responsibility.

---

outcomes that organizations would like to see that may be 5 to 10 years in the future, or further.

A vision should describe the desired future state of the organization, while the mission provides a description of the existing purpose and practice of the firm. A vision to be effective should align with the organizational values, be realistic, be written in concise and understandable language, describe a desirable future, and be clear.

A large, international hospital set as its vision to "become a world-leading institution of excellence and innovation in health care." This required that they prioritize services and designate key centers of excellence for service delivery, and assure that necessary resources would be allocated to these services. On the other hand, there are times when organizations create a vision that may be too complex to be useful for mapping

the organization's future. An eastern U.S. health care system crafted its vision to:

> [C]reate a new standard of community health care, one that combines the personalized, caring environment of the finest community hospital with a commitment to providing the most advanced medical technology and capabilities available to it.

This vision is lengthy and has mostly unrealizable outcomes. A more succinct example is a hospital in the western United States that set as its vision to:

> be the premier regional health care provider to the residents of its service area

Finally, an academic medical center in the southern United States seeks to be recognized as a leading medical center in [the state] and one of the best in the nation. We will be at the forefront of clinical services, medical research and education. With our physician and university partners we will create, teach, and deliver tomorrow's breakthroughs in medical science.

In summary, a vision should motivate and direct an organization. It and the mission should be the foundation of all strategic plans and activities. Leaders should seek to only craft strategies that help fulfill the vision and mission. These two items should be the first and last discussion items of every strategic thinking process. Initially, the vision and mission should be reviewed, the environment analyzed, strategies formulated, and at the end, leaders should confirm that the work aligns and promotes the organizational vision and mission.

# STRATEGY AND HEALTH CARE

The concept of strategic management often centers around achieving competitive advantage over the organization's competitors in the market. There are a number of definitions describing competitive advantage. The organization may achieve competitive advantage by an increase in market power as a result of its actions (Luke, Walston, and Plummer, 2004), improved performance that distinguishes itself from the competition (Porter, 1980), and the implementation of a value-creating strategy not simultaneously implemented by current or potential players (Barney, 1991). Each suggests a competitive business environment of winners and losers in which firms struggle to gain an advantage over their market competitors. In such environments, markets award winners as a result of their relative superior service, pricing, and product innovation that provide consumers greater value. Organizations gain competitive advantage by exploiting their internal strengths in relation to environmental opportunities. As we will discuss, the sources of competitive advantage have been suggested to come from external positioning (Porter, 1980) or organizational resources and capabilities (Barney, 1991).

## What Is Competitive Advantage in Health Care?

Health care, as mentioned, is a very diverse industry containing for-profit, highly competitive pharmaceutical and insurance companies and community-oriented, not-for-profit service providers. Strategic advantage for for-profit firms frequently is based on a "win-lose" perspective. Strategic gain and success depends on finishing ahead of competitors in terms of market share, earnings, or another comparative figure. Health care organizations, especially those that are not for profit and whose mission involves service to vulnerable or disadvantaged populations, may not prioritize gaining a strategic advantage over their competitors as a top organizational goal.

The financial objectives of many health care sectors have evolved over time. Historically, hospitals, nursing homes, and health insurance plans were mostly established for charitable purposes. However, since the 1980s in the United States, health care providers more often have become for-profit businesses. For example, only about 60 percent of hospitals, 30 percent of nursing homes, and 40 percent of health enrollees are managed by not-for-profit companies in the United States today (Alliance for Advancing Nonprofit Health Care, 2009). Health care systems outside the United States, in contrast, exist with greater collaboration than competition. Strategic management literature has suggested that U.S. health care firms focus more on competition for patients than those in other countries. Collaboration appears to be the norm among health care providers in many nations (Commonwealth Fund, 2004). Collaboration and shared responsibility are engendered to reduce duplication and create more efficient care delivery.

Health care experts have argued for and against fostering competition among health care organizations (Hansen, 2008; Muscalus, 2008; Mutter, Wong, and Goldfarb, 2008). Although sufficient income has to be generated by all organizations to survive, fierce competition may not be as effective in health care. Given the high costs associated with the provision of health care, intense competition may simply lower the organization's profits and decrease the quality of service, without reducing the market share of the competitors.

Intense competition also may result in increased duplication and redundancy of services. Actions taken by one organization are frequently copied by competitors, regularly leading to service overcapacity and inefficiencies. For example, in Indianapolis, no hospital dedicated to heart disease existed prior to 2002. However, soon after one hospital announced the construction of a freestanding heart hospital, all other hospitals in the area began development plans for their own heart hospitals. This resulted in three freestanding heart hospitals and one heart hospital that was incorporated in an existing hospital. This duplicated services and increased costs, but did not provide competitive advantage for any organization. A similar instance occurred in the same city a few years earlier, when St. Vincent's Hospital and Community Hospitals announced their merger. Quickly after this announcement, other major players, Methodist Hospital, Riley Children Hospital, and University Hospital, decided to merge and formed a system called Clarion. Ironically, the planned St. Vincent–Community Hospital merger fell apart at the last minute, while the efforts to form Clarion were completed.

## Evolving Strategies

Strategies often evolve and change according to environmental pressures. The pace of change is often dictated by the life cycle of products as well as the uncertainty and "turbulence" in the market. The speed of innovation is extremely rapid for some products and slower for others. Organizations associated with products with short life spans have to move rapidly and form strategic plans of short temporal dimensions. Their strategic plans may cover as little as six months or a very limited number of years. Personal computers and cell phones are two products that have and are experiencing rapid product innovation, requiring short-term strategies.

New technologies can dramatically change the need and provision of services. In health care, rapid technological breakthroughs in the 1900s in pharmaceuticals drastically changed the provision of care of tuberculosis and ultimately closed most tuberculosis hospitals. Also in the 1990s, discoveries in laparoscopic and other tools allowed a significant shift to outpatient surgeries. Likewise, with the use of antiviral cocktails, HIV/AIDS has become a chronic condition that patients live with and manage (using medications) on their own, rather than an acute condition for which patients must be hospitalized. Each required a recognition and evolution of strategies for organizations that were to survive and prosper.

A number of factors affect uncertainty in the environment and therefore strategic planning for an organization:

- Political/legislative changes
- Technology innovation
- Changing customer demand

The pace of change and uncertainty in health care has been spurred on by numerous legislative proposals that have been considered in the past two decades. As the U.S. government

funds over half of health care, and as many of the current health care reform proposals would increase this percentage, the strong political influence in health care in the United States will surely continue. Likewise, technological innovation is rapidly progressing, causing uncertainty. For example, synthetic biology promises to radically change how drugs are discovered, vaccines are produced, and treatment provided (Ball, 2004).

The concept of a business model is a helpful way to see how a firm is organized, creates value, and compares itself to its competitors. A **business model** makes up the core elements of a firm and how it is organized to deliver value to its customers and generate revenues. Many health care users today call for fundamental changes in the business model of health care (Crean, 2010; Lin, 2008; Perkins, 2010). The business model of health care is predicted to have dramatic changes in the future (Jackson, 2008). Health care firms face the challenge to identify when new technology or other factors make conditions right for newer, more efficient ways of providing value, and to modify their business models accordingly.

Business models contain four components, each of which continue to influence one another as the organization begins, evolves, and progresses:

1. Customer Value: A value proposition that better meets a customer's needs in terms of product differentiation, cost, and/or access/availability.

2. Inputs: The combination of resources used to provide the product or service.

3. Processes: The sequence and method resources are combined to deliver the product or service.

4. Profitability: A financial mechanism to recover enough revenue to sustain the provision of the product or service.

Figure 10.5 illustrates the components of a business model where they constantly interact to produce services and evolve. Any or all of these components can be altered to address new challenges.

### *Customer Value*

Different business models provide different forms of value to customers. Customers have differing desires and needs. Some value ease of access and availability, others want low cost, while others seek higher quality. An innovative business model will seek to address those unmet needs. This is usually the first component that is addressed in developing a new business

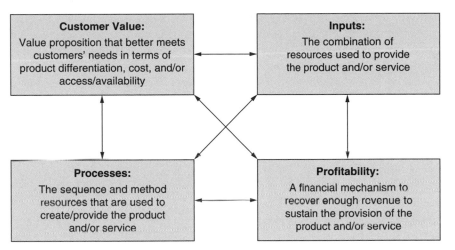

**Figure 10.5** Components of a Business Model.
SOURCE: Delmar, Cengage Learning.

model. For example, retail clinics and generic drugs offer lower prices, while home health provides greater convenience.

## Inputs

The combination and mix of resources used significantly affects the business model. Resources include people, materials, and machines. Companies choose how much and what type of each that will be used. New technology that supplants people is often incorporated into a new business model for the delivery of the product or service. The mix of personnel includes what licenses and skills are used. For example, clinics may utilize nurse practitioners or family practitioners. Anesthesia may be done by nurse anesthetists or anesthesiologists.

## Processes

An organization is composed of many different processes that are ordered to simplify decision making and increase efficiency. These include admissions, financial, and service processes, among many others. Processes can vary. Some hospitals will admit patients directly to their inpatient or outpatient room and may have standardized protocols called clinical pathways to direct how physicians should treat certain conditions. Others simply have patients check in at a centralized location and then transported to their rooms and allow physicians to treat patients as they wish.

## Profitability

Any organization must generate enough revenues to sustain itself. Some mechanism, be it direct payments, insurance, donations, or other means must be found to generate adequate revenues to cover the cost of operation. Enough customers must be found who derive value from the product or services. At the same time, inputs and processes must cost less than the revenues generated. For example, some religious organizations generate revenues from donations, governmental facilities from governmental allocations, and insurance companies from premium payments, and hospitals obtain almost half their revenues from Medicare.

Business models change as both internal and external pressures cause companies to seek different ways to compete and survive. Some argue that the business model of today's leading pharmaceutical companies must change (Pesse, Erat, and Erat, 2006; PricewaterhouseCoopers, 2010). Most large pharmaceutical companies have traditionally owned all functions from research and development through to commercialization. Historically, the business model of this large, complex firm hinged on the ability to do everything within the corporate walls, from identifying promising new molecules in research and testing them in large clinical trials, to generating revenues from sales with extensive marketing and a large sales force who market directly to physicians.

This model relied extensively on "blockbuster" drugs, where a small number of drugs accounted for a very large portion of the pharmacuetical companies' overall revenues. For example, when the patent for Prozac, a widely prescribed antidepressant drug, expired, it accounted for 20 percent of sales for Eli Lilly, the pharmaceutical company manufacturing the drug. Within a year after losing the patent, sales from Prozac dropped over $2 billion a year for the company (Harris, 2004).

It has been predicted that by 2020, there will no longer be a sufficient number of blockbuster drugs to support the current size of drug companies, and that the escalating costs of research and development, including using genetics and biotechnology, in drug discovery will lead to new business models where the drug companies will narrow their core services, increase their alliances, and pursue collaborative agreements (PricewaterhouseCoopers, 2010). Revenue generation will continue to switch from direct sales to physicians to negotiated insurance company contracts, formularies, and governmental agencies based on effectiveness and cost, rather than flashy marketing.

---

## IN PRACTICE: Shifting Business Models – Access to Videos

Renting and watching movies at home have long been a favorite pastime for many on a Saturday night. Twenty years ago, there were thousands of "mom-and-pop" stores that rented videos. Over time, most of these were consolidated into national chains, such as Blockbuster or Hollywood Video. Renting movies requires one to physically visit the store and rent a movie from the inventory on the shelves. The customer had a few days to return it or pay a late fee. A different business model emerged for movie rentals in the 1990s. Direct rental companies sprang up that offered thousands of movie titles and allowed customers to hold movies for any length of time (up to three movies) for a flat monthly charge. Netflix was founded in 1997 by Marc Randolph and Reed Hastings, who had worked together at Pure Software. The site was launched in April 1998 with an online version of a more traditional pay-per-rental model ($4 per rental plus $2 in postage; late fees applied). Netflix introduced the monthly subscription concept in September 1999 without postal charges, and it dropped the single rental model in early 2000. Since then, it has built its reputation on the model of flat-fee, unlimited rentals with no due dates, late fees, shipping or handling fees, or per-title rental fees.

Netflix developed and maintains an extensive recommendation system based on ratings and reviews submitted by customers. The company believes this gives it an edge in competing with online newcomers like Blockbuster Video. On October 1, 2006, Netflix offered a $1,000,000 prize for the first movie recommendation algorithm that could beat its existing algorithm. The Cinematch systems improved the matching between recommendations and customer ratings by more than 10 percent.

Unlike most online on-demand entertainment services, such as Movielink, Netflix's offerings cover a vast range of DVD movies, television series, and games with 80,000 titles. Particularly, Netflix has become noted for its extensive collection of documentary films, Japanese anime, and independent films, titles that are usually hard to find in traditional rental shops. Indeed, in 2008, Netflix offered instant Internet viewing of 10,000 movies and television episodes and a DVD inventory of 100,000 titles (Hansell, 2008).

A competing business model, Redbox, began in 2002, using re-branded kiosks manufactured and operated by Silicon Valley–based DVDPlay. The initial launch included the 140 McDonald's restaurants in the Denver test market. Each kiosk can hold up to 500 DVDs with 70–140 titles, updated weekly. DVDs cost $1 to rent and must be returned the next day or another $1 would be charged. After 25 days, the customer then owns the DVD. Customers can also reserve DVDs online, made possible by real-time inventory updates on the company's website. Redbox Automated Retail LLC was initially funded by McDonald's Ventures, LLC. McDonald's still owns 47 percent of Redbox, with another 47 percent owned by Coinstar. The company surpassed Blockbuster Inc. in 2007 in number of U.S. locations and passed 1 million rentals in February 2008. As of April 2007, the kiosks averaged 49.1 rentals per day and $37,457 a year in revenue.

# The Hospital Business Model

The delivery of medical services has changed rapidly, affecting the way of doing business for many stakeholders and players in the industry. With better technology for diagnosis and treatment and various organizational arrangements for care provision, patients can more readily act as their own advocates, and the increasingly consumerist attitude has led to demands for more privacy, access, and lower costs. The health care workforce has also undergone continuous changes, where nurse practitioners and physician assistants can prescribe certain medications, perform physicals, and other duties in many states. Primary care physicians are now managing patients with mental health needs, where they would traditionally have been referred to psychiatry. Within the industry, new business models have sprung up to include retail health clinics in chain stores (health clinics located in retail stores, supermarkets, and pharmacies for uncomplicated illnesses), medical tourism (travel beyond international borders to obtain health care), specialty hospitals, alternative medicine, and patient-centered medical homes (Berry and Mirabito, 2010; Society for Healthcare Strategy, 2008).

A traditional hospital business model has dramatically overestimated the needs of an average patient while missing some basic concerns. National reports have raised questions about the quality of care provided in hospitals (Institute of Medicine, 2001), and rapidly escalating prices have caused many consumers to seek alternatives. Many hospitals, however, have refined their business models to include outpatient clinics, emergency or urgent care, and expand product lines such as providing physical therapy. In the current environment, hospitals must continue to adapt their business model, which should consider customer value, inputs, processes, and revenue generation, to compete more effectively.

## Customer Value

Traditional hospitals' business models originated in the late nineteenth century as hospitals became the hub for clinical training and scientific research, and the repository of expensive medical technology. Hospitals became the center for the most sophisticated acute-care medical treatment. Hospitals, by having the best technology and medical personnel available, could seek to treat almost any medical problem. Hospitals were initially the only medical facilities that possessed the technology to diagnose and treat serious illnesses. The unpredictability of the medical problems dictated that hospitals needed to employ many specialists to provide value to a wide variety of consumers. Patients gained value by having access to quality care at reasonable costs. The erosion in customer value due to escalating costs has led consumers to access care in alternative settings (LaPenna, 2010).

## Inputs

Inputs included highly professionalized health care personnel such as physicians, nurses, respiratory therapists, physical therapists, pharmacists, dieticians, laboratory technicians, and others. Hospitals also use large quantities of supplies, drugs, and support personnel. New, alternative models vary their inputs to use much less expensive manpower, as in medical tourism, or use innovative technology, such as telemedicine, to transmit health information.

Moreover, inputs vary by the type of hospital. Most community hospitals do not employ their own staff, whereas academic medical centers tend to do so. HMOs, depending on their organizational arrangements, either had staff physicians or contract with individual physicians or medical groups.

## Processes

Jobs have become segregated according to professional expertise, and processes have been developed to dictate how patients are admitted, treated, and released. In health care, work has been "functionally" organized into departments based on skill sets. New business models simplify and change processes to eliminate costly processes and redundant testing. Electronic medical records allow providers to have access to prior patient records, and some procedures are simplified. In addition, many hospitals have employed hospitalists, a physician who coordinates all patients' inpatient care needs, to ensure continuity of care and reduce the likelihood of errors that often occur with multiple handoffs.

## Revenue Generation

In the past, many hospitals were supported by wealthy donors and government funding. With the advent of health care insurance in the mid-twentieth century, insurance payments have become the primary source of hospital revenues, with a small number of people who pay out of pocket. The government, as an insurer, became the biggest payer to hospitals. In 2001, the government accounted for 58 percent of all hospital revenues (Cleverley and Cleverley, 2003). Hospitals are still mostly paid on a per use basis, in that payment received and service utilization have a linear relationship.

A few hospitals owned by HMOs, such as Kaiser Permanente, function contrary to this model, and all revenues are generated by prepayment for the HMO premiums. Hence, within a HMO system, the hospital is a "cost center," and revenue and service utilization would have an inverse relationship.

# EVALUATION OF ORGANIZATIONAL ENVIRONMENT

A critical aspect of strategic planning and strategic thinking is to understand the organization's external and **internal environment** (the conditions and elements within an organization, including employees, management, and culture, that affect the firm's choices and activities). It is important to understand existing and projected environments, as they form the basis of our assumptions and impact the subsequent allocation of resources and strategic direction. Assumptions are propositions that are taken for granted; often with limited evidence (*Merriam-Webster*, 2004). For example, in the past two decades, assumptions were made that hospital care would be rare, being supplanted by outpatient services, that HMOs would control health insurance, and that only integrated health care systems could be successful. Each was shown to be false (Burns and Pauly, 2002). Those organizations that clung too long to such assumptions suffered. Periodic scanning of the organizational environment is essential to uncover changes and to validate our assumptions. Scanning the environment

provides updated information to adjust our assumptions. Organizations should periodically scan the environment to identify changing factors and challenge their assumptions. This scanning should involve examining both the external and internal environments. Frequently, the analyses of the external market have focused on external competition; while the internal assessments have focused on an organization's unique resources and capabilities (Burns, 2002).

## External Evaluation

No organization is immune to the influences of its external environment. The nature of customers and structure of the market directly influence how organizations must compete. Health care is particularly susceptible to the external conditions, including technological innovations, changing customer demands, and governmental regulations. In scanning the external environment, health care organizations should evaluate the following factors:

### Customers

Who are the firm's customers? Are there specific segments by age, gender, income, or geographic locations that use the company's services? Which are increasing? Which are decreasing? Organizations should consider completing customer (patient) origin studies to define what geographic locations their customers come from. For example, the patient origin analysis in Table 10.1 shows that more than half of patients were coming from the Central Region, the

## TABLE 10.1 Hospital Patient Origin Study – 2007 by Region and Gender

| Gender | Eastern Region | Western Region | Central Region | Northern Region | Southern Region | Unknown | TOTAL |
|---|---|---|---|---|---|---|---|
| Female | 1299 | 903 | 5497 | 1176 | 1400 | 397 | 10672 |
| Male | 1054 | 956 | 4721 | 1402 | 1641 | 550 | 10324 |
| TOTAL | 2353 | 1859 | 10218 | 2578 | 3041 | 947 | 20996 |
| Encounter | Eastern Region | Western Region | Central Region | Northern Region | Southern Region | Unknown | TOTAL |
| Female | 12.2% | 8.5% | 51.5% | 11.0% | 13.1% | 3.7% | 100.0% |
| Male | 10.2% | 9.3% | 45.7% | 13.6% | 15.9% | 5.3% | 100.0% |
| TOTAL | 11.2% | 8.9% | 48.7% | 12.3% | 14.5% | 4.5% | 100.0% |

percentage growing from 48.7 percent in 2000 to 57 percent in 2005. While the Central Region saw an increase in the number of patients; the number of patients from the Eastern and Western regions declined significantly. The change in patient volume provides important strategic information to determine adjustments in the development of strategies. These data may trigger questions for further evaluation (e.g., whether other health care facilities have opened in the other regions, whether physicians have changed their referral patterns, which strategic actions are succeeding or failing, etc.).

## Competition

Understanding the competition can also be critical. Organizations should ask the following questions: Who is the competition? What is the nature of competition? What is the level of cooperation and trust among firms? Is the competitive landscape changing? Are there niche players who only compete for segments of the business? Are there new market entries? Are there new exits? Which products and services are more competitive? Are there clusters or competitive strategic groups that compete intensely?

## Other Factors

Health care organizations should also seek to identify other key factors like key referral sources (e.g., key physicians and insurance groups), consumer perceptions of their organization, capacity of competitors (e.g., bed occupancy rates), and price sensitivity for different services and how these may change over time. These factors should have the potential to significantly affect the organization if changed.

# Market Structure

Strategies often vary according to **market structure**. The nature of competition is directly related to the structure and degree of fragmentation of a market. Markets can be categorized, as illustrated in Figure 10.6, into fragmented and consolidated markets. The most fragmented market is **perfect competition**, which is characterized by many buyers and sellers, and many products that are similar and undifferentiated. Markets in perfect competition have few **barriers to entry** (the existence of obstacles that prevent competitors from attempting to enter an industry or market) and prices are generally the means of competition. Markets for agricultural commodities (wheat, corn, soybeans, etc.) often come closest to a perfect competition. Products are homogeneous. Product and pricing

information is known by all, and each individual seller has little or no effect on market prices and must sell at the going rate. Firms often earn only minimal profits. Generic drugs can be considered as close to perfect competition in health care. One generic drug is often seen comparable to another (of the same prescription) and the choice is frequently dictated by price.

The next level of market fragmentation is **monopolistic competition**. This market structure is characterized by a large number of small firms that have similar, but not identical products. There is relative free entry and exit, and knowledge of prices and technology is common. Competition is relatively vigorous, but each firm, depending on the degree of their differentiation, has some control over their prices. General examples would include restaurants and clothing stores. In the United States, physician services are a health care example of monopolistic competition. There are many physicians but minimal competition based on price. Physicians may be differentiated by their office locations, training, and personal relationships with their patients.

An **oligopoly** is a market dominated by a few large companies. The degree of market concentration is very high, with only a few firms dominating the market. Barriers to entry and exit exist; firms are interdependent in that they must take into account the reactions of their competitors when they make decisions regarding pricing and resource allocation. Firms in oligopolies rarely compete on price, but seek to "brand" and differentiate their products on non-price characteristics.

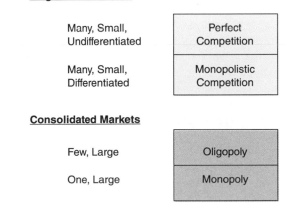

**Figure 10.6** Market Structure.
SOURCE: Delmar, Cengage Learning.

Air travel is an industry where oligopolies exist in both the production of large aircraft (Boeing and Airbus), and air carriers in the United States (United, Delta, American, and Southwest). Many hospital, pharmaceutical, and insurance markets are also oligopolies where firms seek to differentiate themselves and compete in areas of access, quality, and values.

**Monopolies** are fully consolidated markets with only one firm. Monopolists lack competition, as they produce goods or services for which there are not close substitutes. Monopolies often lack incentives to be efficient and maintain high prices. Much of their strategic efforts go into creating barriers to entry to keep potential competitors out of their markets. Water and electric services are often monopolies. Likewise, in many markets, hospitals are monopolies. Most studies have suggested that markets with high hospital concentration (close to monopoly conditions) have also had higher prices (Federal Trade Commission, 2004).

## The Five Forces Framework

**Porter's Five Forces Framework** has often been employed to understand the competitive forces in industries (Figure 10.7). The forces are five common threats from the environment: (1) the threat of new entrants; (2) the threat of substitutes; (3) the bargaining power of suppliers; (4) the bargaining power of buyers; and (5) the threat of rivalry. At the center is the

5 Forces Framework for Industry Analysis

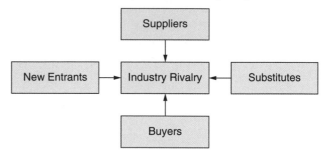

**Figure 10.7** The Five Forces Model for Industry Analysis.
SOURCE: Delmar, Cengage Learning.

intensity of rivalry or competition. Porter (1980) suggests that firms gain competitive advantage by exploiting weaknesses in these five forces, or by adopting strategies that modify these forces and reduce competitive pressures. Together, these forces determine the market structure as previously discussed. As intensity of forces increases, the industry environment becomes more hostile, and overall industry profitability declines. On the other hand, weaker forces allow the creation of monopolist conditions, which can enhance overall industry profits.

---

## DEBATE TIME: Monopoly Power

Monopoly power invokes a negative connotation because being the sole player in the market allows the monopolists to extract higher prices. However, many hospitals in the United States are monopolies. Often times, they exist that way simply because the market in which they operate cannot support another facility, although they can also achieve the monopolistic position through other means. Norman Regional Hospital (NRH), a 288-bed facility, is the only hospital in Norman, Oklahoma. Norman is a growing suburb of Oklahoma City, and the third-largest city in the state with a population of 110,000. NRH's mission is to "provide quality and compassionate health care services and education to our regional community in a responsive, efficient, and safe manner," which is further encouraged by its vision to "improve the quality of life in our regional community." While the number of hospitals in other suburban communities has grown and competition is intense in the state, NRH remains the only hospital in Norman. How has it maintained its monopoly position? In the 1980s, NRH worked with the city of Norman to pass legislation that requires any hospital desiring to enter the market to receive city permission or a "certificate of need." With competitors unable to meet this criterion, NRH has effectively remained the only player in town. NRH has claimed that its quality and costs are much better in the absence of competition. Why do you think NRH can make this claim? Do you agree? To judge their quality and costs, you can go to http://www.ucomparehealth care.com or http://www.hospitalcompare.hhs.gov

## Rivalry

Competitors (rivals) in a market compete for customers and market share. **Rivalry** influences the strategies of firms and determines the overall profitability of the industry. Many factors affect the rivalry in a market. The number and type of firms are significant factors. In an industry where new rivals can enter relatively easily, increasing the number of firms, or where firms can grow in size via merger and acquisition, the industry tends to be more competitive, and firms are less likely to enjoy high average profitability. Rivalry is likely to occur in markets where competitors differ substantially from one to another. For example, markets that have public, community, and private hospitals will face more competition because they offer consumers more choices. Likewise, competition increases as a market becomes less concentrated, or firms control a more equal share of the market. The existence of one (or a few) dominant firms also diminishes rivalry. Hospital markets in the United States exhibit wide variations in their market structures. However, many are monopolies or oligopolies (Luke, Walston, and Plummer, 2004). The pharmaceutical industry has also become more concentrated. The top 10 pharmaceutical companies control almost 59 percent of the world's pharmaceutical sales.

Porter (1980) has suggested that nonmarket structural characteristics also affect the intensity of competition. These include how easily organizational assets may be used outside the industry (asset specificity), amount of fixed costs, degree of product similarity or differentiation, and available excess capacity. Products that are perceived as similar by the consumer become price competitive and stimulate rivalry. In contrast, greater product differentiation means that the organization can charge more for product, thereby extracting higher profits and dampening rivalry. Excess capacity also increases rivalry because it usually results in lower prices, lower profit margins, and therefore a less attractive industry.

Finally, the nature of the sales process can also influence the level of competition. If sales are based on large, infrequent orders, firms will compete more intensely. Similarly, if sales transactions are not very observable and understandable, rivalry will be higher (Burns, 2002).

## Threat of Substitution

The extent and degree of product/service substitution influences the propensity of customers to switch to alternatives. The strength of substitution is tied to customer perception on how well the substitute can match the quality and price characteristics of the original product. Relative price performance, **switching costs** (the cost incurred when a customer changes from one supplier or product to another), and the buyer's propensity to substitute are additional factors that increase the **threat of substitution** (Porter, 1980). In health care, we frequently see the substitution of generics for brand-name drugs. Managed care companies now commonly develop drug formularies and have also created a tiered copayment system, with non-formulary brand-name drugs incurring the highest copayment to encourage the use of the generic drugs. The use of laparoscopic surgery is another example where a less invasive procedure is preferred over traditional open cases for gall bladders, hernias, and appendectomies. Likewise, medications have now all but replaced surgery for treatment of peptic ulcer disease (Kotler, Shalowitz, and Stevens, 2008).

## Buyer Power

A firm's buyers or customers always seek to drive down price and improve quality. Their ability to do so, known as **buyer power**, depends on how much they purchase, how well informed they are regarding the product, and their willingness to experiment with alternatives (Mintzberg, Ahlstrand, and Lampel, 1998). As with rivalry, a buyer's bargaining power is partly dependent on market structure. If, as in the defense industry, there are only one or a few buyers for a given product, the buyer(s) can exert strong influence on the firm's behavior. In health care, medical clinics often will seek to not allow any one insurer provide them a significant portion of their patients. Likewise, hospitals will strive to have more than one or more supplier of important medical goods and equipment.

## Supplier Power

**Supplier power** is the opposite perspective of buyer power. Contrary to buyers, suppliers desire the ability to increase price and minimize quality. Suppliers gain power by the degree of importance of their product or service, when there are few suppliers, and the cost of switching to another supplier is high. For example, there are many vendors of health information systems, but the cost for a company to switch from one system to another is very high, which increases supplier power. On the other hand, some pharmaceutical companies are the only source for special drugs, and are therefore in a position to extract higher prices. For example, the price set by Alexion Pharmaceutical for a year's supply of Soliris, a drug for a rare immune disorder, is $409,500 (Herper, 2010).

### Threat of New Entrants

New entrants threaten markets by potentially decreasing incumbents' market share and increasing price competition. The extent of barriers to entry will influence the number and size of firms within a given market. Some of these barriers are naturally occurring, where others can be enhanced by existing firms as a competitive strategy to maintain and strength their market position (Kotler, Shalowitz, and Stevens, 2008). These barriers include:

- *Economies of scale and high capital requirements.* Incumbent firms might enjoy economies of scale and benefits of learning that may allow existing firms a price and production advantage over new entrants. **Economies of scale** occur when the average cost per unit lowers from increased volumes. High economies of scale tend to exist in industries with significant fixed costs. As volumes increase, the high fixed costs are spread out and the average price per unit declines. For example, hospitals and pharmaceutical companies have very high fixed and capital costs. A firm desiring market entry in these two industries will be at a cost disadvantage to start, as their initial cost per unit will be much higher than that of their competitors until sufficient market share can be achieved. The high amounts of capital required to set up a new facility (e.g., manufacturing) or high research and development costs (e.g., pharmaceuticals) may also impose a barrier for potential new entrants.

- *Access to key resources or distribution channels.* In markets that have scarce, critical resources or high distribution costs, lacking access to key resources or distribution channels can be a significant barrier to entry. In regard to health care providers, this barrier may be the lack of skilled, specialized personnel. Clinics and hospitals, especially in rural areas, often have difficulty recruiting physicians, especially specialists, to their workforce.

- *Government restrictions.* Legal barriers often present barriers to entry. Government restrictions may limit entry through patents, copyrights, and/or requirements for licensure. Industry regulation also causes potential entrants to gain government approval before they can begin offering products or services. Many U.S. states still require "certificate of need" for hospitals, which requires hospitals to obtain state approval prior to initiating a large capital expenditure. Drugs, likewise, must be thoroughly tested and approved by the FDA before they can be sold.

- *Branding.* Marketing advantages are also enjoyed by incumbents as a result of their reputation. Some firms have successfully used their reputation to lower the barriers to entry. For example, many reputable U.S. providers, such as Harvard International, Cleveland Clinic, and Johns Hopkins, have leveraged their "brand" to enter the health care markets in the Middle East (PR Newswire, 2007; The Economist, 2008).

- *Exclusive and/or long-term agreements.* Incumbents with long-term agreements, especially those that are exclusive, create strong barriers to entry. Many managed-care plans establish exclusive arrangements for the provision of psychiatric and chemical dependency problems, making entry into this type of service delivery very difficult (Kotler, Shalowitz, and Stevens, 2008).

- *Excess capacity and threat of retaliation.* If current firms have excess capacity, they are often willing to use price reductions as a strategy. Even the threat of entry will frequently motivate existing firms to lower or maintain low prices. Along with this, incumbents with a credible history of aggressive retaliation will pose an additional barrier to new entrants.

## Evaluation of the Rival Positioning

A company should know and understand its competitors. Determining who is a competitor can be an interesting and sometimes complex process. The concept of "strategic groups" was initially coined by Hunt in 1972, but further developed by Porter in 1980. A **strategic group** is a concept to identify organizations within an industry that have similar business models and/or strategic orientations so that they directly compete with each other. For example, in the restaurant business, there are many different classifications of dining, from fast food to fine dining. McDonalds clearly competes with Burger King and Wendy's, but does not compete with a fine, five-star restaurant. These groups can be distinguished, based on factors such as:

- Price/quality
- Geographic coverage
- Degree of vertical integration
- Product breadth
- Use of distribution channels

# INTERNAL RESOURCES: A SOURCE OF COMPETITIVE ADVANTAGE

Internal resources are a key component of strategic advantage. Resources are of critical importance to ensure the successful implementation of strategies (Barney, 1991; Wernerfelt, 1984).

An organization is a combination of resources, both tangible and intangible. Tangible resources include physical assets, such as equipment, buildings, and technology. According to Barney (1991), these resources may be further classified into three categories: (1) physical capital resources, which include technology, plant and equipment, geographic location, and access to raw materials; (2) human capital resources, which include personnel skill sets, training, experience, judgment, intelligence, relationships, and insights of all organizational participants; and (3) organizational capital resources, which include the organization's formal structure, reporting hierarchy, and formal and informal processes such as planning, controlling, and coordinating systems, as well as informal relations among groups within, between, and among organizations in its environment.

Internal resources are strategically important and may offer sustained benefits in the face of competition. However, to have lasting importance, these resources must be valuable, rare, difficult to imitate, and lack substitutes (Barney, 1991). Obviously, a resource should be valuable to be strategic and needs to be integral to improve a firm's effectiveness and efficiency. A resource should also be rare enough to generate demand and hard to replicate. For example, for many firms, human capital is the critical resource, which can be rare and hard to duplicate. Finally, even if a resource is valuable, rare, and hard to imitate, it may not provide a sustained strategic advantage if it can be easily substituted. Physical assets are less likely to provide sustained strategic advantage, but advantage must be found in the combination of physical, human, and organizational resources. Physical assets are far too easily imitated, and substitutes can be found. For instance, the purchase of the latest imaging machine can easily be imitated by competitors and this service duplicated. Sustained strategic advantage comes when the intangible resources that are hard to duplicate, such as organizational culture, are combined with the tangible (Mintzberg, Ahlstrand, and Lampel, 1998). Culture has been suggested as the most effective and durable barrier to imitation, as it generates unique outcomes and is very difficult to replicate (Barney, 1986). Of course, a positive organizational culture is also very difficult to create. Organizations with strong cultures innovate more, have greater patient satisfaction, and are more able to achieve their goals (Bellou, 2007).

## Evaluating Organizational Capabilities

A value chain analysis can help organizational management evaluate the use of organizational resources and capabilities. Organizational capabilities and delivery capacity can be examined to determine what added value each step produces. Organizational capabilities refer to an organization's skill in combining its resources to produce goods and services. Capabilities can range from simple tasks in daily operations, to complex processes. These capabilities collectively are the activities of an organization's value chain. In other words, these capabilities are organized in a chain of activities that gives the product or service more added value. Traditionally, value chains have primary activities, which include inbound logistics, operations/production, outbound logistics, marketing and sales, and service/maintenance. In examining the use of capabilities, the costs and value drivers for each activity can be examined.

In health care, a value chain assumes a systems approach where there are two subsystems: service delivery and support activities (Figure 10.8). The service delivery subsystem is further divided into pre-service, point of service, and post-service, illustrating where the service is delivered. The support activities consist of organizational infrastructure, culture, resources, and technology. These subsystems support the service delivery system by ensuring the availability of an inviting and supportive environment, as well as a service-oriented culture, sufficient resources and financing, a highly qualified staff, and appropriate information technology (Ginter et al., 2005).

Another common tool for evaluating organizational competitiveness is through a **SWOT analysis**. SWOT (strengths, weakness, opportunities, and threats) is a common analytical tool for evaluating organizational capabilities and to enhance organizational effectiveness and strategic direction (Figure 10.9). The SWOT analysis enables members of the organization to assess all aspects of the organization. These encompass the strengths and weaknesses of the internal organization's capabilities and activities in the areas of organizational culture, structure, access to resources, staffing, operations, external relationships, information technology capacity and function, administrative processes, clinical control processes, and organizational decision making. Through this exercise, organizations may identify areas where they can grow through the agreed upon opportunities and mitigate sources of major threats (Bourgeois, Duhaime, and Stimpert, 1999; Luke, Walston, and Plummer, 2004). Based on results of internal analysis, organizations may develop strategies that would respond to the assessment of their internal strengths and weaknesses, as well as the external opportunities and threats that are present. SWOT analyses are frequently used, as they are very easy to initiate and can involve many participants or stakeholders.

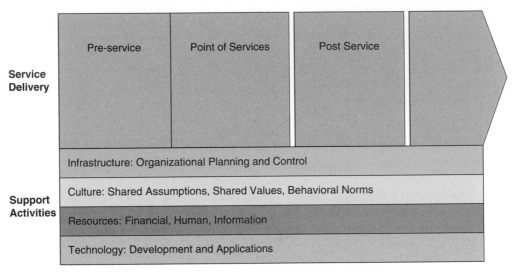

**Figure 10.8** Value Chain.

SOURCE: Adapted from Ginter et al. (2005).

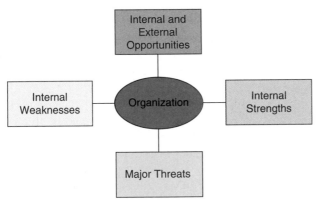

**Figure 10.9** SWOT Analysis.

SOURCE: Adapted from Bourgeois et al. (1999).

However, SWOT has several limitations in that it does not provide trend information, often includes erroneous information, and may not provide clear direction at its conclusion.

# USE OF GENERIC STRATEGIES

Porter (1980) suggested that a firm could obtain strategic advantage by concentrating on either cost or uniqueness/differentiation, and either on a broad or narrow market. These strategies have become known as **generic strategies** whose application is shown in Figure 10.10.

## Low Cost Leadership

This generic strategy calls for being the low-cost producer in an industry for a given level of quality. Some firms have been successful as low-cost leaders. Wal-Mart and Aldi Stores are known for their low prices and acceptable quality. Both companies work on their inputs and processes to maintain very low prices. Generic pharmaceutical companies and retail health clinics also seek to gain strategic advantage from their cost advantage. Factors that allow low cost to work include:

- Vigorous price competition among rivals
- Similar products from rival sellers (products hard to differentiate)
- Most use product in similar ways
- Low switching costs
- High bargaining power with large buyers
- Barriers to entry are low and new entries use introductory low prices to attract buyers

A challenge for any firm in establishing a low-cost position is to assure an acceptable level of quality for its consumers. Quality preferences will vary according to the income, education, and cultural norms of consumers. However, for some products,

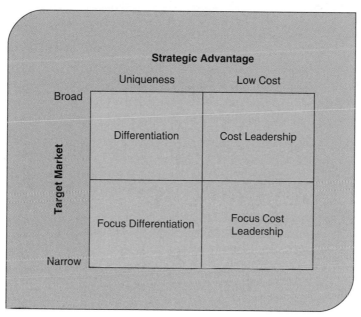

**Figure 10.10** Generic strategies.
SOURCE: Delmar, Cengage Learning.

such as health care, the quality requirements are very high for the vast majority of consumers. Most health care providers that seek a low-cost position have extreme difficulty attracting desirable patients. In the mind of consumers, low cost is tied to low quality for providers in health care. Patients would much rather pay a higher price to obtain high quality.

The challenge of a low-cost position in health care is also related to how insulated many consumers are from the actual cost of health care. Patients with insurance are also mostly protected from the high costs of care, as a result of relatively low fixed deductibles and co-insurance. Rather than having to pay the full charges, insured patients pay a fixed deductible and then generally only a small percent (coinsurance) on charges that have been discounted to the insurance company. Some services, however, are less likely to be covered by insurance, and low pricing can be an effective strategy. Hospitals will often set low prices for normal obstetrical deliveries, physicals, and plastic surgeries. Especially in college towns, hospitals find that prospective parents often shop for best prices. Health care providers may seek to have low-cost positions in these market segments, but realize that patients are not very price sensitive in many other services.

## Differentiation

A differentiation generic strategy requires that the firm provide a product or service that offers unique attributes. These attributes must be valued by customers and perceived to be better than those of the competitors' product. The value may allow the firm to charge a premium price for the product or service. Product differentiation may also be accomplished through products, services, personnel, channel, and image (Kotler, Shalowitz, and Stevens, 2008). Firms may incorporate features that raise product performance or add to what buyers commonly value, such as reliability, durability, ease of use, convenience, cleanliness, safety, and low maintenance. To be perceived as unique, some health care systems are changing facilities to provide "healing gardens," constructing additional hallways to reduce noise, and adding gourmet chefs and room service (Landro, 2007). Organizations can also differentiate products by improving customer service processes, such as simplifying ordering and delivery, and providing maintenance and repair. A company's personnel can also make a difference in their competence, courtesy, reliability, and communication skills. Many health care organizations, including the Mayo Clinic, have initiated service excellence programs that focus on improving the interaction of their employees with patients and families (Frey, Leighton, and Cecala, 2005). Channel differentiation can also distinguish a firm. The extent of coverage, expertise, and performance can be a significant advantage. Health care providers seeking to set up referral clinics in key areas, pharmaceutical firms offering multiple means to deliver medication to patients, and insurance companies forming networks that offer the widest scope of providers all exemplify differentiation strategies.

Image also can be a powerful way to differentiate a product. When competing products or services are similar, buyers may obtain value based on the company's image. A favorable image takes a significant amount of time to build, but can be destroyed very quickly (Armstrong and Kotler, 1999). Image in health care has also become more important. Some health care systems spend millions of dollars per year in advertising. For example, hospitals in Boston, Massachusetts, spent about $20 million on advertising in 2005. "Unlike most advertising, hospital promotions don't trumpet sales or special pricing deals. The focus is on image" (Rowland, 2006). If a strong image and brand name exists, it can potentially be transferred to related products and businesses. For example, entities have partnered with universities because their image has been established in a positive manner. Harvard University has a very recognizable and strong image worldwide. It has used its name to go into related businesses of consulting and publishing with Harvard Medical International, which is a subsidiary of Partners Healthcare System in Boston. Likewise, Hospital Corporation of America pays to use the University of Oklahoma (OU)'s name at the OU Medical Center in Oklahoma City.

## Focused Strategies

Focused strategies, or **market niche strategies**, constitute another category of generic strategies. As shown in Figure 10.10, a focused strategy can be based on either differentiation or cost. The key for a market niche (targeted to a narrow market segment) or focused strategy is that it should be based on some important characteristic, such as population, product line, geographic regions, and political boundaries. Specialist hospitals are an example of organizations that compete in certain market niches. Competitive advantage is achieved by matching an appropriate strategy to the target

market and defining the focus as unique/differentiated or low cost.

## Other Aspects of Strategies

### First Mover Advantage

The **first mover advantage** is a recognized strategic move to gain advantage by being the initial occupant of a market segment or product. This advantage comes from the ability to obtain heightened visibility, technological leadership, or control of crucial resources. First movers often receive extensive free publicity and gain public name recognition and visibility. Sometimes the first mover becomes so prominent that the product becomes associated with the first mover. For example, Kleenex has become synonymous with facial tissue and Xerox with copies. Likewise, in 1954 the first man to break the four-minute-mile barrier, Roger Bannister, has been honored and remembered in athletics, although he placed fourth in the 1952 Olympics and his record lasted just 46 days (Bascomb, 2005).

First movers can also use breakthroughs in research and development to provide strategic advantage. Sustained advantage can be obtained by moving quickly down the learning curve. Apple, for example, has excelled in introducing new technological breakthroughs with their iPhone, iTouch, and iPod. Likewise, pharmaceutical and biotech companies acting as first movers may gain strategic advantage for their innovation through patents and new drugs.

If first movers can gain access to crucial resources and capabilities, they can potentially block other market entrants or place them at a competitive disadvantage. Such crucial resources might be access to patents, superior physical locations, and more competent staff that can be used to solidify their position.

On the other hand, first movers may not be able to sustain their initial gains. Later entrants may be able to imitate or gain a "free ride" on their investments. Also, late movers have the advantage of not sustaining risks of creating new markets and are able to follow set industry standards. Many firms have moved rapidly into a new product with strong financial backing, but lost to later entrants. For example, Prodigy Communications was the first mover in online shopping; Dumont led in selling televisions; Chux was the first mover in disposable diapers; and Ampex in video recorders. All were surpassed by later movers (Shilling, 2007).

## *Product Life Cycle*

All products and services go through phases or life cycles that relate to their level of costs and sales, which have strategic implications. **Product life cycles** occur because of the inherent limited life of any product, as a result of technological advances and adapting consumer preferences. As seen in Figure 10.11, there are four life cycle stages. In the Emerging Stage, there may be only a few firms initially as the technology is developed and explored. Competition remains low, as there may be few substitutes. Sales and profits also remain low in this stage. The Growth Stage sees increasing market entry by competitors as sales grow rapidly. The product has now proven a success, and customers are rapidly adopting it. The Maturity Stage tends to be the most profitable. Sales increase at a slower rate. Competing products at this stage become more similar, which increases the difficulty of differentiating individual company products. Strategically, companies seek to maintain or expand their market share. In the last stage, Declining, the volume of sales drops substantially and firms merge to increase the market concentration, as competition pushes down profit margins. The U.S. health care industry

has been characterized as being in the mature stage with significant competition and governmental regulation (Kepros et al., 2007).

## Portfolio Analysis

In the 1970s, consulting firms developed various methods for analyzing the strategic position of firms. One very popular method is the **portfolio analysis**. This method compares the value of the strategic business units (SBUs) of firms. Components of companies are categorized by their competitive market position and the environmental attractiveness. Various derivations of this concept exist as the BCG's Growth-Share Matrix, which places components of the firm into named quadrants, and the GE/McKinsey Nine-block Matrix. The strategic purpose behind these analyses is to understand which parts of the firm should receive greater capital investment, which should be underfunded, and which perhaps divested (Ghemawat, 2001). These tools assume that economies of scale, market power, and other strategic advantages are directly related to higher relative market share, and that market growth provides the greatest opportunity for firm expansion. Each portfolio tool seeks to:

1. Evaluate the financial viability of a firm's strategic business units

2. Provide direction for strategic decisions among the strategic business units

3. Indicate which businesses should be divested, acquired, and supported

4. Assist in balancing the firm's portfolio between cash producing and cash consuming units (Luke, Walston, and Plummer, 2004)

A company can examine its SBUs by their competitive position and environmental attractiveness (Figure 10.12). This leads to placing the SBU into one of the four quadrants. Such placement then suggests what strategic actions should take place for each SBU, as mentioned above.

Portfolio analysis can be beneficial, especially when funds are scarce. Many health care companies have used it to evaluate and prioritize services to maintain strategic direction (Bess and Bess, 1990).

### Level of Concentration & Competition

| Life Cycle Stage | Concentration | Competition |
|---|---|---|
| Emerging | High | Low |
| Growth | Decreasing | Increasing |
| Mature | Increasing | Moderate to High |
| Declining | High | High |

**Figure 10.11** Life Cycle.
SOURCE: Delmar, Cengage Learning.

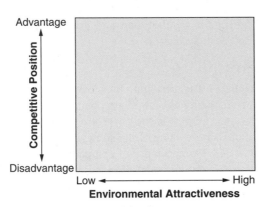
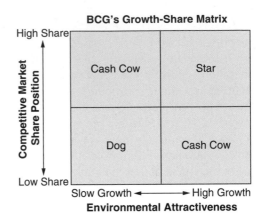

**Figure 10.12** Competitive Positioning.
SOURCE: Delmar, Cengage Learning.

# SUMMARY AND MANAGERIAL GUIDELINES

1. Understand the importance of mission and vision and their relationship to strategy and strategic management. All strategic actions and direction of a firm should be driven by its mission and vision. Leaders should seek to make their mission and vision meaningful by incorporating them into decision making processes.

2. Establish values that are meaningful and that guide actions within the organization. Values should be directly tied to performance and be reflected in annual evaluations.

3. Realize that strategy is more than creating a written plan for the future. Strategy encompasses the ability to analyze the environment, understand potential futures, and allocate resources to strategically position the firm. It involves strategically managing personnel and assets to direct the organization through uncertain times.

4. Understand that good strategies are not static, but evolve over time based upon the experiences and preferences of leaders. Successful organizations must be adaptable, learn from their experiences, and have the agility to evolve.

5. See how a firm's competitive position can change with the change of any of the four components of a business model. The concept of a business model allows leaders to understand the factors that can be individually or jointly altered to improve the competitiveness of an organization. Likewise, it provides a method to analyze competitors to discern how they differ and what potential advantages they might have.

6. Managers should understand different methods for analyzing the firm's environment. Porter's Five Forces Framework provides two means for examining the organization's environment and those factors that affect the level of competition.

# DISCUSSION QUESTIONS

1. Find the mission and values statements for four different hospital types. Do their missions and values reconcile with your expectations for the type of organization? Look at a religiously based organization. Does their mission and values reflect their religious teachings and mission? Now examine a for-profit hospital. Does their mission and values include the need to increase their owners' value and maximize their earnings? Why do you think the missions and values are structured as they are?

2. Health care in the United States has been traditionally a mixture of not-for-profit and for-profit organizations. Do you think that markets where more for-profit firms exist would be inherently more competitive? Why or why not?

3. Business models describe four components of how an organization is organized. They can show comparative differences in a competitive analysis. What is the relationship of strategy and business models?

4. An important aspect of strategic planning is analyzing the internal and external environments. Recently, a large organization completed their environmental analyses only using a very extensive SWOT process. They then used the strengths, weaknesses, opportunities, and threats generated by this process as their environmental analysis. What would be the value of using this technique only? Should other methods also be used? How could data trends be used?

5. There are many firms that have positioned part or all of their products as low cost. Low costs are also commonly thought to equal low prices. Are low costs necessarily the same as low prices? Could a firm have low costs and still have high prices?

6. Large pharmaceutical companies have prospered by owning their discovery, production, and marketing assets and have traditionally made significant portions of their profits from a small number of "blockbuster" drugs. How is the pharmaceutical companies' business model predicted to change? What are the forces that are influencing this change?

7. Porter recommends generic strategies of low cost or differentiation. Is it possible to obtain both at the same time? In health care, is low cost a reasonable strategy? If so, in what circumstances might this be an acceptable strategy?

8. To sustain a competitive advantage, an organization must have resources that are valuable, endure over time, are hard to imitate, and are difficult to find substitutes for. What are some of the common resources in health care that could convey sustained competitive advantage? How do these differ for the different segments of the health care industry? For hospitals? Insurance companies? Pharmaceutical companies? Equipment manufacturers?

# CASE 1: A Strategic Imperative to Merge in an Oligopolistic Market?

In June 1995, George L., CEO of Mack Hospital, was surprised and angered. That morning, his major competitors, Cassid Hospital System and St. Mark's Hospital, had announced plans to merge. Until now, their market area had been an oligopoly, divided into four major quadrants, each area mostly controlled by one of the four major hospitals located in that respective location.

Mack Hospital was by far the largest hospital in the metropolitan area, and the nation, with over 900 beds in service. It was located just off the intersection of two of the busiest freeways just outside of the western portion of the community and dominated the western market. Although centrally located, the hospital had 17 outpatient and ambulatory surgical centers in the suburbs. It also owned and ran a physician-hospital organization (PHO), a network of five community health centers, and an IPA-style HMO, called M-Plan.

St. Mark's Hospital was a religiously affiliated hospital. It had a main hospital with over 700 set-up beds and a satellite smaller hospital, located in the affluent northern part of the community. St. Mark's also owned a network of primary care physician practices and a PHO, and was part owner of a HMO and PPO. The hospital has also joint ventured with its large cardiology groups to provide catheterization laboratories for each group. These two cardiology groups accounted for about 50 percent of St Mark's revenues.

Cassid Hospital System was located in the eastern area and had just over 500 set-up beds. It also owned physician practices, a PPO, and a PHO. They have the only CEO in the area that graduated with an MBA and was seen as highly aggressive.

The last major hospital was St. Francis, another religiously affiliated system that was not affiliated with St. Mark's. They were located in the far south of the community. St. Francis was located in a poorer section of the community and provided just over 400 set-up beds. It also was a part owner in the PPO and HMO that St. Mark's owned and owns primary care physician practices and a PHO.

Other, less dominant hospitals existed, including a 300-bed public hospital in the center of town that had rundown facilities and was the safety net hospital, the only children's hospital in the state also located in the center of the community, a university hospital next to the medical school and children's hospital, and a for-profit women's hospital located in the northern part of the city.

Physician referrals within the community had become increasingly influenced by physician affiliations with PHOs and health systems and their respective financial incentives. Their market also had about 13 percent more hospital beds per 1,000 population than the U.S. average, and its inpatient utilization was about 22 percent higher. Most of the bed capacity was located in the urban core. The community also had about 6 percent more primary care physicians and 17 percent more specialty physicians per 1,000 population than the national average. (Source: Center for Studying Health System Change, 1997)

George L. approached his CFO, Clyde B., and asked, "What in the world are those guys at St. Mark's and Cassid thinking? How can they think they can get away with coming together like that? When they combine their hospitals they will effectively control more than half the metropolitan area. We cannot stand for that!"

Until now, this division of the market had served the hospitals well. Charges were high compared to national averages (one report indicated their average charges were about 30 percent above their neighboring state's charges). They had also been able to keep most major HMOs from deeply penetrating the marketplace. However, in the past three years, managed care had been making progress in influencing the market. About 15 to 20 percent of the commercial insurance market is enrolled in HMOs, but until now, most of these had been owned by one of the top area hospitals. Recently, however, a former BlueCross plan had begun to garner greater market share and threatened the existing, hospital-owned HMOs. Almost all of the area hospitals have been reasonably profitable and had relatively strong financial positions, but had been deteriorating.

## 2000 to 2003 Net Operating Income/Margin for Area Hospitals (Million)

|  | Beds | 2000 | 2001 | 2002 | 2003 |
|---|---|---|---|---|---|
| Mack | 900 | $11.6/1.9% | $12.5/2.0% | $9.7/1.5% | $9.1/1.4% |
| University | 450 | $27.8/7.6% | $4.2/1.2% | $1.1/0.3% | $0.1/0.0% |
| Cassid System | 500 | $8.5/5.1% | $-1.1/-1.5% | $2.3/1.9% | $1.2/1.3% |
| St. Francis | 400 | $1.8/0.4% | $2.4/1.1% | $-3.4/-2.4% | $-1.8/-0.8% |
| St. Mark's | 700 | $16.1/2.9% | $22.1/3.5% | $28.2/4.2% | $12.1/2.1% |
| Safety Net | 300 | $-88.5/-33.3% | $-38.4/-21.8% | $-44.3/-27.2% | $-55.2/-29.6% |
| Children | 220 | $5.5/2.2% | $4.8/1.9% | $-1.3/-0.3% | $1.3/0.8% |

George continued the conversation with his CFO. "If they are going to come together, we will have to do something to protect ourselves. What about combining Mack with the children's and university hospitals? This would still make us the biggest hospital system in the U.S. with the capacity to provide almost every type of medical service and allow us to leverage the new HMOs and keep Cassid's and St. Mark's HMO products from further penetrating our market. Don't you think that we could also get some operational efficiencies this way?"

Clyde was not too certain that this was a good idea. "But, the children's and university hospital are almost downtown and just four miles from Mack! They are also academic facilities and, having worked in one before coming here, I can tell you that physicians and administrators there will have a totally different culture and practice style than we have here. Besides, both hospitals are making money, so why would the state (who owns them) allow them to merge with us? This sounds like a huge headache, but I guess we can't merge with a loser like the safety net hospital or a weak system like St. Francis, though they would let us capture the southern part of our area."

George continued unabated, "Clyde, if they merge we just can't remain by ourselves! Get to work on developing a merger option with these two hospitals."

*Comment:* As in this case, hospitals in oligopoly markets most often divide up their market and do not directly compete against each other. This case demonstrates what can occur when members of an oligopoly deviate from their traditional behaviors. Strategies sometimes become reactive.

### Questions

1. Why is George concerned if the merger of St. Mark's and Cassid occurs?

2. What are the advantages and disadvantages for considering merging with the children's and university hospital?

3. What would happen if the merger of St. Mark's and Cassid did not occur, yet Mack announced their merger? Would Mack be stronger or weaker?

# CASE 2: PhyCor, Inc.

Physician Practice Management Companies and PhyCor, Inc. Physician practice management (PPM) firms grew very rapidly in the late 1980s and early 1990s. PPMs promised to infuse physician practices with needed capital and provide significant cost savings and increased revenues through economies of scale and improved management. They also promised to allow physicians to negotiate better contracts with the emerging HMOs and PPOs. However, by the end of the century, all of the major PPMs had gone out of business or significantly downsized, with their valuations a tiny fraction of prior capitalization. Some, such as MedPartners, declared bankruptcy. Others saw their valuation plummet to almost nothing. What went wrong? This case examines the history of PPMs and the story of PhyCor, one of the prominent players.

PPMs were created in response to the lack of retained earnings and marginal management that existed in many physician practices and the growth of HMOs and PPOs. As a result of increased managed care, physician organizations/medical groups experienced increased costs and lower net revenues. HMOs and PPOs also demanded large discounts from physicians. Capital was also needed to buy out senior partners, install information systems, and change their structures and governance. PPMs with significant venture and Wall Street capital backing purchased prestigious medical groups, consolidated independent practices, and acquired staff clinics being divested by HMOs. Consolidation of PPMs left three large companies by the early 1990s.

Many of the physician practices signed 30- to 40-year management services contracts with the PPMs. These most often specified that physicians would receive a split of revenues after payment of clinic expenses. The lower cost of capital, centralized purchasing, and greater bargaining leverage with insurer organizations were to lower costs and increase revenues.

Phycor, Inc., incorporated in 1988, became by 1995 a medical network management company that managed multispecialty medical clinics and other physician organizations, provided contract management services to physician networks owned by health systems, and developed and managed independent practice associations (IPAs).[1] The company also provided health care decision-support services, including demand management and disease management services, to managed care organizations, health care providers, employers, and other group associations.

---

[1] IPAs are networks of independent physicians who contract together to provide medical services to individuals whose health care costs are covered by health maintenance organizations (HMOs), insurers, employers, or other third-party payors of health care services.

At PhyCor's affiliated clinics, the company implemented a number of programs and services in order to promote growth and efficiency, which included strategic planning and budgeting that focused on, among other things, revenue enhancement, cost containment, and expense reduction. The company negotiated managed care contracts; entered into national purchasing agreements; conducted productivity, procedure coding, and charge capturing studies; and assisted the clinics in physician recruitment efforts. It maintained information processing systems that expanded the clinics' accounting, billing, receivables management, scheduling, and reporting systems capabilities. The company also provided quality improvement initiatives designed to enhance the quality of patient service delivery systems at its affiliated clinics through the maintenance and measurement of performance standards and collection and review of patient evaluations. In addition, it provided operational support through a better practices resource group that focused on assisting clinics or departments within clinics in defining and executing patient services and revenue and expense savings opportunities. Under the terms of existing service agreements, the company typically provided each physician group with the equipment and facilities used in its medical practice, managed clinic operations, employed the clinic's non-physician personnel, other than certain diagnostic technicians, provided capital for expenditures, and received a service fee equal to the clinic expenses it had paid plus percentages of operating income of the clinic (net clinic revenue less certain contractually agreed-upon clinic expenses before physician distributions) plus, in some cases, percentages of net clinic revenue.

PhyCor, which called itself the "Physicians' Corporation" came a long way in five years. PhyCor's revenue soared from $1.2 million in 1988, $136 million in 1992, and $240 million in 1994. It ranked fifth in 1992 on Fortune's list of rapidly growing public companies. The company's long-range goal was to have clinics across the United States.

In 1994, the company owned 22 group practices employing almost 1,200 doctors in 15 states. In 1997, following its disclosure of difficulty in integrating some of its smaller physician practices into bigger groups, the company stock price plummeted. Between September 1997 and September 1998, Wall Street's valuation of the 15 largest PPM firms fell by 64 percent, while the entire industry lost as much as half of its commercial value.

Phycor was undeterred, but wanted to take advantage of the market conditions to gain competitive advantage. They offered $8 billion in stock and debt to buy its much larger competitor, MedPartners Inc., in October 1997. PhyCor's shares fell by more than 10 percent after the deal was unveiled, while MedPartners stock fell even further (45 percent). After a short time PhyCor scuttled its planned purchase of MedPartners, blaming differences on how to run the business of managing physicians' practices. In December 1997, PhyCor also announced that it signed an agreement to purchase Seattle-based CareWise, Inc., a nationally recognized leader in the health care decision-support industry/services, and the company acquired Ontario-based PrimeCare International Inc. on May 1998. The 2,200 general practice and specialty physicians under PrimeCare's management and its Desert Valley Medical Center became part of PhyCor's 20,000-plus physicians and 61 clinics in 29 states.

In 1998, citing industry turmoil, PhyCor announced that they planned not to buy any clinics through 1999. It was a dramatic turn for PhyCor. The company revised downward its earnings estimates for the second half of 1998. PhyCor and other physician practice management companies were plagued by earnings shortfalls, plummeting stock values, and reports of dissatisfied physicians. The PPM companies struggled with declining Medicare rates and an inability to continue growing earnings through acquisitions. The PPMs had also relied too heavily on capitation, a method of payment for services in which doctors or hospitals are paid a fixed amount for each patient, which paid too little. PhyCor stock was down about 74 percent in 1999. The company planned to sell many of its health care clinics, and sold eight such clinics during the fourth quarter, reducing its total number of clinics with the purpose of generating cash and resulting in a smaller company with clinics that were stable and had the ability to grow. Earnings for PhyCor dropped sharply in the last quarter and for the year due to shutdown of several clinics. J. C. Hutts, chairman and CEO of the company, commented, "While we are disappointed by the loss reported in the first quarter, our EBITDA was consistent with our early pronouncements. Our focus this year at PhyCor is to maximize our cash flow. We have identified several assets that we regard as non-strategic and have begun a process to sell these assets for cash."

**5 years price chart**

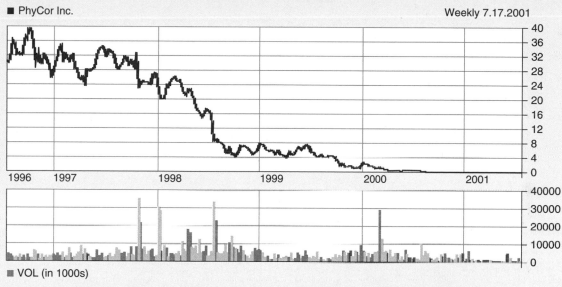

■ PhyCor Inc.                                                    Weekly 7.17.2001

SOURCE: © 2001 Stockpoint Inc. 7.17.2001

PhyCor, which then operated about 48 medical groups with 3,076 physicians in 23 states and managed independent practice associations with nearly 25,000 physicians, had been restructuring or terminating service agreements with nearly all of its multispecialty clinics across the country as it attempted to improve its ailing financial situation. Management contacted most of its 27 clinics to discuss the repurchase of clinic assets from the company by the respective physician groups in connection with the restructuring or termination of the service agreements. Proceeds from the sale of assets were used to retire outstanding debt. The company reported a net loss of $452 million, compared with net earnings of $3.7 million during the same period a year earlier. Analysts said PhyCor paid too much for clinics in some markets that then produced too little revenue, and it suffered from lower reimbursement payments from insurers and from weak productivity at some clinics. As a result of the charges, the company no longer satisfied the minimum net tangible asset listing requirements of the NASDAQ Stock Market and was delisted.

### Questions

1. What was PhyCor's initial strategy and business model?

2. What do you think went wrong with this strategy and business model?

# REFERENCES

Alliance for Advancing Nonprofit Health Care (2009). The value of nonprofit health care. Retrieved August 16, 2010, from http://www.nonprofithealthcare.org/reports/5_value.pdf

American Hospital Association. (2010). Eliminating racial and ethnic disparities. Retrieved August 11, 2010, from http://www.aha.org/aha_app/issues/Disparities/index.jsp

Armstrong, G., & Kotler, P. (1999). *Principles of marketing* (8th ed.). Upper Saddle River, NJ: Prentice Hall.

Ball, P. (2004). Starting from scratch. *Nature, 431*(7009), 624–626.

Barney, J. (1991). Firm resources and sustained competitive advantage. *Journal of Management, 17*, 99–120.

Barney, J. (1986). Organizational culture: Can it be a source of sustained competitive advantage? *Academy of Management Review, 11*(3): 565–665.

Bascomb, N. (2005). *The perfect mile: Three athletes, one goal, and less than four minutes to achieve it.* Mariner Books.

Bellou, V. (2007). Achieving long-term customer satisfaction through organizational culture: Evidence from the health care sector. *Managing Service Quality, 17*(17): 510–522.

Berry, L. and Mirabito, A. (2010). Innovative healthcare delivery. *Business Horizons, 53*(2), 157.

Bess, J. L., & Bess, A. (1990). Hospital portfolio analysis. *Health Care Strategic Management, 8*(5), 10–14.

Bourgeois, L. J., Duhaime, I. M., & Stimpert, J. L. (1999). *Strategic management: A managerial perspective.* Charlottesville, VA: Dryden Press.

Brandenburger, A., & Nalebuff, B. (1997). *Co-opetition.* New York: Crown Business.

Burns, L. (2002). Competitive strategy. In D. Albert (Ed.), A physician's guide to health care management (pp. 46–56). Williston, VT: Blackwell Publishing.

Burns, L., & Pauly, M. (2002). Integrated delivery networks: A detour on the road to integrated care? *Health Affairs, 21*(4), 128–143.

Chaffee, E. (1985). Three models of strategy. *Academy of Management Review, 10*(1), 89–98.

Cleverley, W., & Cleverley, J. (2003). Payment trends achieving stability amid uncertainty: Preparing for future payment policies and practices will require balancing act involving a broad range of revenue-enhancing strategies. *Healthcare Financial Management, 57*(12): 52–58.

Coggins, J. (1990). *Arms and equipment of the Civil War.* Wilmington, NC: Broadfoot Publishing Company.

Collis, D., & Rukstad, M. (2008). Can you say what strategy is? *Harvard Business Review*, 82–90.

The Commonwealth Fund. (2004, May). A 5-nation hospital survey: Commonalities, differences, and discontinuities. Retrieved August 11, 2010, from http://www.commonwealthfund.org/Content/Surveys/2003/2003-International-Health-Policy-Survey-of-Hospital-Executives.aspx

Crean, K. (2010). Accelerating Innovation in information and communication. *Health Affairs, 29*(2): 278–284.

Deloitte and Touche. (2009). Medical tourism report findings. Retrieved August 11, 2010, from http://www.deloitte.com/assets/Dcom-UnitedStates/Local%20Assets/Documents/us_chs_MedicalTourismStudy(3).pdf

DeWeese, D. (1994). *Islamization and native religion in the Golden Horde: Baba Tukles and conversion to Islam in historical and epic tradition.* University Park: Pennsylvania State University Press.

Eicher, D. (2001). *The longest night: A military history of the Civil War.* New York: Simon & Schuster.

Fahey, L. (1999). *Competitors.* New York: John Wiley and Sons.

Fahey, L., & Narayanan, V. K. (1986). *Macroenvironmental analysis for strategic management.* St. Paul, MN: West Publishing Company.

Federal Trade Commission and Department of Justice. (2004, July). Improving health care: A dose of competition: A report by the Federal Trade Commission and the Department of Justice.

Fennell, T. 2005. The next 50 years. *CA Magazine, 138*(3), 45–46.

Frazier, I. (2005). Annals of history: Invaders: Destroying Bagdad. *The New Yorker*, April 25.

Frey, K., Leighton, J., & Cecala, K. (2005). Building a culture of service excellence. *Physician Executive, 31*(6): 40–45.

Ghemawat, P. 2001. *Strategy and the business landscape*. Upper Saddle River, NJ: Prentice Hall.

Ghoshal, S., & Bartlett, C. 1995, Changing the role of top management: Beyond structure to process. *Harvard Business Review, 73*(1): 86–96.

Ginter, P. M., Swayne, L. E., & Duncan, W. J. (2002). Strategic management of health care organizations. Oxford, UK: Blackwell Publishing.

Goodstein, L. D., Nolan, T. M., & Pfeiffer, J. W. (1993). *Applied strategic planning*. New York: McGraw-Hill.

Hansell, S. Netflix to sell a device for instantly watching movies on TV sets. New York Times, May 28, 2010 from http://www.nytimes.com/2008/05/20/technology/20netflix.html?scp=1&sq=netflix%20to%20sell%20a%20device%20for%20instantly%20watching&st=cse

Hansen, F. (2008). A revolution in healthcare. *Review—Institute of Public Affairs, 59*(4), 43–46.

Harris, G. (2004). Despite missteps, Eli Lilly is a hard stock to bet against. *New York Times*, February 25.

Herper, M. (2010). The world's most expensive drugs. *Forbes*, February 22. Retrieved May 11, 2010, from http://www.forbes.com/2010/02/19/expensive-drugs-cost-business-healthcare-rare-diseases.html

Hunt, M. (1972). Competition in the major home appliance industry (Doctoral dissertation). Harvard University, Cambridge, MA.

Institute of Medicine. (2001). Crossing the quality chasm. Washington DC: The National Press.

Jackson, S. (2008). Predicting changes in industry structure. *The Journal of Business Strategy, 29*(2): 54–57.

Kepros, J., Mosher, B., Anderson, C. & Stevens, P. (2007). The product life cycle of healthcare in the United States. *The Internet Journal of Healthcare Administration, 4*(2). Retrieved August 14, 2010, from http://www.ispub.com/ostia/index.php?xmlFilePath=journals/ijhca/vol4n2/product.xml

Kotler, P., Shalowitz, J., & Stevens, R. (2008). Strategic marketing for healthcare organizations. San Francisco: Jossey-Bass.

Landro, L. (2007). Hospitals build a better healing environment. *Wall Street Journal*, March 21, p. D9.

LaPenna, A. M. (2010). "Alternative" healthcare: Access as a revenue source in a consumer-driven market. *Journal of Healthcare Management, 55*(1), 7–11

Lee, O., & Davis, T. R. V. (2004). International patients: A lucrative market for U.S. hospitals. *Health Marketing Quarterly, 22*(1), 41–56.

Lin, D. (2008). Convenient care clinics: Opposition, opportunities, and the path to health system integration. *Frontiers of Health Services Management, 24*(3), 3–12.

Luke, R., Walston, S., & Plummer, P. (2004). *Healthcare strategy: In pursuit of competitive advantage*. Chicago: Health Administration Press.

*Merriam-Webster English dictionary*. (2004). Springfield, MA: Merriam-Webster.

Mintzberg, H., Ahlstrand, B., & Lampel, J. (1998). *Strategy safari: A guided tour through the wilds of strategic management*. New York: Free Press.

Murray, W., Knox, M., & Bernstein, A. (1994). *The making of strategy: Rulers, states, and war*. Cambridge: Cambridge University Press.

Muscalus, R. (2008). Competition and community: Key evolving issues that require careful consideration. *Frontiers of Health Services Management, 25*(2), 25–31.

Mutter, R., Wong, H., & Goldfarb, M. (2008). The effects of hospital competition on inpatient quality of care. *Inquiry—Excellus Health Plan, 45*(3): 263–280.

The $150 million zapper: Does every cancer patient really need proton-beam therapy? (2009, March 16). *Forbes, 183*(5), 62.

Operating profit: Globalisation and healthcare. (2008, August 16). *The Economist, 388*(8593).

Perkins, B. (2010). Designing high cost medicine. *American Journal of Public Health, 100*(2), 223–233.

Pesse, M., Erat, P., & Erat, A. 2006. The network is the customer: Setting the stage for fundamental change in pharmaceutical sales and marketing. *Journal of Medical Marketing, 6*(3), 195–202.

Porter, M. (1980). *Competitive strategy*. New York: Free Press.

PriceWaterhouseCoopers. (2010). Pharma 2020: Challenging business models. Retrieved May 13, 2010, from http://www.pwc.com/gx/en/pharma-life-sciences/pharma-2020/pharma-2020-vision-path.jhtml

Prawdin, M., & Chaliand, G. (2006). *The Mongol empire: Its rise and legacy*. New Brunswick, NJ: Transaction Publishers.

PR Newswire, 2007. Cleveland Clinic enters partnership to manage and operate Sheikh Khalifa Medical City in Abu Dhabi. June 4. New York.

Rowland, C. (2006). Hospitals blitz airwaves with ad campaigns. *Boston Globe*, February 21. Retrieved August 11, 2010, from http://www.boston.com/business/healthcare/articles/2006/02/21/hospitals_blitz_airwaves_with_ad_campaigns

Sawyer, R. (2007). *The seven military classics of ancient China*. New York: Basic Books.

Schendel, D. (1994). Introduction to "Competitive organizational behavior Toward an organizationally-based theory of competitive advantage." *Strategic Management Journal*. 15: 1–5.

Shilling, G. (2007). First mover disadvantage. *Forbes, 179*(13), 00156914, June 18.

Society for Healthcare Strategy and Market Development. (2008). FutureScan 2008: Healthcare trends and implications, 2008–2013. Chicago: Health Administration Press.

Watson, T. (1963). *A business and its beliefs*. New York: McGraw-Hill.

Walter, B. A., & Priem, R. (1999). Business strategy and CEO intelligence acquisition. *Competitive Intelligence Review, 10*, 15–22.

Wernerfelt, B. 1984. A resource-based view of the firm. *Strategic Management Journal, 5*, 171–180.

Wills, B. S. (1998). *The Confederacy's greatest cavalryman: Nathan Bedford Forrest (Modern war studies)*. Lawrence: University Press of Kansas.

# Chapter 11

# Managing Strategic Alliances

Edward J. Zajac, Thomas A. D'Aunno,
and Lawton Robert Burns

## CHAPTER OUTLINE

- **Alliances in Health Care**
- **Types and Forms of Alliances**
- **What Are Alliances Meant to Do?**
- **The Alliance Process: A Multistage Analysis**
- **Frameworks for Analyzing Alliance Problems**

## LEARNING OBJECTIVES

**After completing this chapter, the reader should be able to:**

1. Better understand why strategic alliances are increasing in use, particularly among health care organizations

2. Distinguish between different types or forms of strategic alliances, using a number of dimensions

3. Classify an alliance both in terms of what it looks like and what it is meant to do

4. Understand how alliance motivation is often related to alliance structure and outcomes

5. Identify whether your motivations for a strategic alliance are compatible with those of your alliance partner

6. Think about strategic alliances in terms of the likely stages of development that alliances often experience and the critical issues that you may face at each stage

7. Distinguish between an alliance problem and an alliance symptom and recognize the different implications for managerial intervention

8. Understand both the pros and cons of alliances

9. Identify alliances in health care that work and those that do not work

# KEY TERMS

Alliance Objectives

Alliance Problems

Alliance Process

Alliance Risk

Alliance Symptoms

Control

Cost Reduction

Equity-Based Alliances

Joint Venture

Ownership

Partner Orientation

Pooling Alliances

Revenue Enhancement

Strategic Alliance

Trading Alliances

Turbulent Environment

Uncertainty Reduction

---

**IN PRACTICE:  Hospital Purchasing Alliances: Creating Leverage, Reducing Costs—and Stirring Up Controversy**

Hospitals set up purchasing alliances (also known as group purchasing organizations, or GPOs) starting in 1910. The GPO industry developed throughout the latter half of the twentieth century and consolidated in the 1990s into seven large firms, with lots of regional and smaller players. GPOs exist primarily to pool the purchase of medical-surgical supplies, medical devices, pharmaceuticals, and capital equipment across multiple hospitals to leverage manufacturers, gain lower prices, and thereby reduce hospital costs (Burns and Lee, 2008). Such purchasing alliances are quite common in other industries. Research shows that purchasing alliances reduce input spending anywhere from 10 to 15 percent of costs, consistent with common sense about volume purchasing.

However, in health care, these alliances have become incredibly controversial. The GPOs, for example, have been the subject of four U.S. Senate hearings during 2002–2006 (with another possibly scheduled for 2011), three Government Accountability Office (GAO) reports, and a panel workshop convened by the Federal trade Commission in 2002. Why all the attention? The source of the controversy is a small set of small manufacturers, typically makers of medical devices, who claimed in a series of reports published in the *New York Times* that the GPOs have developed contracts with larger manufacturers that are anti-competitive in nature and therefore exclude them from the market. They claim that hospital efforts to contract for lower prices have the consequence of preventing innovative products from getting to market and thus harming patients.

What is remarkable here is that the anticompetitive practices alleged by the small manufacturers are not attributed to the "usual suspects" in antitrust cases: horizontal combinations of large manufacturers, or vertically integrated combinations of manufacturers and downstream distribution channels. Instead, the practices inhere in what are ostensibly arms-length contractual agreements between groups of hospitals, their purchasing alliances, and the manufacturers who sell medical products. The practices at the center of the controversy do not seem that extraordinary—lower prices for a higher percentage of purchases (committed contracts), lower prices for buying from a single vendor (sole-source contracts) or dual vendors (dual-source contracts), and lower prices for buying a range of products (bundled contracts). Such practices are found in other industries (e.g., customer loyalty programs, McDonald's Value Meal). But in health care, these practices have been under intense public scrutiny.

There have been repeated calls by small manufacturers and their trade association to undercut the funding mechanism for hospital purchasing alliances, which might cause them to cease operation. Managing strategic alliances has become a political hot potato. The GPOs, which used to be faceless and rather unremarkable, have found they have a whole new set of constituents that they did not previously serve, including the U.S. Senate, the GAO, the FTC, small manufacturers, and the press. They have also found themselves playing a lot of defense in Congress, the media, and the courts.

# CHAPTER PURPOSE

There is no doubt that the U.S. health care environment is undergoing major changes that could be characterized as turbulent. As illustrated by the challenges currently facing hospital purchasing alliances, turbulence characterizes rapidly changing environments where: (1) organizations are highly interconnected with one another, and (2) organizations are highly interdependent with the society in which they find themselves (Emery and Trist, 1965).

This emphasis on connectedness and interdependence is an important basis for viewing a specific organization's environment not as some amorphous external force, but rather as the set of other organizations that are interconnected or interdependent with it. This organization, in turn, is part of the environment for the other organizations. In other words, when an organization looks out with concern or anticipation at its **turbulent environment**, what it sees is other organizations looking out at that organization (Shortell and Zajac, 1990).

This conceptualization of organizational environments suggests the need to focus more attention on how specific organizations interact with one another. This chapter emphasizes one such type of interaction—cooperative interorganizational relations. Longest (1990), in discussing what he terms "interorganizational linkages in health care," distinguishes between market transactions, voluntary relationships, and involuntary relationships. We focus most of our attention on those interorganizational relations that are noncoercive and entered into primarily for strategic purposes—that is, that are important to an organization's mission and expected to enhance organizational performance. We term such relationships **strategic alliances**, which are defined as any formal arrangements between two or more organizations for purposes of ongoing cooperation and mutual gain/risk sharing.

# ALLIANCES IN HEALTH CARE

Alliances are often viewed as facing high failure rates; some claim 50 to 80 percent. For example, early research argued that strategic alliances, by their very nature, are risky endeavors (Harrigan, 1985). The cooperative linkages between two or more organizations are viewed as somewhat fragile, exposing each party to the risk that the other party or parties may

not continue to cooperate as expected. The business press has also had a penchant for describing, in detail, particular joint ventures or other alliances that failed. The failure of a cooperative alliance between two organizations often involves considerable drama, as interorganizational cooperation turns to conflict and sometimes litigation.

Although it is very important to recognize the pros and cons of alliances (see Debate Time), we believe that a fixation on the likely failure and inherent riskiness of alliances may be misguided. Specifically, we contend that any assessment of the **alliance risk** should be balanced with an assessment of the expected return or benefit of the alliance in terms of improved financial performance, innovation, and organizational learning, and the opportunity cost of not engaging in a strategic alliance. Regarding the first point, while financial performance is an obvious outcome to consider when analyzing the success or failure of a strategic alliance, it is not clear that it should be considered the most important, direct outcome. For example, innovation may be a driving force behind strategic alliances, and more generally, alliances may be viewed as a desirable way for organizations to learn about new markets, services, and ways of doing business (Zajac, Golden, and Shortell, 1991). These may actually be negatively correlated with financial performance, at least in the short run (Shortell and Zajac, 1988). This issue is discussed in greater detail in the section on how strategic intentions drive alliance activity.

In terms of opportunity cost, the relevant question is not whether an alliance is risky, but rather, which is riskier: going it alone, doing nothing, or engaging in an alliance? Riskiness is not necessarily a problem. For example, the virtues of entrepreneurship are often extolled, despite the high risk and high failure rates involved. Strategic alliances may appear risky when the baseline comparison is not made explicit, but when compared with attempting a *de novo* entry into a new market or ignoring the market altogether, the alliance may actually seem like a relatively low-risk proposition (Shortell and Zajac, 1988). In fact, as subsequently discussed, the creation of a strategic alliance is often motivated by an organization's desire to reduce uncertainty.

The issues just raised are particularly relevant for health care organizations, which have seen an explosion of alliance building in the last few decades (Bazzoli et al., 2000; Olden, Roggenkamp, and Luke, 2002). Alliance building is not limited to hospitals (Alter and Hage, 1993; Zuckerman and Kaluzny, 1991). There are alliances between hospitals and

## DEBATE TIME: Positive and Negative Benefits of Alliances

There are a few facts and many more unknowns about strategic alliances. One fact is that we are witnessing a substantial increase in strategic alliances in health care. An unknown, however, is whether this fact reflects a positive or negative development. An interesting example of an ongoing debate is found in Duncan, Ginter, and Swayne (1992). In this section, we consider some of the arguments swirling around the use of strategic alliances. Kaluzny and Zuckerman (1992) argue on the positive side for alliances, while Begun (1992) offers counterarguments on the negative side. The following list of issues summarizes their points of disagreement.

### Positive

1. Alliances reflect a fundamental shift in how health service organizations do business; namely, a change from thinking in terms of control to thinking in terms of commitment, trust, shared risk, and common purpose.

2. Alliances provide organizations with a way to manage growing complexity and interdependence while maintaining a fair amount of individual organizational autonomy.

3. Alliances enable organizations to transcend the existing organizational inertia that is often created by complexity and vested interests seeking to maintain the status quo.

4. Alliances have been found to be effective in other sectors of our society, and failure to apply these concepts to health services would be a missed opportunity for meeting the challenges in the future.

### Negative

1. Alliances distract organizations from their basic goal, which is to clobber your competitors or at least behave as if you have that need. Managers like the thrill of the competitive chase, and competition creates loyalty and team spirit in an organization.

2. Alliances are essentially a fad whose benefits have been exaggerated, similar to Theory Z, the pursuit of excellence, product-line management, and total quality management.

3. Alliances can lead to collusion between otherwise competing organizations, can lead to legal problems related to antitrust challenges, and are attractive only to lazy organizations that are not interested in competition.

4. The process hassles of initiating and managing alliances are tremendous and costly, and these arrangements are quite fragile.

5. Governing an alliance means governing by committee, which we know to be an ineffective way to run a business. In particular, this problem reduces the speed and flexibility of an organization.

6. Cooperative strategy makes sense for large, multinational firms seeking to enter new and unknown markets or share expensive research and development projects, but not for health care organizations that face well-known local markets and do not need to finance much research and development.

Which of the above perspectives do you favor? How would you justify your position?

physician groups, between hospitals and health maintenance organizations (HMOs), and between hospitals, physicians, and agencies of the federal government (Kaluzny, Morrissey, and McKinney, 1990; Bazzoli et al., 1999; Burns and Pauly, 2002). Nor are alliances limited to providers of care. Alliances known as business coalitions have emerged among buyers of care, that is, employers who band together to increase their effectiveness as purchasers of care for their employees. The variety of possible alliance partners is quite high, given the myriad number of players in the different health care sectors (see Figure 1.1 in Chapter 1) and the number of key relationships between adjacent organizations (see Table 11.1).

**TABLE 11.1 Key Alliance Relationships Between Organizations in Various Health Care Sectors**

| Alliance Relationships within and across Sectors |
| --- |
| **Suppliers and Suppliers** |
| • Pharmaceutical and biotechnology firms (drug development and commercialization) |
| • Pharmaceutical and medical device firms (development of drug-eluting stents) |
| • Medical device and information technology firms (remote monitors) |
| • Medical products firms and wholesalers (key distribution partners) |
| **Suppliers and Providers** |
| • Medical device firms and physician inventors (device innovation) |
| • Medical imaging firms and hospital scientists (imaging advances) |
| • Group purchasing organizations and hospitals (group buying) |
| **Providers and Providers** |
| • Hospitals and physicians (PHOs, MSOs, etc.) |
| • Pharmacies and retail clinics (MinuteClinic, TakeCare) |
| • Hospitals and retail clinics (retail medicine feeder for hospitals) |
| **Buyers and Providers** |
| • Employers and retail clinics (on-site primary care for employees) |
| • Managed care/insurers and hospitals/physicians (pay-for-performance programs) |
| **Buyers and Buyers** |
| • Employers and managed care/insurers (risk-based contracts) |
| • Employers and pharmacy benefit managers (carve out pharmacy benefits) |
| • Employers and business groups (pooled purchasing of health insurance) |
| • Managed care and pharmacy benefit managers (carve out pharmacy benefits) |

The causes for this outburst of activity are not difficult to identify. Perhaps the most important and obvious factor is that health care organizations are experiencing what Meyer (1982) has referred to as a series of "environmental jolts." These are relatively abrupt, major, and often qualitative changes in an environment that threaten organizational survival. Such jolts include increased competition, concern with cost containment, health care reform to reduce the number of uninsured patients, an aging population, and changes to the Medicare program (e.g., Prospective Payment System, Balanced Budget Act, Medicare Modernization Act).

These jolts create great uncertainty for health care managers. Alliances may reflect the reality that it is sometimes better to face life's uncertainties with partners than to go it alone (Kaluzny, Zuckerman, and Ricketts, 2002; Zuckerman, Kaluzny, and Ricketts, 1995). Of course, alliances are but one response to the environmental changes described above. There has also been a marked increase in other types of multiorganizational arrangements, particularly multihospital systems and other forms of horizontal integration (Shortell, 1988; Burns and Pauly, 2002), vertical integration, consortia, and diversification (Clement, 1987). In short, as Starr (1982) observed over 25 years ago, the landscape of the health care field is itself changing: where there were once many small and independent organizations, there are now clusters of organizations, including alliances and other types of multiorganizational arrangements.

# TYPES AND FORMS OF ALLIANCES

Alliances vary in regard to ownership, control, size, governance, and nature of participation.

## Ownership and Control

DeVries (1978) and others (e.g., Starkweather, 1971) have arrayed multi-institutional systems on a continuum of more autonomy to more **control**. However, these rankings often really reflect the degree of **ownership**, with complete ownership being equated with the highest form of control. While it seems reasonable to view ownership as related to control, we argue that this can sometimes be misleading.

For example, it is well known that McDonald's Corporation is very interested in maintaining control over its raw materials to ensure that quality is highly consistent. In dealing with its exchange partners who supply these raw materials, one might therefore expect that McDonald's would prefer an interorganizational arrangement that would involve substantial ownership interest in suppliers in order to have greater control. This is not the case, however. Even with no ownership interests, McDonald's simply communicates its quality requirements to the supplier organizations, and the organizations are typically quick to oblige.

How can this be? Two factors seem to be relevant. The first is obvious. McDonald's, by virtue of its size, enjoys substantial relative power in its relationship with suppliers; McDonald's represents a very large portion of a food supplier's business. This obviates, at least in large part, the need for McDonald's to also own some or all of the suppliers' assets. Ownership and control are essentially separated in this case. The second reason has much less to do with the relative power of the organizations involved and more to do with the establishment of a tradition of mutual gain and cooperation. Specifically, McDonald's has made it a policy to be loyal to high-quality suppliers and to use its size to protect the supplier from dramatic swings in sales revenue. In this way, both parties have incentives to ensure a long-term cooperative relationship—with no ownership interests.

This simplified example is not intended to show that ownership and control are usually unrelated, of course. Rather, the example demonstrates that tight control can exist even in cases where there is no ownership interest. In fact, Bazzoli and her colleagues (1999) analyzed all U.S. hospital systems (i.e., two or more hospitals have a common owner) and alliances (i.e., two or more hospitals agree to work together without common ownership) for the years 1994 and 1995 and found that there were alliances that exercised centralized control over a variety of decisions and systems in which control was decentralized.

Furthermore, it is not at all clear that the pursuit of control through higher levels of ownership should be the paramount consideration in designing strategic alliances. As Li, Zhou, and Zajac (2009) show, an overemphasis on one dimension of alliances, such as the degree of control implied by higher ownership, can lead to negative outcomes on other dimensions of alliances, such as degree of active collaboration between partners. Similarly, one could dimensionalize alliance ownership without direct reference to control by simply considering contractual versus **equity-based alliances**. Contractual alliances, such as preferred buyer-supplier arrangements or licensing agreements, are likely to spell out the terms of partner engagement, including control questions, in legal documents. Equity-based alliances include minority equity investments, which are often observed between large and small firms in the medical device industry, or formal **joint ventures**, in which two organizations give birth to a joint venture "child," with the specific equity percentages agreed upon by the two parent organizations. In these joint ventures, control issues are partly determined by ownership stakes and shareholder vote, but also partly determined by the negotiated joint venture operating agreement.

The lesson emerging from our discussion of ownership and control is that there are many dimensions upon which one can categorize strategic alliances, and that one must exercise caution in interpreting what the dimension really represents and how it relates to other relevant dimensions. We now turn to discussing several additional dimensions upon which one can distinguish one type or form of strategic alliance from another.

## Number of Members

Alliances vary greatly in size. They can consist of two organizations, but they often consist of many more. For example, the Premier health care alliance is a national hospital alliance that now includes 2,300 hospitals. Size makes a substantial difference in several ways. Larger alliances are more difficult to govern because it is more difficult to represent all members on a single board of directors. Larger size may also entail greater diversity among members, which in turn may make it more difficult to find common ground on important issues ranging from alliance strategy (i.e., what are the **alliance objectives**—that is, the overall purpose and goals of the alliance) to the management of alliance programs. Further, even when agreements are reached on alliance strategy and operations, larger size makes it difficult to coordinate members' efforts.

On the other hand, size has virtues. It creates power, as noted earlier. Larger alliances typically have more purchasing power because they can buy in larger volume (assuming, of course, that all members can agree on a particular vendor, which is often difficult). For example, Premier makes $33 billion worth of purchases per year. Similarly, larger alliances have more clout in lobbying at various levels of government. Further, larger alliances can generate capital easier simply from having a larger number of members' fees to collect.

Nonetheless, the costs and benefits of alliance size are difficult to assess in the abstract. What often matters most in determining an effective size for an alliance is its strategic purpose and particular situation. For example, a local or regional hospital network will have a relatively small number of members compared to other hospital alliances. Yet, it may have exactly the number of members it needs for its purpose, which is to provide the local area with a comprehensive service system.

## Governance Structure

In the case of an alliance with two members, it is often not necessary to be concerned about establishing a way to govern alliance activities so as to give them direction. But beyond the simple case of a two-party alliance, governance issues can be considerably complex.

The governing bodies of many alliances, especially hospital alliances, tend to include at least one member from each participating organization, often the director or CEO of the member organization. This practice stems largely from important distinguishing features of alliances; that is, that they are a form of organization in which the members are equal and have a great deal of autonomy.

Further, the boards of health care organizations traditionally have been based on what Fennell and Alexander (1989) term a philanthropic model, which assumes that "bigger is better." In other words, boards were viewed as a key link to the local community and its resources; having more individuals on a board provided a hospital, for example, with greater community support and access to donors. Similarly, we have observed that alliance boards often are large so as to represent various interest groups.

Indeed, as Carman (1992) reports, alliance boards often have physician representatives, board members from participating organizations, and community members as well. Moreover, Carman argues persuasively that alliance boards should not consist entirely of CEOs. He points out that there is enough turnover among CEOs so as to create instability for an alliance if its governance rests only with them (American College of Healthcare Executives, 2009). In contrast, organizational commitment to the alliance is enhanced if it is represented in alliance governance by leaders other than CEOs.

As just noted, however, this means that larger alliances can have boards with dozens of members that, in turn, can make it difficult to achieve consensus and can slow decision making. Of course, large alliance boards can, and sometimes do, have executive committees that consist of a smaller subset of elected members who have the authority to make key decisions. Thus, an important choice for larger alliances is whether to represent all or some members on the alliance board and to determine what kinds of individuals (CEOs, physicians, trustees) should be alliance board members.

## Mandated versus Voluntary Participation

Another important dimension on which alliances vary is whether they are voluntary or mandated by an external group with legal or legitimate authority (Oliver, 1990). Most health care alliances are voluntary. These alliances reflect the efforts of individual organizations to strategically adapt to external changes by choosing to band together. But, it is important to recognize that even voluntary alliances may emerge in large part as a result of external pressure from powerful actors.

A central issue to note in comparing mandated and voluntary alliances is the extent to which the former are characterized more by style than by substance and by instability than by longevity. Scott (1987) argues that mandated forms of organization tend to be adopted only superficially and, as a result, also tend to be short-lived. Many international alliances (including the League of Nations and the United Nations) come to mind in this regard. Superficial compliance with a mandate to form an alliance is especially likely to occur when the participating organizations lack other motives for forming a relationship (Oliver, 1990). In general, managers and other organization members chafe under external constraints and regulation, even when such rules have some merit.

## Discussion

Existing typologies have been useful in documenting and describing the common and different features of a wide range of interorganizational arrangements in health care. However, it is also important to ask what difference an organization should expect to see if it were to choose one form versus another.

In other words, what is the alliance intended to accomplish? For example, Zajac (1986), in an analysis of contract management arrangements, argues that organizations choosing to engage in a similar type of strategic alliance may have widely varying strategic intentions and that expected performance will vary accordingly. In other words, the form of the alliance is not necessarily a good predictor of what the alliance can achieve.

# WHAT ARE ALLIANCES MEANT TO DO?

## Pooling versus Trading Alliances

Most broadly, one can distinguish between **pooling alliances** that bring together organizations seeking to contribute similar resources, and **trading alliances** that bring together organizations seeking to contribute different resources (Doz and Hamel, 1998). This distinction is more precise than the often-made statement that organizations generally seek "complementarities" in alliances. The term *complementarity* suggests differences, but it is important to remember that similarities can often drive alliance activity as well. An example of a pooling or similarity-driven strategic intent for an alliance is one that seeks to gain purchasing power over a supplier or group of suppliers. Such alliances are often seen in health care, in the form of business coalitions (against hospitals) or hospital purchasing alliances (against health care supply organizations).

Examples of a trading or difference-driven alliance are a physician group–hospital joint venture, where each party contributes something distinct to the alliance; a joint venture between two health care supply firms, such as Johnson & Johnson and Merck, where the former is known for its marketing

expertise and the latter for its product development skills; and a hospital-supplier joint venture, where the two parties jointly conduct research on new iterations of the supplier's technology. These examples also highlight how strategic intent can often drive the form of a strategic alliance. Pooling strategies tend to involve more organizations and take the form of federations, consortia, or coalitions; and trading strategies tend to involve fewer (often only two) organizations and take the form of joint ventures, licensing agreements, and related arrangements. Of course, as mentioned, earlier alternative alliance forms can serve similar strategic intent in some cases. For example, a health plan can create a trading alliance with a pharmacy or a benefits management firm, or it may seek to create a consortium of health plans that provides the same service.

## Cost Reduction versus Revenue Enhancement

The strategic intent of alliances can also be examined in terms of their expected outcomes. An emphasis on expected alliance outcomes is relevant for several reasons: The success of an alliance will generally be defined by the degree to which the desired outcomes are achieved; some performance outcomes may be largely incompatible with others; and one alliance partner's perception of the expected outcome may not be shared by that of other partners.

The first and most basic expected outcome refers to financial performance and addresses the issue of whether the alliance is primarily conceived for **cost reduction** or **revenue enhancement**. While this is not to say that the two outcomes are mutually exclusive, there are differences in the challenges for success for alliances, in how one gauges success, and in how cost-reducing versus revenue-enhancing alliances might be organized.

For example, consider a local alliance of four hospitals with historically complementary specialties (or distinctive competencies) that is seeking to increase the volume of patients to be treated in these specialties. Compare this alliance with a similarly sized and similarly located hospital alliance seeking to share the costs of providing indigent care to the local community. One would not measure success the same way, nor would the interaction between partners be the same in the two alliances. One might expect that the alliance motivated by the desire to increase patient volume would require substantial coordination, given that there is a reciprocal interdependence between the partners. In the case of the cost-sharing alliance, one would likely observe a combining of similar resources requiring relatively less active coordination, given that there is a pooled interdependence among the partners (Thompson, 1967).

## Quality, Innovation, and Learning

Another way of classifying the intent of an alliance is the degree to which the alliance seeks to enhance outcomes such as innovation, organizational learning, and quality (Doz and Hamel, 1998; Zajac et al., 1991). These outcomes are distinct from those discussed above in that, while they may lead to revenue enhancement or cost reduction, their relationship to such financial performance measures may be difficult to discern or, in a more extreme case, may be negatively related to financially oriented targets (Shortell and Zajac, 1990).

For example, Zuckerman and D'Aunno (1990) noted that hospitals can increase their reputation for quality by joining a strategic alliance that involves other prestigious organizations. Membership in such an alliance may require only a minor contribution of time, effort, or capital. An interesting feature of such an alliance is that one partner's actions can damage the reputation of another by not delivering the expected level of quality. This suggests the need for appropriate screening of partners in terms of their commitment to quality.

There may also be regional differences in the degree to which membership is prestige-enhancing. One of the authors was involved in a research project on multihospital systems in which a voluntary membership affiliation with a large national, for-profit hospital system was viewed by the local community as an asset to the hospital. The name of the hospital system was proudly displayed at the hospital entrance and on hospital stationery. However, another hospital affiliated with that same system—but located in a different part of the country—made every attempt to downplay that affiliation. No signs were posted with the system name, and no trace of the system could be found on hospital stationery. The reason for this very different treatment? In the first example, the region had many for-profit affiliations, and several of the major hospital chains had their headquarters in that region of the country. In the second example, for-profit hospitals were much less common in the region and were viewed somewhat suspiciously by many in that environment. The point is that, before seeking membership in an alliance for purposes of increasing actual or perceived quality, an organization must be aware of the limits of that benefit.

Other motives driving alliance activity, such as innovation and learning, are also conceptually distinct from other, more straightforward motives. The payoffs from alliances that are driven by innovation and learning motives are often slow to emerge. This requires a particularly high level of partner commitment and patience. An additional factor to consider is that many organizations underestimate the involvement necessary to realize benefits such as innovation and learning. In these alliances, a more substantial personnel flow between partners can often accelerate the learning and innovation process.

## Power Enhancement, Uncertainty Reduction, and Risk Sharing

Power enhancement and **uncertainty reduction** are grouped together because one often has implications for the other. Specifically, alliances can be motivated by an organization's desire to gain influence over, or reduce dependence on, an aspect of the organization's environment. This reduction in dependence may also represent a reduction in uncertainty, although the two are conceptually distinct. An organization might be dependent on another organization, but if the more powerful organization is reliable, then the dependent organization may face little uncertainty.

This perspective can be seen in much of the early literature on interorganizational relations in health care. Longest (1990), for example, views the growth of multi-institutional systems as the result of an "external dependency relationship" between the hospital and its environment. In doing so, Longest is applying the resource dependence perspective to the health care industry (Pfeffer and Salancik, 1978). Longest (1990) uses the term *stabilization strategy* to characterize multihospital arrangements, which he explains are "formulated by people for a hospital that exists in relation to an external environment upon which the hospital is highly dependent."

Uncertainty reduction as an alliance motive can also be compared with a similar, yet distinct, motive: risk sharing. The difference between the two motives is that the former highlights one organization's attempts to reduce its own uncertainty, whereas the latter emphasizes the joint reduction of uncertainty for both (or more) partners. Not surprisingly, the former is equated more with gaining influence of an exchange partner, while the latter is used more in terms of pooling resources to reduce common risk.

---

**IN PRACTICE:** Strategic Alliances between Buyers and Suppliers of Medical Imaging Equipment

---

Over the past 20 years, the manufacturers of medical imaging equipment (e.g., General Electric, Siemens, Philips) have developed strategic alliances with their downstream customers, such as academic medical centers, hospital systems, and large integrated physician groups (Mayo Clinic, Cleveland Clinic). These alliances have sought to transform the traditional buyer-seller relationship from selling more product (supplier goal) and lowering unit product cost (buyer goal) to fostering new product development for sellers and developing solutions to buyers' operational problems.

Imaging equipment manufacturers have developed two types of alliances with providers: research alliances and equipment/service alliances. In the former, the manufacturer contributes equipment (e.g., MRIs, scanners, etc.), research scientists and other personnel, and some research funding to the customer site; the hospital's research personnel work with the manufacturer's scientists on mutually agreed-upon research projects, which typically focus on developing the next-generation technology. Intellectual property may be shared between the two partners, including academic research papers. Manufacturers value these alliances because they allow them to tap the insights and product development capabilities of researchers in academic medical centers, invent the next-generation equipment, and leapfrog their competitors. In the latter, multiyear agreements stipulate technology upgrades, the hospital's service as a clinical show site for the manufacturer's latest technology, and the hospital's access to the manufacturer for their consulting expertise (e.g., GE's lean and Six Sigma techniques). Hospitals seek to tap this expertise to redesign their workflows and reengineer core patient processes. In both cases, the alliances serve as platforms for learning and new capability development on behalf of both partners.

Nevertheless, these alliances are not without their problems and frictions. Primary among these are the amount of time consumed in alliance meetings, the conflict in time horizons of the two partners, turnover in key positions overseeing the alliance as well as among researchers, technical problems with the imaging equipment, and difficulties in migrating solutions developed in one site (one hospital of a multihospital system, one clinical area within that hospital) to other clinical sites. Unlike alliances observed in other industries, these alliances typically have underdeveloped coordinative and governance mechanisms to improve alliance functioning, as well as dedicated alliance personnel on the hospital side.

Overall, these supplier-provider alliances are important for an industry where there has historically been much mistrust between the two parties and little successful alliance formation in the past. Moreover, the two parties in these alliances are large, important stakeholders in the entire health care system and involved in arguably the fastest-rising component of health care spending: imaging procedures. Finally, these alliances constitute a growing set of efforts to enable firms in the health care supply chain to access complementary resources, to promote innovation while also improving quality and efficiency, and ultimately to develop true value chains.

## CEO Rationales for Alliances

Our discussion of the above-mentioned strategic intentions that can drive alliance activity is intended to be illustrative, rather than exhaustive. Indeed, if one were to ask CEOs the question of "Why ally?" it would not be surprising to hear a myriad of broad and narrow reasons as to why their organizations turn to strategic alliances to further their goals. In fact, one survey of CEOs on this question bears out this expectation. Specifically, in a Coopers and Lybrand CEO survey in 1996, U.S. CEOs highlighted the following top reasons for alliance formation:

- Improve competitive position                77%
- Increase sales of existing products          77%
- Create new products or business lines        76%
- Improve operations or technology             71%
- Improve employee skills                      48%
- Decrease cost of existing operations         44%

What this survey also shows, however, is that the reasons for pursuing strategic alliances are likely not mutually exclusive. Returning to a health care example, a business coalition may be formed because it wants to gain influence over local area hospitals, but it also has as its major objective a reduction in the cost of health care that the coalition members have had to pay. Thus, power and cost-reduction motives are both driving alliance formation. Similarly, a joint venture between a hospital and a multispecialty physician group may have as its objective the creation of new innovative services, yet also have the intent of increasing revenues (Longest, 1990).

Understanding the strategic intent of an alliance can be a critical success factor for the alliance (Kale and Singh, 2009). The understanding has several components, including understanding your own motivation for considering an alliance, expressing this understanding to your alliance partner, eliciting and then listening carefully to your partners' expression of their strategic intentions, and examining the compatibility (which could be compatibly similar or compatibly different) of your intentions and those of your partners. The lack of an articulated mission statement is often cited as the root of many failures in organizational strategy. The same is equally if not more true for strategic alliances, particularly given the potential for incompatible intentions across partners.

## Physician-Hospital Trading Alliances

Physician-hospital alliances have spread across the health care system in response to several environmental jolts. The Medicare Prospective Payment System (PPS) altered the financial incentives of hospitals by using fixed, per-case payments but left physician incentives untouched. Because physicians control (directly or indirectly) up to 80 percent of hospital expenditures, hospitals began to develop relationships with their physicians in order to influence their thinking and practice behavior. The rapid increase in managed care (e.g., penetration by HMOs) in the late 1980s and early 1990s provided an additional spur to alliance formation (Olden et al., 2002). As HMOs sought to reduce their inpatient costs (e.g., through lower payments), hospitals looked for ways to cut costs through partnerships with their physicians. Moreover, some HMOs looked to pass on to providers the financial risks for their enrollees. Physicians and hospitals sought to develop alliances to accept and manage this risk. By the mid-1990s, HMO consolidations served to increase managed care's bargaining power over providers in local markets. Providers responded to this threat by forming vertical alliances to pose a countervailing force (Burns et al., 1997). Finally, by the 2000s, hospitals sought out physicians to promote quality improvement and clinical integration.

Physician-hospital alliances take many forms, which contribute to the growing list of acronyms managers must now understand. The two most prominent forms are physician-hospital organizations (PHOs) and integrated salary models (ISMs). PHOs constitute joint ventures designed to develop new services (e.g., ambulatory care clinic) or, more commonly, attract managed-care contracts. ISMs constitute vertically integrated arrangements in which the hospital acquires the physician's practice, establishes an employment contract with the physician for a defined period, and negotiates a guaranteed base salary with a variable component based on office productivity, with some expectation (or anticipation) that the physician will refer or admit patients to the hospital.

Besides PHOs and ISMs, there is now a growing, diverse array of alliance relationships developing between these two parties (Burns and Muller, 2008). The relationships fall into three broad categories: noneconomic integration, economic integration, and clinical integration. Noneconomic integration includes marketing of physicians' practices, medical office buildings, physician liaison programs, physician leadership development, and catering to physicians' technology requests. Economic integration includes the PHO and ISM models above as well as physician recruitment, part-time compensation, leases and participating bond transactions, service line development, equity joint ventures, and funds flow models. Clinical integration, finally, encompasses practice profiling, performance feedback, medical/demand/disease management programs, continuous quality improvement programs, and linkages via clinical information systems.

These alliances are pursued by each party for many reasons, only some of which overlap. Hospitals pursue physician alliances to capture their outpatient markets, to increase their revenues and margins, to improve care processes and outcomes, to increase the loyalty of their physicians, to bolster physicians' practices and incomes, and to address pathologies in the traditional hospital medical staff. Physicians likewise enter these alliances to increase their practice incomes and improve the quality of service to patients. But after this, their goals diverge from those of the hospitals. Physicians also want to increase their access to capital and technology, to increase their control in care delivery, and to increase their own lifestyle satisfaction.

How well have these alliances performed? If success is gauged by provider interest, alliances are doing quite well. There is a plethora of such alliance arrangements with considerable diffusion of several of their forms. Other evidence, however, suggests that alliances have yet to demonstrate their promise. A review of the empirical literature suggests that alliances based on economic integration exert few consistent impacts on cost, quality, or clinical integration. Alliances based on noneconomic integration are widespread but have not been subjected to rigorous academic study. Finally, alliances based on clinical integration are developing with positive, but weaker-than-expected impacts on quality of care (Burns and Muller, 2008).

Why are the results so disappointing, especially given the prevalence of alliances and the attention received in the literature? One reason is the structural form used to implement the alliance. These alliances are typically organized, financed, and controlled by the hospital, with little physician participation. Not surprisingly, physicians balk at partnerships in which they have not participated. A second, related explanation is the lack of infrastructure found in many alliances. Too often, hospitals will develop the alliances as external contracting vehicles to approach the managed-care market, but fail to develop the internal mechanisms that will help the alliance partners to manage risk (Kale and Singh, 2009). Such mechanisms include physician compensation and productivity systems, quality monitoring and measurement, and physician selection (Burns and Thorpe, 1997). Third, the alliances have often served as vehicles to leverage managed care payers, and thus run afoul of antitrust actions taken by the Federal Trade Commission (FTC) and Department of Justice (DOJ) (Casalino, 2006). Fourth, alliances often focus on taking advantage of fee-for-service reimbursement systems and seeking to increase patient and procedural volumes, rather than delivering more appropriate care.

These findings suggest that implementation of the alliance and careful attention to developing its infrastructure is critical for the success of any alliance that physicians and hospitals form. In the absence of the mechanisms discussed above, one would expect alliances to exert little impact on hospital quality and cost of care. In fact, two recent studies have addressed this issue directly. Cuellar and Gertler (2005) and Madison (2004) report that PHO alliances do not lower the cost of care.

Indeed, they may lead to higher prices paid for care (for either the hospital or its physicians) due to the combined bargaining leverage of the two parties in the integrated delivery network (IDN) model. Moreover, there is no evidence that alliances improve quality of care, and in fact, may damage it.

# THE ALLIANCE PROCESS: A MULTISTAGE ANALYSIS

Early studies of alliances focused primarily on why they emerge, how they are structured, and what they do. More attention has been given recently to the **alliance process**— how alliances evolve and behave over time (D'Aunno and Zuckerman, 1987a; de Rond, 2003; Kale and Singh, 2009; Luke, Begun, and Pointer, 1989; Provan, 1984; Sofaer and Myrtle, 1991; Zajac and Olsen, 1993). Based on this work, we develop a life-cycle model that managers can use to understand how alliances develop as they do and what can be done to improve their chances for success (Table 11.2). This model suggests that organizations often move through predictable stages of development, with one or more factors triggering such movement. Further, each stage brings distinctive tasks that alliance leaders and members need to address.

## Emergence: Finding Partners

In the first stage, environmental threats, opportunities, and uncertainty lead organizations with similar ideologies and dependencies to seek out each other. Further, this dance often begins when the potential partners relate to each other symbiotically as well as competitively (Hawley, 1950; Pfeffer and Salancik, 1978). In other words, alliances may be more likely to emerge when potential partners have complementary relationships such that one organization uses some services or products of the other as opposed to the case when two organizations are vying for the same resources. A common example of such complementarity or symbiosis is a rural community hospital that refers cases for tertiary care to an urban teaching hospital. A recent review of 40 studies of alliances concluded that the complementarity of partners not only promotes alliance formation, but also contributes to alliance performance (Shah and Swaminathan, 2008).

Interorganizational exchange processes involve distinct stages (Zajac and Olsen, 1993). For example, in the early stage, each organization engages in the process of projecting exchange into the future and constructing net present valuations of

## TABLE 11.2  A Life Cycle Model of Organizational Alliances in Health Care

| Stages | | | |
|---|---|---|---|
| Emergence | Transition | Maturity | Critical Crossroads |
| Key Factors in Development at Each Stage | | | |
| Environment poses threat to and uncertainty about valued resources | Motivation to achieve purposes of the alliance | Willingness to put alliance interests first | Increased centralization and dependence on alliance motivates members to seek hierarchy or to withdraw from alliance |
| Organizations share ideologies and similar dependencies | Increased dependence on alliance for valued resources | Members receive benefits from previous investments | |
| Examples of Tasks at Each Stage | | | |
| Define purposes of the alliance | Hire or form a management group | Attain stated objectives | Manage decisions about future of the alliance |
| Develop membership criteria | Establish mechanisms for coordination and control | Sustain member commitment | |

alternative exchange relationships on a continuum ranging from markets (i.e., arm's-length transactions with another independent organization), through strategic alliances (i.e., a formal cooperative arrangement between organizations, preserving the independent identity of each partner), and finally to hierarchies (i.e., the merging of two or more organizations into one organization) (Macneil, 1983). Perceptions of what each exchange partner seeks also emerge more clearly, enabling the more precise identification of similarities and differences that can form the basis for mutually beneficial exchange.

Thus, in the early stage, there is preliminary communication and negotiation concerning mutual and individual organizational interests. As a result, the partners learn not only about each other's interests, but also about their compatibility—that is, the fit between their working styles and cultures. An organization's behavior in this stage can set a precedent for future exchange and provide information through which a firm can learn about the expected behavior of its partner. During this phase, initial relational exchange norms are being forged and commitments tested in small but important ways to determine credibility (Macneil, 1983). To summarize, in this initial stage, the purposes and expectations

of the partners are stated, membership criteria are established, and group norms begin to evolve.

Though it is important for expectations to be realistic, it turns out that many young alliances have broadly stated goals that do not necessarily coincide with their activities. This is because goal statements reflect compromises made among members who are, as of yet, not willing to subordinate their interests to those of the group as a whole. Further, broad goal statements may attract other partners, and early members want to have the advantages that popularity typically affords.

Thus, in many cases, the criteria for alliance membership are selective and designed to ensure homogeneity among members. This reduces some of the governance and management problems discussed above. Further, many alliances seek to limit overlap in market areas so as to minimize competition among members and avoid antitrust issues.

At this initial stage, most alliances are not likely to form or hire a management group to direct their activities (D'Aunno and Zuckerman, 1987a), because organizations must initially identify and agree on a set of purposes. Organizations are also reluctant to yield authority and commit resources to a management group. Nonetheless, this is typically what happens in the second stage of alliance development.

## Transition

In this stage, the alliance establishes mechanisms for decision making and overall control of its activities or what is generally termed governance (Kale and Singh, 2009). Governance mechanisms include (1) joint ownership, in which the partners share control of some or all alliance assets; (2) contracts that specify the rights and obligations of alliance partners; (3) informal agreements that rely on trust and goodwill; or (4) some combination of these (Puranam and Vanneste, 2009). Research to date does not suggest that any one of these mechanisms is superior, but rather that it is important to match an approach to governance to the particular needs of an alliance. Informal agreements may work effectively, for example, when the partners know each other well and the alliance activities are not complex or do not involve a high degree of risk. In any case, establishing a governance mechanism may be rocky because, as just noted, organizations are reluctant to grant authority to others or to sacrifice their own autonomy. It is thus critical that alliance managers ensure that their efforts and programs are responsive to members' needs so as to build their commitment to the alliance.

Alliances vary in the extent to which their members are willing to commit resources to initiate and sustain programs and activities. An important weakness of many alliances is their inability to gain adequate commitment of members' resources. For example, there may be free-rider problems in that some members make little commitment but yet can benefit from the investments of others. It is likely that such problems are directly proportional to the value that members perceive in committing resources to the alliance. The more value that members perceive from active participation, the more resources (including autonomy) they are willing to commit to the alliance.

Of course, this leads to a challenging "chicken-and-egg" dilemma. On the one hand, members increase their commitment in proportion to threats from their environment and the alliance's ability to reduce threats and uncertainty. On the other hand, for the alliance to be effective in meeting members' needs, it may require the investment of valued resources from members as well as their willingness to coordinate efforts with each other. At some point, alliances require an investment of resources that are risked by members who have no certainty of return equal to their investment. At this point, trust becomes particularly important.

## Maturity

The third stage of an alliance's life cycle is that of maturity and growth. In this stage, it is critical that the alliance begins to achieve its objectives and aid members in coping with external threats. Such success enables an alliance to continue and to grow. It is also central that members be willing to put the interests of the alliance, at least sometimes, ahead of their own interests. This is necessary because alliances cannot meet the needs of all of their members, at least not simultaneously. Members must recognize that they will not necessarily benefit equally from alliance activities; it is essential, however, that they benefit as equitably as possible.

Successful alliances seem to share two key characteristics at this stage of development: a dedicated manager or group of managers who focus exclusively on alliance work, and processes that enable an alliance to learn from its experience and to build capabilities (Hoang and Rothaermel, 2005; Kale and Singh, 2009). Dedicated alliance managers play several roles. They promote work on important projects, including garnering resources; they signal the legitimacy of the alliance both to its members and to external stakeholders; they monitor performance and progress toward objectives and provide timely feedback to members. Finally, alliance managers may develop tools and processes that enable the alliance to learn from its experience. These processes may include, for example, regular meetings to review factors that have contributed to success and failure in alliance projects. Tools that codify this learning include guidelines, checklists, and manuals that specify best practices and make future projects more efficient and effective.

As alliances seek to attain objectives and sustain member commitment, several issues may arise. For example, alliances that add many members may find it impossible to avoid having members with overlapping market areas. If such overlap does occur, what role, if any, should the alliance play in mediating disputes that may arise among members?

Relationships between the members and alliance managers (if there are any) also become more complex. For example, are new programs initiated through the alliance manager's office, through individual members, or both? If through the alliance office, what happens to similar programs already developed by individual members? For instance, suppose that a hospital alliance wishes to develop an alliance-wide HMO, but some members already have HMOs. Further, are there or should there be incentives for members to produce innovative programs that can be shared by all alliance members? In the absence of such incentives, how will the alliance develop innovations in management or services?

Zajac and Olsen (1993), in their discussion of the development of interorganizational relationships, note that alliances in this stage of development face some particularly sensitive issues because value is not only created, but also claimed and distributed. Surrounding the issue of claiming and distributing value is the question of interorganizational conflict. Explicit or implicit norms for managing the divergence of interest will often arise (Zajac and Olsen, 1993). To the extent that these norms—defined as "shared and reasoned expectations that may arise from agreement or past acts"—emphasize the importance of joint value maximization, this should lead to searches for mutually satisfactory resolutions of conflict situations (Kaufmann, 1987). On the other hand, if these evolving norms do not develop in this way, the pursuit of individual firm interests would lead to an escalation of conflict that could ultimately be destructive to the strategic alliance. The accepted use of conflict-resolution systems can limit the potential damage of interorganizational conflict (Ury, Brett, and Goldberg, 1988).

The continued development of trust is a key issue in this stage of interorganizational exchange. Trust stems from a growing confidence in a firm's expectations of the future (Luhmann, 1979). Schelling (1960) also notes that "trust is often achieved simply by the continuity of the relation between parties and the recognition by each that what he might gain by cheating in a given instance is outweighed by the value of the tradition of trust that makes possible a long sequence of future agreement."

Trust and conflict-management systems are subsets of other relational norms underlying the process exchange over time. These norms include shared expectations of reciprocity between alliance partners and a growing sense of the value of preserving the relationship (Macneil, 1983, 1986). These norms set the tone for the continued execution of either contracts or informal agreements.

## Critical Crossroads

As they evolve into the fourth stage of development, alliances move to what may be a critical crossroads. Up to this point,

members became increasingly dependent on each other for needed resources, and there was growing pressure for greater member commitment to the alliance and more centralized decision making. In many ways, however, these developments run counter to the reasons why many organizations join an alliance. That is, alliances are attractive because they provide a relatively low-cost vehicle to reduce resource dependence while maintaining organizational autonomy. Thus, this stage may be a critical crossroads at which some members conclude that the price of belonging to an alliance is too high and withdraw. Indeed, it appears that at least one hospital alliance collapsed precisely on this point (Ury, Brett, and Goldberg, 1988). In contrast, others may decide that it is necessary to move toward more hierarchical arrangements to gain the full benefits of collective action.

The underlying issue is whether there is sufficient commitment or "glue" to hold alliances together over time (Zuckerman and Kaluzny, 1991). Though there may be common goals, ideologies, values, and inducements that keep members together, alliances typically remain loose arrangements. Can the degree of commitment required of members be secured in the long run? Will members be willing to sacrifice autonomy to allow for greater discipline in decision making? What coordination mechanisms are most appropriate and under what circumstances (Alter and Hage, 1993; Kaluzny and Zuckerman, 1992)? To survive, alliances must balance the need for and benefits of collective action with the need for individual members to retain adequate autonomy.

This critical crossroads represents a reconfiguring stage in the developmental process of a strategic alliance (Zajac and Olsen, 1993). It is usually triggered by reaching the end of the expected duration of the relationship or by changes in the partners' perceived level of the relationship's value. Reconfiguring may imply that an exchange partner will choose to leave, or it may mean that partners will join more tightly together by widening the scope of interorganizational exchange processes. For example, a group of hospitals may move from a shared purchasing arrangement to developing a joint preferred provider network.

With respect to perceived changes in the value of the strategic alliance, such changes may emerge from a new and changing environment or a historical comparison of actual to expected value creation. While this performance gap can lead to a reevaluation (positive or negative) of the interorganizational relationship itself, it may simply lead to a reassessment of the developmental processes. In other words, the reconfiguring stage may not involve a change in the type of strategic alliance per se, but only a change in the process of interaction within the existing strategic alliance. These change options suggest that this stage may loop back to either the emergence stage, where value forecasts are re-specified and strategic motivations are clarified for a new forecast period, or the transition stage, where the forms of exchange are revised and updated based on the continued experiences of the partners. Thus, the process model of strategic alliance development outlined here does not propose a one-way, deterministic path for alliances; indeed, we agree with de Rond (2003), who argued on the basis of several careful case studies of alliances, that their development is often complex and nonlinear. Nonetheless, the model presented here highlights a sequence of likely phases that many alliances may experience and emphasizes a set of critical issues that health care organizations may face at the various stages of alliance development.

# FRAMEWORKS FOR ANALYZING ALLIANCE PROBLEMS

A major difficulty that organizations face in addressing alliance problems is actually their inability to identify the problem correctly. By that we mean that individuals within an organization often do not know, or disagree strongly on, what the problem is, and this is compounded by differences of opinion between partners in alliance problem identification and diagnosis. These disagreements, we contend, can often lead to false diagnoses and the treatment of **alliance symptoms** rather than the root **alliance problems** facing the alliance. These incorrect interventions subsequently lead to greater friction, gridlock, and, ultimately, an increased likelihood of alliance failure (see Case at the end of the chapter). The three simple frameworks offered below are intended to lessen the likelihood of such failure.

## Locating the Problem

If one were to ask several involved individuals why a particular alliance was in trouble, it is possible that one would get a uniform response. In such cases, locating the problem is simple. We argue, however, that such agreement is the exception rather than the norm. Typically there are a host of possible reasons why an alliance might be facing difficulties.

Without some way of organizing these reasons, there may be little hope of remedying the situation. We propose that alliance problems can be viewed as generally falling into the following categories (Johnson, 1986):

- Environmental problems
- Strategy problems
- Structure problems
- Behavior problems

These categories follow a macro-to-micro continuum, but more important for purposes of this chapter, they also tend to follow an uncontrollable-to-controllable continuum.

Consider the problems in health care alliances that require collaboration among professional groups with different training, time horizons, and economic incentives. For example, trading alliances between physicians and hospitals are particularly vulnerable to these difficulties. An analysis of six integrated systems in Illinois suggests that physician-hospital alliances have polarities to be resolved rather than problems to be solved (Burns, 1999). These polarities consist of nine areas in which the integrated system must seek to manage in two directions simultaneously (i.e., pursue the physicians' interests simultaneously with the hospital's interests). For example, the hospital system seeks to expose its physicians to practicing in a risk-based environment; at the same time, it is purchasing primary care physicians who are then given guaranteed salaries for several years—in effect, exempting them from all risk. As another example, the hospital system wishes to become "an organization of physicians," and yet the system is developed and controlled almost exclusively by hospital executives and serves primarily hospital purposes in the short term. For such alliances to be credible to physicians and work effectively, they need to satisfy the interests of both parties simultaneously. In terms of our framework, the problems lie not in uncontrollable environmental issues, or in the basic strategy of deepening physician-hospital relationships, but in the fundamental structural decisions made and the behavioral problems created or exacerbated by those structural decisions. The framework can be particularly valuable in highlighting disagreement as to what fundamental problems are facing a strategic alliance.

### Illustration from U.S. Memories

In 1990, a consortium called U.S. Memories was conceived to provide a secure supply of chips for U.S. computer makers who were unhappy with the occasional shortages and price fluctuations brought on by Japanese chip makers, who controlled almost 90 percent of the DRAM market. This alliance, made up of U.S. chip buyers and a few U.S. chip makers, never got off the ground, as initial players backed out and new players refused to commit resources. Analysts offered several reasons as to why the alliance failed. Some attributed the failure to the fact that, once the temporary chip shortage was over, the alliance had no purpose. Others said it was ill conceived and that the United States could never have competed with the more efficient Japanese chip makers. Some said that not enough players were involved; some said *too many* players were involved; and others said that the deal was not well structured. Finally, some blamed the leader of the consortium, saying that he was not well suited for such a position.

What do we make out of this mess? Could this alliance have been salvaged? Basically, we can start by using the framework above to categorize the myriad of alliance problems into environmental ("the market changed"), strategic ("it was a bad idea from the beginning"), structural ("it wasn't organized correctly"), and behavioral ("we had the wrong person at the top") problems. The point here is that, from a managerial perspective, a person responsible for gathering information about the alliance, processing that information, and making a decision on whether or how to intervene, can begin to piece together problems into useful clusters or categories.

Second, the categories themselves are useful in assessing the degree to which intervention can be effective. For example, after analyzing the categorized reasons, a manager may believe that the primary problem is environmental—that is, the market conditions no longer support the alliance. This is largely an uncontrollable factor and, therefore, suggests that the alliance is not likely to succeed. On the other hand, the manager may believe the primary problem is structural—that the number or composition of the alliance is not right, or that the incentives for participation are inadequate. This is more of a controllable factor and suggests that the alliance can be modified and thus face improved odds for success. In this way, the Environment → Strategy → Structure → Behavior framework can be a useful tool in identifying and diagnosing alliance problems.

## Separating the Root Cause from the Symptom

If you had a rash and were to go to a physician, what would be the first thing the physician would do? Would the physician treat the rash, or first ask a set of questions to discern why you have the rash? Hopefully, the latter approach is the more common. Unfortunately, many organizations involved in strategic alliances take the former approach. There is a problem; let us fix it. This "can do" attitude is laudable in one sense, but potentially reckless (possibly even rash) in another sense. Specifically, when one observes friction in strategic alliances, we argue that the most important response is to first delve more deeply to understand the source of that friction before attempting to treat the problem.

This advice regarding diagnosis before treatment may seem obvious, but it often is not done in alliances. The reason it is often not done stems from alliance partners' unwillingness or inability to put themselves in their partners' shoes. By this we mean that signs of noncooperative behavior from a partner are often viewed with hostility on the part of other partners. The other partners then devise their own response strategy before an analysis or diagnosis is done as to why the partner may appear to be acting noncooperatively. Quite simply, we are stating that the noncooperative behavior is only a symptom of a deeper problem.

The obvious questions then become, "What could the deeper problems be, and how do we treat them?" We propose that there are several classes of problems:

1. Parochial self-interest or cheating behavior

2. Misunderstanding, cultural clashes, and a lack of trust

3. Different assessments, asymmetric investments, and temporary alliance arrangements without a long-term plan

4. Alliance performance ambiguity and low tolerance for such ambiguity

5. Overly optimistic expectations of alliance performance

6. Weak infrastructure and strategic management of the alliance, or lack of alliance experience

These categories, interestingly, match discussions of problems that exist in managing change (Kotter and Schlesinger, 1979). While the categories are not mutually exclusive, they are quite distinct from one another. For example, the first category represents rational, calculative, noncooperative behavior in which one partner knowingly acts in his own interest to the detriment of the other partner. The second type of problem is based less on selfishness than on the absence of accepted and well-developed norms; that is, a trusting relationship between partners has yet to emerge, and cultural clashes dominate.

The third category differs from the first in that, while the first category (i.e., selfish, noncooperative behavior) reflects disagreement on ends and means, the third category reflects agreement on ends but not means. In other words, partners may share the same goal but diverge in their views on how to achieve that goal. They consequently make different investments in the alliance relationship. Fourth, some alliance partners simply feel uncomfortable with the ambiguity and fluidity of alliances. The absence of full control, as is typical in strategic alliances, may not agree with some reluctant partners. The fifth category reflects the partners' initial euphoria with alliance formation without anticipating its subsequent problems, while the sixth category reflects the failure of the partners to sufficiently invest in alliance management and development.

Identifying different categories of problems is in and of itself useful as a way to move beyond the symptom and toward the problem. Treating the problem is the next step, and we propose a simple principle: the treatment should match the problem. Again, while this seems obvious, we find that all too often in alliances the treatment is either insufficient or too harsh. Both of these situations are unfavorable. There are at least 10 ways of dealing with alliance problems:

- Partner selection and due diligence
- Education
- Participation and sharing of alliance management
- Facilitation negotiation
- Swapping capabilities
- Exchange of personnel and information
- Cooptation
- Coercion
- Strategic implementation of the alliance
- Knowledge accumulation

Matching this set of treatments with the set of problems identified earlier represents a step toward effective alliance management (Kotter and Schlesinger, 1979). Consider the case where a partner faces a particularly calculative, self-interested partner. That partner is not lacking information; he knows what the situation is but does not want what his partner wants. In this case, an approach that emphasizes negotiation or cooptation is likely to be more effective than one that emphasizes participation or education. Contrast such a case with a partner whose actions are based on a misunderstanding. Here, negotiation as a response does not address the root problem; education and participation are more appropriate. We invite the reader to draw further matches between problem and treatment.

## Know Thy Partner

A third framework that can be useful in addressing potential and ongoing alliance problems focuses more directly at understanding your partner's "type." Specifically, we suggest that it is a mistake to assume that your partner thinks about your alliance the same way that you do. Ideally, you will know what type of alliance partner you are dealing with at the earliest stages of the alliance. Unfortunately, it is our experience that many times a partner fails to take into adequate account the variety of partner types or **partner orientations** that exist. In our experience, there are five types of partners, ranging from the most desirable to the least desirable; each is discussed briefly below.

### The Cooperative Partner

This partner is primarily interested in maximizing the joint gains in the alliance relationship, and recognizes that such maximization requires attention to what you need to achieve in the alliance. Thus, this partner will work with you in helping you achieve your goals, as well as his own. This is what you hope you have in an alliance partner, but it may be rarer than one thinks. This partner sees the alliance as win-win, and is interested in seeing that both sides win. A major pharmaceutical firm embodies this philosophy with the goal of being "the partner of choice" for biotech firms. This company employs numerous alliance managers who see their role as "omsbudspersons" for the alliance.

### The Quasi-Cooperative Partner

This partner is interested in making sure that you receive just enough value from the alliance so that you will not exit. By providing you with the minimally acceptable amount of value, you still prefer the alliance above other alternatives, but not by much. This relationship is unbalanced in terms of power and dependence, but can be stable, albeit not as rewarding for the weaker party. This partner sees the alliance in terms of keeping you interested, but barely.

## The Indifferent Partner

This partner—for better or worse—is not particularly interested in your strategic aspirations at all. The partner sees the alliance primarily as a vehicle for the achievement of that partner's strategic goals, and you are simply along for the ride. The partner has no objections to your expending effort for your purposes, as long as (1) he does not need to help you do this, and (2) the attainment of his objectives are not impeded as a result. This partner sees the alliance in terms of "I'll get mine, you find yours."

## The Competitive Partner

This partner is worse than indifferent, insofar as he perceives your gains as implying a loss for him, even when really there is no such tradeoff. This person is oblivious to the positive-sum possibilities of the alliance, and very sensitive to the zero-sum aspects. This partner cannot abide any asymmetry in alliance success that might favor you, even if such variation is a natural or short-term occurrence. This partner is so fixated on the relative comparison aspects of the relationship that he sees the alliance in terms of "your gain must mean my loss." Another major pharmaceutical firm had this philosophy, in that managers in this firm viewed a win-win alliance situation as one in which they felt they had "left money on the table." They would often seek to renegotiate win-win alliances.

## The Vengeful Partner

This partner is even worse than a competitive partner, because he is primarily focused on ensuring that you lose, even if he loses, as well. You might not think that such partners exist, and it is unlikely that you would knowingly ally with such a partner; but a partner can develop this orientation when problems in the alliance become personalized and negative emotion plays a larger role. Note that we readily accept the notion of positive emotion in alliances when we claim that trust between partners is a beneficial aspect of an alliance relationship. However, we suggest that when one partner feels that the other has somehow violated that trust, a sense of betrayal emerges that can lead a partner to act irrationally. This partner sees the alliance in terms of "I may lose, but you'll lose more." While this is admittedly rare, several alliances have had protracted legal battles when one party feels that the other party did not act "in good faith."

## Partner Assessment

As you can see, there are multiple partner types, and most of them are not particularly attractive. So, how can you "know thy partner" in advance? First and foremost, you must pay careful attention during the alliance emergence process for cues from your alliance partner that suggest one type versus another. For example, we have observed in working with health care organizations that some alliance partners have little idea what their partners' strategic goals are. A cooperative partner would know this, and a lack of interest in the partner's goals is an early indication that your partner is indifferent, or worse. Similarly, explore with your partner alternative scenarios for the alliance, including some in which you do better initially, and gauge your partner's reaction. If your partner objects to the slightest asymmetries in alliance outcomes, this suggests a problem that will likely emerge again and again.

Finally, assuming you are comfortable with your partner's orientation at the inception of the alliance, you must still be vigilant to changes in that orientation that may arise due to changes in the context of the alliance, whether it be changes in environmental conditions or in personnel. Ideally, this type of "early warning system" will serve you well as the alliance relationship evolves. However, we also encourage you to utilize another valuable feature of strategic alliances: Be sure to have a clear written statement of exit provisions, by which you and your partner can extricate yourselves from an alliance that may no longer be serving its intended valued purpose.

# ALLIANCE CAPABILITIES AND PERFORMANCE DRIVERS

Hundreds of studies in the past two decades have examined factors that can promote and inhibit the success of alliances (Kale and Singh, 2009). We discussed several of these factors above, but it is useful to summarize them here and to consider some key capabilities that alliances need to be successful. Factors that affect alliance success can be grouped into the first three stages of the life-cycle model depicted in Table 11.2: emergence, transition, and maturity.

In the stage of emergence, or alliance formation, three characteristics of partners are critical. Specifically, alliance success depends, as noted above, on the extent to which partners are complementary such that one organization uses some services or products of the other, as opposed to the case when two or more organizations are vying for the same resources. Similarly, alliances will be more successful to the extent that partners are compatible, sharing similar cultures, expectations, and capabilities. A third partner characteristic that seems critical to success is commitment, the extent to which each partner wants to make the relationship work well.

In the next stage of alliance development, or what Kale and Singh (2009) term the phase of governance and design, results from many studies show that alliance success depends on the extent to which partners can find effective and efficient ways to coordinate and control their joint efforts. Three approaches are particularly useful: shared ownership of some or all of alliance projects; contracts that specify the rights and obligations of partners; and goodwill and trust among the partners. Unfortunately, as noted above, research to date does not suggest that any one of these mechanisms is superior, but rather that it is important to match an approach to governance to the particular needs of an alliance.

Finally, in the stage that we term maturity, research results show that alliance success depends on the extent to which mechanisms for coordinating alliance projects (that were established in the transition or design stage) work well and, perhaps more importantly, trust develops among partners. In turn, trust is important because it is more or less inevitable that conflicts or disagreements among partners will occur, and they are more likely to be resolved effectively to the extent that the partners trust each other. Nonetheless, even without high levels of trust, or perhaps especially when trust levels are low, it is important to have mechanisms in place to deal with conflicts or disagreements (e.g., regular meetings that are dedicated specifically to reviewing and resolving potential and actual disagreements). Of course, in the absence of trust, it will be difficult to establish even straightforward mechanisms to deal with disagreements among alliance partners.

Underlying many of the factors noted above are two fundamental capabilities that seem to drive alliances' success. The first is a dedicated manager or group of managers who focus exclusively on alliance work and processes (Hoang and Rothaermel, 2005; Kale and Singh, 2009). For example, one important task for these managers is to monitor performance and progress toward objectives on projects and provide timely feedback to members.

Second, alliances and their members need to be able to learn from their experience and to build additional capabilities as needed. Learning processes may include, for example, regular meetings to review factors that have contributed to success and failure in alliance projects. Further, tools are needed to codify this learning and may include guidelines, checklists, and manuals that specify best practices and make future projects more efficient and effective.

In sum, research on alliances in the past 20 years has produced useful results that can guide managerial action (see the Summary and Managerial Guidelines). Together with the frameworks for analyzing alliance problems introduced above, understanding factors and capabilities that often drive alliance success provides a strong foundation for effective managerial action.

# SUMMARY AND MANAGERIAL GUIDELINES

1. In assessing the risk of forming or entering an alliance, managers should compare the potential costs and benefits of alliances to doing nothing or to alternative strategies that involve going it alone; alliances may well be less risky than other strategies.

2. The form or structure of alliance should follow from its function—that is, what it is intended to do.

3. Managers should consider their options with respect to several important aspects of alliance structure, including ownership and control, number of members, governance structure, and mandated versus voluntary participation.

4. Many of the benefits of control in interorganizational relationships can be achieved without ownership; trust, commitment, and even power may be important substitutes for control based on ownership.

5. Increased size brings greater complexity and often more difficulty in coordinating efforts, but larger alliances tend to be more powerful for certain purposes (e.g., lobbying, purchasing in volume).

6.  Large alliances often need more complex governance structures, and a key issue is who will be represented on an alliance board. It may be a mistake to have only CEOs or executive directors on alliance boards because the interests of other groups may be neglected; further, turnover among top managers is common and may disrupt the alliance if the board has no other types of members.

7.  Mandated participation in an alliance is often less preferable to voluntary participation. Alliances are not likely to succeed if members' only or most important motive for participation is to comply with external demands.

8.  Recognize that alliances can be created to achieve one or more of the following objectives: to pool similar resources (e.g., as in joint purchasing arrangements); to trade dissimilar resources (e.g., as in a symbiotic relationship between a hospital and physician group); to reduce costs; to enhance revenues; to promote innovation, learning, or quality of services; or to enhance power, reduce uncertainty, or share risks among members.

9.  From the above list, it is important to understand your own motives for seeking an alliance and to express these motives to potential or current partners.

10. Similarly, managers need to listen carefully to the intentions of potential or current partners in order to assess compatibility; failure to articulate a shared mission is an important reason for alliance failure.

11. Two kinds of problems are typical when it comes to alliance objectives. First, even though alliance objectives may be shared by members, the objectives may conflict with each other, especially over time. Second, there may be a lack of consensus among members concerning alliance objectives. Both problems highlight the need for effective communication.

12. Recognize that alliances often develop in several stages, each of which brings distinctive threats and opportunities.

13. In the first stage (emergence), it is important to define the purposes of the alliance and select partners accordingly. Clear communication and acknowledgment of interests are critical.

14. After forming an alliance, managers must find ways to coordinate and control activities; this may entail hiring or forming a management group to focus specifically on alliance concerns.

15. As alliances mature, managers are likely to face complex issues about how much individual members must conform to and, indeed, place alliance interests ahead of their own. Further, there may be conflict about how to distribute the benefits (resources) that alliances have generated. Thus, managers need to focus on ways to sustain member commitment through trust, goal attainment, and the use of appropriate mechanisms to resolve conflict.

16. Mature alliances face the task of measuring up to members' original and changing expectations. Such alliances need to rethink their structure and objectives to make sure that they keep pace with members' needs.

17. More specifically, managers can diagnose alliance problems according to whether they are primarily environmental (i.e., stemming from external sources such as shift in market demands); strategic (i.e., concerning the overall purpose and direction of the alliance); structural (i.e., alliance form fits poorly with its purposes); or behavioral (i.e., skills are not adequate for carrying out alliance activities).

18. It is important to match alliance problems with appropriate means to deal with them, ranging from educating members, to negotiating with them, to coercing them.

19. Alliances can be just a management fad—be careful that you are forming one for the right reasons.

20. Recognize that alliances have their costs for managers in terms of time spent in understanding and negotiating with potential and current partners. In fact, alliances can slow decision making and make organizations less flexible—precisely what they are designed to avoid.

21. Select partners and develop ways of relating to them so as to avoid charges of collusion and antitrust problems.

22. Do not let alliance arrangements make your organization lazy and lose its interest in continuous improvement.

# DISCUSSION QUESTIONS

1. Under what circumstances would you agree with someone who said that alliances are very risky?

2. What dimensions would you use to classify the various types of strategic alliances? Why those dimensions?

3. Which alliance motivations do you think are the most compatible with each other?

4. What do you consider to be the likely stages of strategic alliance development? Does every alliance have to go through each stage?

5. What is the difference between an alliance problem and an alliance symptom, and what does this difference mean in terms of managerial intervention?

6. When can you tell if your partner is not likely to have a cooperative orientation?

## CASE: Strategic Alliances in the Pharmaceutical and Biotechnology Industry

In the past two decades, strategic alliances have become an important tool for pharmaceutical and biotechnology firms as they face increased competition, increased public scrutiny of their business practices and profits, and difficulties discovering new products. There is empirical evidence that products developed in strategic alliances have a higher probability of success in Phase II and Phase III clinical trials than products developed independently by either the pharmaceutical or biotechnology firm (Danzon, Nicholson, and Pereira, 2005). Co-development of new drugs via an alliance adds value that outweighs any potential moral hazard problems arising from the two partners sharing development responsibilities (Nicholson, Danzon, and McCullough, 2005). In 2001–2002 alone, there were 923 new (publicly announced) strategic alliances in this industry. This figure includes biotech-biotech, biotech-pharma, and pharma-pharma alliances, and each type offers different benefits to its partners.

For example, in the realm of biotech-pharma alliances, a recent report focusing on licensing alliances between biotech and pharma firms suggests that "the number of biopharmaceutical licensing alliances has remained fairly constant over the past several years, but their value trebled from $30 billion USD to $90 billion USD between 2004 to 2007" (Business Insights. [2009]. *Evolving Trends in Biopharmaceutical Licensing: Deal Assessments, Drivers, and Resistors*. March. Retrieved August 15, 2010, from http://www.globalbusinessinsights.com).

Of the 923 alliances mentioned above, a large number of new alliances (217) occurred between pharmaceutical and biotechnology firms, probably reflecting pharmaceutical firms' needs for access to new products that the smaller, but more research-intensive, biotechnology firms have been generating. These are typically trading alliances that allow pharmaceutical firms to gain access to innovations, while enabling biotechnology firms to gain access to capital, clinical trial expertise, and the marketing capabilities that pharmaceutical firms possess (Danzon et al., 2005). Some support for the view that pharmaceutical firms are using alliances to gain access to technical innovations is found in the fact that almost one-third of the new alliances involved genomics, the path-breaking science that can be used to develop treatments tailored to individuals' genetic types, making them highly effective.

Of course, one can also observe individual biotech-pharma alliances evolving over longer periods of time, as is the case with Gen-Probe and Chiron (now a Novartis company), which began their alliance in 1998 to "develop, manufacture, and commercialize" nucleic acid tests and instrumentation that have been used by blood banks for screening purposes. To date, more than 125 million blood donations have been screened in the United States alone, and "these tests have intercepted thousands of units of blood that were infected with HIV-1, hepatitis C and B, and West Nile virus, thereby preventing life-threatening diseases from being passed along to transfusion recipients" (Novartis Web site, press release, January 27, 2009). A striking feature of the collaboration between Chiron (Novartis) and Gen-Probe is the long-term orientation that both parties shared. The alliance was established in 1998 and was scheduled to expire in 2013, but was recently extended until 2025 (Novartis Web site, press release, January 27, 2009).

Novartis notes in that press release that under the original terms of the agreement, Gen-Probe was responsible for manufacturing costs, while Chiron was responsible for commercial expenses. The companies shared research and development (R&D) costs and shared revenue from the sale of blood-screening assays, and the revenue sharing agreement changed over time, as well.

Note that this very successful trading alliance between the two companies has adapted over the years, with multiple time and scope extensions since its inception. Gen-Probe now looks to Chiron (Novartis) to assist with their globalization efforts, highlighting that alliances are a flexible structure (not a strategy), through which multiple strategic initiatives can be implemented.

Indeed, a high proportion of new alliances (404 of the 923 mentioned above) were between partners who already had an ongoing relationship. New agreements among established partners may signal that the relationship has matured, as indicated in the life-cycle model of alliances presented in Table 11.2.

Interestingly, of the 923 alliances mentioned above, the highest percentage (one-third) occurred between biotechnology firms. This suggests that these relatively small firms found alliances to be an especially important strategy to build the scale (and perhaps scope) needed to compete and perform well. Biotechnology firms may be creating pooling alliances that can allow them to reduce uncertainty and enhance market power.

Finally, it appears that firms are using alliances to enhance their capabilities in key markets. Most new alliances that focused on a specific therapeutic area were focused in the area of oncology, where there is both high demand for new, more effective treatments and the willingness to pay high prices for them (Reuters Business Insight, 2004).

## Questions

1. What do you think are the possible major tensions that exist when a pharmaceutical firm forms an alliance with a biotechnology firm?

2. How would you try to address those tensions?

3. Identify different challenges that exist for maintaining or strengthening an ongoing alliance versus beginning a new relationship.

# REFERENCES

Alter, C., & Hage, J. (1993). *Organizations working together.* Beverly Hills, CA: Sage.

American College of Healthcare Executives. (2009). Hospital CEO turnover, 1981–2008. Chicago: ACHE.

Bazzoli, G. J., Chan, B., Shortell, S. M., & D'Aunno, T. (2000). The financial performance of hospitals belonging to health networks and systems. *Inquiry, 37,* 234–252.

Bazzoli, G. J., Shortell, S. M., Dubbs, N., Chan, B., & Kralovec, P. (1999). A taxonomy of health networks and systems: Bringing order out of chaos. *Health Services Research, 33*(6), 1683–1717.

Begun, J. W. (1992). Cooperative strategies weaken the competitive capabilities of health care organizations. In W. J. Duncan, P. M. Ginter, & L. E. Swayne (Eds.), *Strategic issues in health care management: Point and counterpoint* (pp. 44–50). Boston: PWS-KENT.

Burns, L. R. (1999). Polarity management: The key challenge for integrated delivery systems. *Journal of Healthcare Management, 44*(1), 14–33.

Burns, L. R., & Lee, J. A. (2008). Hospital purchasing alliances: Utilization, services, and performance. *Health Care Management Review, 33*(3), 203–215.

Burns, L. R., & Muller, R. W. (2008). Hospital-physician collaboration: Landscape of economic integration and impact on clinical integration. *Milbank Quarterly, 86*(3), 375–434.

Burns, L. R., & Pauly, M. V. (2002). Integrated delivery networks: A detour on the road to integrated health care? *Health Affairs, 21*(4), 128–143.

Burns, L. R., & Thorpe, D. P. (1997). Physician-hospital organizations: Strategy, structure, and conduct. In R. Conners (Ed.), *Integrating the practice of medicine* (pp. 351–371). Chicago: American Hospital Association Publishing.

Burns, L. R., Bazzoli, G. J., Dynan, L., & Wholey, D. R. (1997). Managed care, market stages, and integrated delivery systems: Is there a relationship? *Health Affairs, 16*, 204–218.

Burns, L. R., Cisneros, E. A., Ferniany, W., & Singh, H. (2010). Strategic alliances between buyers and suppliers: Lessons from the medical imaging industry. In C. Harland and E. Schneller (Eds.), *Handbook of the strategic management of supply*. Newbury Park, CA: Sage Publications.

Carman, J. M. (1992). *Strategic alliances among rural hospitals* (pp. 92–103). Berkeley: Institute of Business and Economic Research, University of California.

Casalino, L. P. (2006). The Federal Trade Commission, clinical integration, and the organization of physician practice. *Journal of Health Politics, Policy and Law, 31*, 569–585.

Clement, J. P. (1987). Does hospital diversification improve financial outcomes? *Medical Care, 25*, 988–1001.

Cuellar, A., & Gertier, P. (2005, January). How the expansion of hospital systems has affected consumers. *Health Affairs, 24*(1), 213–219.

D'Aunno.T. A., & Zuckerman, H. S. (1987a). The emergence of hospital federations: An integration of perspectives from organizational theory. *Medical Care Review, 44*(2), 323–343.

D'Aunno, T. A., & Zuckerman, H. S. (1987b). A life cycle model of organizational federations: The case of hospitals. *Academy of Management Review, 12*, 534–545.

Danzon, P. M., Nicholson, S., & Pereira, N. S. (2005). Productivity in pharmaceutical-biotechnology R&D: The role of experience and alliances. *Journal of Health Economics, 24*, 317–339.

De Rond, M. (2003). *Strategic alliances as social facts: Business, biotechnology and intellectual history*. Cambridge: Cambridge University Press.

DeVries, R. A. (1978). Strength in numbers. *Hospitals: Journal of the American Hospital Association, 55*, 81–84.

Doz, Y. L., & Hamel, G. (1998). *Alliance advantage: The art of creating value through partnering*. Boston: Harvard Business School Press.

Duncan, W. J., Ginter, P. M., & Swayne, L. E. (1992). *Strategic issues in health care management: Point and counterpoint*. Boston: PWS-KENT.

Emery, P., & Trist, E. (1965). The casual texture of organizational environments. *Human Relations, 18*, 21–32.

Fennell, M. L., & Alexander, T. A. (1989). Hospital governance and profound organizational change. *Medical Care Review, 46*(2), 157–187.

Harrigan, K. R. (1985). *Managing for joint venture success*. Lexington, MA: Lexington Books.

Hawley, A. H. (1950). *Human ecology: A theory of community structure*. New York: Ronald Press.

Hoang, H., & Rothaermel, F. (2005). The effects of general and partner-specific experience on joint R&D project performance. *Academy of Management Journal, 48*(2), 332–345.

Johnson, D. E. L. (1986). American healthcare systems. *Modern Healthcare, 16*, 78–82.

Kale, P., & Singh, H. (2009). Managing strategic alliances: What do we know now, and where do we go from here? *Academy of Management Perspectives, 23*(3), 45–62.

Kaluzny, A., & Zuckerman, H. (1992, Winter). Strategic alliances: Two perspectives for understanding their effects on health services. *Hospital and Health Services Administration, 37,* 477–490.

Kaluzny, A., Morrissey, J., & McKinney, M. (1990). Emerging organizational networks: The case of the community clinical oncology program. In S. Mick & associates (Eds.), *Innovation in health care delivery.* San Francisco: Jossey-Bass.

Kaluzny, A. D., Zuckerman, H. S., & Ricketts, T. C. (2002). *Partners: Forming strategic alliances in health care.* Washington, DC: Beard Books.

Kaufmann, P. J. (1987). Commercial exchange relationships and the "negotiator's dilemma." *Negotiation Journal, 3,* 73–80.

Kotter, J. P., & Schlesinger, L. A. (1979). Choosing strategies for change. *Harvard Business Review, 57,* 106–114.

Li, J., Zhou, C., & Zajac, E. J. (2009). Control, collaboration, and productivity in international joint ventures: Theory and evidence. *Strategic Management Journal, 30,* 865–884.

Longest, B. B. (1990). Interorganizational linkages in the health sector. *Health Care Management Review, 15,* 17–28.

Luhmann, N. (1979). *Trust and power.* New York: John Wiley and Sons.

Luke, R. D., Begun, J. W., & Pointer, D. D. (1989). Quasi firms: Strategic interorganizational forms in the health care industry. *Academy of Management Review, 14*(9), 19.

Macneil, I. R. (1983). Values in contract: Internal and external. *Northwestern University Law Review, 78,* 340–418.

Macneil, I. R. (1986). Exchange revisited: Individual utility and social solidarity. *Ethics, 96,* 567–593.

Madison, K. (2004). Hospital physician affiliations and patient treatments, expenditures, and outcomes. *Health Services Research, 39*(2).

Meyer, A. (1982). Adapting to environmental jolts. *Administrative Science Quarterly, 27,* 515–537.

Nicholson, S., Danzon, P. M., and McCullough, J. (2005). Biotech-pharmaceutical alliances as a signal of asset and firm quality. *Journal of Business, 78,* 1433–1464.

Olden, P. C., Roggenkamp, S. D., & Luke, R. D. (2002). A post-1990s assessment of strategic hospital alliances and their marketplace orientations: Time to refocus. *Health Care Management Review, 27*(2), 33–49.

Oliver, C. (1990). Determinants of interorganizational relationships: Integration and future directions. *Academy of Management Review, 15*(2), 241–265.

Pfeffer, J., & Salancik, G. R. (1978). *The external control of organizations: A resource dependence perspective.* New York: Harper & Row.

Provan, K. G. (1984). Interorganizational cooperation and decision making autonomy in a consortium multihospital system. *Academy of Management Review, 9,* 494–504.

Puranam, P., & Vanneste, B. (2009). Trust and governance: untangling a tangled web. *Academy of Management Review, 34*(1), 11–28.

Reuters Business Insight. (2004). Pharmaceutical strategic alliances: Benchmarking 21st century deal-making. Retrieved August 16, 2004, from http://www.the-infoshop.com.

Schelling, T. C. (1960). *The strategy of conflict.* Cambridge, MA: Harvard University.

Scott, W. R. (1987). The adolescence of institutional theory. *Administrative Science Quarterly, 32,* 493–511.

Shah, R., & Swaminathan, V. (2008). Factors influencing partner selection in strategic alliances: The moderating role of alliance context. *Strategic Management Journal, 29*(5), 471–494.

Shortell, S. M. (1988). The evolution of hospital systems: Unfulfilled promises and self-fulfilling prophecies. *Medical Care Review, 45*(2), 177–214.

Shortell, S. M., & Zajac, E. J. (1988). Internal corporate joint ventures: Development processes and performance outcomes. *Strategic Management Journal, 9*, 527–542.

Shortell, S. M., & Zajac, E. J. (1990). Health care organizations and the development of the strategic management perspective. In S. Mick & associates (Eds.), *Innovations in health care delivery: New insights into organization theory* (pp. 141–180). San Francisco: Jossey-Bass.

Shortell, S. M., Morrison, E. M., & Friedman, B. (1990). *Strategic choices for America's hospitals: Managing change in turbulent times.* San Francisco: Jossey-Bass.

Sofaer, S., & Myrtle, R. C. (1991). Interorganizational theory and research: Implications for health care management, policy, and research. *Medical Care Review, 48*, 371–409.

Starkweather, D. B. (1971). Health facility mergers: Some conceptualizations. *Medical Care, 9*, 468–478.

Starr, P. (1982). *The social transformation of American medicine.* New York: Basic Books.

Thompson, J. T. (1967). *Organizations in action.* New York: McGraw-Hill.

Ury, W. L., Brett, J. M., & Goldberg, S. B. (1988). *Getting disputes resolved.* San Francisco: Jossey-Bass.

Zajac, E. J. (1986). Organizations, environments, and performance: A study of contract management in hospitals. Unpublished doctoral dissertation, University of Pennsylvania, Philadelphia.

Zajac, E. J., & Olsen, C. P. (1993). From transaction costs to transactional value analysis: Implications for the study of interorganizational strategies. *Journal of Management Studies, 30*, 131–146.

Zajac, E. J., & Shortell, S. M. (1989). Changing generic strategies: Likelihood, direction, and performance implications. *Strategic Management Journal, 10*, 413–430.

Zajac, E. J., Golden, B. R., & Shortell, S. M. (1991). New organizational forms for enhancing innovation: The case of internal corporate joint ventures. *Management Science, 37*, 70–84.

Zuckerman, H. S., & D'Aunno, T. A. (1990). Hospital alliances: Cooperative strategy in a competitive environment. *Health Care Management Review, 15*(2), 21–30.

Zuckerman, H. S., & Kaluzny, A. (1991, Spring). The management of strategic alliances in health services. *Frontiers of Health Services Management, 7*(5), 3–23.

Zuckerman, H. S., Kaluzny, A. D., & Ricketts, T. C. (1995). Alliances in health care: What we know, what we think we know, and what we should know. *Health Care Management Review, 20*(1), 54–64.

# Chapter 12

# Health Policy and Regulation

**Kristin Madison, Peter D. Jacobson, and Gary Young**

## CHAPTER OUTLINE

- **Federal Policy and Regulation**
- **State Policy and Regulation**
- **Organizational Strategies for Regulatory Compliance**
- **Recent Policy and Regulatory Initiatives**

## LEARNING OBJECTIVES

**After completing this chapter, the reader should be able to:**

1. Recognize why regulations matter
2. Describe the policy and operational context of health care regulations
3. Identify the most important state and federal regulations that affect health care organizations
4. Identify the key regulatory agencies and summarize their current policies
5. Explain how regulatory compliance will affect health care organizations' strategic decision-making
6. Formulate strategies for regulatory compliance
7. Discuss recent policy initiatives that have regulatory implications
8. Evaluate strengths and weaknesses in current regulatory efforts to achieve policy goals

# KEY TERMS

| | |
|---|---|
| Accreditation | HCQIA |
| Anti-Kickback Statute | HIPAA |
| Antitrust Law | Licensure |
| Centers for Medicare and Medicaid Services | Medicare Payment Advisory Commission |
| Certificate of Need | National Practitioner Data Bank |
| Clayton Act | Notice of Proposed Rulemaking |
| Community Benefit Standard | Office of the Inspector General |
| Comparative Clinical Effectiveness | Pay-for-Performance |
| Compliance | Preemption |
| Corporate Integrity Agreement | Recovery Audit Contractor |
| Deeming Authority | Regulation |
| Department of Health and Human Services | Safety Zones |
| Department of Justice | Sherman Act |
| EMTALA | Stark Physician Self-Referral Law |
| ERISA | Tax Exemption |
| False Claims Act | Transparency |

# CHAPTER PURPOSE

The purpose of this chapter is to introduce the key regulatory challenges that managers of health care organizations are likely to encounter. With the increasing intersection between health care delivery and the law, health care executives must confront a wide range of regulatory **compliance** issues that affect how health care institutions operate. By describing the regulatory and policy environment in which health care organizations function, this chapter helps executives understand how regulations are formulated and implemented, as well as how to organize compliance programs and interact effectively with attorneys.

# FEDERAL POLICY AND REGULATION

The health care industry is heavily regulated at both the federal and state levels. By **regulation**, we mean governmental oversight of the private marketplace. This oversight is often intended to increase access, control costs, or improve quality in a world in which market competition may fail to achieve these goals. Regulation can be economic, such as when governments create reimbursement mechanisms or monitor financial arrangements between physicians and health systems; it can also serve a social function, such as when governments require the provision of emergency care regardless of a patient's ability to pay (Shortell and Walshe, 2004). Because federal health care regulations affect so many facets of health care organizations' operations, it is important for managers to understand the nature of these regulations and the agencies that implement them.

## Federal Agencies and Their Oversight

The federal government plays two key roles in health care: payer and regulator. As a payer for health care services, the government makes decisions about the benefits to cover. As a regulator, the government monitors how federal dollars are spent and takes steps to protect the health and safety of the public. These functions are performed through a number of agencies, each with its own distinct responsibilities.

## IN PRACTICE: Physician Price Fixing

*In recent years, many physicians have sought to facilitate negotiations with payers through use of a "messenger model." Structured properly, the model permits independent physicians to efficiently relay information about the fees they are willing to accept. The FTC, however, has taken action against many of these arrangements on the grounds that their activities have extended beyond serving as a messenger, to encompass practices that violate antitrust laws. In these excerpts from a 2003 press release, the FTC describes one physician organization's alleged anticompetitive behavior:*

The Federal Trade Commission has issued an administrative complaint against a group of Texas physicians, charging that they unlawfully restrained competition, increasing the cost of health care for consumers in the Fort Worth area. The FTC alleges that North Texas Specialty Physicians (NTSP) violated federal law by negotiating agreements among its participating physicians on price and other terms, refusing to deal with payors except on collectively agreed-upon terms, and refusing to submit payor offers to participating physicians unless the terms complied with NTSP's minimum-fee standards.

NTSP is a nonprofit corporation funded through fees paid by participating physicians. Organized in 1995, NTSP presently is composed of approximately 600 physicians, of whom approximately 130 are primary care physicians.... A physician may participate in NTSP payor contracts by granting NTSP the authority to arrange for his or her services to be provided to consumers covered by the payors.

The Commission's complaint states that nearly all of NTSP's participating physicians participate in some non-risk contracts. The FTC alleges that, "With respect to these non-risk contracts, NTSP often has sought to negotiate for, and often has obtained, higher fees and other more advantageous terms than its individual physicians could obtain by negotiating individually with payors."

The FTC complaint charges that NTSP's polling practices are illegal. NTSP polls its participating physicians to determine the minimum fee that they would accept for medical services provided pursuant to an NTSP-payor agreement. Once this information is collected, NTSP then calculates the averages of the reported minimum acceptable fees and reports these measures to its participating physicians, confirming to the participating physicians that these will be the minimum fees that NTSP collectively will entertain when negotiating any contract with a payor. The FTC alleges that the exchange of prospective price information among otherwise competing physicians reduces price competition and enables the participating physicians to achieve supra-competitive prices.

The Commission's complaint further charges that NTSP sometimes begins contract discussions with payors by identifying the fee minimums determined by its participating physicians, and states that NTSP will not enter into an agreement with any payor unless the payor agrees to satisfy these fee minimums....

The FTC also alleges that NTSP discouraged payors and participating physicians from negotiating directly with one another....

The Commission's complaint charges that none of NTSP's negotiating practices significantly increase efficiency, because its participating physicians are not integrated in ways that would increase the quality and reduce the cost of health care in the Fort Worth area. The Commission alleges that because of NTSP's practices: price and other forms of competition among the participating physicians were unreasonably restrained; prices for physician services were increased; and health plans, employers, and individual consumers were deprived of the benefits of robust competition among physicians.

*In 2004, an administrative law judge ruled in favor of the FTC, ordering NTSP to cease and desist from engaging in its anticompetitive activities. In response to NTSP's appeal, the full FTC affirmed the judge's decision. NTSP then appealed*

---

**IN PRACTICE:** Physician Price Fixing *(Continued)*

*the FTC's decision to the Fifth Circuit Court of Appeals. In these excerpts from a 2008 press release, the FTC describes the outcome of the case:*

In a unanimous opinion issued on May 14, the U.S. Court of Appeals for the Fifth Circuit affirmed a 2005 Federal Trade Commission decision that found certain activities of North Texas Specialty Physicians (NTSP) violated Section 5 of the FTC Act. In particular, NTSP, a group of independent competing physicians based in Fort Worth, was found to have participated in horizontal price-fixing that was not related to any procompetitive efficiencies. The appellate court's decision fully endorsed the analytical framework applied by the Commission in its decision, which found NTSP's conduct to be "inherently suspect," with no procompetitive justification. . . .

Excerpted from Press Release, Federal Trade Commission (2003, September 17), FTC charges North Texas Specialty Physicians with price fixing. Retrieved March 2010 from http://www.ftc.gov/opa/2003/09/ntexasphysicians.shtm; Press Release, Federal Trade Commission, U.S. Court of Appeals Affirms FTC Decision That Texas Doctors' Group Engaged in Illegal, Anticompetitive Price-Fixing, May 16, 2008, *available at* http://www.ftc.gov/opa/2008/05/ntsp.shtm.

---

The principal federal government agency for health care is the **Department of Health and Human Services** (HHS), under which the Public Health Service and 11 other public health agencies are governed. HHS is dedicated to "protecting the health of all Americans and providing essential human services, especially for those who are least able to help themselves." With over 300 programs, including health and social science research, health information technology, and substance abuse treatment, it represents nearly a quarter of all federal spending (HHS, 2009).

Some of the largest programs in HHS include the **Centers for Medicare and Medicaid Services** (CMS), which manages the Medicare and Medicaid programs; the Food and Drug Administration (FDA), which ensures the safety and efficacy of medical devices, food, drugs, and other biological products; and the National Institutes of Health (NIH), which conducts and supports biomedical research in order to prevent, treat, and cure diseases. Other areas of HHS support specific vulnerable populations within the United States, such as children and the elderly, along with marginalized groups such as Native Americans. Table 12.1 briefly describes the HHS agencies.

### Congressional Committees

Regulatory agencies derive their authority from the legislative branch. Congress and state legislatures often enact broad policy statements, delegating the details to the appropriate regulatory agency. Regulatory agencies must act within the bounds of any specific legislation. For instance, Congress enacted broad language to protect patient privacy under the Health Insurance Portability and Accountability Act (HIPAA), but did not specify how the goals of the act should be accomplished. Congress delegated the details of developing regulatory guidance to the Department of Health and Human Services.

Because Congress delegates authority to federal regulatory agencies, congressional committees play key roles in health care regulation. First, these committees develop and introduce legislation that provides executive branch agencies with the authority to issue regulations. Second, the committees have oversight responsibility for ensuring that the regulatory process is consistent with legislative intent.

In the Senate, the Health, Education, Labor, and Pensions Committee (HELP) has jurisdiction over matters involving health policy. The Senate's Finance Committee contains a health care subcommittee that has jurisdiction over taxation and revenue measures, as well as oversight powers to evaluate existing laws and the agencies that implement them.

In the House of Representatives, the Ways and Means Committee is responsible for taxation, tariffs, and other revenue-generating activities. Its jurisdiction is similar to that of the Senate Finance Committee, but differs in one important way: it only deals with matters related to Medicare, not Medicaid, while the Senate Finance Committee has jurisdiction over both programs. The House Committee on Energy and Commerce contains a subcommittee on health that has legislative oversight over Medicaid, hospital construction, and public health measures.

## TABLE 12.1  Agencies within the Department of Health and Human Services

### The Centers for Medicare and Medicaid Services (CMS)

The Centers for Medicare and Medicaid Services is responsible for managing the provision of government health insurance through the Medicare and Medicaid programs. It works in conjunction with state governments to administer Medicaid and the Children's Health Insurance Program (CHIP).

### Food and Drug Administration (FDA)

The Food and Drug Administration is responsible for ensuring the safety and efficacy of medical devices, food, drugs, biological products, cosmetics, radiation-emitting products, and veterinary products. It also provides education to the public regarding proper nutrition and use of medication, and enforces certain requirements of the Public Health Service Act.

### The National Institutes of Health (NIH)

The National Institutes of Health conducts and supports research into methods of preventing, treating, or curing both common and rare diseases. In addition to engaging in its own internal research efforts, it provides financial support for scientific research to universities and other institutions.

### The Centers for Disease Control and Prevention (CDC)

The Centers for Disease Control and Prevention focuses on "developing and applying disease prevention and control, environmental health, health promotion and health education activities designed to improve the health of the people of the United States." It works with both state and international health agencies to promote health education.

### Agency for Healthcare Research and Quality (AHRQ)

The Agency for Healthcare Research and Quality works to improve the quality, safety, efficiency, and effectiveness of health care in the United States. AHRQ seeks new ways to increase access to care, promote evidence-based medicine, and reduce costs without compromising quality. By conducting, sponsoring, and disseminating research, it enables more Americans to become informed health care decision makers.

### Administration for Children and Families (ACF)

The Administration for Children and Families funds 65 programs to provide assistance to families in areas such as child support, child care, and adoption. Its goal is to promote the healthy development of children and families in order to create empowered communities.

### Administration on Aging (AoA)

The Administration on Aging has a mission to "help elderly individuals maintain their dignity and independence in their homes and communities through comprehensive, coordinated, and cost-effective systems of long-term care, and livable communities across the US" (AoA, 2009). Through the Older Americans Act, it funds state research, demonstration, and training programs dedicated to aging. It also collaborates with CMS through the Medicare program.

### Agency for Toxic Substances and Disease Registry (ATSDR)

The Agency for Toxic Substances and Disease Registry was created in 1980 through the Comprehensive Environmental Response, Compensation, and Liability Act, also known as the Superfund Act. Its purpose is to conduct public health assessments of waste sites, respond to emergency hazardous substance outbreaks, and support research and dissemination of information related to hazardous substances.

**TABLE 12.1**  **Agencies within the Department of Health and Human Services** *(Continued)*

**Health Resources and Services Administration (HRSA)**

The Health Resources and Services Administration is responsible for ensuring that uninsured, isolated, or medically vulnerable populations receive adequate care. It provides direct health care to 24 million people (HRSA, 2009).

**Indian Health Service (IHS)**

The Indian Health Service is focused on ensuring that culturally competent and comprehensive care is provided for American Indians and Alaska Natives. It operates a comprehensive health service delivery system for over 1.9 million people in 562 recognized tribes in 35 states (IHS, 2009).

**Substance Abuse and Mental Health Services Administration (SAMHSA)**

The Substance Abuse and Mental Health Services Administration agency promotes prevention, treatment and rehabilitation of individuals suffering from substance abuse or mental illnesses.

The House and Senate both have appropriations committees, which determine funding for HHS and other health services. The appropriations committees must approve all federal treasury expenditures.

### The Regulatory Process

Agencies carry out their core functions by issuing and enforcing regulations. At the federal level, the Administrative Procedures Act determines the process of promulgating regulations. The process begins when the agency publishes a **Notice of Proposed Rulemaking** in the *Federal Register*. Stakeholders and interested citizens then have a certain time period to submit comments; after reviewing these comments, the agency may choose to revise the regulation. It then publishes the final regulation in the *Federal Register*, along with its responses to the comments. The final regulation is then incorporated into the Code of Federal Regulations.

An alternative approach, negotiated regulation, has become increasingly popular in recent years. In the negotiated regulation process, the regulatory agency meets with the affected industry to develop a regulatory approach that is acceptable to each side to avoid contentious and time-consuming litigation (Jacobson, Hoffman, and Lopez, 2006).

Largely because of the expanding federal investment in health care, the scope and number of regulations have expanded exponentially. At best, the current health care regulatory structure is a fragmented, ad hoc arrangement with overlapping and sometimes inconsistent requirements that can be difficult for health care managers to interpret and implement.

## Medicare and Medicaid Law

If an agency's importance is measured by its budget, then CMS is among the most important federal agencies; the annual outlays of the Medicare and Medicaid programs total in the hundreds of billions of dollars. These expenditures contribute to both the physical health of many millions of individuals and the financial health of many thousands of health care organizations. To understand the importance of Medicare and Medicaid to health care operations, health care managers must understand the programs' coverage policies, their reimbursement mechanisms, and their oversight and administration.

### Medicare

Medicare, created by a 1965 statute, is the federal health insurance program for the elderly and disabled. Today, Medicare is the largest program for financing individual health care: more than 10 percent of the entire federal operating budget is spent on Medicare. CMS administers the program, which covers more than 35 million Americans over age 65 and 6 million individuals with disabilities.

Medicare provides health insurance to three populations: people who are 65 or older, people under 65 with specific disabilities, and people who have end-stage renal disease. It is composed of four distinct parts (A, B, C, and D) that cover different services. Most individuals are automatically eligible to receive benefits when they reach age 65; there is no means-testing for eligibility.

Medicare Part A provides hospital insurance. It covers inpatient care and also skilled nursing facility, hospice, and home health care. Medicare Part A is financed through a payroll tax on employers and their employees. For individuals who paid Medicare taxes during employment (or who have a spouse who paid them), no monthly premium is required for coverage.

Medicare Part B covers some medically necessary services, including outpatient care, home health services, and doctors' services, as well as some preventive care. Automatic enrollment occurs at age 65 for those who are eligible for Social Security benefits or Railroad Retirement Board benefits; it also occurs for those who are under 65 and receive Social Security or Railroad Retirement Board disability benefits. Individuals who have Lou Gehrig's disease are also eligible to receive Part B benefits. Unlike Part A, Part B requires premium payments; however, individuals may choose to opt out of Part B enrollment.

Medicare Part C provides coverage through Medicare Advantage Plans, an alternative to the standard Medicare coverage under Parts A and B. Operated by private insurers, these plans take on a number of forms, including preferred provider organizations and health maintenance organizations. Those who choose to enroll in a Medicare Advantage Plan will have both Part A and Part B coverage through their selected provider. All services covered by Medicare, except for hospice care (which will continue to be available through the traditional Medicare program), must be included in Medicare Advantage Plans. The distinguishing feature of these plans is that they may also offer additional coverage, including hearing, dental, vision, and drug coverage and/or health and wellness programs. Medicare Advantage Plan enrollees pay the Part B premium and may also pay an additional fee to the plan for the extra services provided.

Medicare Part D provides prescription drug coverage through Medicare-approved insurance companies to people with Medicare. It is an opt-in program, and there are variations in terms of what drugs are covered by different plans. Those who are enrolled in Medicare Part A and/or Part B are eligible. Individuals enrolled in Medicare Advantage Plans that do not already include drug coverage can choose to enroll in a Medicare prescription drug plan.

While Medicare covers many services, enrollees are still financially responsible for coinsurance, copayments, deductibles, and products and services that Medicare does not cover. Enrollees who want supplemental insurance to cover these "gaps" may purchase Medigap policies, which are sold by private insurance companies. An enrollee must pay all Medigap premiums.

Medicare enrollee premiums finance only some of the costs of the Medicare program. Medicare Part A is financed through a federal payroll tax, while Part B and Part D are financed in part through general tax revenues. It has been projected that given the current structure of the Medicare program and the taxes that support it, there will be insufficient funds to pay full Medicare Part A benefits by 2019 (Boards of Trustees, 2008). The worker-to-beneficiary ratio is declining, and the growth of the baby boomer population will present additional financial challenges moving forward (Reznik, Shoffner, and Weaver, 2005–2006). It is likely that Congress will need to alter the benefits package, increase taxes, or both in order to maintain the financial viability of the Medicare program.

## Medicaid

Medicaid is a combined federal and state program that provides medical assistance to low-income individuals and families. Largely operated at the state level, it provides care to more than 47 million people, including 24 million children and 13 million elderly and disabled people, at an estimated cost to the federal and state governments of $250 billion per year. Unlike Medicare, Medicaid requires that individuals and families meet certain financial and other eligibility criteria to enroll in the program. The federal government matches state expenditures based on a formula that compares each state's per capita income to the national average.

Medicaid serves three broad purposes. First, it finances health care for families receiving cash assistance through welfare or the Supplemental Security Income (SSI) program. Those who have minimal income and assets and are aged, blind, disabled, or members of families with dependent children fall into this category. Second, it covers low-income children and pregnant women, regardless of their eligibility for cash assistance programs. Third, it provides catastrophic insurance for people whose otherwise-adequate income is consumed by medical bills. Individuals who need nursing home care or other long-term care often fall into this category. In addition, increased coverage has been provided for children through initiatives such as the Children's Health Insurance Program and for disabled individuals through the Ticket to Work and Work Incentives Improvement Act of 1999.

Although these programs vary from state to state, federal statutes and regulations set forth minimum requirements in terms of groups covered and benefits provided. State programs are organized around combinations of categorically needy, medically needy, or special needs groups. Table 12.2 describes some of the categorically needy groups. Medically needy individuals are those who have too much money to be considered categorically needy, such as qualified working disabled individuals. Beyond federally required services, states may offer certain optional services, for which they receive matching federal dollars. Of the optional services, the most commonly offered include prescription drugs (which are offered in all states), dental care, prosthetic devices, hearing aids, and intermediate care facilities for the mentally disabled. States may also seek waivers to offer services in innovative ways.

### Reimbursement

Medicare's reimbursement mechanisms have changed over time. Historically, hospitals that sought to maximize their profits or net revenues from Medicare patients could do so

---

### TABLE 12.2  Categorically Needy Groups

- Families who meet states' Aid to Families with Dependent Children (AFDC) eligibility requirements in effect on July 16, 1996.

- Pregnant women and children under age 6 whose family income is at or below 133% of the Federal poverty level.

- Children ages 6 to 19 with family income up to 100% of the federal poverty level.

- Caretakers (relatives or legal guardians who take care of children under age 18 [or 19 if still in high school]).

- Supplemental Security Income (SSI) recipients (or, in certain states, aged, blind, and disabled people who meet requirements that are more restrictive than those of the SSI program).

- Individuals and couples who are living in medical institutions and who have monthly income up to 300% of the SSI income standard (federal benefit rate).

SOURCE: Retrieved March 2010 from CMS Web site: http://www.cms.hhs.gov/MedicaidGenInfo/Downloads/MedicaidAtAGlance2005.pdf

---

by maximizing the number of services they provided, because Medicare reimbursed hospitals based on their costs. This system contributed to Medicare program cost excesses, however, and Congress ultimately decided to take a different approach.

To maximize their net revenues today, hospitals must consider both Medicare's fixed payment rates and their own costs of providing services. In 1983, Medicare implemented the Prospective Payment System (PPS), a fixed-payment system for inpatient services based on a patient's specific diagnosis. Under PPS, the government pays hospitals for admitted patients according to a formula based on the admitted patient's diagnosis and certain other criteria that are not tied directly to the hospital's actual costs. If the cost of care is less than the payment, the hospital keeps the difference; but if the cost of care is higher, the facility loses money. With PPS, hospitals have an incentive to provide cost-effective care and curtail excessive institutional spending.

In the 1990s, Medicare changed its mechanism for physician reimbursement. Instead of paying usual and customary fees, a practice modeled after commercial insurance reimbursement policies, Medicare adopted a Resource Based Relative Value System (RBRVS) to compensate physicians. In this system, physicians are reimbursed on a fee-for-service basis under a formula based on expected resource use.

Medicare's payment systems for inpatient and outpatient services allow payment for covered technologies. For those technologies that do not fit into a bundled payment category, the Social Security Act requires Medicare to ensure that they are "reasonable and necessary" for diagnosis and treatment. Determining whether to cover the latest technology is an important and highly contested Medicare function.

### Oversight and Administration

Because most health care providers serve Medicare and/or Medicaid patients and accept reimbursement from these programs, they become subject to the rules associated with these programs. These rules relate not just to the reimbursement process, but also to the nature of health care operations. Medicare and Medicaid programs will only reimburse health care organizations that have met specific eligibility requirements, including federal conditions of participation, which impose minimum health and safety standards. Fulfillment of these conditions is determined by a state agency that conducts random and unannounced surveys on behalf of CMS. If a national **accreditation** organization such as the Joint Commission has more stringent requirements, CMS may grant it **"deeming" authority**, which allows it to deem a health care organization as meeting CMS certification requirements.

Thus, while the Medicare and Medicaid programs' primary functions are to increase health care access, they may also significantly influence providers' structures and operations. As described previously, the programs' reimbursement mechanisms affect providers' incentives to control costs. In addition, as described later in the chapter, these programs have recently taken a more proactive approach to encouraging quality improvement through value-based purchasing initiatives. In fact, CMS' mission is not just to provide coverage, but also to "promote quality care for beneficiaries," and its vision is "[t]o achieve a transformed and modernized health care system" (CMS, 2010).

An independent congressional agency, the **Medicare Payment Advisory Commission** (MedPAC), has played a significant role in shaping a variety of Medicare reform initiatives. MedPAC advises Congress on a broad range of issues: "In addition to advising the Congress on payments to private health plans participating in Medicare and providers in Medicare's traditional fee-for service program, MedPAC is also tasked with analyzing access to care, quality of care, and other issues affecting Medicare" (MedPAC, 2010). To the extent that MedPAC's recommendations are translated into legal and program reforms, they may substantially alter the financial and regulatory environments in which health care providers function.

# Food and Drug Law

The Food and Drug Administration (FDA), like CMS, is a federal agency responsible for decisions that have a profound effect on both patients and health care organizations. While CMS exercises its influence primarily through its coverage and reimbursement policies and related rules, the FDA exercises its influence through its regulatory efforts to ensure the safety and efficacy of drugs and medical devices.

The first step in developing a new drug is generally to perform laboratory and animal testing to determine whether it has promise for human use. If so, the developers submit an Investigational New Drug Application to the FDA to obtain approval to conduct clinical trials. After receiving approval, researchers can begin Phase I trials, in which they give the

drug to a small number of people to test its safety and identify its side effects. If a drug's performance in Phase I is sufficiently successful, the drug will then be tested in a Phase II trial, in which researchers study its effectiveness as well as its safety in a larger group of people. In Phase III, the drug is tested on still more people; results are used to assess the drug's benefits and risks and to provide the necessary information for the drug's label.

Drug development may be halted at any stage of clinical trials. If Phase III trials are successfully completed, however, the drug's sponsor can submit a New Drug Application to obtain the necessary FDA approval before marketing the drug. Based on the information supplied in the application, the FDA will weigh the drug's benefits and risks in determining whether the drug is safe and effective for the specified indication. It will also review the drug's proposed label and assess the adequacy of the drug's manufacturing process.

The FDA also regulates medical devices. Depending on the characteristics and uses of the devices, they are classified as Class I, Class II, or Class III devices, with Class III devices being subject to the most intensive regulatory scrutiny. Many Class I devices are exempt from premarket notification requirements, for example, while those seeking to market Class III devices must generally obtain premarket approval, just as developers of new drugs must obtain approval.

## Regulatory Challenges

The FDA faces many regulatory challenges (Merrill, 1996; Slater, 2005); this chapter highlights three. The first challenge is to balance the public demand for speedy access to newly developed drugs against the risk that an accelerated approval process might fail to identify the dangers that new drugs present. More generally, if regulators impose requirements that are too stringent, they will deprive people of access to beneficial drugs; if they impose requirements that are too lax, they will expose people to significant risks of harm.

A second challenge is to ensure continued monitoring of drugs once they reach the marketplace (Lipsky and Sharp, 2001; Slater, 2005). Because some drug risks may emerge only after a drug is used by a large number of patients, it is important to track adverse events that occur after a drug has been approved. In some cases, the FDA asks drug sponsors to conduct Phase IV, or postmarketing, clinical trials designed to permit further assessment of drugs. The FDA also relies on individual reports of adverse events submitted by drug sponsors, physicians, and consumers. Recently, the FDA launched the Sentinel Initiative, which will bring together existing databases from multiple sources, such as medical records and insurance claims databases, in an effort to engage in more systematic surveillance of adverse effects (Platt et al., 2009).

A third challenge is to ensure that information is appropriately disseminated to physicians and patients. With respect to physicians, debate has long surrounded the FDA's policies with respect to a practice known as off-label promotion. The FDA approves drugs for specific indications, but physicians are free to prescribe drugs for other uses. Drug manufacturers, however, are not permitted to promote these off-label uses; federal authorities have recently pursued legal action against a number of manufacturers for illegal marketing practices. The prohibition of off-label promotion may encourage drug sponsors to systematically study off-label uses and seek formal FDA approval for additional indications. At the same time, it may impede the dissemination of data that physicians would find useful in making prescribing decisions.

With respect to patients, the challenge is finding a way to appropriately regulate direct-to-consumer advertising. Regulations require that advertisements for prescription drugs "present a fair balance between information relating to side effects and contraindications and information relating to effectiveness of the drug"; they cannot be "false or misleading with respect to side effects, contraindications, and effectiveness" (21 CFR § 202.1[e][5]). The Division of Drug Marketing, Advertising, and Communications reviews broadcast advertising, but has taken a limited number of regulatory actions against advertisers, eliciting criticism from those who believe that the FDA should engage in more extensive oversight. (GAO, 2002).

## Antitrust Law

Because Medicare and Medicaid law and food and drug law are directed specifically at the provision of health care products and services, it is not surprising that they can be important factors in health care managers' decision-making processes. Other areas of federal law, however, may have a less obvious connection with the health care industry, but nonetheless often play a key role in shaping managerial strategies. **Antitrust law** is one example.

The purpose of the antitrust laws is to promote competition based on the conviction that competitive markets bring

benefits of relatively lower consumer prices, higher output, and greater innovation. Enforcement activity has recently increased in response to substantial merger activity among hospitals and other providers that some policy makers believe has contributed to the growing costs of health care services.

Antitrust laws exist at both the federal and state levels. However, because much of the enforcement activity in the health care industry is at the federal level, we focus here on federal antitrust law. Additionally, most state antitrust provisions parallel what exists at the federal level. There are three primary federal antitrust provisions that apply to the health care industry. Section 1 of the **Sherman Act** prohibits contracts and other agreements that unreasonably restrain trade. This provision applies to situations where individuals or organizations that are in a competitive situation with one another also collaborate to achieve common business objectives. Section 2 of the Sherman Act prohibits activities that are undertaken to obtain or achieve a monopoly. This section is aimed at the conduct of a single entity that undertakes anticompetitive activities to strengthen its competitive position. The third provision, Section 7 of the **Clayton Act**, prohibits mergers, acquisitions, and joint ventures that threaten to substantially lessen competition or are likely to create a monopoly. Because these provisions are broad in scope, over time the courts and antitrust enforcement officials have developed analytic frameworks for deciding when business arrangements and activities constitute violations of the antitrust laws.

Federal enforcement of the antitrust laws is the responsibility of both the U.S. **Department of Justice** (DOJ) and the Federal Trade Commission (FTC). These federal agencies coordinate their efforts in investigating and prosecuting antitrust cases. The Sherman Act permits both civil and criminal sanctions, including imprisonment, whereas the Clayton Act carries civil sanctions only. Also, the FTC can pursue antitrust cases under a provision within its own authorizing statute, Section 5 of the Federal Trade Commission Act, which prohibits unfair methods of competition and unfair or deceptive acts affecting commerce. Although Section 5 is technically even broader in scope than the previously noted antitrust provisions, the FTC typically invokes Section 5 to prosecute arrangements or activities that would otherwise violate the Sherman or Clayton acts.

Of the previously noted antitrust provisions, Section 1 of the Sherman Act has perhaps the greatest relevance to the health care industry. The health care industry is highly diverse, with numerous types of health care providers and other entities who often are in a position to compete as well as collaborate with one another. Some of the earliest antitrust cases in the health care industry involved physicians who were competitors but also agreed to boycott prepaid health plans as a means to protect their fees. More recent Section 1 Sherman Act cases have involved physician networks that have been formed principally to facilitate joint price negotiations on behalf of network members with insurance plans and other payers of health care services. These networks, typically organized as independent practice associations, often comprise physicians who are otherwise competitors but have formed a joint venture to strengthen their negotiating position with payers.

However, Section 1 is not a blanket prohibition on all collaborations among competitors. The courts have long recognized that collaborative arrangements can often have beneficial as well as harmful consequences for competition. Although collaborations involving competitors necessarily impose some limits on competition that can result in harms such as higher consumer prices, they may also generate efficiencies in the participating entities' legitimate business activities or foster innovations that could not possibly be achieved by any one of the entities alone. Accordingly, to decide whether an arrangement is a violation of Section 1, enforcement officials and courts assess whether the benefits outweigh the harms for a given arrangement. Two primary legal standards are applied: per se and rule of reason.

The per se standard is applied to types of arrangements for which it is well established that the arrangement only harms competition. Price fixing is perhaps the best example of such an arrangement. In the case of price fixing, competitors collaborate for the sole purpose of agreeing on certain prices for their services or products so that they no longer are effectively competing on price. For example, consider eight dermatologists who in the past have competed for patients and collectively comprise 80 percent of the dermatologists in a market area. These dermatologists get together to agree on certain prices that they will charge for office visits and other services they provide. As a result, the dermatologists now gain what would likely be considerable negotiating leverage with local health plans for dermatology services. Because such an arrangement entails some degree of harm to competition (because the health plans have to pay higher prices for dermatology services that get passed down to consumers

in the form of higher insurance premiums) but would not produce any efficiencies or innovations, it is treated as per se illegal under the antitrust laws.

The rule of reason standard is applicable when the arrangement has potential for both harm and benefit to competition. Consider the case of physician networks. If joint price negotiation was all that a particular network, one comprised of physicians or physician practices who were otherwise competitors, was designed to accomplish, the arrangement would raise concerns from an antitrust perspective. However, in addition to facilitating joint price negotiations, these networks are often designed to allow physicians to share clinical resources and administrative services that promote the efficiency of their separate practices. The arrangement may also be used to enhance quality of care through shared personnel and clinical resources such as electronic medical records. The resolution of such cases under the rule of reason standard therefore calls for very fact-based examinations as to their net effects on competition. This examination entails a delineation of the affected market in terms of geographic boundaries, number and types of competing physicians within the market, and the degree to which a network is designed to promote efficiencies or quality in patient care.

In addition, although antitrust enforcement officials are most concerned about collaborative arrangements that bring together competitors ("horizontal" arrangements), they also may scrutinize arrangements that involve entities who do not compete directly but rather have ongoing business relationships with each other as suppliers and purchasers ("vertical" arrangements). For example, physician-hospital organizations, which have been organized to enable a hospital and members of its medical staff to jointly negotiate prices with payers, have sometimes fallen under antitrust scrutiny on the ground that they are being used to boycott a health plan or competitively disadvantage certain physicians.

In the health care industry, Section 2 cases are less common but do arise from time to time amid concerns about an entity's ability to thwart competition. One Section 2 case involved an insurance plan that sought to strengthen its competitive position by refusing to contract with a hospital that was owned by a competing insurance plan. In such cases, antitrust enforcement officials look closely at an entity's market power, or its ability to influence prices based on market share. The higher the entity's market share, the more enforcement officials will be inclined to scrutinize any possible anticompetitive actions undertaken by that entity.

Section 7 of the Clayton Act has been most frequently invoked in health care cases for proposed mergers between hospitals or between physician practices. For Section 7 of the Clayton Act, the basic analytic framework applied is similar to that already discussed for Section 1 of the Sherman Act. That is, there is a balancing of potential harms and benefits that may be associated with the merger or other combination of entities. For example, a merger between two hospitals in a six-hospital market may raise concerns about the combined entity's ability to raise prices. At the same time, the combined entity may be able to operate more efficiently than either of the two entities separately due to economies of scale. For such cases, enforcement agencies and courts evaluate the merger's likely effect on the level of competition in the relevant market. Other factors considered include whether the merged entity is likely to be protected from future competition because of certain market entry barriers such as stringent state licensing provisions or certificate of need requirements. The presence of such entry barriers raises the risk that the merger will affect competition in ways that violate Section 7 of the Sherman Act.

Organizations that are planning mergers or acquisitions and meet certain financial criteria are required under the Hart-Scott-Rodino Act to report their plans to the federal government. Once a report is submitted, the federal government has a specified window of time to request additional information and to decide whether it believes the merger or acquisition would be an antitrust violation.

Although antitrust enforcement officials have become increasingly concerned about the anticompetitive consequences of many of the business arrangements now commonplace in the health care industry, they have also recognized that increased antitrust scrutiny may deter providers and other entities from engaging in business arrangements that potentially benefit competition. Accordingly, the DOJ and FTC have jointly issued enforcement guidelines for the health care industry. These guidelines include so-called **safety zones** that outline the factual elements of certain business arrangements they view as acceptable and thus will not prosecute, barring extraordinary circumstances. Two such safety zones relate to physician networks, which, as noted, have been a major source of concern for enforcement officials. For additional guidance, there is also the option of submitting a letter to the DOJ or FTC that outlines a proposed arrangement. An agency's response to such letters is purely advisory but does constitute an important source of additional guidance for industry participants.

## Tax Exemption Law

Like antitrust law, tax exemption law is not necessarily directly targeted at health care organizations, but nonetheless has significant implications for managers' strategic decision making. The U.S. health care industry comprises a relatively large number of organizations that are exempt from paying most if not all taxes, including income, property, and sales taxes. Most such tax-exempt organizations are hospitals. Indeed, the majority of U.S. hospitals are exempt from at least federal income tax. However, some physician organizations, nursing homes and other types of provider organizations have **tax exemptions** as well.

Organizations qualify for federal income tax exemption under Section 501(c)(3) of the Internal Revenue Code, which applies to corporations organized and operated exclusively for religious, charitable, scientific, or educational purposes. Although this provision does not refer to health care specifically as an exempt purpose, most 501(c)(3)-exempt health care organizations have qualified on the basis of having a charitable purpose. Organizations that qualify for a federal tax exemption also are able to issue tax-exempt bonds, which enables them to issue bonds at relatively lower interest rates (and thus reduce their financing costs) because bondholders do not pay federal tax on the interest. The Internal Revenue Service (IRS) is responsible for determinations as to whether an organization qualifies for a Section 501(c)(3) exemption.

In making 501(c)(3) determinations, the IRS applies two tests, one focusing on organizational criteria, and the other focusing on operational criteria. For the organizational test, the IRS examines the applicant's formative documents (e.g., articles of incorporation) as to whether they limit the organization to pursue one or more exempt purposes (e.g., charitable, scientific). All organizations seeking to qualify as a charitable organization must be organized on a nonprofit basis.

For the operational test, the IRS examines the applicant's actual activities relative to three requirements. One is that the organization is operated to achieve an exempt purpose. As discussed subsequently, the IRS has established a **community benefit standard** for assessing whether hospitals are operated to serve a charitable purpose. A second requirement prohibits so-called private benefit and private inurement, which are somewhat complex concepts but essentially mean that the earnings of an exempt organization cannot be distributed to any individual or organization as a form of dividend. The earnings of an exempt organization must be directed to further the organization's exempt purpose. Of course, this requirement does not prevent exempt organizations from paying salaries, even very high ones, to employees needed to carry out the organization's activities. However, the salaries must be in line with what is required to secure individuals with the necessary skills in a given market area. In this vein, all of an exempt organization's business transactions need to be conducted in an arm's-length manner and in accordance with fair market value, or else they jeopardize its exempt status. In recent years, the IRS has been paying closer attention to whether exempt hospitals are meeting this requirement, perhaps in part as a response to high-profile media reports claiming excessively high salaries for hospital chief executive officers and other senior executives (Wangsness, 2009).

The third requirement pertains to political activity by exempt organizations. Specifically, exempt organizations are prohibited from lobbying or otherwise campaigning on behalf of any political candidate. Exempt organizations may engage in lobbying activities to influence legislation or other policy action, but these activities must be limited to less than a "substantial" part of the organization's total activities. The IRS does not apply a quantitative threshold for defining a substantial part, but rather looks at the facts and circumstances of each situation.

The IRS established the community benefit standard in 1969, thereby effectively replacing a standard that had required exempt hospitals to provide services to the poor to the extent of their financial ability. The agency's decision to replace this charity care standard was a response to the recently adopted Medicare and Medicaid programs, which at that time many health policy experts believed would greatly reduce the number of uninsured citizens and thus greatly reduce the need for hospitals to provide charity care. The community benefit standard reflected on the part of the IRS an expanded concept of charitable purpose for hospitals—one encompassing the promotion of health itself rather than strictly the provision of care to the poor.

The community benefit standard consists of several factors: providing charity care to the extent of the hospital's financial ability, operating a 24-hour emergency room, accepting payment from the Medicare and Medicaid programs on a nondiscriminatory basis, extending medical privileges to all qualified physicians in the area, and maintaining a governing board drawn largely from representatives of the community. Although the IRS does not require that an applicant meet all or even any specific combination of these factors, based on past IRS determinations, the presence of a 24-hour emergency room appears to carry considerable weight. Additionally, in recent years, the IRS has also been paying closer attention to governance issues in light of reports that exempt hospitals are increasingly overseen by boards that lack a strong community orientation (Brier and Thompson, 2008; Exempt Organizations, 2009).

Despite the IRS' expanded concept of charitable purpose as formalized in the community benefit standard, in practice it has treated hospitals differently than it does other types of health care organizations. For most other types of health care organizations, the IRS appears to require evidence that the applicant provides care to the poor as part of its activities.

A 501(c)(3) exemption does not necessarily apply to all of the income earned by an exempt organization. Income earned from activities that are unrelated to an entity's charitable purpose may trigger what is known as unrelated business income tax (UBIT). Under UBIT rules, exempt organizations must pay taxes at federal corporate rates on income earned from any activity meeting three criteria: the activity constitutes a trade or business, the activity is regularly carried on, and the activity is not substantially related to the organization's exempt purpose. For example, many hospitals have investment interests in for-profit businesses through either a parent-subsidiary relationship or a partnership arrangement. The income that hospitals earn from these businesses will often qualify for UBIT treatment as their underlying activities are not related to the hospital's exempt purpose—providing hospital services to the local community.

With respect to state income, sales, and property tax exemptions, the overriding issue is also whether the applicant has a charitable purpose. Whereas some states and local taxing authorities grant exemption based on an entity's 501(c)(3) status, others have their own criteria that may require or attach considerable weight to the actual provision of charity care, regardless of whether the applicant is a hospital or another type of provider. A number of high-profile court cases have involved a state's revocation of a hospital's property tax exemption. Tax-exempt hospitals seeking to maximize net revenues or achieve other organizational objectives must remain cognizant of the requirements associated with their tax-exempt status.

# Other Federal Laws and Regulations Affecting Hospital and Health System Operations

While Medicare and Medicaid law, food and drug law, antitrust law, and tax exemption law are all important areas of federal law, many other areas of federal law affect health care providers. Many federal statutes and regulations are relevant for day-to-day operations; executives must develop a culture of regulatory compliance and implement measures to identify and remediate noncompliance. Federal regulations also shape and constrain strategic decision making. Executives must work closely with their attorneys to identify potential regulatory barriers to business arrangements with physicians.

Consider the following questions as you read this section: What organizational strategies would you adopt to ensure compliance with these complex regulations? What disciplinary measures would you recommend for individuals within your organization who fail to comply with applicable regulations?

## *Federal Fraud and Abuse Laws*

The federal fraud and abuse laws prohibit three principal types of conduct. First, the **Anti-Kickback Statute** (AKS) prohibits the knowing and willful solicitation or receipt of remuneration by any person in connection with items or services for which payment could be made by Medicare or Medicaid. While the most obvious violation of the AKS would be a bribe for a referral of a Medicare patient, providers engaged in other kinds of arrangements, such as payments of financial incentives in connection with physician recruitment, may also run afoul of the AKS. Second, the **Stark Physician Self-Referral Law** (Stark) prohibits physicians from referring patients to certain health services providers with which the physicians have a financial relationship. Third, the **False Claims Act** (FCA) prohibits knowingly submitting or causing to be submitted a false claim to the government, such as a Medicare claim for a service different from the one that was actually provided.

The secretary of HHS retains discretion to promulgate regulations to define the scope of these prohibitions and establish specific exceptions. These regulations run for hundreds of pages, with numerous safe harbors (which are defined as arrangements that the regulatory agencies believe are not abusive, and hence are acceptable) and exceptions that are difficult to interpret and apply. So far, HHS has issued three sets of regulations, the last one designed to correct confusion from earlier regulations.

The activities prohibited by the fraud and abuse laws concern policy makers because they provide incentives to deliver more health care than is necessary, increasing the costs of Medicare and Medicaid, and they also expose patients to health risks attributable to too much treatment or poor-quality treatment. Nearly 10 percent of the annual federal health care budget may be lost to fraud and abuse, while federal fraud recoveries total more than $1 billion each year. Because there is a great deal of money involved, the federal government has made fraud and abuse enforcement a primary focus of its regulatory efforts. As a result, the issue is one of ongoing importance to health care executives. Virtually every issue of trade publications, such as *Modern Healthcare*, will have an article discussing various aspects of compliance with the fraud and abuse laws, along with complaints about the government's enforcement policies and the resulting burden.

The HHS **Office of the Inspector General**, with the cooperation of the Department of Justice, dedicates considerable resources to enforcing federal fraud and abuse laws. State authorities may also bring enforcement actions; many states have their own fraud and abuse statutes. Government authorities are not the only entities involved in fraud and abuse enforcement, however. Many FCA suits are initiated not by government entities, but instead by individual employee whistle-blowers pursuant to the *"qui tam"* provisions of the FCA. Individuals who bring *qui tam* actions inform the government of a potential violation and then share in any proceeds the government acquires from a judgment or settlement. Thus, the FCA's *qui tam* provision significantly increases the probability of detection of false claims.

The sanctions associated with statutory violations are significant. They include civil monetary penalties and possible exclusion from participation in Medicare and Medicaid under the Stark Law, AKS, and the FCA, as well as criminal penalties under AKS. Failure to comply with fraud and abuse regulations may also lead the government to impose a **Corporate Integrity Agreement** (CIA), whereby the organization essentially loses control of the compliance process and must adhere to strict governmental oversight.

That all of this imposes a compliance burden on health care providers is clear. What remains uncertain is the magnitude of the burden this regulatory framework places on efficient organizational arrangements. In particular, critics of the current regulations complain that the regulations impede legitimate market arrangements that can advance public policy goals of reducing costs and improving patients' quality of care. Other commentators question whether the fraud and abuse laws "fit" the medical marketplace.

As an example, take the issue of gainsharing, which occurs when physicians and health systems enter into agreements to share cost savings based on certain efficiency and quality-of-care metrics. Initially, OIG stated in an advisory bulletin that gainsharing violated the fraud and abuse regulations. This interpretation was in tension with the policies of the Internal Revenue Service (with respect to tax exemption criteria) and the Department of Justice and Federal Trade Commission (with respect to antitrust enforcement), which encouraged integration and risk-sharing in arrangements between physicians and health systems. Over time, OIG has relaxed its categorical opposition to gainsharing, allowing some arrangements to proceed, as long as they incorporate clear protections against abuse, such as quality-of-care metrics.

Health care executives and physicians have also raised concerns about the impact of fraud and abuse laws on physician payment arrangements and joint ventures between physicians and health systems. To fall within the relevant AKS safe harbor, for example, payment to physicians under personal services contracts must reflect fair market value and cannot be tied to the volume of referrals. Joint ventures must be carefully structured to avoid both the AKS and self-referral laws. The complexity of the regulations governing these and other arrangements may hinder efforts to engage in efficiency-enhancing practices.

Undoubtedly, the government's concern for fraud and abuse is legitimate. Whether it is systematic fraud and abuse that results in the filing of false claims, upcoding for insurance reimbursement, or kickbacks for prescribing pharmaceuticals or ordering durable medical equipment, a regulatory presence to restrain bad behavior is necessary. At the same time, the fraud and abuse regulatory structure suffers from excessive complexity, an undetermined compliance burden, and a lack of empirical evidence to support the current approach.

---

## IN PRACTICE: Physician Recruitment and the Fraud and Abuse Regulations

Health care managers often find themselves in the difficult position of having to navigate through complex and voluminous fraud and abuse laws and regulations. These provisions prohibit many practices, while at the same time creating exceptions and "safe harbors" for others. The safe harbors outline various payment and business practices that, although potentially capable of inducing referrals of business reimbursable under the federal health care programs, will not be treated as offenses under the anti-kickback statute.

Imagine that you are a hospital manager who seeks to expand hospital service offerings by bringing a new physician to your area. Physician recruitment potentially implicates the fraud and abuse regulations. If you are contemplating offering some form of remuneration to the physician, you would first want to consider the requirements of 42 C.F.R. § 411.357. By providing that certain compensation arrangements do not constitute a financial relationship, this federal regulation removes them from the reach of the Stark statute, which applies when a financial relationship exists. The regulation's complex provisions read in part as follows:

. . . the following compensation arrangements do not constitute a financial relationship:

(e) Physician recruitment. (1) Remuneration provided by a hospital to recruit a physician that is paid directly to the physician and that is intended to induce the physician to relocate his or her medical practice to the geographic area

---

**IN PRACTICE:** Physician Recruitment and the Fraud
and Abuse Regulations *(Continued)*

---

served by the hospital in order to become a member of the hospital's medical staff, if all of the following conditions are met:

(i) The arrangement is set out in writing and signed by both parties; . . .

(iii) The hospital does not determine (directly or indirectly) the amount of the remuneration to the physician based on the volume or value of any actual or anticipated referrals by the physician or other business generated between the parties; and

(iv) The physician is allowed to establish staff privileges at any other hospital(s) and to refer business to any other entities (except as referrals may be restricted under an employment or services contract that complies with § 411.354[d][4]).

(2)(i) The "geographic area served by the hospital" is the area composed of the lowest number of contiguous zip codes from which the hospital draws at least 75 percent of its inpatients. The geographic area served by the hospital may include one or more zip codes from which the hospital draws no inpatients, provided that such zip codes are entirely surrounded by zip codes in the geographic area described above from which the hospital draws at least 75 percent of its inpatients. . . .

(iv) A physician will be considered to have relocated his or her medical practice if the medical practice was located outside the geographic area served by the hospital and . . .

(B) The physician moves his medical practice into the geographic area served by the hospital, and the physician's new medical practice derives at least 75 percent of its revenues from professional services furnished to patients (including hospital inpatients) not seen or treated by the physician at his or her prior medical practice site during the preceding 3 years, measured on an annual basis (fiscal or calendar year). For the initial "start up" year of the recruited physician's practice, the 75 percent test in the preceding sentence will be satisfied if there is a reasonable expectation that the recruited physician's medical practice for the year will derive at least 75 percent of its revenues from professional services furnished to patients not seen or treated by the physician at his or her prior medical practice site during the preceding 3 years. . . .

(4) In the case of remuneration provided by a hospital to a physician either indirectly through payments made to another physician practice, or directly to a physician who joins a physician practice, the following additional conditions must be met: . . .

(iii) In the case of an income guarantee of any type made by the hospital to a recruited physician who joins a physician practice, the costs allocated by the physician practice to the recruited physician do not exceed the actual additional incremental costs attributable to the recruited physician. . . .

Before undertaking a transaction that might implicate the fraud and abuse regulations, managers need to discuss the transaction with an attorney to ensure that the business arrangement complies with the relevant regulations. Keep in mind, too, that physician recruitment may also involve other regulatory issues, such as IRS regulations on private inurement and private benefit.

This example is adapted from Gostin and Jacobson (2006).

---

## HIPAA Privacy and Security

Fraud and abuse regulations have affected health care organizations' daily operations for many years, and will likely continue to do so for many more. There is another, newer set of regulations, however, that has emerged over the last few years and promises to become increasingly important as time goes on: privacy and security-related regulations.

In 1996, Congress passed the Health Insurance Portability and Accountability Act (**HIPAA**). As the act's title suggests, many of its provisions are aimed at health insurance plans. For example, HIPAA limits the ability of new employers to exclude coverage for preexisting conditions; this limit applies to conditions that were medically identified at least six months prior to the start of enrollment. If an individual's medical condition developed or was identified within six months prior to enrollment, then the individual may be subject to a preexisting exclusion and therefore not receive coverage, even if it is a chronic illness (DOL, 2010), until either 6 or 12 months (depending on the plan) after employment begins. Coverage for pregnancy, conditions identified through genetic information, and certain newborn and adopted children with medical conditions cannot be excluded. HIPAA also prohibits discrimination against employees and dependent family members with prior medical conditions, offers opportunities to enroll in new plans due to life-changing events, and guarantees certain individuals the ability to access and renew insurance policies (DOL, 2010).

HIPAA's protections expand beyond its regulation of insurance coverage, however, to include privacy and security of health information. Of HIPAA's provisions, it is perhaps these regulations that have had the greatest effect on health care providers. Specifically, these regulations are intended to safeguard the privacy and security of protected health information (PHI), which includes anything that could identify an individual patient. The use of medical records, billing information, and other personally identifiable health data must follow stringent guidelines. Absent specific authorization from patients, protected health information may only be shared for certain purposes, such as provider payment, treatment, and health care operations. Institutions are required to have security measures in place to protect the data from unnecessary dissemination to parties who are not involved in a patient's care and to ensure that contracted entities protect the information as well. Employees must be trained to follow appropriate procedures for protecting health information (HHS, 2010).

From an operational perspective, HIPAA regulations do not require major changes in how providers and staff communicate but, outside of treatment and other specified contexts, permit only the minimum necessary protected health information to be exchanged. The regulations do not define what would constitute the minimum necessary information, but leave it to providers to determine.

Finally, state laws may impose more stringent privacy protections. In that sense, HIPAA sets a floor of privacy protection rather than a ceiling.

## EMTALA

A third statute that affects the daily operations of health care providers is the Emergency Medical Treatment and Labor Act (**EMTALA**) of 1986, which is designed to prevent institutions from denying care to anyone seeking emergency medical treatment, regardless of citizenship, insurance status, or ability to pay. EMTALA's broad purpose is to prevent private hospitals from dumping uninsured patients on hospitals of last resort without first screening and stabilizing them. Hospitals that accept Medicare reimbursement and have emergency departments are subject to EMTALA's two primary requirements (Kamoie, 2004).

First, hospitals must perform an initial patient evaluation. Specifically, the statute states that "if any individual . . . comes to the emergency department and a request is made on the individual's behalf for examination or treatment for a medical condition, the hospital must provide for an appropriate medical screening examination within the capability of the hospital's emergency department . . . to determine whether or not an emergency medical condition . . . exists." Individuals who arrive at the hospital in a location other than the dedicated emergency department must specifically state that they are seeking treatment for an emergency medical condition for EMTALA to apply.

The statute's second requirement is that hospitals stabilize individuals who are determined to have an emergency condition before discharge or transfer to a more appropriate facility. If a hospital elects to transfer, it still has an obligation to mitigate risks to the health of the individual, and in the case of a woman in labor, to the health of the unborn child.

## Health Care Quality Improvement Act

A fourth example of a statute that affects providers' operations is the Health Care Quality Improvement Act (**HCQIA**) of 1986. At the time of its enactment, HCQIA reflected two primary concerns, one relating to weaknesses in existing peer review processes, and the other to the ease with which incompetent physicians were able to move between states without a record of their malpractice experience or professional disciplinary action. HCQIA is designed to address these issues by encouraging physicians to identify and discipline fellow physicians who are incompetent or who engage in unprofessional behavior, so as to improve the quality of care.

HCQIA provides limited immunity to physicians and dentists who engage in the peer review process, mitigating

## Debate Time: Health Care Provider Integration

U.S. health policy reflects a deeply conflicting attitude toward the clinical integration of hospitals and physicians. During much of the twentieth century, there was little or no integration between these two types of providers. Most hospitals maintained a so-called dual structure whereby their medical staff, those physicians who have authority to admit patients to the hospital and use its clinical resources, was organized as a largely separate and self-governed entity. Hospitals and the members of their medical staff rarely collaborated in pursuit of common patient care goals. Indeed, the hospital-physician relationship was predicated largely on the mutual but distinct financial interests of the two types of providers; hospitals relied on physicians for admissions, and physicians relied on hospitals for the equipment and technology that they needed to provide services. This relationship was supported, even promoted, by fee for service reimbursement under which the incomes of hospitals and physicians were tied to the volume of services they provided to patients.

Although in more recent years, several industry forces have motivated hospitals and physicians to collaborate in some areas of patient care, many health care leaders believe that hospitals and physicians continue to function far too independently from each other. The Medicare Payment Advisory Commission, in one of its recent reports to Congress, discussed how the lack of integration between hospitals and physicians translates into a fragmented delivery system that is prone to error, inefficiency, and poor quality of care. Health care leaders have called for hospitals and physicians to collaborate in developing policies and procedures for ensuring continuity of care for patients across clinical settings, sharing expertise and experience for identifying cost-effective medical technologies and devices, and assuming joint financial accountability for managing the care of patients. Toward this end, various policy initiatives have been put forth to create incentives, financial and otherwise, to encourage hospitals and physicians to work more collaboratively to improve patient care.

However, such initiatives are impeded by various U.S. laws and regulations, some of which have been enacted for the very purpose of keeping hospitals and physicians from integrating too closely. In particular, federal fraud and abuse laws impose many restrictions on the ability of hospitals and physicians to form partnerships for sharing financial risks and rewards in the delivery of patient care services, such as through gainsharing arrangements. Hospitals with a federal income tax exemption may jeopardize their exemption when they invest in health care organizations that are controlled by physicians who are members of their medical staff. The antitrust laws also present legal risks for hospitals and physicians that engage in collaborative arrangements as these arrangements can be seen as anticompetitive tactics to strengthen the participants' negotiating leverage with health plans. Although both the Federal Trade Commission and Department of Justice, the two government agencies that are responsible for antitrust enforcement, have encouraged health care providers to integrate clinically to reduce their risk of antitrust violations, the regulatory guidance has not been entirely consistent and, in some instances, has been contradictory to the policies of other government agencies with oversight responsibility for the health care industry. Further, some states have corporate practice of medicine laws that prohibit or otherwise restrict hospitals from employing physicians directly. In light of these legal barriers to collaboration, some health care leaders believe significant legal reforms are a necessary first step for promoting meaningful hospital-physician integration.

So what do you think? An argument in favor of such legal reforms is that many of the previously noted laws are overly broad as they relate to the health care industry and deter hospitals and physicians from engaging in collaborative arrangements that are good for patient care. A counterargument is that wide-scale legal reforms may usher in an era of highly undesirable conduct in the health care industry as some providers exploit legal exemptions and loopholes for their own financial gain rather than to improve patient care.

the risk associated with lawsuits from physicians who face sanctions or loss of staff privileges after formal peer review. HCQIA provides immunity only if the peer review decision was taken: (1) in the reasonable belief that the action was in the furtherance of quality health care; (2) after a reasonable effort to obtain the facts of the matter; (3) after adequate notice and hearing procedures were afforded to the physician involved or after such other procedures as were fair to the physician under the circumstances; and (4) in the reasonable belief that the action was warranted by the facts known after such reasonable effort to obtain facts and after meeting the requirements of (3) above. Most courts have held that bias or malice in the peer review process is irrelevant, as long as those involved in the peer review process made a good-faith effort to ascertain the facts.

HCQIA also establishes the **National Practitioner Data Bank** (NPDB) to store information regarding physicians' and dentists' professional competence and conduct, increasing the accessibility of information about medical liability awards and settlements and peer review sanctions. The data in the NPDB comes from multiple sources, including reports that health care providers are required to make. Health care managers must also consult the NPDB when considering offering staff privileges, and every two years for all physicians with current staff privileges. Note, though, that reports have found that the NPDB is missing data and that it has not been as effective as anticipated.

# STATE POLICY AND REGULATION

While the scope of the federal government's involvement in health care has increased significantly over time, state and local governments have traditionally played a far more central health-related role. State and local governments provide care through public hospitals and clinics, finance care through Medicaid and other programs, and create and enforce health care–related laws and regulations. Whether acting as providers, payers, or regulators, state and local governments can have a dramatic impact on health care delivery, and, ultimately, public health.

As providers, state and local governments have a direct impact on the availability of care. As payers, they affect access and quality through the incentives created by reimbursement policies. They affect access and quality as regulators, too. States' regulations of health insurance, for example, affect both the scope and cost of insurance policies (Jost, 2009). States may limit insurers' ability to turn away applicants, prohibit refusals to renew policies, or regulate premium setting. They may mandate that insurance policies sold within the state include certain benefits, increasing access to the covered providers or services, but also increasing the costs of policies. They may also attempt to ensure access to care through mechanisms such as requirements for external reviews of claims denials.

State regulation also affects public health more generally. In addition to engaging in general health promotion activities, public health departments enforce laws intended to prevent the spread of contagious disease through quarantines or immunization requirements. State laws support public health departments' surveillance efforts through requirements that health care providers report certain injuries and diseases. State agencies regularly become involved in a wide range of public health issues, including foodborne illnesses and environmental health hazards such as lead. State agencies also have responsibility for oversight of the quality and safety of health care facilities. It is in this role that state agencies have the most direct interaction with health care providers.

## Licensure

**Licensure** serves as a primary mechanism by which states regulate the quality of care provided by health care organizations. Many types of health care organizations must secure a license from a state agency before they can begin to operate. The major impetus for state-level licensure of health care organizations was the 1946 Hill-Burton Act. Through this legislation, the federal government made hospital funding available to states but tied the funds to a state's adoption of a hospital licensure statute. Since then, states have expanded their licensure programs to cover more types of health care organizations.

The types of health care organizations required to obtain a license vary somewhat across states. Although all states require licensure for certain types of organizations, namely hospitals and nursing homes, they differ in their treatment of other organizations such as home health agencies, freestanding clinics, and ambulatory surgical centers. States uniformly do not require licensure for physician offices as these entities are not treated as distinct health care organizations, but rather as an extension of the physician practice itself and thus exempt from licensure. Whether or not other entities, such as ambulatory surgical centers, are also extensions of a physician practice, and thus exempt from licensure requirements, has been a source of debate. Ambulatory surgical centers are subject to licensure in many but not all states (American Surgery Center Association, 2010).

In most states, the department of health or a comparable government agency is responsible for the licensure of health care organizations. This is in contrast to the licensure of health care professionals such as physicians and nurses, where responsibility is vested in occupational licensure boards that are largely composed of individuals with the same professional background as the applicants. The state agencies that are responsible for licensure of health care organizations typically subdivide regulatory responsibilities by type of organization, such as hospitals or nursing homes, and these regulatory responsibilities are carried out by state employees who develop expertise as to the relevant licensure requirements and procedures.

For any type of health care organization, the specific licensure requirements and procedures will differ somewhat from state to state. Typically, not all licensure requirements are located in the state authorizing statute itself; the state licensing agency will have responsibilities for issuing additional licensure requirements. In general, licensure requirements tend to focus on structural features of organizations, such as resources and policies, rather than the actual quality provided. For example, state licensing requirements for hospitals typically focus on such characteristics as physical layout, equipment, governance policies, and staffing. Because of this focus on structural features, licensure is often considered to be a minimal form of quality oversight.

All states require as a condition of licensure that an organization undergo a site inspection. In an on-site inspection, state agency personnel visit the organization to observe its campus and review documents and other materials pertaining to licensure requirements. The inspectors will conduct interviews with the administrative and clinical staff regarding the implementation of relevant policies and procedures. At least one inspection will be conducted prior to the time the organization first opens its doors. Subsequent inspections may be announced or unannounced. Also, in some states, certain types of organizations are deemed to be in compliance with licensure requirements if they are accredited by a state-approved accrediting body. For example, in some states, a hospital that is accredited by the Joint Commission is deemed to be in compliance with the state's hospital licensure requirements and does not need to undergo a separate state inspection.

## Certificate of Need Regulation

In many states, a health care facility cannot be constructed, renovated, or expanded without obtaining a **certificate of need** (CON). Existing health care organizations may also need to secure a CON before purchasing major equipment or offering new services. A CON is a form of approval from a state agency, usually the department of public health or a comparable agency, that is responsible for determining whether a need exists for the requested organization, service, or equipment. Thus, like licensure, CON is a regulatory hurdle that must be overcome before a provider can begin to offer services. Numerous empirical studies have examined the effect of CON on health care costs (Conover and Sloan, 1998; Hellinger, 2009). While the results are by no means entirely consistent, the weight of the evidence has not been highly supportive of CON as a form of cost control. CON has also been criticized for being highly politicized in many states and insufficiently transparent.

During the 1970s, almost every state had a CON law because federal policy, specifically the 1974 National Health Planning and Resources Development Act, promoted this type of regulatory mechanism as a form of cost control for health care services. The basic idea was to establish within each state a central planning and regulatory structure for overseeing the use and allocation of health care resources to prevent excess capacity from driving up costs. However, since the 1970s, a number of states have eliminated their CON programs, preferring to approach cost control from the standpoint of market competition rather than relying on a regulatory and central planning structure. Still, as of 2008, 36 states had some form of CON in place (NCSL, 2010).

Among states that have retained their CON programs, there is considerable variation among key program elements, namely the organizations that are covered; the types of projects, equipment, or services for which a CON must be secured; and the expenditure thresholds under which a CON is not required. For example, a state CON program may exempt all projects with an expenditure target of under $200,000.

States also differ in the way they review CON applications. All states require applicants to put forward evidence of need in support of their request that speaks to issues of access, cost, and quality. However, some states require applicants to support their request with a high level of quantitative data and analytic models, whereas other states accept applications that are less formal in their presentation.

## Relationships between State and Federal Law

States' involvement in health-related regulation extends well beyond the insurance, public health, licensure, and certificate of need areas. State law relating to medical negligence is an important consideration for health care providers, for example.

Other state laws, such as those related to antitrust, fraud, or privacy, may exist alongside similar federal laws.

State and federal laws interact in varied ways. For example, as previously noted, states have antitrust statutes that generally parallel federal antitrust statutes. Under the "state action doctrine," however, certain activities that might otherwise be found to violate federal antitrust law are exempted because a state has taken an active role in supervising those activities. State action arguments may be relevant in situations involving seemingly anticompetitive actions of state licensing boards or medical staffs of public hospitals. In addition, providers who turn to state governments for approvals of various forms of collaboration may hope to invoke the state action doctrine (Havighurst, 2006).

**Preemption** principles also affect the interaction between federal and state laws. At the core of preemption analysis is a simple idea: if federal and state laws directly conflict, the federal law applies. (State law may also preempt local laws in the same way.) Preemption may mean that someone who seeks a remedy for an injury under state law, such as the law relating to negligence, may not be able to pursue the claim.

But the forms of preemption are numerous, and the analysis involved is not always straightforward. Litigation involving the federal Employee Retirement Income Security Act (**ERISA**), which imposes minimum requirements on retirement and health benefit plans, illustrates the complexity of preemption issues. The statute itself states that it supersedes all state laws that "relate to" employee benefit plans. Arguably, such laws may include certain statutes intended to encourage employers to expand employee access to health care benefits. Recent federal appeals court cases have come to differing conclusions about whether ERISA preempts state and local efforts to expand access through various forms of employer mandates, such as a mandate that employers spend a minimum amount on health insurance or pay an equivalent amount to the state; one court found a Maryland law preempted, while another rejected a similar challenge to a San Francisco ordinance.

Other ERISA preemption cases have found their way to the Supreme Court. The Supreme Court has ruled, for example, that ERISA does not preempt a state statute requiring health maintenance organizations to permit review of denied claims by independent reviewers. It has also ruled, however, that ERISA preempts certain claims based on a state law permitting

managed care enrollees to sue their plans for injuries resulting from benefit denials.

As these examples make clear, both state law and federal law can have a significant influence over health care entities' activities.

# ORGANIZATIONAL STRATEGIES FOR REGULATORY COMPLIANCE

In view of the numerous regulatory requirements and challenges that hospitals and other health care organizations (HCOs) face, they need to develop strategies for complying with regulatory demands. Noncompliance could result in costly lawsuits and regulatory sanctions that disrupt daily operations. As noted earlier, the imposition of a Corporate Integrity Agreement is very disruptive to the regulatory compliance process. In rare instances, systematic regulatory failures could result in the loss of eligibility for Medicare and Medicaid reimbursement. To avoid such results, it is advisable for health care executives to adopt regulatory compliance practices that are thorough, systematic, and capable of adapting to the continuously changing environment in which HCOs operate.

## Patient Safety

One important strategy for maintaining regulatory compliance involves mitigating risk of harm to patients. The 1999 report by the Institute of Medicine, *To Err is Human: Building a Safer Health System*, stated that between 44,000 and 98,000 deaths could be attributed to preventable medical errors (IOM, 1999). To promote patient safety, HCOs have a responsibility to create and enforce policies that ensure recruitment and retention of competent physicians and other care providers, prevent the spread of infectious disease through safe practices (such as appropriate hand washing), and maintain facilities and equipment properly. Evidence-based practices for safeguarding patients are constantly evolving, and organizations must have a system in place to demonstrate due diligence toward protecting patient safety.

In the event that a patient's safety is compromised as a result of an error or negligence, there are a number of steps an organization could take to protect the institution. First, while care providers and institutions have historically attempted to cover up their mistakes, research has shown that patients are less likely to pursue litigation if they are provided with a transparent care process (Boothman et al., 2009). Although this approach remains controversial because it may increase risk exposure, acknowledging that an error has occurred and demonstrating that the HCO is taking reasonable steps to both mitigate harm to the patient and prevent harm to future patients may deter litigation.

Second, HCOs must report errors to the appropriate state agency and the appropriate accreditation agency, such as the Joint Commission. In 1996, the Joint Commission introduced a sentinel event-reporting policy to help HCOs identify errors and take steps towards preventing future occurrences (Joint Commission, Sentinel events, 2010). The Joint Commission defines a sentinel event as "an unexpected occurrence involving death or serious physical or psychological injury, or the risk thereof" (Joint Commission, Sentinel events, 2010). HCOs are expected to conduct root cause analyses to determine and address the underlying systemic or procedural issues that resulted in the error. Failure to report a sentinel event can result in the loss of accreditation (Joint Commission, Sentinel events, 2010).

Some sentinel events, such as operating on the wrong body part, are known as "never events" (National Quality Forum, 2002). Table 12.3 provides examples of these serious preventable adverse events. Congress has directed HHS to deny Medicare and Medicaid reimbursement for certain specified never events.

## The Role of the Regulatory Compliance Officer

To successfully navigate through the complex regulatory environment, HCOs often appoint a regulatory compliance officer. This individual is responsible for conducting all activities related to regulatory compliance, including educating staff on regulatory compliance protocols through training programs, monitoring compliance, and implementing consistent enforcement policies. Officers also actively respond to compliance violations and seek out opportunities to prevent future violations. In addition to serving as internal monitors, they act as liaisons between HCOs and appropriate regulatory agencies to ensure proper reporting occurs. Collaboration with other departments in the HCO, such as Risk Management, Internal Audit, Employee Services, and Human Resources, is essential to addressing compliance issues as well as fostering the development of a compliance culture.

Regulatory compliance officers must pay special attention to certain areas as a result of their potentially serious consequences for HCOs. Officers often conduct internal audits of practices that might constitute fraud or abuse. For example, Medicare payments to HCOs are based on codes that reflect patients' severity of illness. When upcoding occurs, patients are misrepresented as sicker, thereby allowing an organization to obtain greater compensation for services provided, and placing it at risk for fraud and abuse sanctions.

## TABLE 12.3  Serious Reportable Events (Never Events)

| Event | Example |
|---|---|
| 1. Surgical Events | Wrong surgical procedure performed on a patient |
| 2. Product or Device Events | Patient death or serious disability associated with the use of contaminated drugs, devices, or biologics provided by the HCO |
| 3. Patient Protection Events | Infant discharged to the wrong person |
| 4. Care Management Events | Stage 3 or 4 pressure ulcers acquired after admission to a HCO |
| 5. Environmental Events | Patient death or serious disability associated with an electric shock while being cared for in a HCO |
| 6. Criminal Events | Abduction of a patient of any age |

SOURCE: Adapted from the NQF Web site (NQF, 2002).

A proper internal auditing system will allow for appropriate code assignments and reimbursement commensurate with a patient's disease category.

To deal with issues surrounding improper reimbursement, CMS created the **Recovery Audit Contractor** (RAC) program. RAC audits review improper Medicare payments to correct errors involving both overpayment and underpayment. HCOs should prepare for audits by creating a RAC committee and designating a coordinator. Targeted reviews should be conducted to identify and correct billing areas. Furthermore, coders' knowledge on coding and medical necessity should also be properly evaluated to ensure that they are current (Sheeder and Tonn, 2009).

Due diligence in preparation for such audits is essential for preventing FCA whistle-blower claims concerning an organization's improper conduct. Organizations must have proper policies and procedures to respond to employees who raise compliance concerns.

## Health Care Organizations' Regulatory Challenges

Given the number of regulations under which HCOs must operate, it can be challenging to ensure compliance with all of them. HCOs need to manage quality standards of multiple regulatory agencies and operate transparently, yet also maintain privacy, all at the same time. These potentially conflicting demands can weigh heavily on HCOs' ability to operate.

As a consequence of the complex regulatory environment, HCOs need to invest a considerable amount of resources to ensure compliance. Providers face substantial regulatory paperwork; reporting suspension of physicians' privileges to the NPDB and reporting medical errors to the appropriate body are just two of many examples of reporting requirements.

The costs of noncompliance can be high. For example, if hospitals fail to report suspension of physicians' privileges within 30 days, they will lose the protections against liability that they would otherwise have under HCQIA. In addition, regulatory violations often result in considerable fines.

# RECENT POLICY AND REGULATORY INITIATIVES

Federal, state, and local governments, public and private payers, professional and trade organizations, providers, and others continually search for new ways to improve health care's quality and reduce its cost. This section illustrates a few of the many approaches, both legal and nonlegal, that play important roles in recent efforts to reform the health care system.

For health care managers, familiarity with health reform efforts is important because of their power to transform the regulatory and market environments in which health care organizations operate. Imagine, for example, a proposed law that required the disclosure of a hospital's prices, or mandated reporting of surgery outcomes, or tied Medicare reimbursement to specific quality measures. If you were a health care executive, would you support or oppose such a law? What actions would you take in support of or in opposition to the law? Would you seek to modify the content of the law, and if so, how? If the proposed law were enacted, how might you alter your organization's operations? Consider these questions as you review each of the following examples of recent policy and regulatory reform initiatives.

## Transparency

In most marketplaces, consumers consider the price and quality of available goods and services before making purchasing decisions. This is not the case, however, when it comes to health care. Most patients know little about the price or quality of medical services. This lack of information creates significant hurdles for patient efforts to obtain low-cost, high-quality care. It also undermines the competitive process that might otherwise drive prices lower and quality higher. A number of recent initiatives attempt to address these problems by increasing price and quality **transparency**.

### Prices

Insured patients who are responsible only for fixed copayments or limited coinsurance have little reason to care about medical prices. For the increasing number of patients who are enrolled in high-deductible health plans or who are uninsured, however, health care prices have become critically important. Without price information, these patients will not be able to take financial considerations into account when deciding on a course of treatment. Nor will they be able to choose providers on the basis of price. As a result, providers will have little reason to compete over price.

A number of state governments have responded to the paucity of pricing data (CBO, 2008). In 2003, for example, the California legislature passed a "Payers' Bill of Rights" that mandated that hospitals publicly disclose their charges. Subsequently, it added a requirement that hospitals provide price estimates to uninsured patients upon request. New Hampshire now maintains a Web site that reports the median amounts paid by insurers and patients for a variety of medical services (CSHSC, 2009).

These initiatives may partially remedy patients' pricing information deficit, but unless accompanied by other reforms, they are unlikely to achieve effective competition in health care markets. Patients are not likely to know the precise nature of the hospital services they will require, and even if they do, they will not be able to easily wade through the thousands of items on hospital price lists. In addition, a recent study shows that patients may not always succeed in obtaining hospital cost estimates, despite California's mandate (Farrell et al., 2010). New Hampshire's program may assist patients in learning more about health care costs, but price variation among providers has persisted, suggesting that it has not generated significant patient shopping on the basis of price (CSHSC, 2009). Insurers may provide information about costs or fees, but many enrollees never take advantage of it (Fronstin, 2009). There is also a worry that detailed price disclosure might sometimes raise prices, because it could lead lower-paid providers to seek higher rates or facilitate price coordination among otherwise-competing providers. While price transparency has potential as a tool to encourage more efficient provision of care, the barriers to achieving this potential are considerable (CBO, 2008).

## Quality

Most patients lack information about health care quality, just as they lack information about price. Patients have traditionally turned to friends, family members, and their own physicians for recommendations for health care providers, but have had little access to more systematic assessments of clinical quality. This lack of information hinders patients' abilities to select providers and payers' abilities to compensate providers on the basis of quality. As a result, providers might seek to deliver high-quality care for reasons of professional ethics or regulatory compliance, but might not feel significant reputational or financial pressure to increase quality. In addition, limited availability of quality measures may undermine providers' efforts to assess and improve their own quality.

Governments and other organizations have sought to fill this information void through public quality and safety reporting. Many states, including California, Colorado, Illinois, New York, and Pennsylvania, require hospitals to report health care quality information, while other states require public reporting of errors or hospital infection rates (Madison, 2009; National survey, 2008). Patients in some states can obtain hospital-specific quality and safety information, such as cardiac bypass surgery mortality rates or infection rates, through state-operated Web sites. These legal reporting mandates complement efforts by public and private payers and other organizations to increase public quality information. HHS, for example, provides structure, process, and outcome-based hospital quality measures, as well as measures based on hospital patient surveys, on its Hospital Compare Web site. For-profit companies also provide quality ratings.

Measures of quality of other providers are available, but less common. Medicare, for example, publishes quality ratings for nursing homes. A few states publish physician-specific mortality rates for bypass surgery. California publishes quality ratings for medical groups, as does a Massachusetts-based broad coalition of providers, payers, and others. HHS has begun to collect quality information on a voluntary basis from some physicians, but has not begun to publish it.

Efforts to improve the quality of care through reporting face considerable challenges (Harris and Buntin, 2008; Madison, 2009). Quality measures must be appropriately selected; ideally, they would reflect important dimensions of care without leading providers to neglect unmeasured aspects of care. They must be appropriately designed, so that they accurately capture quality and are not biased by underlying patient illness. Poorly designed measures could encourage providers to try to improve ratings by avoiding sicker patients, while at the same time misleading users about where to obtain high-quality care. They must be appropriately presented, so that users understand them; confusing measures could lead to poor choices of providers (Hibbard and Peters, 2003). They must not be overly burdensome; particularly given the numerous and varied organizations involved in quality reporting efforts, providers may face considerable administrative costs in collecting quality data. Finally, people must use them. Report cards can improve quality only if patients respond by selecting higher-quality providers, or providers respond by increasing their own quality of care.

Some patients use report cards (Harris and Buntin, 2008), and anecdotal evidence suggests that some providers respond to them (Chassin, 2002). But many patients do not use them. Lack of awareness, lack of interest, and illness itself can all serve as barriers to use. In addition, studies have suggested that report cards may have unintended consequences, as providers attempt to improve their ratings by changing the mix of patients they treat, rather than by improving the care they deliver (Dranove et al., 2003; Werner and Asch, 2005). The technical challenges involved in creating measures are formidable, particularly for physicians, who may not treat enough patients to create meaningful measures (Nyweide et al., 2009). Moreover, studies evaluating the early effects of report cards on quality have had mixed results (Fung et al., 2008). Nevertheless, public reporting may become an even more important tool for quality improvement in the future, as reporting technologies improve and familiarity with report cards grows.

## Pay-for-Performance

In recent years, **pay-for-performance** (P4P) has become a widely adopted strategy for improving the performance of health care organizations. In concept, P4P entails linking financial incentives to the accomplishment of assigned performance goals related to efficiency, productivity, or quality. Although there have been various applications of P4P to the health care industry in the past, the last five years have witnessed a substantial interest in applying this concept to quality of care.

Most existing P4P programs follow a similar structure. A typical program focuses on individual physicians, physician groups, or hospitals, as the entities accountable for achieving assigned quality goals. For example, a health plan may assign a set of quality targets for diabetes care to the physician organizations with which it contracts. One of these quality targets may specify that a certain percentage of the group's diabetic patients will receive an annual blood test to monitor for glucose control. The group's score on this and other measures will then be used to compute an incentive payment. The financial incentives can be structured in various ways, including bonuses or fee adjustments.

At present, both the private and public sectors have embraced some form of P4P. Most of the P4P programs on the private side are sponsored by payers, either private sector health plans or employer purchasing groups. There are well

over 150 such programs. In the public sector, many state Medicaid programs have adopted some type of P4P, and, using the label "value-based purchasing," Congress has directed Medicare to adopt P4P as well as part of its reimbursement program for hospitals.

This interest in P4P is in large part a response to a growing body of evidence indicating that the quality of care in the U.S. is suboptimal. Some health policy experts attribute at least part of the quality problem to a lack of provider reimbursement for high quality of care. The promise of P4P is that by linking financial incentives to important quality goals, providers will be motivated to improve quality. Whether this promise is being realized is not entirely clear based on a small but growing body of studies that addresses the impact of P4P on quality (Rosenthal et al., 2005; Young et al., 2007). However, as the health care industry currently has had only limited experience with P4P, it may take several more years before it is possible to sort out the effectiveness of P4P as a strategy for improving quality.

## Specialty Hospitals

Whether or not they achieve their intended effects, laws and regulations often have unintended consequences. The recent growth in specialty hospitals illustrates this point. The federal Stark statute, which is intended to prevent physician self-referrals, contains an exception for physician referrals to hospitals they own when "the ownership or investment interest is in the hospital itself (and not merely in a subdivision of the hospital)" (42 U.S.C. § 1395nn[d][3][C]). This exception permits physician financial support for general hospitals while at the same time blunting the financial impact of a physician-investor's own referrals on his or her investment return. But what if the only services available within the whole hospital were cardiac services? The Stark statute exception would seem to apply, permitting providers to refer despite their ownership interests. The whole hospital exception, along with the profitability of the services involved, contributed to the recent growth of specialty hospitals in areas such as cardiac care (Iglehart, 2005).

Specialty hospitals are controversial. In theory, their narrow focus may help them deliver more efficient and higher-quality care than traditional general hospitals. In addition, their existence may spur competing hospitals to improve their own quality. At the same time, however, physician-owned specialty hospitals are subject to the general concerns underlying the fraud and abuse laws, such as the concern that physician-investors may over-refer patients, increasing costs and perhaps worsening outcomes.

General hospitals are especially worried about the impact of specialty hospitals. Like any organizations facing new competition, they worry about potential losses of net revenues. These losses might be especially high if physician-investors refer patients with generous payers to the specialty hospitals they own, leaving at local general hospitals patients they perceive as money-losers due to either the severity of their illnesses or the identity of their payers. One study found that although specialty hospitals' Medicare patients were not less costly than those of general hospitals, their patients did tend to be less severely ill and were less likely to be insured through Medicaid (MedPAC, 2005). Because nonprofit hospitals' net revenues support the provision of unprofitable services and charity care, the potential loss of these revenues might concern the broader public.

Congress responded to early concerns about specialty hospitals by imposing a temporary moratorium on the use of the whole hospital exception, but this moratorium has expired. Given the uncertainties about both the beneficial and detrimental effects of specialty hospitals, debate continues about how best to respond to their growth.

## Comparative Clinical Effectiveness

As concern about health care costs continues to grow, policy makers continue to look for new ways to control costs. An emerging cost containment strategy is to encourage **comparative clinical effectiveness** research (CER). CER is intended to compare medical treatments and strategies to enable health care providers to determine the most cost-effective clinical treatments. The American Reinvestment and Recovery Act of 2009 introduced a broad economic stimulus package that included provisions to expand CER. Congress allocated $1.1 billion to this endeavor, providing funding to AHRQ, NIH, and HHS.

Each agency involved can use its own discretion in allocating the funds for CER. For example, AHRQ has plans to potentially expand previously developed CER programs, such as the Effective Health Care program, which sets priorities for different health issues and uses a rigorous process to support research activities that meet stakeholder needs. Other agencies are developing plans to identify specific procedures and technologies that have not yet been subject to CER.

A key issue is how the results of CER will affect policy and practice. Physicians may recognize the value of CER, for example, but their behaviors and practices may be slow to change in response (CBO, 2007). In the area of pharmaceutical development, CER could result in policy changes requiring organizations such as drug companies to conduct further clinical trials of their products against alternative treatments to identify superior products in terms of safety and efficacy. With respect to insurance coverage determinations, concerns about whether using CER is tantamount to rationing may limit its use.

While potentially providing substantial assistance in identifying cost-effective clinical treatments, CER remains controversial among physicians and elected officials.

---

## DEBATE TIME: Regulation of Pharmaceutical Promotion

Pharmaceutical companies spend billions of dollars each year to promote products to physicians (Donohue, Cevasco, and Rosenthal, 2007). Pharmaceutical companies advertise in professional journals; make regular visits to physician offices for conversations about their products, a practice called "detailing"; and provide free samples of their products. Pharmaceutical companies may also influence physicians' prescribing efforts through the financial relationships they establish. In addition to distributing small gifts, such as pens bearing logos, pharmaceutical companies have funded catered lunches at physicians' offices; offered payments for advising, consulting, or speaking; and contributed toward the costs associated with continuing medical education and other meetings. One survey showed that over 90 percent of physicians had some sort of relationship with the pharmaceutical industry. More than 80 percent of physicians, for example, received food at their workplace (Campbell et al., 2007).

**DEBATE TIME: Regulation of Pharmaceutical Promotion** *(Continued)*

Studies suggest that pharmaceutical companies' financial ties to physicians may affect prescribing patterns (Rothman and Chimonas, 2008; Wazana, 2000). The changes in prescribing patterns could potentially increase health costs or worsen health outcomes, relative to a world in which fully independent physicians issued prescriptions. The proliferation of financial ties could in the long run reduce patient trust in physicians, potentially undermining treatment relationships.

Concerned about the effects of pharmaceutical company practices, legislators in a few states have imposed restrictions on pharmaceutical marketing. Vermont, for example, now bans most gifts to physicians, while requiring disclosure of payments for speaking, consulting, and research. It also requires that these payments reflect the fair market value of physicians' services. New Hampshire has banned the sale of identifiable prescription data for commercial purposes, including for use in promotional activities, making it difficult for pharmaceutical companies to monitor individual physicians' prescribing patterns and thereby limiting the use of detailing as a promotional tool. Federal laws, too, may sometimes restrict pharmaceutical company practices; for example, federal regulators have emphasized the importance of ensuring that promotional efforts do not run afoul of the anti-kickback statute.

Presumably aware of the likelihood that regulators will act if they do not (Greenland, 2009; Rothman and Chimonas, 2008), physicians have also been adopting policies intended to address concerns about ties to pharmaceutical companies. For example, some academic medical centers have prohibited physicians from accepting meals from pharmaceutical companies, and some health systems have begun to disclose outside payments made to their physicians. Pharmaceutical manufacturers have also revised their own policies. In 2008, Pharmaceutical Research and Manufacturers of America revised its marketing code to ban distribution of promotional pens and mugs to physicians and to prohibit the provision of restaurant meals (but not meals in physicians' offices, which were permitted to continue in certain circumstances), among other changes. Individual pharmaceutical companies have also announced plans to publicly report certain payments to physicians.

Despite these responses to the controversy surrounding promotional practices, the debate continues. Some have advocated federal legislation that would require disclosure of financial ties nationwide, while others have argued that regulation of conflicts of interest has gone too far. What do you think? Would you support federal legislation requiring disclosure of payments made to physicians? If so, what exactly should be disclosed? Should the federal law preempt all state disclosure requirements, or should states be permitted to enact more comprehensive requirements? Would you advocate that more states enact legislation like Vermont's or New Hampshire's? Or do you think that we should abandon our efforts to regulate, relying instead on voluntary efforts to limit any problematic practices? Are you concerned that disclosure regulations might discourage the formation of beneficial relationships between health care professionals and pharmaceutical and medical device companies, such as those that support research, product development, or educational efforts?

# SUMMARY AND MANAGERIAL GUIDELINES

1. State and federal governments have a significant impact on health care delivery through the statutes they enact, the regulations they impose, and the policies they adopt.

2. Governments use varied tools to achieve varied goals. Many governmental initiatives, including FDA regulations, licensure statutes, HCQIA, pay-for-performance programs, and quality reporting programs, are intended to ensure health care quality. Others, including antitrust law, fraud and abuse laws, and certificate of need laws, may in theory help lower health care costs.

EMTALA and the tax code may increase health care access, as do programs such as Medicare and Medicaid. Government initiatives may sometimes achieve several of these goals simultaneously, may achieve one goal but sacrifice progress on another, or, if poorly designed or poorly executed, may achieve no goals at all.

3. Given the large number of applicable laws and regulations, as well as their potential consequences for providers, health care managers must treat regulatory compliance with the importance given to other areas of health care operations. Due diligence is essential, both for internal compliance and responses to governmental inquiries. To ensure that the appropriate attention is devoted to regulatory issues, appoint a regulatory compliance officer who reports directly to the CEO.

4. To ensure ongoing compliance, identify regulatory requirements and develop monitoring procedures for activities that implicate these requirements. Identify troublesome areas that could result in bad publicity or substantial sanctions, and conduct routine audits in these areas.

5. Identify potential violations and establish mechanisms for reporting and correcting them. Determine appropriate internal sanctions for compliance failures and apply enforcement procedures consistently throughout the organization. To increase the likelihood of compliance and reduce the likelihood of legal sanctions, create opportunities for building relationships and resolving conflicts within your organization.

6. Governmental entities continuously experiment with new approaches to achieving policy goals. Health care managers must remain aware of the evolving content of laws, regulations, and policies, because it will necessarily affect day-to-day operations. To ensure continued compliance in a dynamic regulatory environment, maintain lines of communication throughout your organization and create and regularly update training and educational programs.

## DISCUSSION QUESTIONS

1. Identify the major laws and regulations affecting health care organizations. Why is the health care industry so heavily regulated? What are the central goals of these laws and regulations? Who benefits from them?

2. What problems do these regulations present? If you could eliminate one of these laws or regulations, which one would you eliminate, and why? Are there alternative regulatory approaches that would achieve regulatory objectives in a less burdensome way?

3. Critics of formal governmental health care regulation suggest that mechanisms such as self-regulation or accreditation would provide more effective oversight. Do you agree?

4. Nonprofit organizations must meet a community benefit test to take advantage of the federal income tax exemption. Should a facility be allowed to use population health interventions to meet the test instead of the measures noted in this chapter? If so, what measures of population health should the IRS accept?

5. Do you think government entities should devote more resources to developing health care quality report cards? Why or why not?

6. How should we regulate emerging market arrangements, such as pay-for-performance initiatives, and emerging health care providers, such as specialty hospitals?

## CASE: An Ambulatory Surgical Center Joint Venture

David Donaldson is the special assistant to the CEO of Tri-County Hospital, a 350-bed community hospital. Last week, he attended a meeting at which four of the hospital's orthopedic surgeons proposed a joint venture between them and the hospital to establish a freestanding ambulatory surgical center. The proposal they outlined had the following features:

- Tri-County will contribute 70 percent of the capital needed for construction of the facility and purchase of equipment and initial supplies. The other 30 percent will be financed by the surgeons with a bank loan.

- All business issues and questions related to the ambulatory surgical center will be decided by a majority vote of the center's managing directors. Three of the six positions will be occupied by representatives of the surgeons; the other positions will be occupied by representatives of the hospital. The partnership agreement will contain a binding arbitration clause in the event that a decision before the managing directors receives a tie vote.

- The surgeons will receive 65 percent of the profits from the ambulatory surgical center. The hospital will receive the remaining 35 percent.

- The hospital and surgeons will jointly develop a protocol addressing the types of surgical cases that should be handled on an inpatient basis at the hospital versus those that will be referred to the ambulatory surgical center. The hospital will be expected to promote the ambulatory surgical center and encourage medical staff members to make appropriate referrals. Also, profit margin thresholds will be established in advance for the ambulatory surgical center, and as these thresholds are reached, the division of profits between the hospital and the surgeons will be adjusted in favor of the hospital.

As a next step, David plans to prepare a memorandum for the hospital's CEO regarding the proposed joint venture. David generally believes that the CEO should seriously consider the joint venture. Although the surgeons did not say so explicitly, he suspects that if the CEO declines the deal, the surgeons may very well leave the hospital completely and form the ambulatory surgical center on their own. The four surgeons who have proposed the deal account for a substantial percentage of the income the hospital earns from its surgical department. At the same time, David knows the formation of such joint ventures is a complicated matter and requires careful planning to comply with legal and regulatory issues. His initial take on the proposal outlined by the surgeons is that some legal problems in fact may arise.

## Questions

1. Consider what David should say in his memorandum to the CEO about the joint venture. Which laws or regulations might this joint venture violate?

2. What changes, if any, in the proposed arrangement might be needed to keep the ambulatory surgical center in compliance with legal and regulatory requirements?

3. What course of action should David recommend?

# REFERENCES

Administration on Aging (AoA). About AoA. Retrieved March 2010 from http://www.aoa.gov/AoARoot/About/index.aspx

American Surgery Center Association. (2010). The regulation of ambulatory surgery centers. Retrieved March 2010 from http://ascassociation.org/faqs/ascregulations

Boards of Trustees of the Federal Hospital Insurance and Federal Supplementary Medical Insurance Trust Funds. (2008). *2008 Annual Report*. Retrieved March 2010 from http://www.cms.hhs.gov/reportstrustfunds/downloads/tr2008.pdf

Boothman, R. C., Blackwell, A. C., Campbell, D. A., Jr., Commiskey, E., & Anderson, S. (2009). A better approach to medical malpractice claims? A University of Michigan experience. *Journal of Health and Life Sciences Law, 2*(2), 125–159.

Brier, B., & Thompson, A. (2008, June 11). The appropriate role of the Internal Revenue Service with respect to tax exempt organizations good governance issues. *Advisory Committee on Tax Exempt and Government Entities*.

Campbell, E. G., Gruen, R. L., Mountford, J., Miller, L. G., Cleary, P. D., & Blumenthal, D. (2007). A national survey of physician-industry relationships. *New England Journal of Medicine, 356*(17), 1742–1750.

Center for Studying Health System Change (CSHSC). (2009). Impact of health care price transparency on price variation: The New Hampshire experience. Issue Brief No. 128. Retrieved March 2010 from http://www.hschange.com/CONTENT/1095/1095.pdf.

Centers for Medicare and Medicaid Services (CMS). (2010). Overview mission, vision and goals. Retrieved March 2010 from http://www.cms.hhs.gov/MissionVisionGoals/

Chassin, M. R. (2002). Achieving and sustaining improved quality: Lessons from New York State and cardiac surgery. *Health Affairs, 21*(4), 40–51.

Congressional Budget Office (CBO). (2008). Increasing transparency in the pricing of health care services and pharmaceuticals. Economic and Budget Issue Brief. Retrieved March 2010 from http://www.cbo.gov/ftpdocs/92xx/doc9284/06-05-PriceTransparency.pdf

Congressional Budget Office (CBO). (2007). Research on the comparative effectiveness of medical treatments. Retrieved March 2010 from http://www.cbo.gov/ftpdocs/88xx/doc8891/12-18-ComparativeEffectiveness.pdf

Conover, C. J., & Sloan, F. A. (1998). Does removing certificate-of-need regulations lead to a surge in health care spending? *Journal of Health Politics, Policy and Law, 23*(3), 455–481.

Donohue, J. M., Cevasco, M., & Rosenthal, M. B. (2007). A decade of direct-to-consumer advertising of prescription drugs. *New England Journal of Medicine, 357*(7), 673–681.

Dranove, D., Kessler, D., McClellan, M., & Satterthwaite, M. (2003). Is more information better? The effects of "report cards" on health care providers. *Journal of Political Economy, 111*(3), 555–588.

Exempt organizations: IRS releases governance training materials, provides agents with needed exam guidance. (2009, July 30). *BNA Health Law Reporter, 18,* 1009.

Farrell, K. S., Finocchio, L. J., Trivedi, A. N., & Mehrotra, A. (2010). Does price transparency legislation allow the uninsured to shop for care? *Journal of General Internal Medicine, 25*(2), 110–114.

Fronstin, P. (2009). Findings from the 2009 EBRI/MGA consumer engagement in health care survey. Employee Benefit Research Institute Issue Brief No. 337, http://www.ebri.org/pdf/briefspdf/EBRI_IB_12-2009_No337_CEHCS.pdf

Fung, C. H., Lim, Y. W., Mattke, S., Damberg, C., & Shekelle, P. G. (2008). Systematic review: The evidence that publishing patient care performance data improves quality of care, *Annals of Internal Medicine, 148*(2), 111–123.

Gostin, L. O., & Jacobson, P. D. (2006). *Law and the health system.* New York: Foundation Press.

Greenland, P. (2009). Time for the medical profession to act. *Archives of Internal Medicine, 169*(9), 829–831.

Harris, K. M., & Buntin, M. B. (2008). Choosing a health care provider: The role of quality information. Retrieved March 2010 from http://www.rwjf.org/files/research/051508.policysynthesis.qualityinfo.rpt.pdf

Havighurst, C. C. (2006). Contesting anticompetitive actions taken in the name of the state: State action immunity and health care markets. *Journal of Health Politics, Policy & Law, 31*(3), 587–607.

Health Resources and Services Administration (HRSA). About HRSA. Retrieved March 2010 from http://www.hrsa.gov/about/default.htm

Hellinger, F. J. (2009). The effect of certificate-of-need laws on hospital beds and healthcare expenditures: An empirical analysis. *American Journal of Managed Care, 15*(10), 737–744.

Hibbard, J. H., & Peters, E. (2003). Supporting informed consumer health care decisions: Data presentation approaches that facilitate the use of information in choice. *Annual Review of Public Health, 24,* 413–433.

Iglehart, J. K. (2005). The emergence of physician-owned specialty hospitals. *New England Journal of Medicine, 352*(1), 78–84.

Indian Health Service (IHS). Introduction to IHS by Dr. Yvette Roubideaux. Retrieved March 2010 from http://www.ihs.gov/PublicInfo/PublicAffairs/Welcome_Info/IHSintro.asp

Institute of Medicine (IOM). (1999). *To err is human: Building a safer health system.* Washington, DC: National Academies Press.

Jacobson, P. D., Hoffman, R. E., & Lopez, W. (2006). Regulating public health: Principles and application of administrative law. In R. A. Goodman, R. E. Hoffman, W. Lopez, G. W. Matthews, M. A. Rothstein, & K. L. Foster (Eds.), *Law in public health practice* (2nd ed.). New York: Oxford University Press.

The Joint Commission. Facts about patient safety. Retrieved March 2010 from http://www.jointcommission.org/PatientSafety/facts_patient_safety.htm

The Joint Commission. Sentinel Events. Retrieved March 2010 from http://www.jointcommission.org/SentinelEvents/

Jost, T. S. (2009). The regulation of private health insurance. Retrieved March 2010 from http://www.nasi.org/sites/default/files/research/The_Regulation_of_Private_Health_Insurance.pdf

Kamoie, B. (2004). EMTALA: Dedicating an emergency department near you. *Journal of Health Law, 37*(1), 41–60.

Lipsky, M. S., & Sharp, L. K. (2001). From idea to market: The drug approval process. *Journal of the American Board of Family Practice, 14*(5), 362–367.

Madison, K. (2009). The Law and Policy of Health Care Quality Reporting. *Campbell Law Review, 31*(2), 215–255. Retrieved March 2010 from http://www.law.campbell.edu/lawreview/articles/31-2-215.pdf

Medicare Payment Advisory Commission (MedPAC). About MedPac. Retrieved March 2010 from http://www.medpac.gov/about.cfm

Medicare Payment Advisory Commission (MedPAC). (2005). Physician-owned specialty hospitals. Retrieved March 2010 from http://www.medpac.gov/documents/Mar05_SpecHospitals.pdf

Merrill, R. A. (1996). The architecture of government regulation of medical products. *Virginia Law Review, 82*(8), 1753–1866.

National Conference of State Legislatures (NCSL). CON-Certificate of need state laws. Retrieved March 2010 from http://www.ncsl.org/IssuesResearch/Health/CONCertificateofNeedStateLaws/tabid/14373/Default.aspx

The National Quality Forum (NQF). (2002). Serious reportable events in healthcare: A consensus report. Retrieved March 2010 from http://www.qualityforum.org/WorkArea/linkit.aspx?LinkIdentifier=id&ItemID=1221

A national survey of medical error reporting laws. (2008). *Yale Journal of Health Policy, Law, and Ethics, 9*(1), 201–286.

Nyweide, D. J., Weeks, W. B., Gottlieb, D. J., Casalino, L. P., & Fisher, E. S. (2009). Relationship of primary care physicians' patient caseload with measurement of quality and cost performance. *Journal of the American Medical Association, 302*(22), 2444–2450.

Platt, R., Wilson, M., Chan, K. A., Benner, J. S., Marchibroda, J., & McClellan, M. (2009). The new sentinel network – Improving the evidence of medical-product safety. *New England Journal of Medicine, 361*(7), 645–647.

Reznik, G. L., Shoffner, D., & Weaver, D. A. (2005–2006). Coping with the demographic challenge: Fewer children and living longer. *Social Security Bulletin, 66*(4). Retrieved March 2010 from http://www.ssa.gov/policy/docs/ssb/v66n4/v66n4p37.html

Rosenthal, M. B., Frank, R. G., Li, Z., & Epstein, A. M. 2005. Early experience with pay-for-performance: From concept to practice. *Journal of the American Medical Association, 294*, 1788–1793.

Rothman, D. J., & Chimonas, S. (2008). New developments in managing physician relationships. *Journal of the American Medical Association, 300*(9), 1067–1069.

Sheeder, F. E., & Tonn, K. L. (2009). Is your organization prepared to respond to burgeoning compliance and enforcement trends? Be proactive and perform a status assessment. *In-House Counselor, 15*(2): 7–9.

Shortell, S. M., & Walshe, K. (2004). Social regulation of healthcare organizations in the United States: Developing a framework for evaluation. *Health Services Management Research, 17*(2), 79–99.

Slater, E. (2005). Today's FDA. *New England Journal of Medicine, 352*(3), 293–297.

United States Department of Health and Human Services (HHS). About HHS. Retrieved March 2010 from http://www.hhs.gov/about

United States Department of Labor (DOL), Employee Benefits Security Administration. Frequently asked questions about portability of health coverage and HIPAA. Retrieved March 2010 from http://www.dol.gov/ebsa/faqs/faq_consumer_hipaa.html

United States General Accounting Office (GAO). (2002). FDA oversight of direct-to-consumer advertising has limitations. Retrieved March 2010 from http://www.gao.gov/cgi-bin/getrpt?GAO-03-177

Wangsness, L. (2009, March 4). Nonprofit hospitals targeted on leader pay. *Boston Globe*, 1.

Wazana, A. (2000). Physicians and the pharmaceutical industry: Is a gift ever just a gift? *Journal of the American Medical Association, 283*(3), 373–380.

Werner, R. M., & Asch, D. A. (2005). The unintended consequences of publicly reporting quality information. *Journal of the American Medical Association, 293*(10), 1239–1244.

Young, G. J., Meterko, M., Beckman, H., Baker, E., White, B., Sautter, K. M., ...Burgess, J. F. (2007). Effects of paying physicians based on their relative performance for quality. *Journal of General Internal Medicine, 22*(6), 872–876.

# Chapter 13

# Health Information Systems and Strategy

Karen A. Wager and Mark L. Diana

## CHAPTER OUTLINE

## LEARNING OBJECTIVES

**After completing this chapter, the reader should be able to:**

1. Discuss the factors that are contributing to the widespread adoption and use of health information technology, including electronic health records (EHRs)

2. Define the major components and functions of an EHR system

3. Discuss the major barriers to EHR implementation and strategies that are being employed to overcome them

4. Describe the process a health care organization generally goes through when planning and implementing health information technology, including EHR systems

5. Understand the importance of aligning health information technology (IT) plans with the overall strategic plans of a health care organization

# KEY TERMS

| | |
|---|---|
| **Electronic Health Record (EHR)** | **Personal Health Record** |
| **Electronic Medical Record** | **Project Management** |
| **Health Information Exchange (HIE)** | **Regional Health Information Organization (RHIO)** |
| **Health Information Technology** | **Systems Development Life Cycle (SDLC)** |
| **HITECH Act of 2009** | |

---

**IN PRACTICE:** Successful Use of Health Information Technology

In 2010, the Healthcare Information Management and Systems Society (HIMSS) and American Society for Quality (ASQ) recognized 16 health care organizations nationally for their use of health information technology (IT) to improve patient safety. Six of the awardees were identified as "Tier 1" organizations that addressed the Joint Commission's National Patient Safety Goals in their innovative use of health IT. Awardees, and the successful outcomes they experienced, included:

- Bassett Health Network, Cooperstown, New York
    - On-time first surgical case starts increased by 35 percent
    - Operating room suite turnaround times decreased from 45 minutes to 25–30 minutes
    - Case supply costs decreased $200 per case
    - Documentation of hand off communication between providers during surgery went from 50 percent to 97 percent within a three-month period (Brooks, 2010).
- Eastern Maine Medical Center, Bangor, Maine
    - Significant reduction in number of patients receiving transfusions, pre- and post-CPOE
    - Blood acquisition costs reduced by 25 percent (Hartz and Gross, 2010)
- Mercy Des Moines–Mercy Heart Hospital, Des Moines, Iowa
    - Implemented radio frequency identification (RFID) in catherization laboratory, an inventory management system
    - Resulted in reduction of manual tasks allowing staff to spend more time with patients
    - Received a 568 percent return on investment, improved charge capture (Wilson, 2010)
- Queens Long Island Medical Center, Queens, New York
    - Diabetes-related mortality decreased by 21 percent
    - Quality of diabetic care improved by 4 percent
    - Health care cost reduced by $18,000 per patient
    - Physician productivity increased by 20 percent (Queens-Long Medical Center, 2010)
- Greater Rochester Independence Practice Association, Rochester, NY
    - Prescription-related phone calls reduced by 80 percent
    - Patient complaints reduced by 50 percent
    - Renewals decreased from one week to 24 hours
    - Improved quality of documentation and compliance (Electronic prescribing, 2010)

**IN PRACTICE:** Successful Use of Health Information Technology *(Continued)*

- University of Rochester Medical Center, Rochester, NY
  - More than 90 percent of cases have electronic signature of records
  - Patient documentation completed at time of discharge
  - High physician satisfaction with remote access (Williamson, 2010)

Visit the Stories of Success! Web site (http://www.himss.org/storiesofsuccess/caseStudies.asp) to read more about each of these organizations. Describe the organization, the problem they initially faced, and the IT strategy used to assist the organization in improving patient safety and efficiency. What factors contributed to the organization's success? What barriers did they face? How might the lessons learned from these cases be useful to others?

# CHAPTER PURPOSE

In today's health care environment, no health care management book would be complete without a chapter on health information systems and strategy. Health care leaders must ensure that their information systems technology plans are well aligned with the overall strategic plans of the health care organization. Investing in health information technology, particularly new clinical information systems such as electronic health records (EHR), can have a profound impact on the organization, including the medical staff, nurses, other clinicians and staff, and the patients they serve. Many health information system projects are known to fail despite well-formulated and strategic plans. Project failures may be due to unmet expectations, uncontrolled changes in the project's scope, insufficient buy-in, or inability to effectively manage change. The purpose of this chapter is to provide the reader with an overview of what is happening at the national level to promote the adoption and use of electronic health records; in addition, there is a discussion of some of the barriers to EHR use and strategies for overcoming them. The chapter focuses on the process a health care organization generally undergoes when attempting to effectively implement and evaluate health information systems technology.

# HISTORICAL OVERVIEW AND TODAY'S HEALTH INFORMATION TECHNOLOGY LANDSCAPE: A NATIONAL PERSPECTIVE

Twenty years ago, the Institute of Medicine published a landmark report that outlined the numerous problems inherent with paper-based medical record systems and called for the widespread adoption of electronic health record (EHR) systems (Institute of Medicine, 1991). Back then, such systems were also referred to as computer-based patient records (CPR). Studies had shown that paper-based medical record systems can lead to medical errors and duplication of services; in addition, they are often incomplete, illegible, and frequently unavailable when and where the information is needed (Burnum, 1989; Hershey, McAloon, and Bertram, 1989). Computer-based record systems could provide an electronic record of the patient's care, and therefore make an abundance of information instantly available to multiple care providers, improving their decision-support capabilities, providing them with alerts and reminders, and giving them access to knowledge aids and the latest research findings. The computer-based patient record could essentially "follow" a patient throughout his or her lifetime, and instantly track all relevant health, mental and social well-being information electronically (Institute of Medicine, 1991). However, if we progress forward to today, we find that EHR adoption rates are low despite the many benefits to be gained from using them.

What has happened since then? It depends how one defines and measures health information technology adoption. We have seen a great deal of technological advances in Web-based technologies and wireless personal devices, including the cell phone (for example, remote monitoring from the home is now possible via a cell phone). Consumers are far more active in the management of their own care, with the Internet serving as their personal library of health information. Social networking (including the use of blogs, wikis, etc.) has created new ways for patients with similar conditions to connect with one another. We have also seen health care organizations and providers invest in a host of clinical applications designed to help ensure patient safety, improve quality, and increase efficiency. Such systems include laboratory, radiology, and pharmacy information systems, medication administration systems using bar-coding technology, computerized provider order entry (CPOE), and other clinical ancillary systems. However, despite the advances and uses of information technology and the implementation of these applications, U.S. health care organizations still lag behind in the adoption and use of EHR systems (Wager, Lee, and Glaser, 2009).

Three U.S. presidents have called for the widespread adoption of EHR systems since the IOM report was first published. Most recently, President Obama moved that every American should have an EHR by 2014. Consequently, the American Recovery and Reinvestment Act of 2009 (ARRA) (also known as the stimulus act) includes a significant section known as the Health Information Technology for Economic and Clinical Health Act, or **HITECH Act**. The HITECH Act sets forth a plan for advancing the appropriate use of health information technology to improve quality of care and establish a foundation for the electronic exchange and use of health information systems (Blumenthal, 2009). Included in the HITECH Act are Medicare and Medicaid incentives for hospitals and eligible practitioners to implement certified EHR systems in a way that fully integrates these tools into the care delivery process and leads to meaningful use. The Office of the National Coordinator for Health Information Technology, led by Dr. David Blumenthal, has been allocated over $21 billion in stimulus funding to achieve this goal; this is the largest investment ever in federal funds to help spearhead the widespread deployment of EHR systems, including funding for workforce development and health care IT training. Before we explore the factors that have contributed to the need for the adoption and use of EHR systems, as well as some of the major barriers to widespread deployment, we should begin with a review of key terms and definitions.

# TERMS AND DEFINITIONS

**Health information technology** is a general term that is often used to describe a broad range of technologies for transmitting and managing health information for use by consumers, providers, payers, insurers, and others interested in health care (Blumenthal and Glaser, 2007). For our purposes, we will focus on technologies that are particularly relevant to processing, storing, and sharing data about patients. Examples include clinical information systems that are generally used to diagnose, treat, and report on patient clinical findings—such as laboratory, radiology, or pharmacy systems; computerized

provider order entry; bar-coding medication administration systems; and EHRs—as well as administrative systems that have more to do with the business and operational side of the encounter or visit (such as scheduling, billing, and registering patients). Both administrative and clinical functions may integrate into an EHR.

The terms **electronic medical record, electronic health record**, and **personal health record** are commonly found in the literature today and are often used interchangeably. For our purposes, EMR and EHR are essentially the same in functionality, except that an EHR conforms to nationally recognized interoperability standards that enable it to exchange information *across* organizational boundaries. For example, hypothetically, if physician John Doe had in his office an EHR system that adhered to industry connectivity standards, he would be able to share clinical data about a specific patient on a secure network with a Brownville Memorial Hospital across town that also has an interoperable EHR system. In contrast, EMR systems can share information within a single health care organization, but not across organizational boundaries.

Unlike EMR or EHR systems, which are managed by the health care organization, a personal health record (PHR) is generally managed and controlled by the patient or consumer. It may include both health and wellness information, such as an individual's diet, exercise, and daily routine. The consumer decides who has access to the information and thus controls the content of the record. PHRs are in earlier stages of development than EMRs and EHRs; however, with the growth of the Internet, social networking, blogs, and other Web-based technologies, consumers are already assuming a much more active role in managing their own health care. Companies such as Google and Microsoft, as well as major health insurers, also offer consumers the opportunity to maintain their own safe and secure online PHR. Some organizations are integrating PHR data with EHR data to have a complete picture of the patient's health information (Halamka, Mandl, and Tang, 2008). From a strategic perspective, both EHRs and PHRs have enormous potential to enable organizations to transform how they deliver health care services, communicate with patients, and engage patients in managing their care more fully.

There are eight main functions of an EHR as defined by the IOM (see Table 13.1). The first four are core functions: an EHR is able electronically to collect and store data about patients,

**TABLE 13.1  Functions of an EHR System as Defined by Institute of Medicine**

| Core Functionalities | Other Functionalities |
|---|---|
| *Health information and data:* Includes medical and nursing diagnoses, a medication list, allergies, demographics, clinical narratives, and laboratory test results | *Electronic communication and connectivity:* Enables those involved in patient care to communicate effectively with each other and with the patient; technologies to facilitate communication and connectivity may include e-mail, Web messaging, and telemedicine |
| *Results management:* Manages all types of results (for example, laboratory test results, radiology procedure results) electronically | *Patient support:* Includes everything from patient education materials to home monitoring to telehealth |
| *Order entry and support:* Incorporates use of computerized provider order entry, particularly in ordering medications | *Administrative processes:* Facilitates and simplifies such processes as scheduling, prior authorizations, and insurance verification; may also employ decision-support tools to identify eligible patients for clinical trials or chronic disease management programs |
| *Decision support:* Employs computerized clinical decision-support capabilities such as reminders, alerts, and computer-assisted diagnosing | *Reporting and population health management:* Establishes standardized terminology and data formats for public and private sector reporting requirements |

SOURCE: IOM Committee on Data Standards for Patient Safety (2003).

supply that information to providers on request, permit providers to directly enter orders into the computer, and provide health care professionals with advice in making decisions about a patient's care (e.g., alerts, reminders, clinical decision support) (Blumenthal and Glaser, 2007). The other four functions of an EHR will enable **health information exchange (HIE)** across organizational boundaries and more fully engage the patient in his or her own care through home monitoring and telehealth. Telehealth is the use of technology to deliver or monitor health care services at a distance. Administrative processes, such as prior authorizations and benefits/insurance verification, will occur automatically and greatly simplify what are now labor-intensive processes. In addition, public and private health reporting will become standardized.

HIE can take different forms, but most policy makers have focused on **Regional Health Information Organizations (RHIOs)** as the primary model to drive information exchange (Adler-Milstein, Landefeld, and Jha, 2010). RHIOs generally bring together unaffiliated stakeholders with clinical data (such as physician practices, labs, hospitals, and pharmacies) and set up the infrastructure for the HIE. Although there

have been a number of RHIOs established, all in various stages of development, a number of them have failed due to lack of financial sustainability (Adler-Milstein, McAfee, and Bates, 2008). Adler-Milstein and her colleagues conducted a national survey of RHIOs in mid-2008 to examine the factors associated both with becoming operational and with financial viability. They found that RHIOs that exchanged a narrow set of data with a broad group of stakeholders were more likely to become operational. In addition, securing funding from participants early in the process helped RHIOs become more self-sustaining (Adler-Milstein, Landefeld, and Jha, 2010).

# FACTORS DRIVING DEMAND FOR HEALTH IT AND CURRENT ADOPTION RATES

Few would argue that the U.S. health care system is not in need of reform. Health care costs are high, quality is uneven, a growing number of Americans are at risk of losing their health insurance or being denied coverage due to preexisting conditions, and an increasing number of Americans are uninsured or underinsured. Reducing medical errors and making our health care system "safer" remains a priority. Although the EHR is not the end-all in solving our health care problems, it is viewed as a means of improving quality of care, the health of populations, and the efficiency of health care systems (Blumenthal, 2009). Studies over the past 30 years have demonstrated that EMR-type systems can lead to important quality- and efficiency-related benefits, particularly in improving adherence to evidence-based practice guidelines, enhanced surveillance and monitoring, and decreased medical errors (Bates, 2005; DesRoches et al., 2008; Hillestad et al., 2005; Institute of Medicine, 2001; Ornstein et al., 1991). However, Chaudhry and colleagues found in their systematic review of the literature concerning studies of EMR-type systems that the majority of the work in this area has been limited to a handful of academic medical centers that have developed in-house systems over the past few decades (Chaudhry et al., 2006). It is not known if these same results would be found in community-based facilities with commercially developed EHR systems. Several recent studies indicate the national impact of EHRs on hospital and ambulatory care quality and costs have been mixed (Himmelstein, Wright, and Woodhandler, 2009; Kazley and Ozcan, 2008; Zhou et al., 2009). As EHR systems are becoming more widely deployed, further research into their impact on quality, efficiency, and overall health care costs will be needed.

## ADOPTION RATES OF HEALTH INFORMATION TECHNOLOGY

Current adoption rates of EHRs in U.S. hospitals and physician/ambulatory care settings are relatively low. Approximately 8–15 percent of hospitals are estimated to have fully operational EHR systems (AHA, 2007; Jha et al., 2009). Hospitals that are more likely to have an EHR are larger teaching hospitals, those that are part of a hospital system, or hospitals that are located in urban areas. Adoption rates in physician practices are not any higher; a recent national study found that only 4 percent had a fully functional EHR system, and 13 percent reported having a basic system (DesRoches et al., 2008). However, physicians who practice in groups of more than 50 are more likely to have a fully functional EMR system.

## BARRIERS TO ADOPTION AND STRATEGIES FOR OVERCOMING THEM

Despite the benefits that can be gained from implementing health information technology, there are a host of barriers. The most frequently cited barrier is cost (DesRoches et al., 2008; Jha et al., 2009; Kausal et al., 2009). Upfront costs for purchasing a system can be substantial, as well as the financial and human resources needed to maintain and support the system. Purchasing and installing an EHR system are estimated to range from $15,000 to $50,000 per physician (Bodenheimer and Grumbach, 2003; Miller et al., 2005; Miller and West, 2007). For small hospitals and physician practices, it is difficult for them to come up with the necessary capital to invest in EHR systems. Other barriers to adoption include misalignment of incentives, unclear return on investment, lack of availability of staff with adequate expertise in information technology (Jha et al., 2009), privacy and security concerns, and issues with interoperability (Andersen et al., 2005). Health IT projects also do not have a strong track record of success. According to Kaplan and Harris-Salamone's (2009) review of the literature, between 40 and 70 percent of health IT projects are often not successful. How one defines system failure can vary, but a common definition in health care is one that has significant budget and time overruns, fails to achieve the goals intended, and outright termination of the project before completion (Glaser, 2005). Therefore, it is important for health care managers to appropriately ensure that any major health information technology investment is well aligned with the overall strategic plans of the organization and therefore worth the investment and effort.

Much is happening at the national level to assist physicians and hospitals in adopting certified EHR systems that meet industry standards. The overarching goal is that providers will not simply adopt EHR technology, but will use the technology as a tool to accomplish five major health outcome policy priorities:

1. Improve quality, safety, and efficiency, and reduce health disparities
2. Engage patients and families in their health care
3. Improve care coordination
4. Improve population and public health
5. Ensure adequate privacy and security protections for personal health information (EHR Incentive Program, 2010).

To that end, care goals and measures have been established for eligible professionals and hospitals. Those that can demonstrate that they meet or exceed the measures/standards will receive incentive payments through the Medicare and Medicaid programs. Although the details of the proposed legislation are beyond the scope of this chapter, additional information can be found in the January 13, 2010, issue of the *Federal Register* (EHR Incentive Program, 2010).

In the section that follows, we describe the process that an organization should go through in managing the planning, implementation and evaluation of a health care information system.

# STRATEGIC ALIGNMENT

It is fundamentally important that an organization recognize the benefits of aligning its IS function with its organizational strategy; this recognition can be influenced by the role played by the chief information officer (CIO) (Chun and Mooney, 2009). The impact of this role on strategic alignment takes place primarily through the reporting relationship to the CEO. A direct reporting relationship of the CIO to the CEO reflects a fundamental view by executive management that the information systems (IS) function of the organization has strategic value. Further, a direct reporting relationship enhances the ability of the CIO to view the IS function in a strategic manner through participation in high-level strategy sessions and discussions with other executives. Conversely, an indirect reporting relationship, where the CIO reports to an intermediary such as the chief financial officer (CFO) or the chief operating officer (COO), reflects a view of the IS function as primarily a cost center with little, if any, strategic impact (Chun and Mooney, 2009).

There has been an ongoing debate over the strategic value of IS for a number of years (Carr, 2003; Lacity and Hirschheim, 1993). The premise that information systems do not have strategic value to an organization stems from a view of IS as a utility-like commodity similar to electricity. The argument is that such commodities only level the playing field among organizations, but they do not impart a strategic advantage (although their absence leads to a marked disadvantage). Fundamental to this view is the thought that once an organization has figured out how to use IS to improve the way it performs, other organizations can readily imitate them and achieve the same performance improvement.

The alternate view is that IS can provide a strategic advantage to organizations precisely because it is not commodity-like. Lacity and Hirschheim (1993) addressed this issue (a decade before Carr wrote his provocative piece) by pointing out that an organization's information needs are idiosyncratic, unlike utility requirements. How often does an organization need to communicate with its electric supplier to discuss changing business requirements? This is particularly relevant to health care organizations, where large numbers of individual patient encounters generate highly idiosyncratic information. Furthermore, this makes the ability of one organization to successfully imitate another and achieve the same results highly unlikely. Indeed, the difficulty in doing so under certain conditions is the basis for the ability to achieve strategic advantage according to the resource-based view (Barney, 1991).

The two extremes of this debate miss the fundamental issue that IS consists of a number of different components, some of which may be commodity-like and others of which may not be. Feeny and Willcocks (1998) developed a framework for a high-performing IS function within an organization that recognizes this distinction. Their framework categorizes certain capabilities as important for the organization to be able to stay informed of its demand-side needs and its IS investments; these capabilities include such things as governance, management, business strategy, and information architecture. Other capabilities are of little or no strategic value and can be minimized or outsourced; these capabilities include such things as building and operating the technical infrastructure (e.g., the datacenter and telecommunications) and systems acquisition or development. What this amounts to is the idea that the activities with strategic impact—the "what do we do and how do we do it" activities—remain within the organization, while those with little or no strategic impact—the execution of the strategy—can be done either internally or externally.

Central to this approach to organizing the IS function is the belief that IS serves as a means of achieving the goals of the organization, rather than IS being an end in itself. Indeed, the Lacity and Willcocks model focuses largely on the relationship between the IS function and the business needs of the organization, and they were not the first or only ones to do so (Boynton, Jacobs, and Zmud, 1992; Brown and Magill, 1994; Martin et al., 2005). There are a number of models for organizing the IS function, just as there are for the organization as a whole, and there has been much debate over the best way to align the IS function with the rest of the organization. This debate has tended to follow two general approaches.

The first approach is the idea that the structure of the IS function should mirror that of the organization. If the organization is highly centralized, than the IS function should be also. The second approach is the idea that the IS function should be organized around the various activities for which it is responsible, similar to a functional arrangement. This trend has resulted in an approach that is best characterized as federated, which in some ways mirrors the strategic nature of the IS activities. Enterprise-wide, commodity-like functions, such as e-mail and network services, are centralized, and activities requiring some level of customization, such as applications and support services, are decentralized. The federated approach also has the benefit of improving the ability of the IS organization to develop relationships with the business managers within the organization, and therefore become more aware and focused on the IS needs of the business.

# CRITICAL SUCCESS FACTORS

The ability to align the IS strategy with the organizational strategy is a key factor for the successful adoption of HIT.

There are a number of ways an organization can make strategic decisions about what kind of IS capabilities it needs in order to achieve its goals and objectives. Among these are the standard strategic planning tools, including analysis of the internal and external environments and the identification of strategic opportunities and threats. Such activities should result in a set of long- and short-term goals and objectives for the organization. The development of goals and objectives may be impacted by the availability of new technology that enables new ways of doing things, which requires a thorough and thoughtful assessment of the potential of emerging technologies.

Organizational strategies can drive the development of IS strategies and result in a set of IS goals and objectives that are explicitly linked to higher-level goals and objectives. This is an explicit approach to strategic alignment that would require, for example, any IS proposal to demonstrate a clear link to the organization's goals and objectives. This approach may be used regardless of how alignment is achieved, but it is sometimes problematic, particularly for infrastructure types of projects. For example, it may be difficult to link an enterprise-wide network upgrade to specific goals and objectives, but such an upgrade could have a significant impact on the success of other IS projects.

## DEBATE TIME: Does IT Offer a Competitive Advantage?

An article in the Harvard Business Review in 2003 titled "IT Doesn't Matter" challenged the idea that information technology could gain a competitive advantage at the firm level. The premise of the argument was that IT is what the author called an infrastructural technology, similar to railroads and electricity, as contrasted with proprietary technologies. Infrastructural technologies have more value when shared than when used in isolation in an attempt to gain a competitive advantage. The argument is that early in the development of infrastructural technologies, they may appear as proprietary technologies because of restricted access or a lack of standards, and so convey some advantage over competitors. Similarly, some companies may gain a unique insight into potential uses of the new technology, or into market changes that may come about as a result of it, and be able to get a step ahead of the competition. Such advantage is temporary, though, as the technology becomes commoditized and is available with the same capabilities and at much reduced cost to everyone (the author argues that there is no more perfect a commodity than a byte of data). Because of this argument, the author suggests three new rules for IT management. Develop an argument for and against each of these rules in health care.

1. Spend less on IT.

2. Follow, rather than lead (do not be on the "cutting edge").

3. Focus on vulnerabilities, not opportunities.

SOURCE: Adapted from Carr (2003).

## IN PRACTICE: SunHealth Case Study

Two years ago, the senior leadership team at SunHealth Medical Center engaged in a strategic planning process that resulted in a refined mission statement and a set of strategic priorities for the organization. SunHealth's mission is to improve the physical, emotional, and spiritual health of all individuals and communities they serve; to provide care with excellence and compassion; and to work with others who share their fundamental commitment to improving the human condition. Their strategic priorities are:

1. To improve patient safety and quality

2. To foster a patient-centered environment whereby patients are actively engaged in their own care and partners in the care process

3. To improve care coordination and efficiency

As part of the strategy discussion, the CEO, Mary Lewis, felt it was important to explore the ways in which IS/IT might help SunHealth achieve their strategic objectives. SunHealth is a nonprofit, community-based, integrated delivery system comprised of three community hospitals in the Southeast. It also includes a large physician practice plan, a cancer center, a women's health center, and a wide range of ancillary and rehabilitation services. Soon after the initial strategic planning discussions took place, SunHealth recruited a new chief information officer (CIO), John Martin. John holds an undergraduate degree in computer science, a master's in industrial engineering, and has over 15 years of experience in working with IT and health care professionals in the selection and implementation of IS projects. John agreed with Mary that the organization's IS plans should be well aligned with the overall strategic plans of the organization—and he quickly found himself at the leadership table.

After many discussions and given the strategic priorities of SunHealth, the leadership team recommended moving forward with the selection and implementation of an electronic health record (EHR) system. (Note: The leadership team was comprised of the CEO and CIO, as well as the chief financial officer, the chief nursing officer, and the chief of the medical staff). They felt that an EHR would improve patient safety, decrease medical errors, and help ensure that providers were using evidence-based medicine. They also envisioned that by allowing patients to view their records through a PHR or patient portal, the patients would become more involved in their own care. This could help them achieve their goal of creating a patient-centered environment and improve care coordination and efficiency.

However, the team was concerned about doing too much at once. Based upon John's prior experience, he recommended that the EHR system be selected and implemented using a phased approach with a series of applications introduced over time:

Stage 1: Clinical documentation for nurses and all ancillary staff members

Stage 2: Medication administration using bar coding technology

Stage 3: Computerized provider order entry (CPOE)

Stage 4: Physician notes

This approach was eventually accepted and approved by the leadership team and the board. It was just the beginning of a series of milestones and challenges, with the final goal of a fully implemented EHR yet to be realized.

Once the EHR vendor was selected and the phased approach for implementing the various applications was determined, John established a governance structure for the project. There was a senior-level Steering Committee that oversaw the entire project, and individual project managers that managed each stage of the project. An overall project manager was also appointed. Melissa Drake was selected to serve in this role. She had been a critical care nurse for 10 years before being lured away to work on IT-related projects. Melissa is well respected in the organization, has a sense of the big picture, and is able

---

**IN PRACTICE: SunHealth Case Study** *(Continued)*

---

to delegate fairly well. She is also fairly well organized, although she does tend to forget details and often laughs at herself that she needs a full-time secretary to keep her straight. It is easy for her to overcommit, as she also serves as the controller for the IT department and manages all IT contracts with vendors.

Other key members of the Steering Committee include the chief medical informatics officer, medical staff director, chief nursing officer, CIO, and director of pharmacy. The hospital is a teaching hospital and uses residents, so the expectation is that the residents will be entering orders directly when the hospital gets to the CPOE phase of the implementation. Buy-in by the residents will be critical. The medical staff director, Dr. Paul Long, is rather quiet and reserved. He sees the value of the EHR, but has been very busy and not able to attend many of the Steering Committee meetings. He also admits he has not written an order in 10 years. His residents write all orders for him.

One of the main tasks of the Steering Committee was to establish an overall time frame and sequence for implementing the various applications. As problems or major challenges arose, John or Melissa would bring these issues to the attention of the Steering Committee for deliberation and discussion and changes would be made to the master calendar, as appropriate. The Steering Committee also kept a pulse on how things were going in terms of training, resource allocation, staffing, and whether too much change was occurring at once. If priorities had to shift or additional people needed to be brought in, the Steering Committee serves in this capacity.

As of this date, SunHealth has completed phases 1 and 2, and is currently in phase 3. They have implemented CPOE in one of their hospitals and are in the process of rolling it out to the other two. The rollout of CPOE has been fairly successful, although it has gone in live in the new hospital—with strong physician leaders. Melissa is concerned that the same success might not happen in the other hospitals, where the physicians are older and tend to be less engaged in the project. The Steering Committee estimates it will take another year before this phase of the project is completed, and they can begin work on the final phase in moving on to physician notes. As with any project, numerous requests and changes for enhancements have been made. Only those that have patient safety implications are acted upon immediately. All others are being prioritized and considered as time permits.

---

Other approaches can also link directly to an organization's strategic outlook. For example, an organization may be committed to continuous improvement, which could be reflected in an IS strategy of continuous improvement in processes and management. Also, as suggested earlier, the development of an IS strategy may be driven by fundamental views about the nature of competition and the role of IS in facilitating competitive advantage (Wager, Lee, and Glaser, 2009).

Successful strategic alignment should result in a set of IS projects that the organization has identified as important to its strategic direction or for sustaining existing capabilities. This portfolio of projects typically includes pending requests, projects approved but not begun, and projects that are in progress. This portfolio of IS projects should be managed by an executive-level team that includes both senior business and IS executives. This team prioritizes projects in the portfolio and determines which project to fund in the current period,

which to fund later, and which will have to wait. In this way, the strategic direction of the organization is linked directly to the ongoing IS projects.

In order to be successful in HIT adoption, the strategic-level questions must eventually give way to questions of execution. In other words, an organization must move from the "what and why" to the "how" of adopting HIT. One advantage of achieving strategic alignment is that it tends to lead to another critical factor in the success of IS projects, which is executive-level and clinical-leadership support. High-level support for IS projects not only communicates to the rest of the organization that they are serious about adopting the system in question, but it also increases the chances of having the necessary resources dedicated to the project. Executive leadership can allocate the financial and human resources needed to increase the chances of project success. These resources should be directed toward critical activities such as user involvement and training, change management, and incentive programs.

It is crucial to understand that information systems are not simply collections of computers and software (that is, a better description of information technology). An information system includes the data, processes, people, information technology, and the way these factors interact to collect, process, store, and present information that supports the organization (Whitten and Bentley, 2005). They are generally complex systems, and therefore it is critical to approach their acquisition, implementation, and management with proven methodologies. The obvious analogy is architecture. Architects have perfected a methodology for successfully completing highly complex projects. Anyone who has worked with an architect to build a house or a hospital has been exposed to at least parts of this methodology (see Zachman, 1987) for an early description of this analogy. One should no sooner attempt to build a complex information system without a methodological approach than they should try to build a hospital without one.

## Systems Development Life Cycle

One important methodology is the **systems development life cycle (SDLC)**. The SDLC is a generic methodology for selecting, acquiring, implementing, and maintaining a system. There are a number of such methodologies, each with its own strengths and weaknesses. Generally, the SDLC includes definition (planning), construction (analysis, design, and testing), implementation, and maintenance phases. The SDLC improves the chances that the health care organization selects the correct application or system for its needs and the probability of a successful implementation.

A generic SDLC places a great deal of emphasis on the definition or planning phase. Generally, this begins with a feasibility analysis, which includes economic, operational, and technical feasibility assessments. The product is a 10- to 20-page document that includes an executive overview and recommendations, a description of what the system would do and how it would operate, an analysis of its costs and benefits, and a development plan. If the decision is made to move ahead, the next step is the "requirements definition." The requirements definition is arguably the most important part of the project. It focuses on logical design—processes, data flows, and data interrelationships—instead of the specific physical implementation. The product is a system

requirements document that includes a detailed description of inputs and outputs and processes used to convert input data to outputs, formal diagrams, and output layouts, a revised cost-benefit analysis, and a revised plan for the remainder of the project.

The requirements definition serves as the basis for the construction phase, whether the system is to be developed internally or acquired from an outside vendor. In the latter case, it severs as the basis for the development of criteria for the evaluation of existing vendor products. If the system is to be acquired from a vendor, the requirements definition also forms the basis for the development of a request for proposal (RFP) document that vendors respond to by indicating how their product meets the requirements. It is crucial to recognize that the development of system requirement is a crucial activity regardless of whether the organization intends to build its own system or acquire it from a vendor. In either case, the requirements definition serves as the basis for system selection or development, and for evaluation.

The activity of developing the requirements definition involves a systematic approach using a variety of tools. Typically, the approach begins with a high-level logical definition of the existing system, whether it is manual, automated, or a combination of both. This description tells what the system currently does, but not how it does it. The next step is a physical description of the existing system, which describes how the system does what it does. Documenting the as-is system is necessary, even if the existing system is manual. How else do we know what work processes need to be done? How do we know what data we need to support the process if we do not document it, and how will we transfer the data to the new system if we do not know how it is stored in the old system? For these reasons, we include both logical and physical models in this analysis. This phase is where we should begin to ask questions about why the process is done as it is, and if there might not be a better way to do it. If the activities in the definition phase are done well, it will pay off in all other phases of the SDLC. The cost of finding and fixing a mistake in the definition phase is significantly lower than in the construction or implementation phases.

The construction phase of the SDLC includes system design, building, and testing. There are also a number of specific methodologies with their associated tools for these activities. It is important to understand that while a vendor may have done many of these activities in developing their product, there may still be the need for modifications to the vendor's product. This occurs because a vendor must develop a generic product in order to appeal to a wide variety of customers, so it is unlikely that any vendor product will provide all of the required functionality of the new system defined in the RFP (based on the requirements definition). In this case, the organization has essentially three choices: (1) modify the vendor product, (2) modify their work processes, or (3) live with the differences. For this reason, it is important for the organization to identify, either in the requirements definition or the RFP, which functionality is critical. For example, the organization may prioritize functionality as "have to have," "nice to have," and "can live without," and so have a basis for determining the best fitting vendor product and the need for package modifications.

The implementation phase can be approached using several strategies. At one end is the parallel strategy, where the old system continues operating while the new system is implemented. The systems are run in parallel until everyone is using the new system and no one is using the old system. The problem with this strategy is it may be difficult to get people to move to the new system when they can keep using the old one. At the other end is the cutover or "big bang" strategy, where the old system is turned off and the new system turned on at one time. This is considered a risky strategy by some, and generally leads to a drop in productivity until people are used to using the new system and the work processes associated with it. In between these two approaches are the pilot strategy and the phased strategy. The pilot approach involves implementing the new system in a subunit and identifying any problems or bugs before implementing across the entire organization. The idea is to limit the problems to a small portion of the organization, and reduce or eliminate them before implementing everywhere else. This strategy can also help to illustrate to the organization the ability to be successful with the new system. A phased strategy is essentially a series of pilots in one unit after another until the entire organization is converted.

The SDLC, however, has been criticized for its tendency to not handle system changes and backlogs particularly well, and to be slow. There are modifications and new approaches (e.g., object-oriented design and analysis) that some claim to be better at these aspects of managing the life cycle. The point here is not to endorse a particular SDLC methodology, but to stress the importance of adopting and using such a

methodology. An organization's familiarity and expertise with a methodology may be as important as the specific choice of methodology.

## Project Management

The ability of an organization to successfully implement project management has a significant impact on the success of IS projects. **Project management** is a discipline of its own that is not specific to IS projects, but that is crucial to the success of any complex project. Certainly not every IS project is complex enough to warrant a full-fledged project management team, but on projects of any reasonable complexity, mangling the project management will seriously jeopardize its success. An organization that excels at project management stands a much better chance of successfully adopting HIT than one that does not.

Once the executive team defines the IS portfolio of funded projects, project management becomes crucial to the success of the project. The first step to initiating an IS project is developing the project charter. The charter should detail the project's objectives, scope, and intended results. Many of the inputs from the definition phase of the SDLC will be used to develop the project charter, including the feasibility analysis and requirements definition.

The next key step is identifying the project manager. The project manager can be either a business manager or an IS manager, depending on both the need for technical expertise and the degree to which the project will affect the business unit. Project managers' characteristics can affect the success of projects, including a range of nontechnical skills such as leadership, communication, organizational, and team-building skills; this is particularly true when there are high levels of change and uncertainty associated with the project (Martin et al., 2005).

Two other key roles present in successful project management teams are the project sponsor and the project champion. The project sponsor is the business manager that is financially responsible for the project. This person should have participated in the development of the project proposal and the feasibility analysis. Once the project begins, he or she provides the funds for the project and oversees the project to ensure the benefits are realized. The sponsor may also be responsible for providing members of the project team, and for making other personnel that are not formal members of the project team available for activities such as defining the as-is system, providing end-user feedback on screen designs or prototypes of the new system, and system testing. The business sponsor needs to free up these personnel along with the project team members so they can provide the level of effort required to make the project a success; this means the sponsor needs to be at a high enough level of the organization to have the authority to make such decisions. For large projects that involve multiple business processes, this may mean that the project sponsor should be the CIO or the CEO.

The project champion needs to be an individual with (1) a high degree of credibility among those within the organization who are most likely to be affected by the new system, and (2) the ability to continually communicate the vision and benefits of the new system; for example, the project champion could potentially be a business manager. It is also possible for the project sponsor to fill this role, but often the demands on the sponsor's time make it difficult or impossible, so therefore the champion is often someone other than the sponsor. In health care organizations, a physician who advocates the use of HIT can fill this role, as long as he or she is seen as credible among other physicians and clinicians and is good at communicating the vision within the organization. The project champion role is not always formally designated, nor does it need to be for the champion to be successful.

Project planning includes developing a project schedule, budgets, and staffing. These activities are critical and interrelated, and weaknesses in one area can negatively affect the others. The project schedule includes a work breakdown analysis, which identifies the phases and sequences of tasks and the time to complete each. A master schedule is developed from this breakdown, and project milestones, dates for achieving them, and the specific resulting products of each are identified. The budget can be developed using either a top-down or bottom-up approach. Once a master schedule is developed, a bottom-up approach, where cost elements are estimated from the lowest-level tasks and aggregated up for a total project cost estimate, is appropriate. In early stages this may not be possible, and a top-down approach can be used. Staffing involves identifying the skills needed to complete the project tasks and the individuals who collectively have those skills, and assigning them to the project.

An additional critical piece of successful project management is change management, or the ability to successfully introduce change to individuals within organizations. One might get the impression from the discussion so far that implementing information systems is a difficult process. The difficulty stems not only from the complexity of the system and the technology, but also from its impact on the organization. This includes the way people do their work and the political implications of work being done in different ways that are often introduced by new systems. When people within organizations are faced with the prospect of significant change, they often consciously or unconsciously engage in tactics that prevent or delay the completion of the project. Such tactics may include withholding people or resources including designating staff to the project that are unqualified, raising new objections about project requirements, or expanding the size and complexity of the project.

Most approaches to change management are based on the work of Lewin (1947), Schein (1999), and Kotter (1995). The Lewin/Schein model has three stages: unfreezing, moving, and refreezing. Kotter expanded these to eight stages, but they generally mirror the three stages of Lewin and Schein. Unfreezing involves persuading individuals within the organization that there is a need for change and motivating them to make the change, which also requires creating a safe environment for the change to take place. Moving requires that the individuals within the organization acquire the knowledge, skills, and abilities to function in their new roles, which requires time and resources. Refreezing happens when the new way of doing things becomes the norm within the organization. Incentives to reinforce the new behaviors help to establish them as the norm. Kotter (1995) has emphasized that the refreezing process may not be as desirable as once thought. The idea behind this is that an organization needs to be ready to change regularly.

The three main activities most helpful in successfully managing change in IS projects are communicating, training, and providing incentives (Martin et al., 2005). These activities can be related back to the three stages of the Lewin change model. Effective communication helps to make the case for the need to implement the new system and do things in a new way (unfreezing). Providing adequate training assists people in gaining the new skills required to function in the new system (moving). It is easy to underestimate training requirements. Providing incentives for adopting and using the new system helps to institutionalize the new system and establish new norms (refreezing).

# ASSESSING HIT PERFORMANCE AND VALUE

A chapter of health information systems and strategy would not be complete without some discussion of the assessment of system performance. If we accept the notion that IS can support the strategic goals of the organization, and if we go about managing it with the expectation that it will support those goals, it makes sense that we should evaluate how well our IS has done. This is a more difficult proposition than it may seem at first, however. This is partly because the nature of IS varies, as discussed previously, from enterprise-wide infrastructure technologies to department-specific clinical information systems. How does one assess the value of laying fiber-optic cable related to the strategic goals of the organization? Further, the performance of these systems in terms of achieving strategic value may hinge more on their collective performance than their individual performance. For example, analyzing the ability to integrate and share data across laboratory, pharmacy, radiology, and provider order entry systems may have a greater impact than evaluating each system alone.

One key to a meaningful assessment of IS performance is to choose the correct metric or metrics for assessment. For example, not all IS projects will yield a positive return on investment (ROI), but if the system is designed to enable achievement of a strategic goal of the organization, the ROI of that system is not the appropriate metric, even if it were positive. This is complicated by the fact that many information systems have diverse value propositions within and across proposals. A single system can potentially improve service and productivity, reduce cost, and generate revenue, while other proposals under consideration may cost significantly more or less and have widely differing risks and benefits. This is not to say that formal financial analysis of proposals and implemented systems is not warranted, but that such an analysis may not be the only or the best measure of the outcome of an IS investment.

In order for the organization to assess the impact of IS on the ability of the organization to achieve its strategic goals, the organization must link its IS investments to its organizational strategy. Without this linkage, the IS function may be performing at a high level but doing the wrong things, or it may be that the IS function is supporting the overall strategy, but

that strategy may be the wrong one. The Agency for Healthcare Research and Quality (AHRQ) has developed a useful toolkit for evaluating IT projects (Cusack et al., 2009). The evaluation process begins with defining the goals of the project and the goals of the evaluation itself, which should include a discussion of who the intended audiences are for the evaluation.

The next step in the evaluation process is to link the project goals to outcome measures. This linking should be explicit and a range of outcome measures should be considered, both quantitative and qualitative. The key is to choose valid measures that will allow you to determine how well the project is meeting its stated goals. Examples of types of measures include clinical outcomes, clinical process measures, provider adoption, provider attitudes measures, patient adoption, patient knowledge, patient attitudes measures, workflow impact measures, and financial impact measures. It can also be beneficial to consider measuring barriers and facilitators related to the implementation, since that information may be useful when undertaking similar projects.

Once measures are chosen, they should be assessed for validity, importance, and feasibility. Linking the potential impact of the project on the measure can assess validity; the greater the potential impact on the measure, the more suitable the measure is for evaluating the project. Similarly, rate each measure on its importance to the stakeholders, or to those who will receive the evaluation report. Lastly, determine the feasibility of obtaining the data necessary for the measure. Be sure to consider the required sample size when assessing feasibility. Even if the measure is feasible to obtain, it may require too large a sample size to be feasible (e.g., observing rare events such as patient deaths). Once you have this information, you can choose the final measures for the project. Those measures that are both high in importance and highly feasible are sure candidates for inclusion on the evaluation. Those that are low in importance and not feasible to measure are likely to be excluded, while those in the middle can be considered in order of importance and feasibility.

Lastly, choose the study design, including an assessment of its cost. The study design should include both a timing approach and data collection strategies. In general, timing means a study can be either retrospective or prospective. Prospective studies typically are more expensive to conduct, but they are also a stronger design than retrospective studies. The types of data collection also affect the cost of the study.

Conducting manual chart reviews or observing clinician behavior is more costly than obtaining secondary data already being collected. Once all of these activities have been concluded, an overall evaluation plan should be developed. The plan should include all of the components discussed.

Health IT projects are largely costly investments, with often widely varying impacts. They are difficult to implement in any industry setting, but perhaps more so in health care.

Such costly investments are difficult to justify without a clear understanding of the impact throughout the organization. A solid evaluation plan that is an integral part of the project from the beginning provides a means of assessing such impacts, and of the overall value of the project. This information can be invaluable when considering whether to engage in future projects and in an organization's ability to successfully conduct such projects.

# SUMMARY AND MANAGERIAL GUIDELINES

1. The demand for access to quality, complete, and accurate health information where and when it is needed has never been greater. Federal legislation has been enacted that creates financial incentives for eligible providers and hospitals to become meaningful electronic health record (EHR) systems users in an effort to finally make EHR systems a reality. States will play a pivotal role in ensuring that health care providers can participate by sharing information through a health information exchange.

2. Health care leaders should stay current on the latest federal rules, regulations and standards related to the adoption and meaningful use of EHR systems. Key resources include:

   - Office of the National Health Information Coordinator (ONC). http://healthit.hhs.gov/portal/server.pt?open=512&objID=1204&parentname=CommunityPage&parentid=1&mode=2&in_hi_userid=10741&cached=true

   - Agency for Healthcare Research and Quality: http://healthit.ahrq.gov/portal/server.pt

   - Centers for Medicare and Medicaid: http://www.cms.hhs.gov/

   - Healthcare Information Management and Systems Society: http://www.himss.org

   - American Health Information Management Association: http://www.ahima.org

   - American Medical Informatics Association: http://www.amia.org

3. Investing in EHR (or other types of health information systems/technology) is not something that should be taken lightly. It is critical that the information systems plans are well aligned with the overall strategy plans of the health care organization.

4. Leading organizations will generally employ some type of standardized methodology for guiding the selection and implementation of any new information system, particularly large complex systems. Using a systems development life cycle (SDLC) methodology with four phases—(1) planning, (2) requirements definition, (3) construction phase, and (4) implementation phase—is an example of one.

5. Project management, clinician buy-in, and governance are also key to success. Every major health information systems project should include an evaluation of its impact on the organization and the goals it was intended to achieve.

# DISCUSSION QUESTIONS

1. Did the EHR seem to be well aligned with SunHealth's overall strategic plan? Explain your rationale.

2. Does Melissa Drake appear to possess the qualities and characteristics of an effective project manager? Why or why not? What other qualities might be important for a project manager in a case such as this one?

3. Evaluate the composition of the Steering Committee. Do you feel it has adequate representation? Explain. What do you think its role should be in the project? Is its charge clear?

4. How might SunHealth measure the value gained from implementing EHR? The systems impact on achieving the organization's strategic goals?

# CASE: The Wilmington Blood Center

*The following case was originally written by James Decker, a doctoral student in the executive health administration and leadership program at the Medical University of South Carolina. The case has been edited for educational purposes. It is used with permission.*

One of the greatest challenges facing Wilmington Blood Center is the selection and implementation of a new computer system to replace the existing computerized donor tracking system. The current system is somewhat dated and lacks the functionality that will be critical in the future. While the decision is an important one and necessary for sustainable organizational success, it will also require a substantial financial commitment and would place additional stress on an already tight budget.

## Organizational Description

Wilmington Blood Center is a private, not-for-profit blood center located in the Midwest. Established nearly 40 years ago, it is the sole supplier of blood and blood products for 35 hospitals within a 15-county service area. It has limited financial resources upon which to make capital investments, and 98 percent of its operational and capital costs are financed by blood supplier processing fees charged to its client hospitals.

While Wilmington Blood Center has enjoyed steady and consistent growth over the past 40 years, every facet of its operations, including the management of donor information, must adhere to the strict blood product safety regulations established by the U.S. Food and Drug Administration (FDA). The FDA conducts routine inspections so as to assure compliance with standards related to donor recruitment, screening and registration, phlebotomy and collections, lab testing, labeling, and distribution. Accurate and detailed records of each area of the blood center must be maintained in accordance with prescribed FDA standards.

## Information Systems

Perhaps Wilmington's greatest organizational weakness is the fact that the current computer system used for tracking donors and donor information is over 20 years old and close to being obsolete. The system, known as Trakker, is one which was custom built internally by a consultant programmer. Although once state of the art, Trakker's functionality and capabilities are not up to current industry standards. The technology of the system platform is no longer supported, and the programmer, while still on retainer by the organization, is nearing retirement.

Trakker is a database platform from a relatively small company, which functions primarily in the UNIX and custom-mainframe environment. Certain aspects of Trakker rely on FoxPro, a legacy database and development platform that is no longer in general use. Since this is a somewhat rare system by today's standards, finding people with the skill set to support Trakker is extremely difficult and expensive. With the impending retirement of the consultant, there is growing concern regarding how the system might be supported in the future and the risk to the organization in the event that he is no longer available.

It is envisioned that it will become increasingly difficult to keep Trakker operational in an ever-evolving technological environment. Trakker utilizes technologies and processes that are gradually being phased out of contemporary information systems because of security concerns and limitations of such legacy systems. Trakker is a relatively unsecure platform running on a personal computer, and from a hardware standpoint, is not able to take advantage of advances in computing technologies that have been made since its inception.

## The Challenge

There are several commercially available systems on the market that have specific applications to the blood banking industry. Advantages to replacing Trakker with another system are:

- Most new systems run on an Oracle platform, thus making use of commonly used technology for which there would be available personnel with the appropriate skill set for system support.

- Commercially available systems would already be 510K compliant; therefore, they would function in accordance with FDA regulations.

- A new system could be configured so as to communicate with other peripheral systems (i.e. donor recruitment, financial reporting, lab testing, etc.) with sufficient network security layers, redundancy, and firewall protection.

- The new system would be able to utilize current and future advances in technology so as to improve functionality and storage of information.

The obvious obstacles to overcome will be:

- Hardware and software licensing costs are estimated to be in the $1 million to $1.5 million range, creating a major capital budgeting challenge.

- A trained professional would need to be hired in an Information Technology Management capacity to assist with implementation and ongoing technical support.

- Annual operating costs, estimated at $125,000, would need to be budgeted to account for additional personnel and system support from the vendor of choice.

- System configuration, data transfer, and initial training will place additional duties on all members of the management team.

- All user groups throughout the organization would need to participate in time-consuming training, thereby affecting productivity.

## Questions

1. Assume you were the CEO of Wilmington Blood Center, what process would you use to replace the current system? Who would be involved? Who do you think should lead the effort? Include your rationale.

2. Once a preferred vendor and product is chosen, what steps would you take to implement the new system? How might you ensure that the implementation process is managed effectively so as to protect the interests of the organization and ultimately lead to a successful installation? What do you anticipate will be your greatest challenges? How will you evaluate success of the project?

# REFERENCES

Adler-Milstein, J., Landefeld, J., & Jha, A. K. (2010). Characteristics associated with Regional Health Information Organization viability. *Journal of the American Medical Informatics Association, 17*, 61–65.

Adler-Milstein, J., McAfee, A., & Bates, D. W. (2008). The state of regional health information organizations: Current activities and financing. *Health Affairs, 27*, w60–w69.

American Hospital Association (AHA), ed. (2007). Continued progress: Hospital use of information technology. Chicago: AHA.

Andersen, G. F., Hussey, P. S., Frogner, B. K., & Waters, H. R. (2005). Health spending in the United States and the rest of the industrialized world. *Health Affairs, 24*(4), 903–914.

Barney, J. (1991). Firm resources and sustained competitive advantage. *Journal of Management, 17*(1), 99–120.

Bates, D. W. (2005). Physicians and ambulatory electronic health records. *Health Affairs, 24*(5), 1180–1189.

Blumenthal, D. (2009). Stimulating the adoption of health information technology. *New England Journal of Medicine, 360*(15), April 9, 1477–1479.

Blumenthal, D., & Glaser, J. P. (2007). Information technology comes to medicine. *New England Journal of Medicine, 356*(24), 2527–2534.

Bodenheimer, T., & Grumbach, K. (2003). Electronic technology: A spark to revitalize primary care? *Journal of the American Medical Association, 290,* 259–264.

Boynton, A. C., Jacobs, G. C., & Zmud, R. W. (1992). Whose responsibility is IT management? *Sloan Management Review, 33*(4), 32–38.

Brooks, K. V. (2010). The use of perioperative information technology to improve quality of patient care and operating efficiency in an academic teaching hospital. Retrieved August 18, 2010, from http://www.himss.org/storiesofsuccess/docs/tier1/BassettHealthNetwork.pdf

Brown, C. V., & Magill, S. L. (1994). Alignment of the IS functions with the enterprise: Toward a model of antecedents. *MIS Quarterly, 18*(4), 371–403.

Burnum, J. F. (1989). The misinformation era: The fall of the medical record. *Annals of Internal Medicine, 110,* 482–484.

Carr, N. G. (2003). IT doesn't matter. *Harvard Business Review, 81*(5), 41–49.

Chaudhry, B., Wang, J., Wu, S., Maglione, M., Mojica, W., Roth, E., ...Shekelle, P. G. (2006). Systematic review: Impact of health information technology on quality, efficiency, and costs of medical care. *Annals of Internal Medicine, 144*(10), 742–752.

Chun, M., & Mooney, J. (2009). CIO roles and responsibilities: Twenty-five years of evolution and change. *Information and Management, 46,* 323–334.

Cusack, C. M., Byrne, C. M., Hook, J. M., McGowan, J., Poon, E., & Zafar, A. (2009). Health information technolgy evaluation toolkit. Rockville, MD: Agency for Healthcare Research and Quality.

DesRoches, C. M., Campbell, E. G., Rao, S. R., Donelan, K., Ferris, T. G., Jha, A. ... Blumenthal, D. (2008). Electronic health records in ambulatory care—a national survey of physicians. *New England Journal of Medicine, 359*(1), 50–60.

EHR Incentive Program. (2010). Edited by M. a. M. Programs. *Federal Register.*

Electronic prescribing significantly and measurably improves the quality and efficiency of patient care in a teaching-hospital's outpatient medical clinic. (2010). Retrieved August 18, 2010, from http://www.himss.org/storiesofsuccess/docs/tier1/RochesterGeneralHealthSystem_Tier1.pdf

Feeny, D. F., & Willcocks, L. P. (1998). Core IS capabilities for exploiting information technology. *Sloan Management Review, 39*(3), 9–21.

Glaser, J. P. (2005). More on management's role in IT project failure. *Healthcare Financial Management, 59,* 82–89.

Halamka, J. D., Mandl, K. D., & Tang, P. C. (2008). Early experiences with personal health records. *Journal of the American Medical Informatics Association, 15*(1), 1–7.

Hartz, C. E., & Gross, I. (2010). The impact of education and computerized provider order entry (CPOE) on standardization and reduction of blood transfusions in a community hospital. Retrieved August 18, 2010, from http://www.himss.org/storiesofsuccess/docs/tier1/EasternMaineMedicalCenter.pdf

Health information technology: Initial set of standards, implementation specifications and certification criteria for EHR technology. Interim final rule. (2010). *Federal Register.*

Hershey, C. O., McAloon, M. H., & Bertram, D. A. (1989). The new medical practice environment: Internists' view of the future. *Archives of Internal Medicine, 149,* 1745–1749.

Hillestad, R., Bigelow, J., Bower, A., Girosi, F., Meili, R., Scoville, R., & Taylor, R. (2005). Can electronic medical records transform health care? Potential health benefits, savings, and costs. *Health Affairs, 24*(5), 1103–1117.

Himmelstein, D. U., Wright, A., & Woodhandler, S. (2009). Hospital computing and the costs and quality of care: A national study. *American Journal of Medicine.*

Institute of Medicine. (1991). *The computer-based patient record: An essential technology for health care.* Edited by R. Dick and E. Steen. Washington, DC: National Academy Press.

Institute of Medicine. (2001). *Crossing the quality chasm: A new health system for the 21st century.* Washington, DC: National Academy Press.

IOM Committtee on Data Standards for Patient Safety. (2003). Key capabilities of an electronic health record system. Edited by T. N. A. Press. Washington, DC: Institute of Medicine.

Jha, A. K., DesRoches, C., Campbell, E. G., Donelan, K., Rao, S. R., Ferris, T. G., ... Blumenthal, D. (2009). Use of electronic health records in U.S. hospitals. *New England Journal of Medicine, 360*(16), 1628–1638.

Kaplan, B., & Harris-Salamone, K. D. (2009). Health IT success and failure: Recommendations from literature and an AMIA workshop. *Journal of the American Medical Informatics Association, 16*(3), 291–299.

Kausal, R., Bates, D. W., Jenter, C. A., Mills, S. A., Volk, L. A., Burdick, E., ...Simon, S. R. (2009). Imminent adopters of electronic health records in ambulatory care. *Informatics in Primary Care, 17,* 7–15.

Kazley, A. S., & Ozcan, Y. A. (2008). Does hospital electronic medical record use increase health care quality? An examination of three clinical conditions. *Medical Care Research and Review, 65*(4), 496–513.

Kotter, J. P. (1995). Leading change: Why transformation efforts fail. *Harvard Business Review,* March–April, 59–67.

Lacity, M. C., & Hirschheim, R. (1993). *Information systems outsourcing: Myths, metaphors, and realities.* Chichester, NY: John Wiley & Sons.

Lewin, K. (1947). Frontiers in group dynamics. *Human Relations, 1,* 5–41.

Martin, E. W., Brown, C. V., DeHayes, D. W., Hoffer, J. A., & Perkins, W. C. 2005. *Managing information technology.* Fifth ed. Upper Saddle River, NJ: Prentice Hall.

Miller, R. H., & West, C. E. (2007). The value of electronic health records in community health centers: Policy implications. *Health Affairs, 26*(1), 206–214.

Miller, R. H., West, C., Brown, T. M., Sim, I., and Ganchoff, C. (2005). The value of electronic health records in solo or small group practices. *Health Affairs, 24*(5), 1127–1137.

Ornstein, S. M., Garr, D. R., Jenkins, R. G., Rust, P. F., & Arnon, A. (1991). Computer-generated physician and patient reminders: Tools to improve population adherence to selected preventive services. *Journal of Family Practice, 32*(1), 82–90.

Queens-Long Medical Center improves quality and physician satisfaction with EHR backbone and patient centered Medical Home initiative. (2010). Retrieved August 18, 2010, from http://www.himss.org/storiesofsuccess/docs/tier1/QueensLongIslandMedicalGroup.pdf

Schein, E. H. (1999). *The corporate culture survival guide: Sense and nonsense about culture change.* San Francisco: Jossey-Bass.

Wager, K. A., Lee, F. W., & Glaser, J. P. (2009). *Managing health care information systems: A practical approach for health care management* (2nd ed.). San Francisco: Jossey-Bass.

Whitten, J., & Bentley, L. (2005). *Systems analysis and design methods* (7th ed.). New York: McGraw-Hill/Irwin.

Williamson, M. (2010). Facilitating safe and efficient patient handoff using a home-grown e-signout system that is integrated with other hospital systems. Retrieved August 18, 2010, from http://www.himss.org/storiesofsuccess/docs/tier1/Univ_Rochester_Tier1.pdf

Wilson, L. (2010). Patient safety improvements through real-time inventory management. Retrieved August 18, 2010, from http://www.himss.org/storiesofsuccess/docs/tier1/MercyHeartHospital.pdf

Zachman, J. A. (1987). A framework for information systems architecture. *IBM Systems Journal, 26*(3), 276–292.

Zhou, L., Soran, C. S., Jenter, C. A., Volk, L. A., Orav, E. J., Bates, D. W. & Simon, S. R. (2009). The relationship between electronic health record use and quality of care over time. *Journal of the American Medical Informatics Association, 16*(4), 457–464.

# Chapter 14

# Consumerism and Ethics

Ann Leslie Claesson

## CHAPTER OUTLINE

- **Consumerism: Concepts and Challenges**
- **Health Care Reimbursement and Consumerism**
- **The Role of Consumers in Health Management**
- **Retail Medicine**
- **Ethical Considerations in Health Care**

## LEARNING OBJECTIVES

**After completing this chapter, you will:**

1. Identify key concepts of consumerism and how they impact health care
2. Define consumer-driven health care and its impact on the health care environment
3. Identify different types of health care reimbursement that are a result of the consumer-driven health market
4. Understand the interrelationship between retail medicine, consumer's choice, and health marketing
5. Understand the role of social networking in consumer-driven health care
6. Comprehend the influence of Microsoft and Google's investment in PHRs on the health care environment
7. Differentiate different ethical principles and how they are demonstrated in health care

# KEY TERMS

Autonomy

Belmont Report

Beneficence

Bioethics

Confidentiality

Consumer-Driven Health Care

Consumer-Driven Health Plan (CDHP)

Consumers

Consumerism

Convenient Care Association (CCA)

Convenient Care Clinic

Electronic Health Record (EHR)

Fidelity

Flexible Spending Accounts or Arrangement (FSA)

Health Insurance Portability and Accountability Act (HIPAA)

Health Reimbursement Account (HRA)

Health Savings Account (HSA)

High Deductible Health Plan (HDHP)

Human Subjects

Institutional Review Boards (IRBs)

Justice

Medical Savings Accounts (MSA)

Nonmaleficence

Office for Human Research Protections (OHRP)

Personal Health Record (PHR)

Privacy

Retail Medicine

Research

---

## IN PRACTICE:  Consumer-Driven Markets

Richard pauses from his morning run to upload cardio data to his iPod from the sensor in his Nike running shoe. He then sends today's fitness data directly to his online Nike+ account where it will be stored for future use and possible integration into his personal health record at Microsoft HealthVault.

Across town, Patti, a health care manager for an integrated health care system, checks her lab results online and receives an e-mail reminder for an upcoming doctor's appointment. Her employer offers a High Deductible Health Plan (HDHP), which includes options for health care reimbursement arrangements (for health services not covered by the plan) and a wellness option. Jennifer has chosen to utilize the wellness option and is tracking her exercise and weight loss on a "tethered PHR" based out of her hospital system. She then checks the PatientsLikeMe Web site for new information in the ALS and fibromyalgia blogs before she goes to lunch.

The above situations are examples of applications targeting the consumer-driven health care movement. Consumers are choosing to take more responsibility for their own health and wellness and expect increased access to health information from a variety of sources. Advances in technology and telecommunications have contributed to enhanced expectations and needs by consumers for rapid access to health information and services, instant communications, and customer satisfaction. Health care environments need to remain current in the latest health information technology, treatment advances, and consumer needs in order to remain competitive. Consideration of health-related advances and applications such as Personal Health Records (PHRs), health network sites (e.g., PatientsLikeMe) and changes in health care reimbursement structures (e.g., HDHP) contribute to an increased awareness of health and wellness by consumers. Consumers have changed the face of health care in today's marketplace and will continue to do so in the near future.

# CHAPTER PURPOSE

The purpose of this chapter is to provide information and resources concerning the role of consumerism and ethics in our health care environment. In the past few decades, our society has seen a shift toward a greater emphasis on consumerism and how consumer decision making can impact health care service delivery. Consumers play a more important role in negotiating and maintaining their own health care as well as what services are required to fulfill their needs.

Ethical scenarios and choices have become de rigueur in many health care environments, with issues such as end-of-life decisions, health care disparities (who gets the care?), birth control and right-to-life, and religious/cultural preferences in health care treatments. Hence, ethical decision making and health care could easily take up an entire chapter on its own. For the purposes of this chapter, we will focus on the interrelationships between consumerism and ethics and how these relationships can impact effective health care delivery.

The chapter will begin with an exploration of consumerism, key concepts and challenges such as shared decision making, transparency, HIPAA, and consumer-driven marketing. Next, we will examine how the health care reimbursement market has changed due to an increased emphasis on the role of the consumer-driven health care, and the expanded role of the consumer in health care management and personal wellness. The concept of retail medicine and its influence on the current and future health care market will be the fourth area of discussion. Finally, the chapter will conclude with ethical considerations in health care, key concepts, challenges, and guidelines for health care managers and consumers.

# CONSUMERISM: KEY CONCEPTS AND CHALLENGES

Health care has traditionally been considered a provider or medical-driven environment with an emphasis on medical services provided by physicians according to predetermined, quantitatively tested research and methods. Recent trends and advances in health care treatment, increased use of technology, higher demands and expectations by consumers, and a change from the acute-care model to the chronic-care

model due to the aging population has contributed to a shift toward a more consumer-oriented or **consumer-driven health care** system.

As the population ages and the Baby Boomer Generation retires, increased pressure is placed on Generations X and Y to fill the expectations and roles set by the previous generation. Due to recent advances in health care treatment and technology, people are living longer with more chronic diseases as a daily part of their lives (Cahan and Lancashire, 2008, March 27; Federal Interagency Forum on Aging-Related Statistics, 2008, March). This has caused a shift from the acute-care to the chronic-care model (Saver, 2006). The change in demographics and socioeconomics, shortage of health care professionals, this shift toward a more chronic care model for health care service delivery, and increased consumer expectations have provided impetus for alternative forms of health care, including a more consumer-driven health care system that caters to the specialized needs and well-being of individuals, groups, populations, and payers.

With increased access to the Internet and health care–related education, **consumers** expect care to be delivered in different settings. For instance, care that was once delivered in the hospital is increasingly being offered (particularly for our aging population) at home in the name of wellness (Saver, 2006). Health care recipients are no longer merely "clients" or "patients" who accept the health care provider's decisions as their treatment; instead, they are active participants in their own health care decision making.

Traditional approaches to health care service delivery in the United States have been paternalistic in nature. As such, services given to patients were decided upon without significant input from them concerning their needs or expectations. With the advent of the consumer-driven health movement, more health care consumers are rejecting this paternalistic approach and demanding greater choice and control over health care decisions and treatment choices. If their needs are not met they do not hesitate to complain to elected officials or use litigation to express their dissatisfaction (Ranson, E. R., et al., 2008). A report by the Kellogg Foundation noted that 65 percent of health care consumers felt they should have control over health care decision making (Ranson, E. R., et al., 2008).

Customer satisfaction has been a recognized marker for quality in many industries, and particularly in health care.

Consumers have grown accustomed to e-commerce, service guarantees/warranties, 1-800-number information call centers, and higher standards for quality in many products and services. Health care is expected to be no different with the same level of high quality, instant service, and customer satisfaction (Ranson, E. R., et al., 2008). The U.S. health care system has not kept pace with other industries in this need to maintain customer satisfaction and loyalty. The consumer-driven health movement has provided the momentum for a fundamental change in our health care environment, and health organizations and providers are moving toward a more customer-friendly, consumer-driven product: consumer-driven health care.

## Consumers, Consumerism, and Economics

The *Oxford English Dictionary* (OED, 1989h) defines a **consumer** as "a person who uses up a commodity; a purchaser of goods or services, a customer," as opposed to one who produces goods or services (producer or provider). Consumer expectations are what drives a market, in particular our current health care system. Consumers' expectations and perceptions of what should be available, accessible, convenient, and safe are primary indicators of who and what is successful in today's economy.

**Consumerism** has been defined as "doctrine advocating a continual increase in the consumption of goods as a basis for a sound economy" or "advocacy of the rights of consumers" (OED, 1989h). Consumer-driven health care is health care that is directly motivated and impacted by what its consumers expect and demand. Today's health care consumer expects and demands high-quality, safe, and accessible health care services. They research health problems, and they seek information and second opinions on diagnosis and treatment options through available media and personal networking such as online support groups (PatientsLikeMe), social networking sites (Facebook, Twitter), disease-specific associations, public service and government Web sites, alternative/complementary medicine, and other health care professionals.

## Key Principles of Health Care Consumerism

A number of key concepts have been identified regarding health care consumerism. Havlin, McAllister, and Slavney (2003) referred to consumerism in health care as a strategy that encourages and enables people to take charge of their personal health through: (1) knowledge of their current status and needs; (2) informed decision making; (3) wise use of health care dollars; and (4) confident and active participation in their own health care decisions and treatment choices. Potter (1988) recognized five basic principles needed for a consumer-driven market structure that can also be applied to health care: access, choice, information, redress, and representation. Consumers need to have access to services and products, accurate information to assist them in making informed choices, a method for communicating dissatisfaction with service or product choices, and some process to ensure that their interests are represented to decision makers impacting their well-being and welfare (Potter, 1988).

Bachman (2006) noted in his report "Healthcare Consumerism: The Basis of a 21st Century Intelligent Health System" that our health care environment was moving toward a more demand-control model influenced by specified economic forces. This concept aligns health care more closely with consumer purchasing behaviors seen in other industries. He identified six "mega-trends" that impact the demand-control model, one of which is consumerism:

1. Personal responsibility
2. Self-help, self-care
3. Individual ownership
4. Portability
5. Transparency (right to know)
6. Consumerism (empowerment) (Bachman, 2006)

In addition to these six mega-trends, Bachman also noted five key "building blocks" of health care consumerism that are important for health care managers to consider:

1. Personal accounts (FSAs, HRAs, HSAs)
2. Wellness/prevention and early intervention programs
3. Disease management and case management programs
4. Information and decision support programs
5. Incentive and compliance reward programs (Bachman, 2006)

## Shared Decision Making and Transparency

Consumer awareness of service/product quality and cost are key drivers of transparency in health care. Many people are more aware of the price of a new cell phone or automobile than health care services that they depend upon for their own well-being and health status (Goodman, 2006). As health care insurance reimbursement options now include **consumer-driven health plans (CDHP)** such as **High Deductible Health Plans (HDHPs)**, flexible spending accounts (FSA), and **Health Reimbursement Accounts (HRAs)**, employees are being asked to take more responsibility for their own health care needs. As more employees are being asked to make choices in their health care coverage, the question remains: do they have the information to effectively make these decisions?

In order to make informed choices, certain health care information needs to be readily available and *visible* to the public. Therefore, our health care environment needs to become more *transparent* in its approach to information utilization and access. Though this does suggest the need for several reforms, a move towards increased transparency does not mean that all health information should be made pubically available. A number of regulations and legislation exists to protect individual health information, such as the Health Insurance Portability and Accountability Act (HIPAA) and the Patient Safety and Quality Act.

*Access to* and *an understanding of* available health care information is a requirement for consumers to make informed health care decisions (Potter, 1988).

# Health Information Privacy

## Consumers versus Providers: Users of Published Information

Transparency in health care has brought about a plethora of information on health, wellness, treatment options, and disease management. Conventional and nonconventional forms of medicine are frequented by health consumers often on a daily basis. Increased access to information and communication through a variety of formats (e.g., the Internet, social networking, media advertisements, and personal contacts) has brought about questions such as "What information should be made available?" and "To whom?"

## HIPAA and the "Need to Know"

As advances in technology and telecommunications began to change the face of our health care environment, concerns over the privacy of health information, portability of insurance

and utilization, and exchange of electronic data became primary focuses of concern. In 1996, the **Health Insurance Portability and Accountability Act (HIPAA)**, Public Law 104-191, was enacted by Congress to combat waste, fraud and abuse in health care (U.S. Department of Health and Human Services, n.d.; Maryland Department of Mental Health and Hygiene, 2007). It became effective in 1997 with a Privacy Rule finalized in 2002.

The HIPAA legislation specifies regulations for the privacy of personal health information, portability of health insurance, and the organization of the interchange of electronic data for certain financial and administrative operations (Maryland Department of Mental Health and Hygiene, 2007). HIPAA rules limited the use and disclosure of personal health information by "covered entities" who qualified on a "need-to-know" basis according to HIPAA criteria. These "covered entities" include health plans (e.g., individual, group, and government insurance plans), health care providers (e.g., physicians, dentists, and other providers, hospitals, health care organizations, and "any other person or organization that furnishes, bills, or is paid for health care"), and health care clearinghouses (e.g., health care billing services, health information management systems) who conduct standard health care transactions electronically (U.S. Department of Health and Human Services, n.d.).

HIPAA also included Administrative Simplification (Title II, Subtitle f of HIPAA), which required the U.S. Department of Health and Human Services (HHS) to adopt national standards for the use of electronic health information such as unique health identifiers, code sets, and health care transactions (U.S. Department of Health & Human Services, 2009). The HIPAA Privacy Rule and Security Rule are enforced by the HHS Office for Civil Rights. Additional information pertaining to the HIPPA Administrative Simplification can be found at 45 CFR Parts 160, 162 and 164. (U.S. Department of Health & Human Services, 2009).

Another federal regulation that protects the privacy and disclosure of personal health information is the Patient Safety and Privacy Act (PSQIA). Passed in 2005, the PSQIA created a voluntary reporting system pertaining to data utilized in patient safety and health care quality concerns (U.S. Department of Health and Human Services, n.d.). The PSQIA ensures federal protection for patient safety data and enforces civil money penalties for violations of patient safety confidentiality.

Health care consumers and managers should be aware that while HIPAA does provide protection and privacy for personal health information, it pertains only to those entities listed in its criteria (health care providers, health plans, and health-clearing houses). Many online health-related services and locations are not included under the HIPAA regulations, including personal health information uploaded to online Web sites, support groups, social health networks (e.g., PatientsLikeMe, CureTogether) or **personal health records** (e.g., Google Health or Microsoft's HealthVault). While these online vendors do have compliance agreements, which consumers sign prior to participation, they are not considered covered entities; hence there is no recourse via HIPAA protection for consumers or uses of these online services (Stewart, 2009).

# HEALTH CARE REIMBURSEMENT AND CONSUMERISM

Today, consumers are demanding more input into choices regarding health and wellness, and the consumer-driven health movement is in full swing. The movement has been propelled by consumers' revolt against organized methods for cost-containment and limitations on health services and treatment options that have been commonplace in the era of managed care. Although managed care proposed to control health costs by managing resource allocation and access to care, many people rebelled against these constraints, resenting HMO organizations and the health providers who participated in them (Robinson and Ginsburg, 2009). HMOs offered a comprehensive benefit design, a limited provider network, and a means of capping health expenditure with an emphasis on medical management, but also imposed limits on care through the use of precertification, second opinions, and exclusion of treatment for specified populations (Robinson and Ginsburg, 2009).

Consumer-driven health care movement has fostered changes to health plans and approaches to health care reimbursement. Health care expenditures have increased due to advances in technologies, treatments, pharmaceuticals, and the public's expectations for rapid, quality health care that is cost effective, accessible, and understandable. Other drivers of health care cost are the aging workforce, move to more of a chronic disease model than an acute care model, consumer demand for life-enhancing or life-sustaining therapies, drug

company direct-to-consumer advertising, and increased health risks in the population due to stress, obesity, smoking, high blood pressure, diabetes, heart disease, and a lack of personal responsibility in self-care and wellness (Havlin, McAllister, and Slavney, 2003). People make daily choices that impact their own health and well-being. Interventions that target individual choices and expectations are appealing to the public, particularly in our current socially connected society.

## Consumer-Driven Health Plans (CDHPs)

**Consumer-driven health plans (CDHPs)** are designed to allow the employee greater choice in their health care, thus enabling them to be wise consumers (Patterson, 2004). These plans conribute to collective decison making in health care with more responsibility on the employee. CDHPs are deigned specifically to enable consumers greater input into their plan and wellness choices. These plans: (1) provide more information to aid in the selection of providers, treatment options and facilities; (2) offer greater choices in services; and (3) may allow the employee to design their own health plan, including benefits covered, deductible, co-pay, and providers. It is common for CDPHs to offer quality evaluations of health care providers as well as to provide health coaches or designated specialist coaches for specified health conditions (Patterson, 2004). Additional features of CDHPs that are appealing to the modern consumer are 100 percent preventative care and saving accounts that may be carried over to traditional PPO health plans (Havlin, McAllister, and Slavney, 2003).

A number of characteristics of enrollees in consumer-driven health plans have been identified from the 2009 EBRI/MGA Consumer Engagement in Health Care Survey. This annual survey reports nationally representative data concerning consumer-driven health plans and high-deductible health plans (Fronstin, 2009). Information on consumer behavior, attitudes, and impact of the health plan were identified, which is of particular importance to health care managers who are considered redesigning existing services and programs.

Four percent of the population (five million adults aged 21 to 64 with private insurance) participated in CDHPs in 2009, an increase from 3 percent in 2008 (Fronstin, 2009). HDCP enrollment inceased to 13 percent (16.2 million people) in 2009 from 11 percent in 2008. When compared with individuals enrolled in traditional health plans, individuals enrolled in CDHPs were:

1. More likely to demonstrate cost-conscious behaviors

2. More likely to engage in wellness programs

3. More likely to realize financial incentives for healthy behaviors

4. Less likely to have a health problem

5. Less likely to smoke

6. More likely to exercise

7. Less likely to be obese

8. More likely to have a higher household income and be highly educated (Fronstin, 2009).

CDHPs members are more likely to be proactive in determining the coverage available in their health plan, ask for a generic drug as opposed to a brand name, talk with their physician regarding treatment options and choices, develop a budget to manage health care costs, and use online cost-tracking tools (Fronstin, 2009).

## High Deductible Health Plans (HDHPs)

One form of consumer-driven health plans are **High Deductible Health Plans (HDHPs)**. These health plans offer a broad provider network, limited involvement with medical management, higher deductibles and lower premiums (Robinson and Ginsburg, 2009). Minimum annual deductibles for HDHPs as noted by the IRS for the year 2010 are:

- Self-coverage only: $1,200 (minimum deductible); $5,950 (maximum deductible and other out-of-pocket expenses)

- Family Coverage: $2,400 (minimum deductible); $11,900 (maximum deductible and other out-of-pocket expenses) (Department of the Treasury, Internal Revenue Service, 2008).

Typical deductibles for HDPHs range from $500 to tens of thousands of dollars. Health care is paid for by the enrollee until the deductible has been met. Additional benefits include optional participation in Health Savings Accounts (HSAs) or Health Reimbursement Accounts (HRAs). For basically healthy individuals who expect limited health care expenses per year, HDHPs may be a viable option.

HDHPs focus on the premise that health insurance should function similarly to other forms of insurance; covering high-cost,

unpredicted, and catastrophic health needs, but not necessarily providing coverage for everything. They have also been referred to as "catastrophic" health insurance (Treasury, U.S., 2008). Predictable and low-cost health needs are the responsibility of the individual to finance. The structure of HDHPs generally includes an account where pretax monies can be set aside for these predictable low-cost health expenses through a Health Savings Account (HSA) or Health Reimbursement Arrangement (HRA) (Robinson and Ginsburg, 2009). In order to be eligible for HSAs, individuals must be enrolled in an HDHP (Treasury, U.S., 2008).

Generally, HDHPs provide exceptions for preventive care such as well baby/well-child services, certain health evaluations, immunizations, weight loss and smoking cessation programs, routine prenatal care, and specified screenings (Treasury, U.S., 2004). Under these guidelines, preventive care generally does not include treatment of existing conditions, but rather stresses the early identification of new conditions that may require treatment (Treasury, U.S., 2004).

Survey results published by the America's Health Insurance Plans (AHIP) noted a modest increase in HDHP plan enrollment from 400,000 in September 2004 to more than 6.1 million in January 2008. Still, these numbers remain relatively small when compared to total enrollment of individuals in private health insurance (Robinson and Ginsburg, 2009). The percentage of employers who offered a HDHP with HSA or HRA option increased to 13 percent in 2008 from 4 percent in 2004; however, only 8 percent of those with employment-based health coverage were participating in such products in 2008 (Robinson and Ginsburg, 2009).

While consumer-driven health plans such as HDHPs are increasing in popularity, the dominant forms of employer-based health coverage continue to be various forms of managed care, with HMOs maintaining 20 percent of coverage and PPOs accounting for 58 percent of employer-based health coverage in 2008 (Robinson and Ginsburg, 2009). Robinson and Ginsburg (2009) also noted that average deductibles for PPOs averaged around $560 for a single coverage and $1,812 for HDHPs members.

## Reimbursement Accounts for Non-Covered Health Expenses: HSAs, MSAs, FSAs, and HRAs

Historically, health care plans have not included coverage for all health services. Optional savings accounts were established where qualified individuals could deposit pretax monies to use on specified health-related expenses. These accounts may be linked directly to other health plans such as an HDHP. Examples of these types of health-related savings accounts include **Flexible Spending Accounts or Arrangements (FSAs)**, Health Savings Accounts (HSAs), Medical Savings Accounts (MSAs), and Health Reimbursement Arrangements (HRAs). These types of accounts offer tax advantages to assist in offsetting health care expenses (Department of the Treasury, Internal Revenue Service, 2008).

Before 2004, these financial health accounts were the creation of the IRS regulatory processes, were employer-funded only, and called **Health Reimbursement Accounts** or **HRAs** but the name may be changed due to the labeling of each individual vendor (Patterson, 2004). These accounts may also be referred to as a Personal Care Account and were funded by the employer only. The balance in the account can be carried over, or "rolled over," annually (Patterson, 2004). Starting in 2004, a new type of medical carryover account, the **Health Savings Account (HSA)**, was established by the Medicare Prescription Drug, Improvement, and Modernization Act (Patterson, 2004). These accounts can be funded by the individual, the employer (with employee pretax monies or through an employer-provided cafeteria plan), or another individual on the behalf of the account owner (IRC section 125; TASC, 2008b). Participation in an HDHP was required, and the account was able to be carried from employer to employer. HSAs can also receive rollovers from Archer MSAs (Department of the Treasury, Internal Revenue Service, 2008; Patterson, 2004). This change in IRS restrictions on spending in these types of accounts was a key factor in the consumer-driven health movement. The IRS Code (IRC) Section 125 now allowed employees to carryover unused monies from year to year for noncovered health expenses as opposed to FSAs, where all monies must be spent annually (Patterson, 2004).

## Health Savings Accounts (HSAs)

HSAs are tax-exempt financial accounts used to reimburse medical expenses not covered under existing health plans. These noncovered medical expenses include periodical health evaluations (annual visits), routine prenatal and well-child care, smoking cessation programs, obesity/weight-loss programs, health screenings (e.g., cancer, heart

disease, infectious diseases, substance abuse, mental health conditions, pediatric conditions, etc.) (Department of the Treasury, Internal Revenue Service, 2008; TASC, 2008b).

Requirements for participation in a HSA are as follows: participation in a HDHP and no other health coverage except for certain specified areas (such as long-term care, accidents, vision care, dental care, liabilities under workman's compensation, tort or other liabilities incurred via property requirements, etc.), not enrolled in Medicare, and not being claimed as a dependent on another individual's tax return (Department of the Treasury, Internal Revenue Service, 2008). Benefits of HSAs include that contributions are tax-exempt and can be made by the individual, another individual on the owner's behalf, or the employer. Monies accrued in the HSA do not need to be spent during a single year, and can be rolled over on an annual basis, and the HSA is "portable"—you are able to take it with you when changing employers or leaving the workforce (Department of the Treasury, Internal Revenue Service, 2008).

## Medical Savings Accounts (MSAs)

Archer **Medical Savings Accounts (MSAs)** are another type of tax-exempt financial account created to offset noncovered medical expenses for self-employed individuals or employees in small businesses (fewer than 50 workers) since their creation in 1997. Requirements for participation in MSAs include employment (or spouse of employee) in a small employer that maintains a HDHP; or self-employment (or spouse of self-employed person) (Department of the Treasury, Internal Revenue Service, 2008).

Benefits for MSAs are similar to those for HSAs (see Table 14.1). Contributions are tax-exempt and can be made by the individual owner (or an individual on the owner's behalf) or by the employer, but not by both during the same year (Department of the Treasury, Internal Revenue Service, 2008). Like in the HSA, monies accrued in the MSA do not need to be spent during a single year and can be rolled over on an annual basis. Also like in the HSA, you are allowed to move your MSA with you when you change employers or leave the workforce (Department of the Treasury, Internal Revenue Service, 2008). Contributions to Archer MSAs are limited by the employee's income and annual deductible limits (Department of the Treasury, Internal Revenue Service, 2008).

Another type of Archer-designated Medical Savings Account is the Medicare Advantage MSA. Medicare

**TABLE 14.1  Financial Reimbursement Accounts for Non-Covered Health Expenses**

| Account Type | Participation in HDHP | Tax considerations | Monies can be rolled over annually | Contribution type | Who establishes account | Portable? |
|---|---|---|---|---|---|---|
| HSA | Yes | Tax-deductible contributions; employer contributions are pretax and excluded from gross income | Yes | Individual or employer; both in same year allowed | Self or employer | Yes |
| MSA | No | Tax-deductible contributions; employer contributions are pretax and excluded from gross income | Yes | Employer or self, but not both | Employer | Yes |
| FSA | Optional | Tax-deductible contributions; employer contributions are pretax and excluded from gross income | No | Employer-funded through voluntary salary reduction agreement | Employer | No |
| HRA | Yes | 100% tax deductible for employer; tax-free for employee | Discretion of employer | Employer-funded | Employer | No |

Advantage MSAs are a tax-exempt trust arranged through financial institutions such as insurance companies or banks. They can only be funded by Medicare and the monies used to pay for medical expenses accrued by the account holder who is a Medicare enrollee (Department of the Treasury, Internal Revenue Service, 2008). Participants must be enrolled in a HDHP that meets Medicare guidelines and be enrolled in Medicare.

## Flexible Spending Arrangements (FSAs)

Flexible Spending Arrangements (FSAs) are a blanket term for financial accounts where pretax monies are held to be used for reimbursement for noncovered medical expenses. Contributions to FSAs are generally made by the employer through a voluntary salary reduction arrangement with the employee (Department of the Treasury, Internal Revenue Service, 2008). Employers can offer FSAs in addition to other benefits or as a part of a cafeteria plan. Employees do not have to participate in other health plans, and they can decide to participate only in an FSA if they so choose (Department of the Treasury, Internal Revenue Service, 2008).

A requirement of the FSA is that all monies held in the account must be spent annually; the balance could not be carried over from year to year (Department of the Treasury, Internal Revenue Service, 2008; Patterson, 2004). Self-employed individuals do not qualify for FSAs. Reimbursement for medical expenses through FSAs may occur through employer-sponsored debit cards, credit cards, and stored-value cards (Department of the Treasury, Internal Revenue Service, 2008).

## Health Reimbursement Arrangements (HRAs)

Health Reimbursement Arrangements (HRAs) are financial arrangements that are used for reimbursement of substantiated medical expenses. These substantiated or qualified medical expenses are determined by the employer and may include deductibles, co-payments, coinsurance, prescription medications, dental and vision expenses, or other noncovered medical expenses (TASC, 2008a).

HRAs are employer-funded with pretax monies only, but they cannot be funded through an employer-employee salary reduction agreement as with FSAs (Department of the Treasury, Internal Revenue Service, 2008; TASC, 2008a). They are generally offered in combination with High Deductible Health Plans (HDHPs). All contributions to the HRA are 100 percent tax deductible for the employer and tax-free for the employee, which makes them an attractive consideration for many individuals and families with identified noncovered annual medical expenses.

The use of unused monies in the HRA can be carried over annually, partially carried over, or required to be spent annually at the discretion of the employer (Department of the Treasury, Internal Revenue Service, 2008; TASC, 2008a), and are subject to COBRA laws. Reimbursement for noncovered medical expenses may be through the use of employer-distributed debit cards, credit cards, or stored-value cards (Department of the Treasury, Internal Revenue Service, 2008; TASC, 2008a).

For additional information on Health Savings Accounts and other health plans (Publication 969: Health Savings Accounts and Other Tax-Favored Health Plans), visit http://www.irs.gov/pub/irs-pdf/p969.pdf

# THE ROLE OF CONSUMERS IN HEALTH MANAGEMENT

By the year 2030, the Baby Boomer Generation will be age 65 or older, which will significantly impact the economic and workplace structure of this nation. The age-65-and-older population is predicted to increase to 88.5 million by 2050, which is double the current number in 2008 (38.7 million) (Bernstein and Edwards, 2008). In addition, the age-85-and-older population will have tripled from 5.4 million to 19 million between the years 2008 and 2050. How will the face of health care change as the Baby Boomer Generation retires and other generations assume the responsibilities for our fast-paced, demanding health care market? What is the impact of the aging Baby Boomer Generation, increasing diversity in our patient and health care populations, and increased responsibilities on Generations X and Y?

## Personal Health Management: Key Concepts and Responsibility

Societal changes have influenced how Americans perceive their health and wellness status. Technology, instant messaging, and instant communications have contributed to the public's expectations of instant service, customer satisfaction, and a more prominent role in their own health care. The public is more aware of health concerns and the personal responsibility required in maintaining health and well-being.

Reports by the Institute of Medicine (IOM), the U.S. Census Bureau, and Health People 2010 have escalated the public's awareness of the health status of the American people and identified issues of concern, including prevalence of obesity and overweight, diabetes and cardiac disease, cancer and health care disparities, and lack of access to health service and treatment options. New technologies and advancements in medicine and pharmaceuticals have contributed to increased longevity. As longevity increases, so does the propensity for chronic disease and the need for self-help and self-care in order to achieve quality of life. Key areas for improvement for the American population include: obesity and weight loss, increased exercise, health eating and nutrition, regular health screenings for diseases such as heart disease, diabetes, high blood pressure, and certain types of cancer and genetic diseases.

Ten leading health indicators were identified by Healthy People 2010 as key areas of concern in the U.S. population at the beginning of the 21st century (Healthy People 2010, n.d.) (Table 14.2). Each indicator is directly linked to Healthy People 2010 objectives. Each indicator and objective was chosen on its ability to be measured (available data to measure progress), its importance as a public health issue, and its ability to motivate the public to action (Healthy People 2010, n.d.).

Why are these Leading Health Indicators important for health care managers? Since many of these areas have been targeted by media and specific private and publicly funded health care initiatives, gaining awareness of what the U.S. public as consumers is looking for can assist health care managers in tailoring their organizational and departmental goals to fit those needs.

## Wellness and the Consumer

While the public is taking more responsibility for its own health and wellness, not everyone has embraced or can embrace the need for self-improvement or personal responsibility. Technology has increased access to information for many, but what does the public do with that information once received? Differences in socioeconomic status and language barriers have contributed to lack of understanding and often lack of access to health care services for certain population groups. Health care managers who work with these populations should be aware that differences in culture or socioeconomic status do not mean that health and wellness are not areas of concern. Strategies for health and wellness promotion that may

work in one population or culture may not work in another. Health information disseminated via social networking sites (e.g., Twitter, MySpace, Cyworld or Facebook), by the Internet or the use of personal health records (e.g., Microsoft's HealthVault, Google Health) may be effective for certain populations or age groups, whereas television advertisements, telephone calls and personal interaction may be better techniques for other populations and age groups. Consumer-driven healthcare seeks to tailor offerings to fit the population served including health and wellness choices with respect for culture and traditional viewpoints and methods.

Health information technology has changed the way in which medicine and health care is delivered. Health information technology (HIT) can be defined as the computer-based storage, usage, retrieval and sharing of health care information, data and knowledge for communication and decision-making purposes (Cohen and Stussman, 2009). Examples of HIT include electronic medical or health records (EMRs/EHRs), personal health records (PHRs), health networks (PatientsLikeMe), social network sites, telecommunications (iPhone, Blackberry) and personal data storage devices (PDAs, eBook, iPad).

A report on health information technology use among U.S. men and women aged 18–64 by Cohen and Stussman (2010) noted that 74 percent of adults in the United States use the Internet, with 61 percent using the Internet to search for health or medical information. Cohen and Stussman's report is based on preliminary estimate findings from the National Health Interview Survey (NHIS) from January through June 2009. Additional results show:

- Forty-nine percent of adults accessed a Web site with specific information on a medical condition or problem

- Adults aged 18–49 are more likely to use HIT than older adults

- Among those 18–64 years of age, women were more likely than men to look up health information on the Internet (58.0 percent versus 43.4 percent), request a prescription refill on the Internet (6.6 percent versus 5.3 percent) or communicate with a health care provider via e-mail (5.6 percent versus. 4.2 percent).

What does this mean for health care professionals and health care managers? Health information technology is being used by more adults to access health information and to communicate with health providers. Health care managers who chose to embrace health information technology and

## TABLE 14.2 Healthy People 2010 Leading Heath Indicators

| Physical activity | Mental health |
|---|---|
| Overweight and obesity | Injury and violence |
| Tobacco use | Environmental quality |
| Substance abuse | Immunization |
| Responsible sexual behavior | Access to health care |

SOURCE: For additional information on the Healthy People 2010: http://www.healthypeople.gov/LHI/lhiwhat.htm

telecommunications in their practice and health care service delivery will enhance their appeal to consumers, particularly younger generations and those who are technologically savvy.

## Social Network Sites and Health Management

*Social networking* has become a household word and a common method of communication for many people. *Social networking* is done through *social network sites* (SNS), which are defined as "web-based services that allow individuals to (1) construct a public or semi-public profile within a bounded system, (2) articulate a list of other users with whom they share a connection, and (3) view and traverse their list of connections and those made by others within the system" (Boyd and Ellison, 2007). While social networking (implying the initiation of a relationship or place to meet) may occur on these sites, it is generally not the primary focus of many of these sites; rather, they provide a medium for their users to verbalize and make their social networks visible and expressive to others (Boyd and Ellison, 2007). Many users of large SNS already have an extended social network and use these sites as a means of extending communication within their existing network.

Social network sites are used by individuals to connect with others based on common interests, language, political or religious views, and racial, sexual, ethnic, or nationality-based identities (Boyd and Ellison, 2007; Stewart, 2009). Sites may vary in the extent to which they cater to diverse audiences or how they incorporate new information and communication tools (e.g., blogging, mobile connectivity ability, or photo sharing). Social network sites are not exclusively a U.S.-based phenomenon. They have gained popularity globally, such as: Friendstar (Pacific Islands), Orkut (Brazil and India), Mixi (Japan), LunarStorm (Sweden), Hi5 (smaller Latin American countries, South America, Europe), and Bebo (United Kingdom, New Zealand, Australia) (Boyd and Ellison, 2007).

What does this mean for consumer-driven health care and health care managers? Social networks have contributed to increased public awareness of health and wellness issues and have been used as media to disseminate information to larger numbers of people.

Social marketing has been utilized by the public sector to elicit the interest of the public in policy and governmental issues by aligning key issues and initiatives with the needs of the people (Stewart, 2009). Applying social marketing techniques to health care, with its emphasis on understanding people and their needs, and using this understanding to design interventions, may be a good strategy for appealing to the consumer-driven health care market (Stewart, 2009).

One example of social marketing can be seen in the popularity of health social network sites and personal health records (PHRs). Health social networks are a type of social network that links users to common health or medical themes or areas of interest such as Lou Gehrig's Disease (PatientsLikeMe) or genetics (23andMe) (Stewart, 2009). Users of health social networks may be linked together through common personal experience, shared health information, blogs, or shared camaraderie.

Health networks and personal health tracking was made popular by Nike with the introduction of its Nike+ Web site in April 2008, and the use of running shoes with sensors implanted in them to gather and transmit fitness data through its Web site to monitor performance. The data can be uploaded via an iPod to the Nike+ Web site (http://nikerunning.nike.com) (Stewart, 2009). A number of other sites have emerged to track and monitor cardio, fitness, and health data as well as providing jogging routes, sharing information, and establishing support groups centered around specific health activities or situations, such as DailyStrength (support groups) and Organized Wisdom (connection between health accurate information and consumers) (Stewart, 2009). PatientsLikeMe was formed as a network centered on ALS and has since expanded to 19 disease states and behavioral conditions. PatientsLikeMe and other sites such as MediHelp and CureTogether utilize basic information common to all social network sites plus simplified data entry forms where users can manually enter health data and treatment details (e.g., dosage and side effects of treatments) to share with others on the site. In this way, users can see what has and has not worked for others in similar situations and disease stages (Stewart, 2009). Examples of health social networks include: PatientsLikeMe (http://www.patientslikeme.com), CureTogether (http://www.curetogether.com), and 23andMe (http://www.23andme.com).

## Electronic Health Care Records

### *Electronic Medical Health Records (EMR/EHR) versus Personal Health Records (PHR)*

One of the most common forms of health information technology (HIT) is the Electronic Health Record (Robert

Wood Johnson Foundation, 2008). The terms **Electronic Health Record (EHR)** and Electronic Medical Record (EMR) have been used to describe health or medical information that is stored, utilized, retrieved, or shared electronically. The Health Information Management System Society (HIMSS) defines electronic health records as:

> [A] longitudinal electronic record of patient health information generated by one or more encounters in any care delivery setting. Included in this information are patient demographics, progress notes, problems, medications, vital signs, past medical history, immunizations, laboratory data, and radiology reports. (Allan and Englebright, 2000)

It is important to remember that EHRs are developed and maintained by health care organizations (e.g., clinic, hospital, physician's office) as a record of care rendered at that facility at that point in time. They are not a complete record of all care provided to an individual over all venues of time (Allan and Englebright, 2000).

Medical records were initially designed by physicians as a means of documenting and storing information regarding patient encounters. They were designed around the premise of meeting the needs of the physician, and contained information that physicians deemed important, though not necessarily everything the patient considered important (Robert Wood Johnson Foundation, 2010). The first EHRs appeared in the 1960s, but most of the current EHR versions are based on clinical care projects such as COSTAR (Computer Stored Ambulatory Record, developed by Harvard), HELP (Health Evaluation through Logical Processing, developed by the Latter Day Saints Hospital at the University of Utah), CHCS (Composite Health Care System—Department of Defense), and DHCP (De-Centralized Hospital Computer System—Veteran's Administration) (Allan and Englebright, 2000).

As health information technology became more prevalent, medical records began to be digitalized and information transferred to electronic files for use by physicians, nurses, and hospital staff. Benefits of the Electronic Medical Record include larger storage capacity (electronic versus paper files), easier access for patients to view their records (through intranet and online Web portals), and easier transferability of records and data sharing (per HIPAA criteria) (Robert Wood Johnson Foundation, 2010). EMR Web portals can be internally accessed through the organization's intranet or externally accessed via online Web portals using predetermined authorization codes and access protocols. As access to personal health information via electronic medical and health records and organizationally based Web portals increased, individuals began to recognize the value in having accessible personal health information.

## Personal Health Records (PHR)

As utilization of health information technology and Internet access became *de rigueur* for consumers and health care professionals in the United States, it became evident that access to such health information might assist consumers in their personal wellness efforts and contribute to increased personal responsibility for health care decision making (Robert Wood Johnson Foundation, 2010). Consumers began to question why they could not see their medical information alongside other information they considered valuable when making health choices. The option of using their own medical or health information in areas they considered important, such as weight or exercise tracking, monitoring of chronic conditions, or personal wellness initiatives, led to the development of the **Personal Health Record** or **PHR**.

PHRs are electronic Web-based repositories for personal health information, whereas electronic health records reside in a hospital or health care organization's database. With PHRs, consumers decide what health information will be provided, where it comes from, and who has access to it (Stewart, 2009). PHRs can be freestanding or tied to institutions (tethered) (Robert Wood Johnson Foundation, 2010).

Some larger health care systems have moved toward further integration of tethered PHRs that include basic features of electronic health records plus wellness and personal health management options (Stewart, 2009). For example, Kaiser Permanente has launched a tethered PHR incorporating aspects of medical history, accessing test results, e-mail communication with physicians, prescription refills, scheduling options, and tracking of personal information such as diet and exercise (Stewart, 2009).

Freestanding PHRs draw their information from varied sources of patient data instead of being linked directly by a tethered system. Examples of freestanding PHRs include Dossia, WebMD, Revolution Health, Google Health, and Microsoft's HealthVault. Freestanding PHRs require consumers to enter health information manually; however for users of Dossia, there is the option to choose to automatically pool information from insurance claims, laboratory tests, or physician medical records into their PHR through the utilization of Indivo, an open infrastructure (Stewart, 2009).

Some differences between PHRs and Electronic Medical Records (EMRs) or health records include privacy concerns, record design and maintenance responsibilities, reason for record development, and ability to move through the PHR or EMR system and accomplish tasks. While some tethered PHRs may provide access to health information and even some limited messaging within the system, they are still limited by what and where information can be accessed and communication exchanged (Robert Wood Johnson Foundation, 2010).

Some barriers exist regarding the full implementation of health information technology; hence the expansion and full capabilities of personal health records. Systemic barriers identified by the Robert Wood Johnson Foundation in their *Project HealthDesign* and research on personal health records (2010) included: (1) a fragmented state of the current health care system; (2) diversity of health care data; (3) interoperability and technical difficulties related to the sharing of health data; and (4) the current reimbursement system (Robert Wood Johnson Foundation, 2010).

Lack of coordinated use of HIT, with electronic health records in particular, throughout the U.S. health care system is one area that impedes acceptance and utilization of PHR. Just how prevalent is the use of Electronic Health (Medical) Records by health providers in the United States? A report by the Robert Wood Johnson Foundation on "Health Information Technology in the United States: Where We Stand, 2008" (2008) made some interesting findings:

- Thirteen percent more physicians were utilizing Electronic Health Records (EHR) since 2006

- There was no significant difference in quality noted between users of EHRs and nonusers of EHR

- Health care providers who worked with vulnerable populations tended to be less likely to use EHR than other providers

- A number of developed nations were ahead of the U.S. in their utilization of EHR with some moving toward universal adoption of HER

One of the primary constraints in the full utilization of EHR by physicians is the cost. Estimates on the cost for EHR installation for a physician or physician practice are $60,000 (Robert Wood Johnson Foundation, 2010).

Another area of concern pertains to how health care providers are reimbursed for their services. Under the current system, online advice is not a reimbursable commodity. Pay-for-performance has contributed to a piecemeal system where certain behaviors and actions are reimbursed, such as office visits and patient treatment activities, whereas rendering advice or consultation in non-traditional formats such as online do not fit within current regulations. Paul Tang, MD, chair of the national advisory committee for *Project HealthDesign*, stated:

> Giving people advice in an online fashion is not reimbursable in today's world . . . Even though it will prevent a complication because you're reaching someone earlier, and it can prevent an office visit, which is obviously much more expensive, . . . [the] limitations of the current reimbursement system create a disincentive to use this efficient patient-empowering tool. (Robert Wood Johnson Foundation, 2010)

Privacy can also be a concern with the use of personal health information in PHR platforms. Web-based applications that are not under the jurisdiction of health care providers raised some privacy concerns by consumers, policy makers, and consumer advocates. The Health Insurance Portability and Accountability Act (HIPAA) regulates and provides protection for health information used by "covered entities" (health care providers who transmit health information electronically, health plans, and health care clearinghouses) (Stewart, 2009). PHRs are not covered under HIPAA privacy regulations, and there are currently no laws monitoring or protecting personal health information in these formats. While vendors of PHRs such as Google Health and Microsoft's HealthVault have volunteered to comply with current privacy laws, there is no legal recourse for consumers who feel they have had their privacy violated or intruded upon (Cushman, n.d.; Robert Wood Johnson Foundation, 2010; Stewart, 2009).

For users of current platforms of PHRs and health network sites, consumers should use discretion of who has access to their private health information. "Private" may no longer be equal to confidential under these circumstances (Stewart, 2009). Consumers who are familiar with online banking or social network sites such as Twitter or Facebook are aware of the level of privacy that is currently available. However, discretion over personal health information use, who has access to this data, and what they can do with it may entail stronger information management systems and privacy that are currently available. Advice for consumers and health care managers who supervise employees who use these types of platforms is to caution users to reconsider what they share and what remains private.

# RETAIL MEDICINE

## Key Concepts

**Retail medicine** has been described as health care services that are provided in "retail settings" or nonhospital,

nontraditional medical environments (Nash, Jacoby, and Murtha, 2008). Examples of retail medicine include minor emergency health care clinics, **convenient care clinics**, lasik centers, dental clinics, and cosmetic services (Hilgers, 2005). Emphasis on the customer as the consumer of services has changed the health care environment toward a more market-based, sales-oriented approach to health care service delivery.

People's lives have become more complicated. Many find themselves immersed in multiple roles such as parent, child, spouse, employer, employee, caretaker, student, friend, colleague, or expert that come with increased expectations and requirements. Increased access to information, knowledge, and communication via the media, the Internet, social networking,

---

**IN PRACTICE: Microsoft and Google Investments in PHRs**

The consumer-driven health care movement has caused consumers to be more aware of health needs and expectations. Consumers are taking more responsibility for their own health and wellness and are turning to health network sites (e.g., CureTogether) and Personal Health Records (e.g., Google Health, Microsoft's HealthVault) to assist them in this venture (Froomkin, 2008; Robert Wood Johnson Foundation, 2010; Stewart, 2009).

Microsoft and Google are two leading vendors in Personal Health Records (PHRs). Personal Health Records are individual health records that are owned and controlled by the patient, not a health care facility or health provider (Stewart, 2009). The patient decides what is included and who has access to the information. PHRs are usually Web-based and stored on health-related Web sites that provide PHR platforms such as Google Health and Microsoft's HealthVault.

Google Health uses a Continuity of Care (CCR) record, which is a type of standardized health record developed by a collaboration of health care advocacy groups, health providers, and regulators (Stewart, 2009). By choosing this type of health record, Google Health expects that the information contained will be of value to its users and what health care providers hope their patients will track themselves. Information can be either manually entered or imported from a number of partnered sources, such as An Vita Health, Inc., or Medi Connect (Stewart, 2009). One major advantage of PHRs is that your record stays with you even if you change doctors, employers, or health plans.

While Google began its ventures into PHRs in 2006, announcing the advent of Google Health in February 2008, Microsoft released its HealthVault PHR application in October 2007, partnering with 40 health care organizations such as Johnson & Johnson and the American Heart Association (Anonymous, 2008; McBride, 2008; Stewart, 2009). HealthVault's PHR platform is based on a need to house large amounts of information and health-related transactions. HealthVault is accessed through a Windows LiveID and has additional search capabilities through "Live Health Search." Another interesting feature of HealthVault is its capability to upload information from personal and medical devices such as blood-glucose monitors, heart rate monitors, bathroom scales, and over 50 Wi-Fi- and Bluetooth-enabled devices (Stewart, 2009).

Both Google Health and Microsoft HealthVault have partnered with additional health clinics, pharmacies, and other health-related groups (e.g., Cleveland Clinic, CVS Pharmacy, Quest Diagnostics) (McBride, 2008; Robert Wood Johnson Foundation, 2010). While Google Health and Microsoft HealthVault have volunteered to comply with curent health information privacy standards, HIPAA regulations do not cover health data stored in these PHR sites; hence consumers should use discretion when considering what to upload and who really has access to their personal health information.

and personal interaction has caused people to become more aware of and sophisticated in their perceptions of what health services are available and what *they* expect. The use of instant messaging, PDAs, cell phones, and e-mail has become a way of life for many Americans.

Health care consumers expect health services to be readily available when needed, in easily accessible locations, staffed by health care professionals current in the latest treatments and diagnostic procedures, and to be cost effective. Many consumers have a basic understanding and recognition of many non-life-threatening health conditions such as ear infections, urinary tract infections, and influenza. As the pace and stress of their lives increases, rapid accessibility to care and treatment for these routine health concerns becomes a market need. Hilgers (2005) noted that retail medicine and health services usually contain at least one of the following characteristics: (1) price competition and marketing emphasis on cost-effectiveness; (2) mass marketing techniques through multiple media formats; (3) corporation of health services via larger multistate organizations; and (4) the targeting of health needs that are not considered to be life-threatening or serious. As customer expectations continue to rise, service providers—especially those who provide health care–related services—must adapt to the needs of their customer base. Retail medicine is one answer to the expanding consumer need for health services.

## Choices and Challenges in Retail Medicine

### Convenient Care Clinics (CCC)

One form of retail medicine that caters to the diagnosis and treatment of non-life-threatening conditions are retail health care clinics often referred to as minor emergency clinics, "doc-in-a-box," urgent care clinics, or **convenient care clinics**. These clinics tend to be located in high-volume areas such as retail outlets or shopping malls. They may be associated with pharmacies or with large chain department or consumer stores such as Wal-Mart, Target, CVS, or Walgreens. This type of medical clinic has been referred to as "Wal-Mart medicine" due to the proximity of the health clinic inside a Wal-Mart, Target, or other large consumer store. Convenient care clinics, minor medical or minor emergency clinics, and their parent organizations do display some of the characteristics noted by Nash, et al. (2008) such as corporation of health services via larger multistate organizations, targeting needs that are

not considered to be life-threatening, use of mass-marketing techniques targeting consumers who frequent the stores they are located in, and generally not taking insurance.

These retail clinics or convenient care clinics offer walk-in services for a limited scope of medical conditions from minor sore throats and ear infections to preventative services such as flu shots, vaccinations, and health screenings (Nash, Jacoby, and Murtha, 2008). They are usually staffed by advanced practice health professionals such as nurse practitioners (NPs) or physicians assistants (PAs).

Many of the convenient care clinics are members of the **Convenient Care Association (CCA)**. The CCA is an organization of health care systems and companies that offer accessible, cost-effective, quality health services located in retail-based environments (Convenient Care Association, 2008). Executive management for the CCA is provided by a nonprofit public health institute, the Public Health Management Corporation (PHMC).

The first convenient care clinic opened its doors in 2000 in Minneapolis—St. Paul, Minnesota, operated by QuickMedX. Its services were limited to a very small number of illnesses operating on a cash-only basis (Convenient Care Association, 2008). By 2008, CCA member clinics had increased to approximately 1,200 clinics operating in 32 states. Ninety-five percent of the convenient care retail clinics were noted to be CCA members in 2008 (Convenient Care Association, 2008) with more than 3.5 million patients treated (Convenient Care Association, 2008; Nash, Jacoby, and Murtha, 2008).

Despite their rise in popularity, many consumers are left wondering: Is convenient care quality care? How do I know whether the care I receive is up to quality industry standards? Some health care professionals and organizations have questioned the quality of care delivered at retail and convenient care clinics and consider them to be controversial in regards to clinical care (Nash, Jacoby, and Murtha, 2008). Other traditional-based practitioners and health organizations view the impetus of retail medicine as a threat to health care quality and safety by removal of patients from traditional medical practices and services (e.g., hospital- and physician office—based). The Convenient Care Clinic Association requires its member clinics to implement national guidelines and standards for health care quality and safety in assisting clinical providers with their health care decision making (Convenient Care Association, 2008; Nash, Jacoby, and Murtha, 2008).

## Complementary, Integrative, and Alternative Medicine Considerations

Complementary and alternative medicine (CAM) refers to health and medical practices that are not considered to be part of conventional Western medicine or standard care. Conventional medicine or "standard care" is defined as medicine that is practiced by a medical doctor (MD) or doctor of osteopathy (DO) (conventional medicine) or by allied health professionals such as registered nurses or physical therapists (standard care) (MD Anderson Cancer Center, 2009; Medline Plus, 2009). Other terms for conventional medicine are Western medicine, mainstream medicine, or allopathy (MD Anderson Cancer Center, 2009). Alternative medicine pertains to "therapeutic choices taken in place of traditional medicine used to treat or ameliorate disease" (MD Anderson Cancer Center, 2009). Complementary medicine is therapies and practices used to "complement" or be used in addition to Western or allopathic medical choices or treatments (MD Anderson Cancer Center, 2009). CAM therapies may include mind-body interventions (e.g., meditation, prayer, music therapy), biologically based and herbal treatments (e.g., herbal medicine or plant therapies), manipulative and body-based therapies (e.g., massage, reflexology), or energy therapies (e.g., Reiki, qi gong, Therapeutic Touch) (MD Anderson Cancer Center, 2009).

The consumerism movement in health care compounded by changes in socioeconomic status and insurance coverage has increased the demand for the availability of retail and complementary and alternative medicine choices (Hilgers, 2005; Wolsko et al., 2000). Reasons why consumers may choose to utilize complementary and alternative medicine include economics, poor results from conventional medical treatments, negative experiences with traditional Western medical practitioners, unpleasant side effects for pharmaceutical therapies, or personal views and perceptions of health that are not in alignment with traditional Western medical choices (Barnett, 2007).

## Concierge Medicine and Global Competition

Concierge care is an additional form of medical care delivery that caters to the wealthy and upper middle classes. Consumers who can afford to pay for special health services with personalized benefits may choose concierge care over other forms of traditional, alternative, or retail medicine. Second opinions, precertification and long waiting lists are some of the reasons why the wealthy may choose to select the convenience and instant access of concierge care, even if it means going outside the United States to get it.

Concierge care is not dependent upon insurance reimbursement, and consumers may pay an additional fee of $1,500 per individual or up to $20,000 per couple for personalized health care services. Services provided may include same-day appointments, home visits, provider accompaniment to emergency rooms, and after-hours accessibility via pagers or cell phones. This extra fee is in addition to co-payments or deductibles designated by insurance companies (Nash et al., 2008). The concept of concierge care has also been extended globally where health care providers and physicians (many of whom are U.S.-trained) offer specialty services in other countries for a designated fee structure. Surgical procedures, radical oncology treatments, cosmetic reconstruction, and fertility clinics are a few of the services provided by these health clinicians. Conventional Western, non-Western, and alternative medical therapies can be found in various locations nationally, such as Arizona and Illinois, or globally for those who are able and willing to afford them. There has always been some sort of a concierge care trade for upscale medical services, but the recent trend for a more consumer-based approach to health care increased the potential for this particular market in meeting the real or perceived needs for a knowledgeable, informed, and fiscally sound public.

# ETHICAL CONSIDERATIONS IN HEALTH CARE

## Key Concepts

The very nature of health care and health care systems evokes certain ethical concerns and considerations for the health care manager. Consumerism and the increasing demands of consumers as active participants in their health care decisions may cause controversies between ethical decision making and treatment options. Does everyone have the right to all treatment options? Should the truth always be told even if it jeopardizes a patient's health or well-being? What key ethical principles are frequently seen in health care decision making, and are they the same for all organizations and industries? These questions reflect some of the ethical concerns raised in health care environments.

In this section, we will explore the ethical considerations inherent in health care, particularly those that are impacted by the expanded consumer role. Consider how consumers have impacted ethical decision making and how choices can impact quality patient care in health care environments. How will these change the interrelationship between ethics and consumerism in the next decade or two? What will be changed and what will remain the same?

**Ethics** has been a topic of examination, critique, and discussion throughout history. Leading figures as Socrates and Hippocrates have debated merits and controversies inherent in the study of ethics, logic, and human behavior. As science and medicine continued to evolve and expand, new perspectives on societal obligation, behavior, and moral considerations began to emerge. Professional standards and codes of conduct were developed as guides for professional morality and ethical behavior. The medical and health care fields are somewhat unique in respect to certain moral and ethical expectations. Health care professions are expected to comply with general moral/ethical principles to "do good" (beneficence) and "do no harm" (nonmaleficence) to others. The Hippocratic Oath (OED, 1989f), taken by physicians, is an embodiment of the principle of nonmaleficence and requires physicians to "do no harm" to their patients and others in their professional practice, but does not recommend the principle of veracity (truth telling) in professional dealings (Beauchamp and Childress, 2009). Hence, many of the initial codes of conduct for medicine and health care have been revised over the years as societal views and expectations changed. Key moral/ethical principles that pertain directly to health care relationships that will be discussed in this section are: respect for autonomy, privacy, confidentiality, fidelity, veracity, nonmaleficence, beneficence, and justice.

## Autonomy

**Autonomy** relates to the freedom to follow or act according to one's own will (OED, 1989a). Personal autonomy pertains to self-rule or self-governance where the individual, organization, institution, or entity is free from limitations or control by others. This includes the capacity to adequately understand and have access to information needed to make meaningful decisions (Beauchamp and Childress, 2009). The majority of ethical theories pertaining to autonomy and respect for autonomy encompass two primary elements: liberty (freedom from controlling factors or influences) and agency (the capacity for intentional choices and actions) (Beauchamp and Childress,

2009). Therefore, when a physician, individual, or institution is respectful of autonomy, they display a respect for the rights of others to hold personal views and to make choices based on their own system of values, beliefs, and mores. Respect for others, with particular emphasis on personal autonomy, is evidenced in the Patient's Bill of Rights, and the patient's ability to obtain, understand, and make informed decisions (consent) for procedures and other health-related choices.

Conflicts in autonomy can be seen in ethical dilemmas concerning competence, informed consent, or assumptions of control over others (certain family and organizational situations). Beauchamp and Childress (2009) note that respect for autonomy includes acknowledgment of the value and decision-making rights/capacity of others; hence, disrespect for autonomy may be seen as disrespectful actions, attitudes or behaviors that demean, insult or do not include attention to autonomous rights of others.

## Privacy

The principle of **privacy** relates to the right or choice of being alone, undisturbed, or free from public attention or intrusion (OED, 1989i). Privacy in health care and medicine also pertains to freedom from intrusion of others, especially concerning personal choice, protection from outside interference or observation, and a reasonable expectation of isolation or seclusion without access of self by others (Beauchamp and Childress, 2009). Privacy issues have been a cause of concern in health care for a number of years, such as public controversy over abortion or family planning, child rearing, relationships, and other areas of personal choice. An example of the expectation of privacy can be seen in *Griswold v. Connecticut* (1965), where the right to protection of information and privacy from the government and others concerning contraception was upheld. (Beauchamp and Childress, 2009).

Five types of privacy have been identified that have relevance to health care: (1) informational privacy, (2) physical privacy, (3) decisional privacy, (4) proprietary privacy, and (5) relational or associational privacy. Informational privacy is emphasized in bioethics and rights to access of certain information. Physical privacy pertains to physical and personal space. Decisional privacy relates to personal choices and decision making. Proprietary privacy is concerned with "property interests in the human person" (Beauchamp and Childress, 2009), and relational or associational privacy pertains to expectations of intimate relationships and family where decisions are made in relation to others (Beauchamp and Childress, 2009). Examples of conflicts concerning privacy and privacy issues seen in health care include invasion of privacy and physical space without the consent of the individual, unauthorized access to personal information, or a lack of respect and privacy concerning personal decisions in intimate/close relationships such as friends, spouses or physicians.

## Confidentiality

Confidentiality is closely related to the principle of privacy. The term confidential has been defined as an expectation of a certain privacy and non-disclosure regarding information relayed to another person (OED, 1989d). **Confidentiality**, therefore, pertains to the nature of a confidence or confiding of secrets or private information from one to another. Inherent in the concept of confidentiality is the expectation that the information confided will remain secret between the confider and confide whether this understanding is implicit (implied) or explicit (specifically stated) and the person to whom the information was entrusted agrees to not disclose it to anyone without the permission of the confide (Beauchamp and Childress, 2009).

Breaches of confidentiality and privacy are closely related. The primary differences between the two are that a breach of confidentiality occurs when an individual (organization or institution) who received confidential information discloses (or fails to protect) it without the permission of the first party (Beauchamp and Childress, 2009). Issues of confidentiality occur in the disclosure of personal health information and the right to privacy and confidentiality of private health care information is protected by HIPAA regulations for covered providers

It is important to note, as stated earlier, that the HIPAA requirements do not pertain to what the impact is on privacy and confidentiality through the use of Electronic Health Records (EHRs) and Personal Health Records (PHRs). As mentioned earlier, Electronic Health Records are protected under the HIPAA regulations, whereas personal health information that is provided to Web sites, social networking groups, or Personal Health Records such as Microsoft's HealthVault or Google Health is not.

Information housed in EHRs can generally be considered private and confidential due to their protection under HIPAA. Although this may not always be the case as with Farrah Fawcett and Brittany Spears, whose private medical information was leaked to the press by a health care employee at the UCLA Health System (Dissent, 2008 in phiprivacy.net;

Silverman, 2009; UCLA Media Relations, 2008). Privacy and confidentiality of health care information (real or presumed) should be considered by consumers (e.g., individuals and groups) who may choose to use one form of health record maintenance over another.

## Fidelity

The principle of **fidelity** refers to the concept of being faithful, loyal, or honest (OED, 1989e). Fidelity also pertains to the obligation to honor commitments. In health care, fidelity pertains to relationships between individuals such as between a health care professional or physician and a patient. Conflicts can occur when there are cross obligations or instances of divided loyalties (Beauchamp and Childress, 2009). Conventional physician-patient relationships tend to place the patient's interests first; therefore, behaviors that are in contrast to what can be conceived as the patient's best interest may be construed as conflicts of fidelity. Health care providers or managers may encounter conflicts of fidelity regarding multiple allegiances to other colleagues, institutions, religious beliefs, funding agencies for research studies, or patients (Beauchamp and Childress, 2009).

## Veracity

Veracity concerns truth-telling or the quality of truthfulness (OED, 1989j). It is assumed in health care that information and relationships will be truthful and honest. Beauchamp and Childress (1989) identified three components that are inherent in the concept of veracity that pertain directly to health care: (1) respect for others; (2) fidelity, promise-keeping, and contract; and (3) health professional–patient relationships based on trust. Relationships between health care provider and patients are based on trust and the assumption that the provider will act in the best interest of the patient. When this does not occur, violations of fidelity in the patient-provider relationship can occur, which can escalate to larger ethical situations that may come to the attention of the health care manager or director.

Examples of possible conflicts of veracity in health care include nondisclosure of pertinent health information to patients such as a potentially terminal disease or impending death. Interestingly enough, a number of health-related standards and guidelines, such as the Hippocratic Oath and Declaration of Geneva of the World Medical Association, do not recommend veracity in professional relationships (Beauchamp and Childress, 1989). The American Medical

Association's medical ethics principles did not support the principle of veracity or truth-telling to patients until 1980, when physicians were encouraged to "deal honesty with patients and colleagues" (Beauchamp and Childress, 1989) with an added revision in 2001 stating that physicians should be honest in all their professional interactions and interrelationships.

## Nonmaleficence

**Nonmaleficence** relates to the duty to "not inflict harm on others" (Beauchamp and Childress, 2009). Obligations of nonmaleficence pertain to *intentionally reframing from doing* (or nonparticipation in) actions or behaviors that would hurt others. This includes potential for causing harm as well as placing another into a risk for harm. An example seen in health care would be to not cause pain and suffering or demean others (Beauchamp and Childress, 2009). Negligence is an example of an infraction of nonmaleficence that can be seen in health care. Negligence is the absence of care or treatment that is given or that which is below the expected standards of care in the profession or specialty area (Beauchamp and Childress, 2009). Conflicts related to the principle of nonmaleficence frequently seen in health care can be related to religious beliefs and traditions; withholding (withdrawing) life support, treatments, and technologies used to sustain life; extraordinary (and ordinary) medical treatments; and euthanasia/death (Beauchamp and Childress, 2009).

## Beneficence

**Beneficence** is closely related to the principle of nonmaleficence in that beneficence pertains to the obligation to do good, prevent or remove harm, and to act in a kind or benevolent manner (OED, 1989b; Beauchamp and Childress, 2009). Obligations of beneficence, as opposed to nonmaleficence, contain positive requirements for action, may not provide reasons for legal punishment for noncompliance, and are not required to be followed impartially (Beauchamp and Childress, 2009).

Three key aspects of the principle of beneficence that are expected in professional relationships and health care interactions are: (1) prevent harm or evil; (2) remove harm or evil; and (3) promote and do good. Health care is essentially a "helping" profession in which individuals choose to try to make a difference in a caring manner to others. Many health care organizations are based on an altruistic approach to health and wellness with a love and compassion for the human condition. Other terms for beneficence that have

been used in relation to health care professionals are mercy, kindness, and charity (Beauchamp and Childress, 2009).

## Justice

The Oxford English Dictionary Online (1989) defines **justice** as "the quality of being (morally) just or righteous," including just conduct, integrity, and conformity to a moral right or reason. Other words associated with justice are rightfulness, fairness, correctness, and propriety. Justice can take many forms. Distributive justice relates to fair and equal distribution as defined by society. Criminal justice is concerned with the fair (just) infliction of punishment for criminal acts, and rectificatory justice deals with breaches of contracts or malpractice issues (Beauchamp and Childress, 2009). Some beliefs pertaining to distributive justice that can be seen in health care interactions are the concept of equal shares— distribution according to need, effort, contribution, merit or free-market exchange (Beauchamp and Childress, 2009). Health care disparities, treatment accessibility, and equal employment opportunities are examples of some of these conflicts that can be seen in health care and that the health care manager may encounter.

## Clinical Bioethics: Rights and Responsibilities

**Bioethics** is the discipline concerned with ethical questions and actions in medicine and biology (OED, 1989c). It differs from other forms of ethics in that bioethics concentrates on issues found in medicine such as clinical treatment, end of life, and research concerns and situations. Clinical bioethics departments and considerations can be found at a number of universities and government entities nationally and internationally. The Department of Bioethics at the National Institutes of Health was established in 1996 and is divided into three key areas of interest: health policy, human subjects' research, and genetics (National Institutes of Health, n.d.). Additional information on these three areas may be obtained at: http://www.bioethics.nih.gov/home/index.shtml.

## Research Considerations and Human Subject Protection

Ethical considerations also pertain to clinical research and study in health care. Research standards, guidelines, and regulations have been established that delineate criteria for research study design and participation by human subjects.

Biomedical and behavioral clinical research, especially pertaining to human subject participation in health care facilities, is overseen by Institutional Review Boards (IRBs) and certain governmental agencies such as the Office for Human Research Protections (OHRP).

**Institutional Review Boards (IRBs)** are administrative entities established by institutions to protect the ethical rights of human subjects who participate in research conducted under their supervision (OHRP, Jurisdiction of the Institutional Review Board, n.d.). Institutional Review Boards have the capacity to review research protocols, require modifications or disprove research activities as specified under federal and local institutional policy. They determine whether the clinical situation presented is considered to be research and if it involves human subjects. The regulatory definition of **research** is "a systematic investigation, including research development, testing and evaluation, designed to develop or contribute to generalizable knowledge" [Federal Policy §___.102(d)], and **human subjects**, as they pertain to research, are defined as "living individual(s) about whom an investigator (whether professional or student) conducting research obtains (1) data through intervention or interaction with the individual, or (2) identifiable private information" [Federal Policy §___.102(f)] (OHRP, Jurisdiction of the Institutional Review Board, n.d.).

The **Office for Human Research Protections (OHRP)** is a branch of the U.S. Department of Health and Human Services that provides leadership regarding protection of human subjects involved in research activities. The OHRP oversees and safeguards the rights, welfare and wellbeing of human research subjects through regulatory oversight, education, advice on bioethical and regulatory issues, and clarification of existing ethical requirements and standards of conduct (OHRP, 2005, September). The Office for Human Subjects Protections also offers a guidebook for IRBs which contains valuable resources for IRB formation, new review committee members, basic considerations for IRB review and institutional administration. The IRB guidebook can be found at: http://www.hhs.gov/ohrp/irb/irb_guidebook.htm.

A seminal publication that has been instrumental in the establishment of federal regulations for human subject protection is the **Belmont Report**. The Belmont Report is a result of work by the National Commission for the Protection of Human Subjects of Biomedical and Behavioral Research in the 1970s with revisions by the Department of Health and Human Services (HHS) in the late 1970s and early 1980s for the protection of human subjects 45 CFR part 46 (OHRP, 2008, November 13). The report by the National Commission entitled "Ethical Principles and Guidelines for the Protection of Human Subjects Research" was renamed the Belmont Report in 1978 after the Belmont Conference Center where the commission initially met when working on the report (OHRP, 2008, November 13). Three interrelated ethical principles are outlined in the Belmont Report that pertains to biomedical and behavioral research: respect for human persons, beneficence and justice (Figure 14.1). These three principles are the foundation for HHS human subject protection regulations.

The information contained in the Belmont Report and subpart A of 45 CFR part 46 led to the creation of a code of conduct for the protection of human subjects called the "Common Rule." This was created in 1991 by HHS and 14 other federal agencies and departments (OHRP, 2008, November 13). The Belmont Report remains an integral resource for human subject protection education for researchers and IRBs that involve human subjects. Additional information on 45 CFR part 46 can be obtained at http://www.hhs.gov/ohrp/humansubjects/guidance/45cfr46.htm, and the Belmont Report can be found at http://www.hhs.gov/ohrp/humansubjects/guidance/belmont.htm.

Training in human subjects protection is a requirement for researchers in biomedical, behavioral, and other health care–related fields. The Collaborative Institutional Training Initiative (CITI) provides Web-based education and training in human subjects protections including biomedical modules and education. CITI is a joint venture between the University of Miami and the Fred Hutchinson Cancer Research Center and was made available to subscribing institutions in 2000. Additional information on the CITI training initiative may be obtained at: https://www.citiprogram.org/aboutus.asp?language=english.

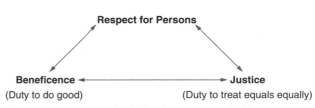

**Figure 14.1** Key Principles for Human Subjects Protection from the Belmont Report.

SOURCE: Delmar, Cengage Learning.

## Patient Rights

The rights of patients in health care have been implied for many years, but it was not until 1973 when the American Hospital Association (AHA) approved the use of the Patient's Bill of Rights that health care providers and organizations began to define what these rights were. The original version of the Patient's Bill of Rights (American Hospital Association, 1992/1998) contained 12 conditions that were expected on the behalf of the patient, many of which echo many of the ethical principles noted in this section.

1. Right to considerate and respectful care.

2. Right to obtain current, relevant, and understandable information concerning diagnosis, treatment, and prognosis.

3. Right to make decisions regarding the plan of care and to refuse treatment to the extent permitted by the law and organizational policy.

4. Right to have an advance directive or designate a surrogate decision maker.

5. Right to every consideration of privacy.

6. Right to expect confidentiality of information and communication.

7. Right to review records pertaining to his or her medical care with explanation (or interpretation) of said records and information.

8. Right to expect reasonable response to the patient's request for appropriate and medically indicated care and treatment according to the organization's capacity and policies.

9. Right to ask and be informed of business relationships among the organization and other internal or external stakeholders that may influence the patient's care and treatment.

10. Right to consent or refuse to participate in research studies that affect care and treatment and to have those research studies or activities fully explained.

11. Right to expect reasonable continuity of care when appropriate and to be informed of available and realistic patient care options when hospital care is no longer appropriate.

12. Right to be informed of organizational policies and practices that pertains to the patient's care, treatment and responsibilities.

Although the AHA Patient's Bill of Rights was revised in 1992, it was still considered to be difficult to read and understand by most Americans (Gardner, 2010). Efforts toward increased communication and comprehension between provider and patient, the AHA again revised the Patient's Bill of Rights and shortened it to a brochure entitled "Understanding Expectations, Rights, and Responsibilities." This brochure includes six rights written in plain language which include "high quality hospital care, a clean and safe environment, involvement in your care, protection of your privacy, help when leaving the hospital," and "help with your billing claims" (American Hospital Association, 2003).

Other health and medical organizations and advisory groups have developed their own versions of the Patient's Bill of Rights. The President's Advisory Commission on Consumer Protection and Quality on the Health Care Industry under President Clinton issued a 1997 interim report defining a Patient's Bill of Rights in Medicare and Medicaid emphasizing three goals, seven sets of rights, and one set of responsibilities (U.S. Department of Health and Human Services, 1999, April 12). Additional information on this version of patient rights can be found at: http://www.hhs.gov/news/press/1999pres/990412.html. These revised patient rights expanded existing expectations to include access to emergency services, care without discrimination, right to speedy complaint resolution, and additional patient responsibility and involvement in their own health and welfare (U.S. Department of Health and Human Services, 1999, April 12).

## Ethics and the Health Care Manager

The role of the health care managers or director can vary according to job description and level of responsibility over others. However, all health care managers and directors, regardless of their level, type of facility, or geographic location should function in an ethical and competent manner.

A number of issues impact ethical management in health environment, such as reimbursement issues, organizational change and behavior, situations related to clinical and behavioral research studies, fiscal needs, and public/consumer pressure. Managed care and the move toward pay-for-performance can contribute to questionable behaviors on the part of health care providers, third-party reimbursement organizations, and expectations (versus reality) of patients regarding service delivery and payment.

Temptation to not always act in an ethical manner can become prevalent if an organization does not require high standards for quality and ethics. While societal examples of unethical behavior such as that seen by leaders in Enron, WorldCom, and Tenet Health Care may not be enough to dissuade leaders or health professionals to avoid ethical temptation, it is important that high professional standards for ethical and professional conduct be set and followed in order to establish and maintain an ethically competent organization. Just as high-quality standards in compliance with industry standards is important from a regulatory and public-perception standpoint, the method by which a facility or organization regulates its ethical standards can be equally important, especially in this age of consumer-driven health care.

Some ways in which health care managers and directors can work to ensure ethical practices at the organizational level have been identified by Hofmann and Nelson (2001):

1. Refuse temptation to incorporate or excuse inefficient business practices through rationalization (e.g., not-for-profit agencies do not need to fully comply with progressive or aggressive policies and procedures).

2. Ensure that your organization's mission, vision and values statements are fully understood by all staff, and that decisions and actions made are consistent with these statements.

3. Involve physician, board, and management in significant change efforts that may impact the organization's role in the community.

4. Assess all possible effects (positive and negative) on the community before starting competitive strategies.

5. Assess and evaluate all potential ramifications (economic, non-economic, internal and external) of eliminating programs or services beforehand.

A number of useful tools and resources are available for managers and leaders concerning ethical behavior and practice. Specific health-related organizations such as the American College of Surgeons, the American Medical Association, the American Organization of Nurse Executives, the National Center for Healthcare Leadership, and the American College of Healthcare Executives provide specific guidelines and resources for ethical practice. For example, the National Center for Healthcare Leadership (NCHL) has a Leadership Competency Model that can be used to guide the design and development of health care management academic programs. This model

(version 2.1) contains 26 competency areas (with five or six levels of attainment) such as accountability, professionalism, change leadership, community orientation, and human resource management (NCHL, 2006). Ethics and ethical behavior are emphasized in *L18.4—Understanding the Basics of Organization Governance* ("Understands governance practices, including board relations, committee structure, and fiduciary, *ethics*, and clinical review responsibilities"); and *L19—Professionalism* ("The demonstration of *ethics*, sound professional practices, social accountability, and community stewardship. The desire to act in a way that is consistent with one's values and what one says is important.") (NCHL, 2006). Another tool provided by NCHL is a leadership self-assessment test, which leaders can take to determine their current status in the leadership development schemata. Information regarding NCHL and the leadership self-assessment may be obtained at: http://www.nchl.org and http://nchl.org/static.asp?path=2852,3241.

The American College of Healthcare Executives has an ethics self-assessment instrument (http://www.ache.org/newclub/career/ethself.cfm) as well as an ethics toolkit (http://www.ache.org/ABT_ACHE/EthicsToolkit/ethicsTOC.cfm) and other useful resources for health care managers and leaders. For additional information on ethical behavior in business and practice for health care environments including biomedical and behavioral research, review the following links:

American College of Healthcare Executives: http://www.ache.org

America College of Surgeons: http://www.facs.org/

American Medical Association—The Council on Ethical and Judicial Affairs: http://www.ama-assn.org/ama/pub/category/4325.html

American Organization of Nurse Executives: http://www.aone.org/

Center for Practical Bioethics: http://www.practicalbioethics.org/

Institute for Global Ethics: http://www.globalethics.org/

IRB Forum: The Institutional Review Board—Discussion and News Forum: http://www.irbforum.org

Office for Human Research Protections (OHRP): http://www.hhs.gov/ohrp

The Petrie-Flom Center for Health Law Policy, Biotechnology, and Bioethics: http://www.law.harvard.edu/programs/petrie-flom

## DEBATE TIME: Ethical Dilemmas for Health Care Managers

An ethical or moral dilemma has been defined as a situation where an individual's obligations require two or more possible pathways or alternatives, but only one is possible (Hamric et al., 2009). Ethical dilemmas (or conflicts) occur in health care environments on a daily basis. The ability to recognize a potential conflict with possible intervention to prevent the conflict from advancing to a dilemma is a valuable skill for the health care manager's professional toolkit. Table 14.3 contains examples of possible health-related ethical conflicts or dilemmas. See which ones you can identify with and what strategies you could use to intervene or prevent the situation from advancing into a more serious situation.

### TABLE 14.3  Health Care Conflicts and Ethical Principles

| Ethical Principle | Definition | Ethical Issue for Consideration |
|---|---|---|
| Autonomy | Duty to respect individual rights of "personal liberty, values, beliefs and choices" | Shirley's daughter tells you that her father is "old and doesn't know what he is doing." She will be making his decisions for him and is taking him off of two of his medications |
| Nonmaleficence | "Duty not to inflict harm" | Joe Smith increases Jerome Terrell's pain medication because he can't stand to see the child suffer due to a sickle cell crisis. Jerome becomes unconscious and lapses into a coma. |
| Beneficence | "Duty to do good and prevent/remove harm" | Sue Jacobson, a 34-year old woman with metastatic breast cancer, has a hip fracture and is waiting in the emergency room to be seen. You are walking through the ER on your way to a meeting when you see Sue reaching for her purse on a bedside stand just out of her reach. She is about to roll onto the floor. |
| Formal Justice | "Duty to treat equals equally" | Miguel and Roxanne are patients of yours with the same diagnosis of multiple sclerosis (MS). There is an experimental drug that proposes to reverse signs and symptoms and reduce pain in MS patients. Both Miguel and Lin are moaning in pain, the same age, and at the same stage of MS. You have only enough of the drug for one person. |
| Veracity | "Duty to tell the truth" | Dr. Fred has just diagnosed Mrs. Olsen with advanced ovarian cancer. Her prognosis is four months at the most. Since Dr. Fred likes this patient and she is old (89 years old), he decides to not "upset her" and keeps her diagnosis to himself. |
| Fidelity | "Duty to honor commitments" | Roger is a health care provider who is employed under an integrated health care system. The organization has told him not to continue treating Baby X because the insurance carrier has denied the last two months' worth of claims. Baby X is 4 months old, and you have been his only health care provider since birth. You promised his mother that you would look after him just before she died in childbirth. While you are committed to the health care organization that employs you, you made this promise to Baby X's mother. |

**DEBATE TIME: Ethical Dilemmas for Health Care Managers** *(Continued)*

**TABLE 14.3 Health Care Conflicts and Ethical Principles** *(Continued)*

| Ethical Principle | Definition | Ethical Issue for Consideration |
|---|---|---|
| **Confidentiality** | "Duty not to disclose information shared in a trusted manner" | "She told me not to tell anyone, but I know I can trust you"—conversation overheard in the elevator at a large metropolitan medical center between two nurses you know. The person they are discussing turns out to be your boss's wife. What do you do? |
| **Privacy** | "Duty to respect limited access to individuals" | Sarah works in medical records. She learns that her son's girlfriend, Raquel, is an inpatient on the psychiatric floor. She decides to "sneak a peek" at Raquel's medical records to see why she is there; after all, her son's welfare may be at stake! |

SOURCE: Adapted from Beauchamp and Childress (2009).

# SUMMARY AND MANAGERIAL GUIDELINES

1. Technological advances, changes in societal communication, and access to information have contributed to the consumer-driven health care movement. Consumers expect different modes of health care delivery, access to understandable information, involvement in their health care decisions, and high quality and satisfaction with health services and health providers.

2. Consumer-driven health care has contributed to increased individual expectations and has fueled new markets and applications such as retail medicine, electronic medical and personal health records, and personalized health reimbursement and insurance models.

3. Personal health information is protected by HIPAA regulations, but this applies only to "covered entities" (e.g., health care providers, health plans, and health care clearinghouses). It is important for health care managers and leaders to keep in mind that not all health information is covered under the HIPAA regulations such as health networking sites (e.g., PatientsLikeMe, CureTogether) or personal health records (e.g., Google Health or Microsoft's HealthVault).

4. Health Plans and employer-sponsored health care reimbursement have moved toward a consumer-driven model that encourages the use of High Deductible Health Plans or HDHPs. These plans generally have optional health accounts for noncovered health expenses that participants have the option to participate in. While many of these plans are still considered part of the managed care model, health care managers need to be aware of the criteria of these health plans from the standpoint of the limitations and extent of reimbursement coverage for organizations, health providers, and employees.

5. Ethical behavior and standards are vital components of effective high quality health care organizations. Awareness of key ethical principles, common occurrences of specific ethical conflicts and how their organization regulates compliance with ethical standards are vital aspects of the health care manager's professional role. Important ethical principles to understand include: autonomy, privacy, confidentiality, fidelity, veracity, nonmaleficence, beneficence, and justice.

6. Bioethical considerations in clinical and behavioral research impact the success and quality of an organization and are a reflection of the leadership staff. Adherence to human subjects protections standards and ethical behavior in research and organizational activities are required and monitored by Institutional Review Boards (IRBs), and federal agencies such as the Office of Human Research Protections (OHRP), the National Institute of Health (NIH), and U.S. Department of Health & Human Services (HHS).

# DISCUSSION QUESTIONS

1. How has the consumer-driven health movement impacted health care service delivery?

2. What is the impact of Bachman's "five building blocks of healthcare consumerism" for health care managers?

3. How do HIPAA regulations protect the public's privacy in regards to electronic medical records (EMRs), personal health records (PHRs), and health information used in social health networking groups (e.g., PatientsLikeMe)?

4. How have Consumer-Driven Health Plans (CDHPs) and High Deductible Health Plans (HDHPs) changed health care service reimbursement and health insurance expectations?

5. What is the difference between Health Savings Accounts (HSAs), Medical Savings Accounts (MSAs), Flexible Spending Arrangements (FSAs), and Health Reimbursement Arrangements (HRAs)?

6. What is retail medicine, and should it be of concern to health care managers and leaders in for-profit and not-for-profit environments?

7. Why has retail medicine become popular with consumers? How can health care managers and organizations leverage retail medicine concepts to enhance current service delivery practices in non-retail environments?

8. How do Electronic Medical Records (EMRs) and Personal Health Records (PHRs) differ? How are they similar?

9. Consider Google (Google Health) and Microsoft's (HealthVault) impact on the consumer-driven health movement and the public's need to participate in their own health care. What are the pros and cons of this type of consumer health application? What barriers to expansion of this concept do you foresee in the near future?

10. How can consumers become more involved in their own health care? What products and resources are available for people who wish to take control of their health or monitor chronic disease states from home?

11. Name five key ethical principles that impact the health care environment. What examples of each are commonly seen in health care and why?

12. How do nonmaleficence and beneficence differ, and why are they important in health care?

13. Why do IRBs exist, and how do they impact biomedical, behavioral, and clinical research activities?

14. Do all health care organizations and providers need to comply with the Patient's Bill of Rights? Why or why not?

15. Should health care providers always tell the truth to their patients, even if the truth may cause pain or distress?

# CASE: Consumer-Driven Changes for the ABC Health Options Clinic

Robert has been made the new director of the ABC Health Care Options Clinic in Phoenix, Arizona. The clinic is a large, freestanding, multi-specialty clinic providing general and specialty health services to the southeastern Phoenix area. It has been in existence since 1963, with 53 physicians and 10 multi-physician groups. The Internal Medicine (IMP), Family Practice (FMP) and OB-GYN (OGP) groups are the largest and have a history of exerting the most control in the clinic's affairs.

Before he took early retirement, the previous director began a plan to make the clinic more "consumer-friendly," incorporating new additions such as mandatory electronic medical records based on a tethered system, Saturday office hours, and two freestanding satellite minor emergency and primary care clinics in southeastern Phoenix to assist with the uninsured and underinsured population groups. In the last meeting, the chiefs of staff for each of the three primary physician groups expressed their opinions regarding some of the new changes, particularly the satellite clinics for the uninsured and under-insured populations. Dr. Smee, chief of staff for IMP, was concerned that this would bring in "an unfavorable sort into our clinic," decrease their fiscal solvency, and increase the liability. Whereas Dr. Loo, chief of staff for FMP, felt that this was a good way that the clinic can impact the issue of lack of access to care and would increase their ability to provide quality health care to all, but was wary of how the clinics would be staffed particularly over the weekends.

Dr. Rodriguez, an endocrinologist specializing in diabetes care, stated concern about the tethered electronic medical record system, which is proposed to be linked with Google Health and HealthVault. Her primary concern was the safety of the information and presumed privacy of health information in personal health records that would be linked to the clinics records. Drs. Blue and Green from rheumatology and orthopedics felt that this push to increase the clinic's public image and consumer appeal is a good strategy, and one which could increase the clinic's ability to remain competitive. Mary Johnson, the lead nurse practitioner from the family practice group, felt that the move toward a more consumer-friendly system and increasing access to care for all was a good move and stated that she and six other NPs were willing to staff the satellite clinics on Saturdays on a rotating basis.

For the last two weeks, Robert has been reviewing all the meeting notes and interviewing representatives from the physicians in each clinic. While the majority of the physicians and groups were in favor of the changes, the Internal Medicine group (IMP) was opposed to the changes and felt threatened by any new change to their accustomed routines.

Robert has called an all-clinic meeting on Friday to discuss these changes and how they will impact the routine of the clinic or if they should be done at all. As he ponders his situation, he has to decide what the best choices are.

## Questions

1. What are the key problems?

2. How will these consumer-driven changes affect the clinic overall? Per physician group?

3. Are the tethered medical records a good idea?

4. What ethical concerns have been expressed by the physicians that could impact the success (or failure) of these new changes?

5. Are the satellite clinics such a good idea? What will their impact be on the clinic financially? Will one group bear the majority of the financial obligation and liabilities for this population?

# REFERENCES

Allan, J., & Englebright, J. (2000). Patient-centered documentation: An effective and efficient use of clinical informatin systems. *Journal of Nursing Administration , 30*(2), 90–95.

American Hospital Association. (1992–1998). *AHA—Patient bill of rights. American Hospital Association Mandatory Advisory.* Retrieved January 19, 2010, from http://www.patienttalk.info/AHA-Patient_Bill_of_Rights.htm

American Hospital Association. (2003). *Understanding expectations, rights, and responsibilities.* Retrieved January 19, 2010, from http://www.aha.org/aha/content/2003/pdf/pcp_english_030730.pdf

Anonymous. (2008). Microsoft offers online health records. *Information Management Journal, 42*(1), 19.

Bachman, R. E. (2006). *Healthcare consumerism: The basis of a 21st century intelligent health system.* Retrieved November 30, 2009, from http://www.healthtransformation.net/galleries/wp-consumerism/Healthcare%20Consumerism%20-%20 The%20Basis%20of%20a%2021st%20Century%20Intelligent%20Health%20System.pdf

Bandman, E., & Bandman, B. (2002). *Nursing ethics through the lifespan* (4th ed.). Upper Saddle River, NJ: Prentice Hall Pearson Education, Inc.

Barnett, H. (2007). Complementary and alternative medicine and patient choice in primary care. *Quality in Primary Care, 15,* 207–212.

Beauchamp, T. L., & Childress, J. F. (2009). *Principles of biomedical ethics* (6th ed.). Oxford: Oxford University Press.

Bernstein, R., & Edwards, T. (2008, August 14). *An older and more diverse nation by midcentury.* Retrieved November 22, 2009, from http://www.census.gov/Press-Release/www/releases/archives/population/012496.html

Boyd, D. M., & Ellison, N. B. (2007). Social network sites: Definition, history, and scholarship. *Journal of Compuer-Mediated Communication, 13*(1), article 11.

Brinkmann, J. (2004). Looking at consumer behavior in a moral perspective. *Journal of Business Ethics, 51*(2), 129–141.

Busch, S. H., Barry, C. L., Vegso, S. J., Sindelar, J. L., & Cullen, M. R. (2006). Effects of a cost-sharing exemption on use of preventive services at one large employer. *Health Affairs, 25*(6), 1529–1536.

Cahin, V., & Lancashire, J. (2008, March 27). *Older Americans 2008: Key indicators of well-being, press notes.* Retrieved November 12, 2009, from http://www.agingstats.gov/agingstatsdotnet/main_site/default.aspx

Christianson, J. B., Ginsburg, P. B., & Draper, D. A. (2008). The transition from managed care to consumerism: A community-level status report. *Health Affairs, 27*(5), 1362–1370.

Cohen, R. A., & Stussman, B. (2010, February). Health information technology use among men and women aged 18-64: Early release of estimates from the National Health Interview Survey, January–June 2009. Retrieved February 2, 2010, from http://www.cdc.gov/nchs/data/hestat/healthinfo2009/healthinfo2009.htm

Collaborative Institutional Training Initiative (CITI). (n.d.). About the Collaborative Institutional Training Initiative. Retrieved January 19, 2010, from http://www.citiprogram.org/aboutus.asp?language=english

Convenient Care Association. (2008). About CCA. Retrieved August 6, 2010, from http://www.ccaclinics.org/

Costello, D. (2008). A checkup for retail medicine. *Health Affairs, 27*(5), 1299–1303.

Cushman, R. (n.d.). *Primer: Data protection and the personal health record.* Retrieved January 19, 2010, from http://www.projecthealthdesign.org/media/file/primerdata_protection.pdf

Department of the Treasury, Internal Revenue Service. (2008, November 25). *Health savings accounts and other tax-favored health plans.* Retrieved December 30, 2009, from http://www.irs.gov/pub/irs-pdf/p969.pdf

Dissent. (2008, April 2). UCLA staffer looked through Farrah Fawcett's medical records. Retrieved May 31, 2010, from: http://www.phiprivacy.net/?p=189

Dixon, A. (2007). Personal responsibility for health and healthcare. *Consumer Policy Review, 17*(6), 256–260.

Domaszewicz, A. S. (2007). Personal responsibility in health benefits: Looking backward, looking forward. *Benefits Quarterly, 23*(2), 18–24.

Dutta-Bergman, M. J. (2003). Developing a profile of consumer intention to seek out health information beyond the doctor. *Health Marketing Quarterly, 21*(1/2), 91–112.

Dutta-Bergman, M. J. (2004). The readership of health magazines: The role of health orientation. *Health Marketing Quarterly, 22*(2), 27–49.

Federal Interagency Forum on Aging-Related Statistics. (2008, March). *Older Americans 2008: Key indicators of well-being.* Retrieved November 22, 2009, from http://www.agingstats.gov/agingstatsdotnet/Main_Site/Data/2008_Documents/OA_2008.pdf

French, J., Blair-Stevens, C., McVey, D., & Merritt, R. (2010). *Social marketing and public health: Theory and practice.* Oxford: Oxford University Press.

Fronstin, P. (2009). *Findings from the 2009 EBRI/MGA consumer engagement in health care survey.* EBRI Education and Research Fund. Employee Benefit Research Institute (EBRI).

Froomkin, A. M. (2008). *The new health information architecture: Coping with privacy implications of the personal health records revolution.* Retrieved January 19, 2010, from http://www.projecthealthdesign.org/media/file/social-life-info-15.pdf

Galvin, R. S. (2007). Consumerism and controversy: A conversation With Regina Herzlinger. *Health Affairs, 26*(5), w552–w559.

Gardner, A. (2010). *Patient's bill of rights too tough to read.* Retrieved January 19, 2010, from http://www.healthfinder.gov/news/newsstory.aspx?docID=624592

Goodman, J. C. (2006, March 29). *Transparency in health care.* Retrieved December 30, 2009, from http://www.ncpa.org/pub/ba548

Grossman, J. M., Zayas-Cahan, T., & Kemper, N. (2009). Information gap: Can health insurer personal health records meet patient's and physician's needs? *Health Affairs, 28*(2), 377–389.

Hamric, A. B., Spross, J. A., & Hanson, C. M. (2009). *Advanced nursing practice* (4th ed.). St. Louis, MO: Saunders Elsevier.

Havlin, L. J., McAllister, M. F., & Slavney, D. H. (2003, September). How to inject consumerism into your existing health plans. *Employee Benefits Journal,* 7–14.

Healthy People 2010. (n.d.). *What are the leading health indicators?* Retrieved January 19, 2010, from http://www.healthypeople.gov/LHI/lhiwhat.htm

Herzlinger, R. (2004). Consumer-driven health care: Taming the health care cost monster. *Journal of Financial Service Professionals, 58*(2), 44–48.

HHS.gov. (n.d.). *Value-driven health care home.* Retrieved December 30, 2009, from http://www.hhs.gov/valuedriven/

Hilgers, D. W. (2005). The rise of retail medicine: Adding new complexity to the practice of health care law. *National CLE conference.* Snowmass: Law Education Institute.

*HIPAA White Papers and Glossary.* (2009). Retrieved December 31, 2009, from ohio.gov: http://hipaa.ohio.gov/glossary.htm

Hofmann, P. B. (2001). Serving and competing ethically. In P. B. Hofmann, *Managing ethically: An executive's guide* (pp. 159–160). Chicago: Health Administration Press.

Hofmann, P. B., & Nelson, W. A. (2001). *Managing ethically: An executive's guide.* Chicago: Health Administration Press.

Kolar, R. (2008). A consumer revolution in retail medicine: Where is it heading? *HFM (Healthcare Financial Management), 62*(6), 46–48.

Kotabe, M., & Helsen, K. (2008). *Global marketing management* (4th Ed.). Hoboken, NJ: John Wiley & Sons, Inc.

Labig, C. E. (2009). Bad measures don't make good medicine: The ethical implications of unreliable and invalid physician performance measures. *Journal of Business Ethics, 88*, 287–295.

LaGesse, D. (2009). Moving your health records to the Web. *U.S. News and World Report, 146*(2), 75.

Laing, A., & Hogg, G. (2002). Political exhortation, patient expectation and professional execution: Perspectives on the consumerism of health care. *British Journal of Management, 13*(2), 173–189.

Longo, D. R., & Everett, K. D. (2003). Health care consumer reports: An evaluation of consumer perspectives. *Journal of Health Care Finance, 30*(1), 65–71.

Lutz, M. A. (2008). The "Dismal Science"—Still? Economics and human flourishing. *Review of Political Economy, 20*(2), 163–180.

Maryland Department of Mental Health and Hygiene. (2007, June 13). *What is HIPAA?* Retrieved December 30, 2009, from http://www.dhmh.state.md.us/hipaa/whatishipaa.html

McBride, M. (2008). Google Health: Birth of a giant. *Health Information Technology, 29*(5), 8–9.

MD Anderson Cancer Center, University of Texas. (2009). *About complementary/integrative medicine.* Retrieved December 29, 2009, from http://www.mdanderson.org/education-and-research/resources-for-professionals/clinical-tools-and-resources/cimer/about-complementary-integrative-medicine/index.html

Medline Plus. (2009, December 30). *Complementary and alternative medicine.* Retrieved December 31, 2009, from http://www.nlm.nih.gov/medlineplus/complementaryandalternativemedicine.html

The MITRE Corporation. (2006, April). *Electronic health records overview.* Retrieved January 19, 2010, from http://www.ncrr.nih.gov/publications/informatics/EHR.pdf

Myers, J., Frieden, T. R., Bherwani, K.M., & Henning, K. J. (2008). Ethics in public health research: Privacy and public health at risk: Public health confidentiality in the digital age. *American Journal of Public Health, 98*(5), 793–801.

Nair, K. V., & Valuck, R. J. (2004). Consumer Responses to a Pharmacy Benefit Report Card. *Jorunal of Health Care Finance, 31*(1), 55–72.

Nash, D. B., Jacoby, R., & Murtha, M. (2008, July 14). *Retail medicine and the quality of care.* Retrieved December 31, 2009, from http://www.medpagetoday.com/Columns/10113

National Institutes of Health. (n.d.). *Bioethics.* Retrieved January 19, 2010, from http://www.bioethics.nih.gov/home/index.shtml

Neupert, P., & Mundie, C. (2009). Personal health management systems: Applying the full power of software to improve the quality and efficiency of care. *Health Affairs, 28*(2), 390–392.

Office of Human Research Protections (OHRP). (2005, September). *Office of human research protections, fact sheet.* Retrieved January 19, 2010, from Office of Human Research Protections, U.S. Department of Health & Human Services: http://www.hhs.gov/ohrp/about/ohrpfactsheet.htm

Office of Human Research Protections (OHRP). (2008, November 13). *The Belmont report.* Retrieved January 19, 2010, from http://www.hhs.gov/ohrp/belmontArchive.html

Office of Human Research Protections (OHRP). (n.d.). *History of human subjects protection system.* Retrieved January 19, 2010, from http://www.hhs.gov/ohrp/irb/irb_introduction.htm

Office of Human Research Protections (OHRP). (n.d.). *Jurisdiction of the Institutional Review Board. In the Institutional Review Board guidebook.* Retrieved January 19, 2010, from http://www.hhs.gov/ohrp/irb/irb_chapter1.htm

Ostergen, K. (2006). The Institutional construction of consumerism: A study of implementing quality indicators. *Financial Accountability & Management, 22*(2), 179–205.

Oxford English Dictionary. (1989a). *Autonomy.* Retrieved January 19, 2010, from http://www.oed.com/cgi/entry/50015226?single=1&query_type=word&queryword=autonomy&first=1&max_to_show=10

Oxford English Dictionary. (1989b). *Beneficence*. Retrieved January 19, 2010, from http://www.oed.com/cgi/entry/50020270?single=1&query_type=word&queryword=beneficence&first=1&max_to_show=10

Oxford English Dictionary. (1989c). *Bioethics*. Retrieved January 19, 2010, from http://www.oed.com/cgi/entry/50022316?single=1&query_type=word&queryword=bioethics&first=1&max_to_show=10

Oxford English Dictionary. (1989d). *Confidential*. Retrieved January 19, 2010, from http://www.oed.com/cgi/entry/50046956?single=1&query_type=word&queryword=confidentiality&first=1&max_to_show=10

Oxford English Dictionary. (1989e). *Fidelity*. Retrieved January 19, 2010, from http://www.oed.com/cgi/entry/50084378?single=1&query_type=word&queryword=fidelity&first=1&max_to_show=10

Oxford English Dictionary. (1989f). *Hippocratic oath*. Retrieved January 19, 2010, from http://dictionary.oed.com/cgi/entry/50106410/single=1&query_type=word&queryword=hippocratic&firts=1&max_to_show=10

Oxford English Dictionary. (1989g). *Justice*. Retrieved January 19, 2010, from http/www.oed.com/cgi/entry/50124865/query_type=word7queryword=justice&first=1&max_to_show=10&sort_type=alpha&result_place=1&research_id=eUe9-9fXtzj-8471&hilite=50124865

Oxford English Dictionary. (1989h). *Oxford English Dictionary Online* (2nd ed.). Oxford, UK: Oxford University Press.

Oxford English Dictionary. (1989i). *Privacy*. Retrieved January 19, 2010, from http://www.oed.com/cgi/entry/50188914/signle=1&query_type=word&queryword=privacy&first=1&max_to_show=10

Oxford English Dictionary. (1989j). *Veracity*. Retrieved January 19, 2010, from http://www.oed.com/cgi/entry/50276176?single=1&query_type=word&queryword=veracity&first=1&max_to_show=10

Patterson, M. P. (2004). Defined contribution health plan to consumer driven health benefits: Evolution and experience. *Benefits Quarterly, 20*(2), 49–59.

Paul, I. R. (2008). *Part III—Administartive, procedural, and miscellaneous: Health savings accounts*. Retrieved December 29, 2009, from http://www.treas.gov/press/releases/reports/notice200859.pdf

Potter, J. (1988). Consumerism and the public sector: How well does the coat fit? *Public Administration, 66*(2), 149–164.

Ransom, E. R., Joshi, M. S., Nash, D. B., & Ransom, S. B. (Eds.). (2008). *The healthcare quality book. Vision, strategy, and tools* (2nd ed.). Chicago: Health Administration Press

Robert Wood Johnson Foundation. (2008). *Health information technology in the United States. Where we stand 2008*. Retrieved January 19, 2010, from http://www.rwjf.org/files/research/062508.hit.exsummary.pdf

Robert Wood Johnson Foundation. (2008, June). *Health information technology in the United States*. Retrieved January 19, 2010, from http://www.rwjf.org/pr/product.jsp?id=31831

Robert Wood Johnson Foundation. (2009, June 17). *Round one final report*. In Project HealthDesign: Rethinking the power and potential of personal health records. Retrieved February 2, 2010, from http/www.projecthealthdesign.org/media/file/Round%20One%20PHD%20Final%20Report6.17.09.pdf

Robert Wood Johnson Foundation. (2010). *Feature: The power and potential of personal health records*. Retrieved January 19, 2010, from http://www.rwjf.org/pioneer/product.jsp?id=49988

Robinson, J. C., & Ginsburg, P. B. (2009). Consumer-driven health care: Promise and performance. *Health Affairs, 28*(2), w272–281.

Robinson, J. C., Casakino, L. P., Gillies, R. R., Rittenhouse, D. R., Shortell, S. S., & Fernandes-Taylor, S. (2009). Financial incentives, quality improvement programs, and the adoption of clinical information technology. *Medical Care, 47*(4), 411–417.

Robinson, J. (2005). Managed consumerism in health care. *Health Affairs, 24*(6), 1478–1489.

Saba, V. K., & McCormick, K. A. (2006). *Essentials of nursing informatics* (4th ed.). McGraw-Hill Professional.

Saleem, H. T. (2003, December 19). *Health spending accounts.* Retrieved December 30, 2009, from http://www.bls.gov/opub/cwc/cm20031022ar01p1.htm

Saussy, P. F. (2004). Health care costs: Back to the fundamentals. *Journal of Financial Service Porfessionals, 58*(3), 35–37.

Saver, C. (2006). Nursing—today and beyond. *American Nurse Today, 1*(1), 18–25.

Shmuel, J. (2009, January 1). Microsoft, Telus launch e-health software. *Telegraph-Journal,* B1.

Silverman, S. M. (2009, May 11). Farrah Fawcett breaks her silence. *People* magazine; Time, Inc. Retrieved May 31, 2010 from http://www.people.com/people/article/0,,20278026,00.html

Stewart, D. (2009). Socialized medicine: How personal health records and social networks are changing healthcare. *EContent, 32*(7), 30–35.

Tai-Seale, M. (2004). Voting with their feet: Patient exit and intergroup differences in prosperity for switching usual source of care. *Journal of Health Politics, Policy & Law, 29*(3), 491–514.

Thomas, R. K. (2005). *Marketing health services.* Chicago: Health Administration Press.

Thompson, C. J. (2006). Benefits, consumerism and an "ownership society." *Benefits Quarterly, 22*(2), 7–14.

Thompson, M., & Checkley, J. (2006, Second Quarter). Employer-driven consumerism: Integrating health into the business model. *Benefits Quarterly, 22*(2).

Total Administrative Services Corporation (TASC). (2008a). *What is a health reimbursement arrangement (HRA)?* Retrieved December 30, 2009, from http://www.tasconline.com/businessresourcecenter/hra.html

Total Administrative Services Corporation (TASC). (2008b). *What is a health savings account?* Retrieved December 30, 2009, from http://www.tasconline.com/businessresourcecenter/hsa/index.html

Treasury, U.S. (2004, March 30). *Treasury issues additional guidance on health savings accounts (HSAS).* Retrieved December 29, 2009, from http://www.treas.gov/press/releases/js1278.htm

Treasury, U.S. (2008, November 19). *HSA frequently asked questions: The basics of HSAs.* Retrieved December 29, 2009, from http://www.ustreas.gov/offices/public-affairs/hsa/faq_basics.shtml

UCLA Media Relations. (2008, April 2). UCLA health system statement on report about Farrah Fawcett's medical records. UC Regents. Retrieved May 31, 2010, from http://newsroom.ucla.edu/portal/ucla/fawcett-48120.aspx?id=

U.S. Department of Health & Human Services. (2009, December). *Health information privacy: HIPAA administrative simplification statute and rules.* Retrieved December 31, 2009, from http://www.hhs.gov/ocr/privacy/hipaa/administrative/index.html

U.S. Department of Health and Human Services. (n.d.). *Patient Safety and Quality Improvement Act of 2005 statute and rule.* Retrieved December 30, 2009, from http://www.hhs.gov/ocr/privacy/psa/regulation/index.html

U.S. Department of Health and Human Services. (n.d.). *Summary of the HIPAA privacy rule.* Retrieved December 20, 2009, from http://www.hhs.gov/ocr/privacy/hipaa/understanding/summary/index.html

Wolsko, P., Ware, L., Kutner, J., Lin, C-T., Albertson, G., Cyran, L., Schilling, L., & Anderson, R. J. (2000). Alternative/complementary medicine: Wider usage than generally appreciated. *The Journal of Alternative and Complementary Medicine, 6*(4), 321–326.

# Chapter 15

# Globalization and Health: The World Is Flattening

Jon Chilingerian, Eilish McAuliffe, and John R. Kimberly

## CHAPTER OUTLINE

- **Introduction**
- **How Flat Is the World of Health Care?**
- **The Flow of Patients across International Borders**
- **The Flow of Health Workers across Borders**
- **The Flow of Policy Instruments and Management Practices across Borders**
- **Additional Considerations**

## LEARNING OBJECTIVES

After completing this chapter, the reader should be able to:

1.  Explain how this increasing interconnectedness is playing out in the world of health and health care
2.  Understand how flows across national borders have changed
3.  Define medical tourism
4.  Describe the evolution and effect of patient flows on comparative advantage
5.  Describe the effect of health worker mobility on health systems
6.  Describe the flow of policy instruments and managerial practices across borders
7.  Appreciate the managerial and policy implications of health care globalization

# KEY TERMS

Antiretroviral Therapy (ART)

Brain Drain

Comparative Advantage

Diagnosis-Related Groups (DRGs)

General Agreement on Trade in Services (GATS)

Gini Index

Global Health Workforce Alliance (GHWA)

Globalization

Infant Mortality Rates

Joint Commission International (JCI)

Kohl and Dekker Cases

Managed Migration

Medical Tourism

Medical Innovation

Migrant Remittances

Millennium Development Goals (MDGs)

Model for End Stage Liver Disease (MELD)

Network of Organ Sharing (UNOS)

Not-Invented-Here Syndrome (NIHS)

Patient Classification System

Prospective Payment

Retrospective Reimbursement

Reverse Innovation

---

**IN PRACTICE:  A Country Case Study on the Partnership between Abu Dhabi and the Cleveland Clinic in the United States***

Abu Dhabi is the capital of the United Arab Emirates, a federation of seven Emirates. A modern city set on the Arabian Gulf, it is hydrocarbon-based—with 9 percent of the world's oil reserves and 5 percent of the world's natural gas. With a population of 1.5 million, of which 400,000 are nationals, the majority of the other 120 nationalities are expatriates, and 98 percent are younger than 65. All UAE nationals have a government-funded, mandatory health insurance provided by a public or private option. In the Emirates, 25 percent of the population suffers from diabetes, and 85 percent of breast cancer cases are diagnosed late. The leading causes of death are cardiovascular disease (20 percent) and motor vehicle accidents (16 percent). A large number of the population has been diagnosed with eye disease, musculoskeletal disease, cancer, hypertension, and obesity. Although 19 of the 33 hospitals in the UAE are located in Abu Dhabi, by 2025 demand for beds will increase 180 percent. Many of the acute-care services are oversubscribed; historically cardiology, oncology, psychiatry, urology, cardiac surgery, neurosurgery, orthopedic surgery, and thoracic surgery have had long waits. Consequently, many Emiratis travel overseas to obtain access to world-class health care; each year the government spends 25 percent of their health budget sending patients to other countries to obtain medical care. To stem the flow of patients abroad, one of the government's global targets is to create health care services that meet and exceed international standards.

One of the catalysts for change in Abu Dhabi is Mubadala Development Company PJSC. Established and owned by the government, the company's strategy is built on the management of long-term, capital-intensive investments that deliver strong financial returns and tangible social benefits for the Emirates. They partner with "best-of breed" international organizations, attracting world-class experts to help diversify the economy in several business units such as aerospace,

---

* Note: Information for this case study was based on 2008 and 2010 interviews with Mr. Mark Erhart, executive director of Mubadala's health care unit, and 2009 interviews with Ziad Fares, formerly with Mubadala. The information was also sourced on December 22, 2009, from the Cleveland Clinic's Web site, Cleveland Clinic Abu Dhabi Night, retrieved from http://my.clevelandclinic.org/departments/abudhabi/video.aspx

---

**IN PRACTICE:** **A Country Case Study on the Partnership between Abu Dhabi and the Cleveland Clinic in the United States** *(Continued)*

---

infrastructure, real estate and hospitality, and health care. (A full list is available at http://www.mubadala.ae). Mubadala Healthcare, under executive director Mark Erhart, has formed alliances with leading international health care organizations, including Cleveland Clinic and Johns Hopkins Medicine International of the United States and Imperial College London. In 2012, construction will be completed on Cleveland Clinic Abu Dhabi (CCAD), a state-of-the-art 364-bed multispecialty hospital.

Under the executive leadership of Dr. Andrew Fishleder, CCAD will attempt to replicate the culture and best practices of the Cleveland Clinic. The organizational model will be Cleveland's physician-led multispecialty approach with a shared vision of achieving "outstanding patient experiences," "superior clinical outcomes," and "improved quality of life for the people." The hospital in Abu Dhabi will be a spectacular state-of-art facility. The patient rooms will not be cold and sterile; the rooms will be beautiful, with comfortable modern couches for family and guests. The majority of patients (70 percent) will come from Abu Dhabi, 20 percent from the other Emirates, and 10 percent from the surrounding countries—Saudi Arabia, Kuwait, Oman, Bahrain, and Qatar. Given the population, 55 percent will be UAE national citizens and 45 percent will be expatriates and medical tourists.

The CCAD hospital will be highly focused, with service lines: divided into five institutes and six departments. The concept of an Institute was pioneered by Cleveland Clinic and can be best illustrated by the Heart and Vascular institute. To break down the usual silos, cardiology, vascular medicine, and vascular surgery, cardiac surgery will be physically located and formally arranged in one unit. The five institutes will be: (1) Digestive Disease (colorectal and gastroenterology), (2) Heart and Vascular, (3) Neurosciences (neuroscience and neurosurgery), (4) Ophthalmology, and (5) Respiratory and Critical Care. The six departments will be: Anesthesiology, Laboratory Medicine/Pathology, Radiology, Emergency Medicine, Medical Subspecialties, and Surgical Subspecialties.

Patient care will be managed by salaried, Western-trained, U.S. board-certified or equivalent specialists assisted by physicians without admission or operating theatre privileges. They plan to have well-integrated IT platforms and electronic medical records (EMR) aligned with state of the art clinical support services and a delivery system built on a patient-centered model. Physicians and other employees will receive six months of training on process flows, order entry, and EMR. All employees will get annual employee reviews and strong support for training and development including utilization of a state of the art simulation center. Cleveland Clinic's goal is to bring world-class medical care to the people of the world wherever possible.

# CHAPTER PURPOSE

The chapter will introduce the idea that the world of health care is globalizing (or becoming flatter), but that we are really only at the beginning stages of this process, a process that is likely to accelerate with the passage of time. In this chapter, we will present three case illustrations of how flows of various kinds across national borders are changing the landscape of health care. This first case will explore the variables that can affect the number of patients traveling out of their local region or country to obtain health care services somewhere else. In the second case illustration, we explore the extent of this misdistribution of health professionals, the financial implications, and its impact on middle- and low-income health systems. The third case in the chapter examines the spread of patient classification systems in general, and DRG-based systems in particular, from the United States, where the first model was developed and implemented to a number of countries around the globe. The chapter will conclude with a discussion of the managerial implications of globalization for health care organizations.

# INTRODUCTION

We live in a time in which we are increasingly aware of what is going on in other parts of the world. CNN brings us live reports from the conflicts in Iraq and Afghanistan; the labels in our clothing tell us they were made in China or Honduras or Malaysia; the fruit we eat in winter we discover was grown in Chile; we receive e-mails instantly from colleagues in Australia or Israel; Facebook connects us with "friends" in Russia or in Japan as quickly as those next door. So we are more aware than ever before of both the existence and the significance of the world outside our own borders, and of the importance of understanding both the scope and the implications of interconnectedness.

Our purpose in this chapter is to examine how this increasing interconnectedness is playing out in the world of health and health care. In so doing, we have to make some choices about what to include and what to leave out, so let us be clear about what this chapter will not cover. It will not examine the epidemiological structure of disease around the world. Prevalence of various diseases varies from one region or locale to another, but this is not our focus. The chapter will not cover the etiology of disease around the globe, although this is certainly interesting and important. Last, it will not provide a descriptive status report of health and illness around the globe, although this, too, is interesting and important. Rather, it will explore the way in which many aspects of health and health care are globalizing—that is, how things are changing in health care as the potential for global interconnectedness expands.

# HOW FLAT IS THE WORLD OF HEALTH CARE?

"The world is flat," pronounced Thomas Friedman in his best-selling book published in 2005. By this he meant that a variety of forces were leveling the playing field of commerce around the globe and that, as a consequence, significant economic opportunities were opening up for countries such as China and India, countries that, by and large, had previously been inwardly focused.

These forces, the so-called "flatteners" he identified, were the collapse of the Berlin Wall, which allowed people and firms on both sides of the wall to become part of the economic mainstream; the broadening of access to the Internet and the proliferation of digitization; the emergence of software protocols that permitted the design and publication of documents that could be both sent and read anywhere; the advent of collaboration on online projects; the proliferation of outsourcing; the transfer of manufacturing and other business processes "offshore," that is to another country where cost economies could be realized; the streamlining of supply chains that was enabled by new technologies of both an information and logistical nature; the development of what he called "insourcing," whereby Company A's employees perform a variety of services for Company B, above and beyond the principal one; the explosion of information availability enabled by the development of powerful search engines such as Google; and the commercialization of a variety of personal digital devices that enable access to this information anytime and in any place. Friedman argued that together, these forces have reinforced one another and have transformed the world of commerce by opening up new opportunities on a truly global scale and enabling countries that had previously been relatively isolated from the economic "mainstream" to join in.

Friedman's work has both admirers and critics. Pankaj Ghemawat (2007), for example, argues that while the forces that he discusses are certainly present, Friedman exaggerates their importance, as much of the world of commerce involves transactions that are essentially local. Alan Rugman and Chang Oh make a similar argument in their critique of what they call "Friedman's Follies" (Rugman and Oh, 2008).

Whether one agrees with Friedman or thinks he has pushed his basic arguments too far, there is no question that his book has provoked much reflection and debate, and we find it useful to use his metaphor as a springboard for our analysis of globalization in health care. Just how flat is the world of health care?

The fundamental question that must be addressed in examining globalization in any domain, including health care, is how flows of various kinds—both legal and illegal—across national borders have changed. A hallmark of increasing **globalization** is the increasing openness of national borders to flows of goods and services, financial and human capital, information, and expertise. In the domain of health care, we would point specifically to flows of investment capital; of patients; of physicians, nurses and other health workers; of medical technology; of pharmaceutical products; of policy tools and initiatives; of a variety of types of information and expertise; and of diseases such as H1N1, HIV/AIDS, etc., across national borders as indicators to use in examining how health care is globalizing. To the extent that these flows are increasingly common and increasingly significant as measured by their frequency and volume, we can conclude that the process of "flattening" is accelerating.

We should be clear that we are not making the case that flattening per se is good and more flattening is better. Certainly, flattening is not an unmitigated blessing. Flows that are welfare-enhancing in some countries have the opposite effect in other countries. Some flows are mutually beneficial, and, as we will argue later, some are of dubious legal and ethical value.

As of the year 2010, our view is that the world of health care is globalizing (or becoming flatter), but that we are really at the very early stages of this process, a process that is likely only to accelerate with the passage of time. We illustrate this view with three examples, one looking at patient flows across borders, one examining health worker flows across borders, and a third tracing the flow of policy instruments across borders. In each case, we present evidence that these flows are increasing, which is a testimony to some of the ways in which flattening in health and health care is taking place. We conclude with some examples of cross-border flows that are cause for concern and that illustrate a dark side to globalization.

# THE FLOW OF PATIENTS ACROSS INTERNATIONAL BORDERS

A decade ago, if you were sick, health care service options were perceived as "peculiarly and tenaciously local" (Cortez, 2008); today, people are increasingly willing to travel to other countries to obtain health care services (Chilingerian and Savage, 2005; Cortez 2008; Schroth and Khawaja 2007). Nowadays, individuals who require advanced surgical procedures are able to go on the Internet, search by country or medical specialty, and find an international smorgasbord of "best care" accredited hospitals and world-class physicians. In addition to sophisticated medical services at international destinations, medical travelers may also find door-to-door concierge services, patient ambassadors, and five-star hotel services as well as big cost savings. In this section, we examine the flow of patients around the globe—a trend that has been called **medical tourism**.

Medical tourism is about seeking value in any or all of the following ways: more comprehensive care, more advanced care, more specialized care, less costly care, improved quality,

and better access and patient experiences. Porter (1987) argues that "the global competitor can locate activities wherever comparative advantage lies, decoupling comparative advantage from the firm's home base or country of ownership." **Comparative advantage**, when applied to health care, refers to the discovery and deployment of significant differences in a nation's cost, quality, or access such that a medical or surgical procedure, health activity, or service creates patient value. Consequently, a care program for lung cancer or organ transplantation could become a "power offering" to anyone, anywhere in the world.

Travel in search of medical services is not a new phenomenon. The royals, retirees, rich, and famous have done this for generations. What is new, however, is the realization that both low- and high-GDP countries that have efficient, high-quality, technologically advanced health care organizations can attract medical tourists and achieve comparative advantage. Conversely, both low- and high-GDP countries also have inefficient, low-quality, technologically weak health care organizations with long waits or poor service attitudes, and these countries will therefore lose some of their patients to other countries.

To illustrate the "big cost savings," one study found that the average weighted price of a procedure in the United States was $10,629, versus $1,410 for other accredited international destinations (Keckley and Underwood 2008). One 53-year-old American traveled to India to replace both hips and one knee for a total out-of-pocket cost of less than $30,000 (Comarow 2008). This price included all hospital charges, physician fees, ancillary services, airfare, visas, and other miscellaneous expenses—easily a price that is substantially below what he would have paid out of pocket in the United States.

When one marketing director for an American business coalition heard about American patients going abroad, he organized a due diligence mission, investigating both quality and prices from U.S. facilities and abroad. His leadership team reached a dramatic conclusion:

> We came to believe that quality of care in facilities credentialed by the Joint Commission International (JCI) in foreign countries, and in India in particular, is as good as or better than that in the United States, and offers a 70–80 percent cost differential in many cases. (Douglas, 2007)

Some third-party payors in the United States have reached similar conclusions. For example, Blue Cross and Blue Shield of Wisconsin, Florida, California, and South Carolina have pilot programs to send patients to India, Mexico, and Thailand (Keckley and Underwood 2009). The globalization of health care means that if hospitals or physicians refuse to negotiate their prices with patients, insurance companies, and sick funds, their patients might cross borders.

## Size of the Global Market: Inbound and Outbound Patient Flows

A literature review reveals that there are neither definitive studies nor very accurate estimates of the size of the global market for medical travelers. The data on medical travelers often comes from tourism boards, newspaper accounts, and government estimates of hospital claims, social media, stakeholder media, or hospital Web sites. Estimates often include expatriates obtaining acute and primary care in their current locations, outpatient visits, visitor emergency cases, and tourists obtaining alternative medical care such as acupuncture.

A study by Ehrbeck, Guevara, and Mango (2008), which excluded expatriates, emergencies, traumas, cosmetic surgeries, and outpatient visits, estimated the size of the global acute market to be between 60,000 and 85,000 people. Although the market is much smaller than previously reported, the study predicts it will grow into a multibillion-dollar global industry. That study found five reasons for medical travel to an international destination for acute care: (1) better quality (40 percent); (2) the most advanced technology (32 percent); (3) quick access (15 percent); (4) lower costs for medically necessary procedures (9 percent); and (5) lower costs for discretionary procedures (4 percent).

What becomes clear is that 87 percent of acute medical travelers want good quality and fast service rather than low costs. An obvious conclusion is that a key factor for global competition is a provider's clinical reputation, defined in terms of (1) outcomes; (2) technological backup; and (3) use of the most advanced medical procedures.

## The Growing Rivalry for Inbound International Patients

Although these temporal changes in patient flows have not received much attention because they have been difficult to track, global rivalry for patients appears to be heating up. Since 1998, nearly 150 international hospitals have been accredited by the **Joint Commission International (JCI)** (Timmons, 2009). Countries like Abu Dhabi, Belgium, Costa Rica,

Cuba, India, Israel, Mexico, Poland, Singapore, South Korea, Taiwan, Thailand, and Malaysia are becoming major players (Al-Hammouri, 2009; Benveniste, 2008; Fleni, 2008; Heyman, 2008; Keckley and Underwood 2009). Not unlike the Olympics, the health care playing field is leveling, allowing both high- and low-GDP countries to compete for each other's patients.

Many Asian countries report a large number of medical tourists. In 2006, Malaysia claimed to have more than 300,000 tourists annually, India 450,000, Singapore 410,000, and Thailand 1.2 million (Keckley and Underwood, 2008). Bumrungrad Hospital, in Thailand, claims it treats many if not most of the non-Thai medical tourists, treating more than 400,000 non-Thai medical tourists annually, of whom nearly 40,000 are inbound patients from the United States (Woodman 2008).

The difference between inbound and outbound medical tourism can have a significant effect on economy (Chilingerian and Savage, 2005; Fried and Harris, 2007). In 2007, 750,000 Americans received health care abroad and spent $2.1 billion, whereas the 400,000 international patients who came to the United States spent $5.0 billion (Keckley and Underwood 2009). That sounds like the United States came out ahead. However, an outbound American patient represents a loss in revenue. Conservative estimates of the revenue that would have been generated if the 750,000 patients had received care in the United States were $15.6 billion versus the $5 billion from the inbound patients (Keckley and Underwood 2008).

On the one hand, international inbound patients (flowing to the United States) are projected to grow to only 500,000 by 2017; on the other hand, U.S. outbound patients are projected to be 1.6 million. The projected increase in the number of outbound American medical tourists represents a potential $30.3 billion to $79.5 billion spent overseas for medical care, resulting in a revenue loss of anywhere between $228.5 billion to $599.5 billion for the United States (Keckley and Underwood 2008).

What we learn by observing patient flows around the world is that medical tourism may be a "disruptive innovation" that deserves more clinical and managerial attention (Garman 2008).

## Understanding the Outbound Patient Flows

Table 15.1 helps us to visualize the global flow of acute patients around the world (Ehrbeck, Guevara, and Mango 2008). Patients who travel can come from countries with high per capita GDP

## TABLE 15.1 Global Trade Routes for Acute Care Patients by Point of Origin

| | From Africa | From Asia | From Europe | From Latin America | Middle East | North America | From Oceana |
|---|---|---|---|---|---|---|---|
| To Africa | 0% | 0% | 0% | 0% | 0% | 0% | 0% |
| To Asia | 95% | 93% | 39% | 1% | 32% | 45% | >99% |
| To Europe | 4% | 1% | 10% | 0% | 8% | 0% | 0% |
| To Latin America | 1% | 0% | 5% | 12% | 0% | 26% | <1% |
| To Middle East | 0% | 0% | 13% | 0% | 2% | 7% | 0% |
| To North America | 0% | 6% | 33% | 87% | 58% | 27% | 0% |
| To Oceana | 0% | 0% | 0% | 0% | 0% | 0% | 0% |

SOURCE: Adapted from Ehrbeck, Guevara, and Mango (2008).

or low per capita GDP. Latin American countries (87 percent) and the Middle Eastern countries (58 percent) favor travel to North America. North America favors travel to Latin America (26 percent) and Asia (45 percent). Oceana (99 percent), African (95 percent), and Asian countries (93 percent) favor travel to Asia. Finally, European travelers are divided between North American (33 percent) and Asian countries (39 percent). So a strong health care infrastructure with excess capacity gives some countries a disproportionate share of the patient flow, and consequently a comparative global advantage.

Studies have also found that patients who went to places like India, Singapore, and Thailand were mostly satisfied with the care (Ehrbeck, Guevara, and Mango 2008; Woodman 2008).

There are several factors that may affect a patient's willingness to travel out of their country to seek heath care: clinical reputation of the local and national providers; an individual's ability to afford the total cost of care abroad; and the value to the patient when the perceived sacrifices are considered in relation to the perceived benefits. Medical tourists can be categorized into five groups (Alsagoff 2005; Chilingerian and Savage, 2005).

### Wealthy Patients from High GDP Countries that Lack Comprehensive Health Services

According to Alsagoff (2005), the number of infant deaths per 1,000 live births is highly associated with degree of local health care infrastructure. In general, countries with high per capita GDP have low **infant mortality rates** (Alsagoff, 2005). There are also outlier countries. For example, Qatar, Bahrain, and United Arab Emirates have a higher per capita GDP. All of these countries have fewer than one million indigenous people, but higher infant mortality rates—14 infant deaths per 1,000 live births (Alsagoff, 2005). Although the problems may be more complex, the presence of a rich population and the absence of adequate health care facilities may lead to medical travel. Some countries, like Abu Dhabi, are taking this very seriously. (See the In Practice, "A Country Case Study on the Partnership between Abu Dhabi and the Cleveland Clinic in the United States.")

### Patients from Countries with Large Disparities between Rich and Poor

Using the **Gini Index** to measure income disparities between rich and poor countries (i.e., values > 35), Alsagoff (2005) examined the relation between infant mortality rates and income disparities. This approach identified countries that may have inadequate health care or social services, but mainly targeted countries with large income disparities between rich and poor. He identified Turkmenistan, Jordan, Malaysia, Vietnam, the Philippines, Pakistan, Indonesia, India, China, and other countries that likely have wealthy patients who travel for medical care, since they cannot get technically advanced or comprehensive care within their own country.

### Patients from High GDP Countries with Relatively Expensive Health Care Services

The United States and Japan have excellent and comprehensive health care systems; however, they are very expensive. Apollo Hospitals of India offer very low cost and immediate access for people who want to avoid the lengthy waits that often accompany the higher cost alternatives. Table 15.2 displays the cost advantages of traveling to other countries for health care. An American patient who has no health insurance can fly to India and have a coronary artery bypass graft for 10 percent of the average U.S. price—paying only $7,000 versus $70,000 dollars for the procedure. U.S. medical travelers can also go to Panama and pay $5,500 for a hip replacement versus $33,000 in the United States.

### Patients from Countries with Long Waits

From time to time, patients living in high-GDP countries with government-sponsored national health systems can experience difficulty getting access to all medical services across the continuum of patient care. As health care expenditures keep rising, governments try to limit spending. When services are underfunded, and patient demand exceeds the capacity constraint, the result is overutilization, bottlenecks, and longer wait times for all services.

Lengthy waits can be psychologically and physically damaging to older patients. For example, a study conducted in Scotland of older people needing hip and knee replacements found that patients with urgent cases were waiting as long as 30 months, and nonurgent cases waited as long as 78 months (Roy and Hunter, 1996). These patients experienced great pain, mobility restrictions, an inability to go out or climb stairs, and one-fourth had been forced to retire. A Canadian study of patients waiting for hip and knee replacements found that some patients had been waiting up to three years (36 months) (Williams, Llewellyn Thomas, Arshinoff, Young, and Naylor, 1997). In another study, cataract patients from Canada, Denmark, and Spain were asked if they would be willing to pay out of pocket to shorten their wait times (Anderson, Modrow, and Tan, 1997). Approximately 38 percent of the Canadians, 17 percent of the Danes, and 29 percent of the Spanish were willing to pay $500 for a shorter wait.

In July 2002, the British Medical Association conducted a survey of 2,000 adults in the United Kingdom. These citizens, entitled to free care from the National Health Service (NHS), were asked how far they would be willing to travel if they faced a lengthy wait for health care services. More than 40 percent were willing to travel outside the United Kingdom; 15 percent would travel anywhere in Europe, and 26 percent would travel anywhere in the world (Beecham, 2002).

In 2003, the average wait for inpatient surgery in the national health service programs was more than 200 days (Chilingerian and Savage 2005). One patient from Canada facing a lengthy

### TABLE 15.2  Cost Comparison of Selected Procedures in 2008

| Procedures | United States* | Medicare** | India | Thailand | Singapore | Malaysia | Panama |
|---|---|---|---|---|---|---|---|
| Coronary Artery Bypass Graft | $70–$133 | $18.6–$23.6 | $7.00 | $22.00 | $16.00 | $12.00 | $10.50 |
| Hip Replacement | $33–$57 | $10–$12 | $10.00 | $12.70 | $12.00 | $7.50 | $5.50 |
| Knee Replacement | $30–$53 | $10–$12 | $9.00 | $11.50 | $9.60 | $12.00 | $7.00 |
| Gastric Bypass | $35–$52 | $7.9–$9.8 | $9.30 | $13.00 | $16.50 | $12.70 | $8.50 |
| Prostate surgery (TURP) | $10–$16 | $3–$3.7 | $3.60 | $4.40 | $5.30 | $4.60 | $3.20 |

\* Average hospital charge
\*\* CMS Payment
$= lowest price
SOURCE: Adapted from Woodman (2008) and Comarow (2008).

one-year wait for a hip replacement went to India, was treated immediately, and paid a total of $4,500 for the entire procedure versus an average price of $15,000 or more in Western Europe or the United States (Solomon, 2004). Some people from England, Canada, and other parts of the world are willing to become medical tourists because their perception of value includes such factors as spending less time in pain and the high quality of life that results, in relation to the perceived sacrifice of leaving home and paying out of pocket. Patients dissatisfied with the quality of the health care services offered by their country, but unable to pay any out-of-pocket costs, had to accept the inconveniences rather than fight. In Europe, a 1988 ruling by the European Court of Justice gave citizens of Europe the right to travel abroad to receive health care. The now famous **Kohl and Dekker cases** established that health care resources should be treated as any other part of the European Union economy with regard to the free movement of goods and services. Patients can seek treatment across borders unless the same treatment can be provided more conveniently within their own country. European patients are no longer held hostage by their local providers.

The threat of outbound medical tourists has elicited competitive responses from some countries. In England, the National Health Service (NHS), for example, has responded by setting explicit targets and performance standards with penalties, and also has conducted many experiments to reduce wait times and create competitive pressures. By 2009, significant progress had been achieved, and the average wait time for acute care was 8.6 weeks, and 4.6 weeks for outpatients (Cumming, 2009).

### Patients Seeking Better Outcomes, Highly Focused Care, or Extraordinary Service Experiences

If we measure a global health care organization by geographic distributions of sales (i.e., patient care delivered outside the country), some health care organizations would qualify as more "internationally developed." Although most hospitals that promote international patients have fewer than 10 percent of their patients from foreign countries, there are some interesting exceptions. Bumrungrad Hospital in Bangkok, with five-star hotel services and accreditation from the Joint Commission for International Accreditation, annually treats 400,000 international patients from 154 countries, accounting for 37 percent of its patient revenues (Intel Corporation, 2004). The hospital offers deluxe rooms, VIP and royal suites,

laptop computers, a swimming pool, and a fitness center, and is within walking distance of Bangkok's most prestigious restaurants, shopping, and entertainment venues.

A large number of patient-centered, integrated health care organizations are attracting patients across national borders because they offer high quality and high efficiency. A good example of a focused clinic offering quality and efficiency is the Canadian hernia hospital, Shouldice. The hospital claims that only 56 percent of its patients are Canadian; most of the rest are from nearby, English-speaking United States (42 percent), while the remaining 2 percent come from Europe (Urquhart and O'Dell, 2004). Factors that might attract medical tourists to a hospital specializing in hernias, for instance, include the excellence in outcome and strong clinical reputation; high patient satisfaction; low-cost, one-standardized-care process; and excellent relationships among patients and hospital staff. These factors might be measured by low recurrence and complication rates, patients' satisfaction with and recommendations of the facility, average cost per case, limited delays between diagnosis and treatment, optimal involvement of patients in care process, short wait times once admitted, excellence in food and pleasing décor, and trusting, long-term relationships with other patients and hospital staff.

## Managerial Implications of Patient Flows

When health care organizations depend on patients from abroad, the environment can become more problem-filled. There are unstable incidents and events, alarming trends, and lots of ambiguous information to manage. Geography, global economics, and politics expose health care management to many risks and uncertainties. A few years ago, oncology patients from Oman and cardiology patients from Abu Dhabi traveled to get health care. However, when credible providers came on site to Oman and Abu Dhabi, medical travel dropped more than 50 percent.

In 2000, patients from the Persian Gulf states reportedly spent approximately $27 billion to obtain care abroad (Alsagoff, 2005). In 2001, the United States received 44 percent of all acute patients from Middle Eastern countries. Following the events in New York on September 11, 2001, entry to the United States from the Persian Gulf region became very difficult and time consuming. Subsequently, U.S. hospitals lost between $750 million and $1.25 billion in international patient revenues from just two countries, Saudi

Arabia and the United Arab Emirates (Landers, 2002). In 2002, the United States' share of Middle East patients dropped from 44 percent to 16 percent, and in 2003 and 2004 it dropped further, from 16 percent to only 8 percent. International patients who formerly went to U.S. destinations like the Mayo Clinic or John Hopkins discovered health care in Thailand, Malaysia, and India (Chilingerian and Savage, 2005).

In the past, the incumbent providers developed their name brands by having a strong clinical reputation built over long periods of time (sometimes decades). Today, information is moving much faster thanks to the Internet, social and stakeholder media, and new institutions that bring credibility to a destination. For example, accreditation from the JCI can quickly bring legitimacy to a provider (Ehrback, Guevara, and Mango 2008). New JCI-accredited organizations, such as Health Travel Media, publish information to guide medical tourists, legitimize new brands, and routinize the global flow of patients.

Nevertheless, a decision to go out of the country for care is made by individual patients (and their families) with unmet needs. The flow of patients abroad depends on perceived value of medical travel in relation to the perceived sacrifices. The perception of sacrifice can be driven by local and global events that influence perceptions of air safety, transportation costs, national rivalry for patients, the global economy, national moods, and health policies and politics that influence barriers to entry. Many of these factors are out of the control of hospital managers.

## Managerial Challenges to Outbound Patient Flows

The flow of patients out of their country to obtain an organ transplant raises ethical questions, especially about efficacy and safety. In 2010, 15,000 U.S. patients were on wait lists for a liver transplant out of approximately 105,000 Americans on the **Network of Organ Sharing (UNOS)** transplant registry. Liver candidates are triaged based on a **Model for End Stage Liver Disease (MELD)** scoring system that ranges from a score of 6 for the earliest stages of their liver disease to 40 for the most critically ill. One study estimated that some 400 Americans jump their queue and travel out of the United States to avoid the wait (Schiano and Rhodes, 2010). Often they come back home for follow-up care, which requires expensive immuno-suppressant drugs.

A study carried out by two physicians reported that their patient, HQ, was on the list for one year. During that time his MELD score went from 18 to 21 (see Schiano and Rhodes, 2010). HQ visited the People's Republic of China and received a transplant two weeks after arriving. In China, the organs of executed prisoners are used for transplantation. HQ came back to the United States and checked in to a U.S. hospital for follow-up care. On the one hand, the America Society of Transplantation has a policy that optimal care will be provided to patients, even if they sought their transplant abroad. On the other hand, should the U.S. government take a position against the exploitation of donors and, in particular, the practice of taking organs from executed prisoners or paid living donors?

Medical tourism raises ethical issues and can even involve false advertising or fraud. Some treatments are experimental, offering large risks and only modest benefits. For example, in the United States, some stem cell treatments are available only in clinical trials, and some patients may not be eligible, whereas such stem cell treatments may be available in other countries.

The lesson is that targeting the market for medical travelers has risks. To attract international patients requires substantial investments in buildings, equipment, service processes, and people who can "delight" patients. There is growing rivalry among nations to attract medical tourists with no long-term guarantee of sufficient numbers. Hospitals and clinics that want to serve medical tourists must also recruit "world-class" clinical talent at a time when there is a global shortage of skilled professionals such as nurses, physicians, therapists, pharmacists, and others. The flow of these health workers across borders may be one of the most serious global health care issues and is addressed in the next section.

# THE FLOW OF HEALTH WORKERS ACROSS BORDERS

Technological and **medical innovation** coupled with an aging population has increased the demand for health care worldwide. Countries are finding it difficult to keep pace with these changes, and many countries are experiencing shortages of health human resources. As the labor market becomes more globalized and health professionals become more mobile, countries are looking beyond their national boundaries to recruit the skills and expertise to meet their health care delivery needs.

There has always been an imbalance in the distribution of health workers (akin to the broad imbalance in resource availability). The increasing demand for health workers and the ability of high-income countries to offer more attractive remuneration packages has exacerbated this maldistribution—a phenomenon known as the **brain drain**.

In this part of the chapter, we explore the extent of this maldistribution of health professionals, the financial implications, and its impact on middle- and low-income health systems. We explore the variety of coping mechanisms put in place to reduce the impact of the shortages, giving examples of Human Resources initiatives from several countries. We also consider the broader implications for how we should staff our health systems of the future. The section concludes with specific implications that managers and leaders of health care need to consider as they face the challenge of staffing their health delivery system in an ethical, cost-effective, and efficient manner.

## Health Worker Mobility

In an increasingly globalized labor market, national health systems can no longer rely on the commitment of graduates to work within their own country, and so must look to the international labor market to meet their demands for health professionals. It has therefore become common for high-income countries to recruit their health labor force from middle- and low-income countries. This health worker migration first became an issue for African countries in the postcolonial period, when developing countries were starting to expand their health services and to train their own nationals to deliver these services. These developments coincided with the rapid expansion of health systems in high-income countries and a shortage of health professionals to meet service requirements. Thus opportunities opened up for health care workers in search of better pay and enhanced career opportunities to work in these countries, and the term "brain drain" was coined to describe the large-scale movement of health professionals from low-income to high-income countries (Bach, 2004). This process has been facilitated by the growth of free trade blocks, reinforced by service sector liberalization that arose from the **General Agreement on Trade in Services (GATS)** (OECD, 2002). For example the European Union has established an inclusive model of mutual recognition of qualifications in which registered nurses or midwives are free to work in any member state. Bach claims that the migration of health workers is distinctive because it is strongly influenced by the regulatory frameworks of individual governments that control the training, recruitment, and deployment of health professionals; such frameworks giving rise to particular national patterns of migration (2003). However, this centrality of government regulation also provides greater scope for policy interventions that address migration of health workers, as we discuss later in this chapter.

## The Scale of the Flow

The establishment of accurate data on the flows of health workers presents a challenge, given the different classification, regulation, and registration systems for health professionals in every country. As Clemens and Pettersson (2007) point out, no comprehensive and systematic bilateral database of the international flows of people for all countries exists. All high-income countries collect occupation-specific data on people who arrive in the country, but most do not do so for people who depart the country, making high-frequency, occupation-specific data on bilateral gross migration flows impossible to compile (Clemens and Pettersson, 2007). However, identifying the stock of health workers in different regions of the world gives us some sense of the inequities that exist in the distribution of health workers. Africa carries 25 percent of the world's disease burden, yet has only 1.3 percent of the world's health workers (Commission for Africa, 2005). The health personnel to population ratio in Africa has always lagged behind the rest of the world, falling far short of the WHO (World Health Organization) minimum standard of 2.3 trained health workers per 1,000 population (230 per 100,000). The sub-Saharan average was 15.5 physicians for 100,000 people, 73.4 nurses per 100,000 people, 30.9 midwives per 100,000 people and 1.1 pharmacists per 100,000 people in 2002. In contrast, the average among the Organization for Economic Co-operation and Development (OECD) countries was approximately 311 physicians and 737.5 nurses per 100,000 people in 2002. On average, African countries have about 20 times fewer physicians and 10 times fewer nurses than high-income countries. Even compared to other emerging countries, SSA numbers are strikingly low. For India, Korea, Singapore, and Vietnam, in the early years of the last decade, the average number of physicians per 100,000 people was estimated at 106.3; for nurses it was 220.4 (Liese, 2004).

Clemens and Pettersson (2007) estimate that approximately 65,000 African-born physicians and 70,000 African-born professional nurses were working overseas in a high-income country in the year 2000. This represents about one-fifth of

African-born physicians in the world, and about one tenth of African-born professional nurses. The fraction of health professionals abroad varies enormously across African countries, from 1 percent to over 70 percent according to the occupation and country.

Also, it is estimated that 10 percent of Canada's hospital-based doctors and 6 percent of the total health workforce in the UK are South African (Padarath et al., 2003). A study by Hagopian et al. (2004) analyzed the numbers, trends, and characteristics in the migration of physicians trained in SSA to the United States. A total of 179,978 (23.3 percent) of the 771,491 active nonfederal physicians in the USA in the year 2002 received their medical qualification in another country. The largest proportion of these (115,835 physicians) originate from SSA, a number that represents more than 6 percent of physicians practicing in SSA.

## Impact on African Health Systems

It is widely acknowledged that Africa's health systems are struggling to meet the population health needs of their citizens. The **Millennium Development Goals (MDGs)**, adopted by the United Nations in 2000, are eight major goals for reducing extreme poverty, reducing child mortality rates, fighting disease epidemics such as AIDS, and developing a global partnership for development. The target date for the achievement of these goals has been set at 2015. Three MDGs are most directly related to health:

Goal 4: Reduce child mortality.

Goal 5: Improve maternal health.

Goal 6: Combat HIV/AIDS, malaria and other diseases.

The Joint Learning Initiative (JLI), a network of global health leaders, launched by the Rockefeller Foundation, suggested that on average, countries with fewer than 2.5 health care professionals (counting only doctors, nurses, and midwives) per 1,000 population failed to achieve an 80 percent coverage rate for deliveries by skilled birth attendants or for measles immunization (Chen et al., 2004). The 57 countries that fall below this threshold, and which fail to attain the minimum 80 percent coverage level, are defined as having a critical shortage of health workers. Of the 46 African countries, 36 are estimated as having a critical shortage. Analysts estimate that in the best-case scenario for 2015, Tanzania, for example, would only reach 60 percent of their estimated supply needs, whereas in Chad, the need would be 300

percent greater than the available supply (WHO, 2006). The JLI report (2004) indicated that the low–health worker density in some countries has already had a major impact on maternal and child mortality. African countries, especially in SSA, have a very low density health workforce, compounded by poor skill mix and inadequate investment in training and development (Chen et al., 2004). Liese et al. (2003) argue that the proportion of health personnel to population has stagnated or declined in nearly every African country since 1960. According to Kalanda et al. (2004), "In most developing countries which are affected by HIV and AIDS, lack of human resources is arguably the most limiting factor in providing **antiretroviral therapy (ART)** and running health systems in general." Furthermore, in 2004, it was estimated that the United States would require an additional one million nurses to meet the shortfall from its own training programs up to 2014 (EQUINET, 2004). It is estimated that across the United States, United Kingdom, Canada, and Australia, over a quarter of medical and nursing staff are foreign trained (Organisation for Economic Cooperation & Development, 2002). Among the countries that attract African health workers in relatively large numbers are the United States, United Kingdom, Canada, Australia, France, Spain, Portugal, Belgium, and South Africa (attracting workers from other African countries). Between 2001 and 2002, Awases et al. of the World Health Organization interviewed 2,382 doctors, nurses, and other health professionals in six African countries. Each person declaring an intention to emigrate was asked for his or her preferred destination. Out of this group, 89.3 percent in Cameroon, 91.8 percent in Senegal, and 94.6 percent in South Africa listed one of the previously mentioned nine countries. It is clear that these nine countries play a significant role in depleting the resources of struggling health systems. South Africa is an interesting case, as it plays two roles: being poached (losing health workers to US/UK institutions, etc.) and doing the poaching (attracting health workers from its poorer neighbors in Lesotho, Malawi, Zimbabwe, etc.).

Experts have suggested that individuals with tertiary education are the most likely to emigrate, and those who emigrate are also those most likely to be institution builders (Kapur and McHale, 2005a, 2005b). This results not only in gaps in the delivery of care, but also in the development of services. Active recruitment by high-income countries tends to focus on attracting the most experienced health professionals. Other researchers have argued that the gap in experienced health workers, coupled with the increased output of newly graduated health professionals, is creating its own difficulties for health systems (McAuliffe et al., 2010). The shortage of experienced health professionals raises concerns about training, clinical supervision, and ultimately the quality of care (McAuliffe et al., 2010). WHO makes the link between supervision and performance, suggesting that supervisory visits that are strictly administrative and viewed as punitive have limited positive effects and could have negative effects on an organization; this contrasts to supervision that is supportive, is educational, and helps to solve specific problems; such supervision may improve motivation and performance (WHO, 2006). Good supervision made a difference in staff motivation and performance between public hospitals and autonomous quasi-government hospitals in Ghana (Dovlo et al., 1998). An additional impact identified in a study by Troy et al. (2007) is that the health workers who remain in low- and middle-income countries are faced with increased workloads and rising stress levels because of the depleted numbers. This has led to increased sick leave and absenteeism, further de-motivating the remaining staff. As an indication of the seriousness of the problem, one director of nursing from South Africa, in an attempt to ease the nurses' workload and stress, asked them to lower their standards so that they could complete more work in less time (Troy et al., 2007).

Human resources are at the core of any effective health system—the delivery of care is managed through it. In SSA, the reduction in health workers, at a time of increasing health demands, is at a crisis point and is seriously undermining potential advances not only in antiretroviral (ARV) rollout for HIV/AIDS, but also in the provision of the most basic primary care services.

## Financial Implications

The exodus of health workers from low- and middle-income countries continues to maintain and increase the dependence of those countries on more developed nations—ironically, the nations to which health personnel migrate. The recruitment of the best-qualified health personnel from low-income countries, at no training cost to the recipient countries, is increasingly being recognized as unethical. Almost 50 percent of doctors trained to work in Africa leave to work abroad (EQUINET, 2004). With an estimated cost of US$60,000 for training a general medical practitioner in the Southern African Development Cooperation (SADC) region, outflows from the region to more "developed" countries amount to a $500 million reverse subsidy per annum (EQUINET, 2004). Martin, Abella, and Kuptsch (2006) assert that South Africa is "suffering" from a "brain drain" of doctors and nurses with a financial loss of over US$1 billion. UNCTAD has estimated that the United States has saved US$3.86 billion as a consequence of importing 21,000 doctors from Nigeria alone.

Clemens and Pettersson (2007) suggest a relationship between the loss of professionals and economic and political stability. Angola, Congo-Brazzaville, Guinea-Bissau, Liberia, Mozambique, Rwanda, and Sierra Leone all experienced civil war in the 1990s, and they found that all had lost more than 40 percent of their physicians by 2000. Kenya, Tanzania, and Zimbabwe all experienced decades of economic stagnation in the late twentieth century and, by its end, each had lost more than half of its physicians. By contrast, countries with greater stability and prosperity—Botswana, South Africa, and pre-collapse Côte d'Ivoire—managed to retain their doctors (Clemens and Pettersson, 2007).

However, some argue that the movement of workers from low-income to high-income countries is positive for the source countries as well as the host countries. Pritchett (2006) argues that "the gains to people in poor countries from labor mobility are enormous compared to everything else on the development agenda." Pritchett cites estimates that if rich countries were to permit a mere 3 percent increase in the size of their labor force by easing restrictions on labor mobility, the benefits to citizens of poor countries would be $305 billion a year—almost twice the combined annual benefits of full trade liberalization ($86 billion), foreign aid ($70 billion), and debt relief (about $3 billion in annual debt service savings). Pritchett argues that demographic forces for greater international labor mobility are being slowed by immovable anti-immigration ideas of rich-country citizens. He highlights the difficult political and ethical issues that the movement of people across national borders presents to the current system and proposes breaking the gridlock through policies that support development while also being politically acceptable in rich countries. These include greater use of temporary worker permits, permit rationing, reliance on bilateral rather than multilateral agreements, and protection of migrants' fundamental human rights.

One of the positive financial implications of labor migration from low-income to high-income countries is the value of remittances to families in low-income countries. **Migrant remittances,** defined as the transfer of funds from migrants to relatives or friends in their country of origin, have become an increasingly important feature of modern economic life. Indeed, remittances are now recognized as an important source of global development finance (DFID, 2006). They not only supplement the incomes of families, but also provide a much-needed source of foreign exchange to these countries. The report of a study of UK migrants undertaken by the Department for International Development (DFID) in 2006 states that "international remittance flows by migrant workers are huge and growing, with remittance flows perhaps exceeding development aid and without doubt playing a substantial role in alleviating poverty in recipient countries" (DFID, 2006). The report cites three factors to explain this trend:

- Remittance flows are now the second-largest source of external funding for development countries (foreign direct investment being the largest)

- Remittances are one of the least volatile sources of foreign exchange for developing countries

- Remittances are expected to rise significantly in the long term (DFID, 2006)

The recognition that remittances are playing an important role in supporting families in low-income countries has resulted in international organizations, bilateral donors, and nongovernment organizations taking initiatives to better understand the nature and scope of migrant remittances and to identify ways of maximizing their development impact in countries of origin.

In addition, international migration has been used to stimulate economies in some low-income countries. The export of contract labor as a strategy for stimulating domestic market conditions is a primary feature of Philippine economic policy (Matejowsky, 2006). Since the 1970s, millions of Filipinos have responded to slow economic growth at home by taking advantage of nonpermanent job opportunities abroad. There are also considerable benefits to be gained, should the migrants return to their home countries. They usually return having improved their education and expanded their skill sets, and bring with them an international network that they can tap into for ongoing support and development.

## International Response

Increased awareness of the scale of health worker migration and the belief that migrant health worker flows will continue have shifted the attention of governments towards the concept of **managed migration**—a term that signals attempts to link international migration to the health policy goals of individual states and to regulate the flows of health workers in a way that is beneficial to both source and destination countries (Bach, 2003). The practice of recruitment agencies in high-income countries actively encouraging migration has been heavily criticized because of its impact on low-income countries. These countries are effectively utilizing scarce resources of low-income countries to educate health professionals, only for high-income country health systems to reap the benefits. There have been calls for a tax or compensation payment by countries who recruit large numbers of health workers from countries that can ill afford to lose them. Attempts have been made to develop international recruitment guidelines, but these have been fraught with difficulty and have had little impact on the management of international migration of overseas nurses (Buchan, 2006). The Commonwealth Code of Practice has a strong emphasis on mutuality of benefits for both countries: "Many developing Commonwealth countries have expressed the view that recruiting developed countries should in some way compensate source countries for the loss of personnel trained at great expense. Compensation may be in a variety of ways such as building capacity in training institutions" (Bach, 2003).

According to Bach (2003), this was "a step too far" for Australia, Canada, and the UK, and they declined to sign the Code because of the statements on compensation. As such codes and guidelines are not mandatory, many countries have chosen not to follow them, and therefore, at best, they serve to highlight good employment practices when adhered to.

Bilateral agreements between countries such as policies on return, the incorporation of ethical codes of practice into national recruitment practice, and measures to cap the numbers of internationally recruited health workers entering countries have met with limited success. The UK National Health Service ended its active recruitment of staff from sub-Saharan Africa in 2001. However, this has not entirely stemmed the flow, and some writers are calling for more radical measures to address the problem. Alkire and Chen urge that high-income countries' migration policy "should adopt 'medical exceptionalism' based on moral and ethical grounds." Kapur and McHale caution against "poaching" health workers from developing countries and claim that the case is "obvious" for "restraint" in the recruitment of doctors and nurses. Labonte et al. (2006), in a study of Canadian policy makers, found that reducing pull factors by increasing domestic self-sufficiency and reducing push factors by strengthening source country health systems have the greatest policy traction in Canada. The **Global Health Workforce Alliance (GHWA)** partnership was established in 2006 to identify and implement solutions to the global health workforce crisis. It assists countries with their efforts to develop and implement plans for scaling up the health workforce. It brings together a variety of actors, including national governments, civil society, finance institutions, workers, international agencies, academic institutions, and professional associations in addressing the crisis.

## National Level Responses

Individual countries, alarmed by the scale of emigration from their health systems and the devastating impact this has had, have begun to take serious measures to address their human resources crisis. Some have suggested that countries themselves can reduce the outflow of health workers by improving incentive packages, human resource management systems, and availability of training (Dovlo and Martineau 2004), although the ability to achieve these improvements may require international coordination.

The prospect of financial gain is believed to be a pivotal factor in the decision to migrate. In order to counteract this, many African countries have introduced top-up salaries and other kinds of benefits and allowances for some cadres of health workers. Namibia is reported to be offering generous end-of-service payments, and subsidized house-owning schemes and car ownership. In Ghana, the government has increased incomes, especially for physicians. Nigeria also introduced a separate duty allowance structure for physicians. Botswana introduced 30 percent overtime allowance for nurses and 15 percent for physicians. Other countries such as Kenya, South Africa, Zambia, Malawi, Tanzania, and Mozambique have increased salaries of various cadres of health workers in an effort to retain them. While countries such as Thailand and Ireland have had some degree of success in persuading physicians who have migrated abroad to return home by providing monetary incentives and research funds, as well as services and assistants (Pang et al., 2002), it has been argued that providing monetary incentives alone will not alter migration significantly, considering the enormous wage differentials in the source and recipient countries (Vujicic, 2004). Most SSA countries cannot compete with the financial incentives of overseas countries, but it has been

argued that nonfinancial incentives, which have been found to be important in motivating health workers, can be used to supplement these financial incentives. Indeed, growing evidence suggests that other factors in the work environment may also be acting as strong push factors. Workload and staff shortages are contributing to burnout, high absenteeism, stress, depression, low morale, and de-motivation, and these factors are responsible for driving workers out of the public sector (McAuliffe et al., 2010; Sanders and Lloyd, 2005). Poor working conditions are reported to seriously undermine health system performance by thwarting staff morale and motivation, and directly contributing to problems in recruitment and retention (Troy, Wyness, and McAuliffe, 2007; WHO, 1996). Financial incentives are only one part of a much more complex picture of motivational factors and perceived fairness and management support in particular are important motivators (McAuliffe et al., 2009).

One strategy being used to alleviate health worker shortages and to improve access and quality of health services is task-shifting, or the delegation of tasks that would traditionally fall within the scope of practice of doctors or nurses to other health workers who have undergone shorter periods of training (see "In Practice. A Country Case Study on Ethiopia's Flooding and Retention Strategy"). These cadres have different titles in different countries, but are commonly referred to as midlevel workers or non-physician clinicians. Midlevel workers are health care providers who have received less training and have a more restricted scope of practice than professionals. These workers, in contrast to community or lay health workers, however, do have a formal certificate and accreditation through their countries' licensing bodies (Lehmann, 2008). Mullan et al. (2007) identified non-physician clinicians (NPCs) in 25 of 47 countries in sub-Saharan Africa, although their roles varied widely between countries. In nine countries, numbers of NPCs equaled or exceeded numbers of physicians. In general, NPCs' training cost less than a physician's, and lasted for an average period of 3–4 years post secondary school. All NPCs do basic diagnosis and medical treatment, but some were trained in specialty activities such as caesarean section, ophthalmology, and anesthesia. Many NPCs were recruited from rural and poor areas, and worked in these same regions (Mullan, 2007). Non-physician clinicians deliver health services in low-, middle-, and high-income countries. For example, more than 300,000 non-physician clinicians practice alongside

## IN PRACTICE: A Country Case Study on Ethiopia's Flooding and Retention Strategy*

Ethiopia is a federal government, comprising nine regional states, two city administrations, 624 districts and 15,000 villages. Federal Ministry of Health data from 2006 showed that 85 percent of the population, or 77.3 million persons, lived in rural areas. It is estimated that 60 percent to 80 percent of the country's health problems are due to largely preventable communicable diseases such as malaria, pneumonia, and TB. HIV/AIDS is also a growing problem. Ethiopia suffers from an acute shortage of health workers at every level, and rural areas have been particularly chronically underserved. The government's Health Sector Development Program, which began to be implemented in 1997, is focused on achieving the health-related Millennium Development Goals (MDGs), and on providing comprehensive and integrated primary care services, mainly at community-based health facilities. One of the program's eight components is to expand the supply and productivity of health personnel. The initial focus was on community-level provision, with the initiation of the Health Extension Worker (HEW) Program in 2004. This program aims to improve primary health services in rural areas through an innovative community-based approach that focuses on prevention, healthy living, and basic curative care. It introduced a new cadre of health worker, Health Extension Workers (HEWs), and defined a package of essential interventions for them to deliver from village health posts. Female high school graduates are recruited and trained for one year (candidates must have completed grade 10 in school, need to be from the local community, and speak the local language). They are trained to deliver a package of 16 preventive and basic curative services that comprise four main components: hygiene and environmental sanitation; family health services; disease prevention and control; and health education and communication. The program has deployed 30,000 new HEWs to work at local health posts and is well advanced in achieving this.

A second initiative is the Ethiopia Public Health Training Initiative (EPHTI)—a partnership between the Ethiopian government ministries of Health and Education, The Carter Center, seven Ethiopian universities, and other nongovernmental organizations—aims to improve the quality of pre-service training to health science professionals within Ethiopia. Because the biggest hurdle to better health in Ethiopia is the lack of access to health personnel, the mission of EPHTI is to build a team of qualified health care workers across the country, especially in underserved rural populations. EPHTI has three primary goals:

- Assist Ethiopians in developing their own training and educational health learning materials
- Strengthen the teaching capacity of Ethiopian university faculty members
- Improve the campus teaching and learning environments of Ethiopian health sciences universities.

In 2005, EPHTI began to implement the Accelerated Health Officer Training Program in Ethiopia. The health officer is the leader of the community-based health center professional staff, and the program's objective is to train 5,000 health officers by 2010. Health officers provide clinical services at health centers and manage both the health center and world health offices. Five universities and 20 hospitals are involved in the training program. The majority of students in the training program were practicing nurses who received basic science education in the first year, followed by two years of tailored instruction at a training hospital. By mid-2008, more than 900 had graduated, and 3,168 were under training.

The Ethiopian government is to be commended for its novel approach to addressing the health worker shortage. Although the initiative is on target and there are signs that the health indicators for the country are improving, the real question is whether the country can retain these newly trained cadres in the country, but more particularly in the remote rural areas, and achieve an equitable distribution of health care workers across this vast nation.

---

* Information for this case study was sourced from the Ethiopia's Ministry of Health Web site, Carter Center, and WHO GHWA's Country Case Study: Ethiopia's Human Resources for Health Programme. Retrieved from http://www.who.int/workforcealliance

physicians in the USA (Cooper, 1998). There is growing evidence from many African countries for the clinical efficacy (Chilopora et al., 2007; Pereira et al., 2007) and economic value (Kruk et al., 2007) of these midlevel cadres, particularly in the provision of emergency obstetric care. One particularly interesting case study is the use of the midlevel cadres in Ethiopia (see "In Practice: A Country Case Study on Ethiopia's Flooding and Retention Strategy"). This initiative, although progressing well, is not sufficiently advanced to assess the true impact on the availability of health services or on the country's health indicators. If successful, however, it will raise interesting questions about the wisdom of attempting to populate low-income countries with Western-trained, expensively produced doctors.

Some countries have continued to produce highly trained doctors and nurses but have adopted a strategy of overproduction. The Philippines has, for more than a decade, been exporting its degree-level nurses to many countries throughout the world. The government has deliberately adopted this strategy of overproduction in the belief that the country would benefit both from remittances of their emigrants and from the additional expertise and knowledge of returning migrants. This strategy has certainly been welcomed by countries that have benefited from this large pool of nursing staff—e.g., Canada, the United States, Ireland, and the United Kingdom. However, interviews with directors of nursing in the Philippines showed that, while acknowledging these benefits to the emigrant nurses, their concerns on the detrimental effect on nursing and the health systems in their own country were noticeable: "The nurses that migrate from low and middle income countries tend to be experienced and highly skilled." (Troy et al., 2007).

Cuba also presents an interesting case (see In Practice: "A Country Case Study on Cuba's Internationalist Principle and the Latin American Medical School Program"). When faced with a critical shortage of doctors following the revolution, it began not only to overproduce, but to change the very nature and structure of medical training in an attempt to engender values of solidarity and loyalty to local communities in its new medical graduates. Health indicators in this country have shown huge improvements, and Cuban doctors have assisted many low-income countries to build their supply of medical manpower. Again, this could be seen as a challenge to the traditional model of training and deployment of health professionals to staff our health systems.

## The Implications for Health Care Managers

As we have shown above, migration of health workers has increased over the past several decades, and there are many indications that it will continue to be a feature of the landscape for the foreseeable future—the world is indeed flattening for health workers. Some of these migration flows are predictable, others less so. An example that serves to highlight this is the case of nurses migrating from the Philippines to Ireland. Earlier we described the strategy of overproduction that was adopted by this country in the 1990s. In the late 1990s, Ireland had a critical shortage of nurses and began to recruit hundreds of Filipino nurses to fill gaps in the services. They came, they settled, and their families followed them. Ireland considered its problem solved until it was discovered that those who had been in the country for 4–5 years were moving on to the United States or Canada in search of higher salaries and greater opportunities for skill development. South Africa experiences similar problems with unpredictable migration flows. At the service delivery level, coping with this unpredictability requires careful manpower planning, matching supply with current and predicated future demand. It is no longer sufficient to expect domestic labor markets to fulfil the needs of service delivery. Recruiting beyond one's own national boundaries is inevitable (and desirable from the perspective of the health professional who wishes to travel and broaden his or her clinical expertise).

In an era of ever-increasing health care demands, all health systems need to be strengthened and further developed. However, such development needs to be conducted with due cognizance of health as a basic human right—entitling everyone to affordable health care regardless of their means or their address. If the international mobility of highly skilled workers is likely to increase, what of the future of developing countries already experiencing substantial losses and struggling to provide basic health care for their populations? Lowell and Findley (2001) in a report synthesizing the International Labor Office's research, advise that immigration policies of developed countries should facilitate movement; yet, they should incorporate mechanisms that encourage developing country economic growth.

> Developed countries might: encourage temporary and return migration; restrict recruitment from at risk countries; establish best practices; regulate recruitment agencies; establish bilateral agreements; and standardize GATS commitments. (Lowell and Findley 2001)

**IN PRACTICE: A Country Case Study on Cuba's Internationalist Principle and the Latin American Medical School Program***

The devastation caused in Central America and the Caribbean in 1998 by hurricanes George and Mitch prompted Cuba to send 1,000 Cuban doctors to volunteer in the disaster areas. The scale of the disaster and the impact for populations without healthcare led the Cuban government to a decision to offer Cuban medical teams for longer-term assistance to strengthen local health systems and to open a medical school in Cuba offering 10,000 scholarships to students from those countries. This became the Comprehensive Health Program (CHP).

By 2007, more than 3,000 foreign doctors had graduated from this school. Government-to-government agreements have expanded the program to 27 countries, and in the case of the United States, attracted students even in the absence of a bilateral agreement. The program is distinctive in its underlying mission to train doctors to serve local communities by combining population-based public health principles and prevention with clinical medicine. Students are placed in polyclinics (the basic unit of the system, which serves a population of 25,000–30,000) to work with local Cuban communities even in their basic science years. The focus of the training is bio-psycho-social; individual, family, and community. This prepares students well for working in resource-poor settings where the close association between poverty and ill health means that health professionals must have a good understanding of the economic, social, cultural, and environmental determinants of health in order to be effective. The Cuban principle is that "medicine as merchandise has not—and will not—guarantee health for the world's poor majorities" (Frank et al, 2008). Health professionals must believe in health as a human right and must be prepared to make sacrifices to deliver on this right.

Along with this large-scale training of doctors, Cuba also trained auxiliary personnel, such as nursing auxiliaries and health technicians, to serve in the rural areas and to meet the changing needs of the health system. Marquez (2009) writing in the *Lancet*, claims that "The development of a diversified workforce has been crucial for the provision of free-of-charge services along the continuum of care, particularly ambulatory services in polyclinics . . . The system's community healthcare approach has allowed the placement of a doctor trained in primary care and a nurse in every neighborhood (serving about 150 families)."

Cuba now has one of the best doctor-to-population ratios in the world and has better health indicators than countries that have substantially higher per capita spending on health.

As discussed earlier, there are many ways in which high-income countries can help strengthen low-income-country health systems, from monetary (recruitment tax paid to source country) to capacity building (contributing to source-country training, exchange of staff and expertise, etc.) methods. The migration of health workers has also led to questions about how health workers can be retained; happy health workers tend to stay in jobs longer. Understanding and improving the motivation of health workers is a key task for any health care manager, regardless of context or scarcity of resources. Creating an environment that attracts and retains health professionals has become a focus of many low-income countries' attempts to stem the brain drain.

However, the hard reality is that, at the global level, there is an insufficient supply of health professionals to meet current service demands. This reality prompted Ethiopia and several other African countries to adopt alternative methods of staffing their health systems. Shorter training, more specialized training, task shifting to lower cadres, etc., are all features of these environments. This formula seems to be working.

* Materials for this case study were sourced from: Presentations at the Global Forum for Health Research, Havana, and November 2009. Marquez, M. (2009). Health-workforce development in the Cuban health system, *Lancet, 374,* Issue 9701, pp. 1574–1575; Frank, M., & Reed, G. (2008) Doctors for the (Developing) World: Training physicians for global health, *MEDICC Review.* Retrieved August 5, 2010, from http://www.medicc.org/publications/medicc_review/0805/spotlight.html

Does this suggest that it might be time to change how we staff our health systems in high-income countries? Are some professionals overtrained for the work that they do? Can we afford to continue training health professionals for periods of 5–10 years, or is this now a luxury we can no longer afford? With increasingly sophisticated technological and medical diagnostic aids, how important is the human element in the process? These questions about health care worker mobility will be debated as health care demand continues to grow.

We have focused on patients and health care workers as two examples of how interconnectedness is playing out in the world of health and health care. Turning now to our third and final illustration, we describe new policy instruments and management practices that are spreading from country to country.

# THE FLOW OF POLICY INSTRUMENTS AND MANAGEMENT PRACTICES ACROSS BORDERS

On April 1, 1983, the first **patient classification system** (PCS) used for paying hospitals for services they provided was adopted by the U.S. Congress. As Kimberly et al. (2008) state, "For the first time a payer—in this case Medicare—had a way of comparing the outputs of one hospital with those of another as a basis for paying hospitals in a standardized, consistent fashion for the 'products' they produced. This system is a policy instrument whose impact on management practices in hospitals and other health care facilities has been profound."

## What Is the Policy Instrument in Question?

The patient classification system that was adopted by Congress, known as **Diagnosis-Related Groups**, or DRGs, was developed by a team of researchers at Yale University in the late 1970s. The lead researchers, Robert Fetter and John Thompson, were trained in industrial engineering and nursing, and brought an industrial engineer's mind-set to the analysis of hospital performance—a mind-set that placed a premium on standardizing production processes and applying basic cost accounting principles to those processes. If you did not know how much it cost to produce whatever product(s) you were producing, how could you ever know how to price them in a way that ensured that your revenues would exceed your costs? This logic was completely foreign to the world of health care management in a time when hospitals would justify higher costs by asserting that their patients were sicker and therefore cost more to treat. Fetter and his team reasoned that case mix differences from one hospital to the next were important in determining costs. Patients with similar illnesses should incur similar costs for treatment, and if patients were classified correctly by diagnosis (and if the resources necessary to treat them were correctly specified), it would be possible to determine what a treatment costs and then pay hospitals accordingly. Furthermore, hospitals could be funded through **prospective payment** or **retrospective reimbursement** on the base of what they charged. This would lead to significant improvements in efficiency at the hospital level, and result in significant cost savings at the national level.

The logic underlying the development of the DRGs was truly revolutionary at the time, and, once the system was adopted by Congress, it forced hospitals to adopt management practices that would allow them to understand their costs; it put incentives in place for hospitals to manage themselves more efficiently than they ever had in the past. They knew in advance what they would be paid for a whole range of procedures. If they were able to deliver a given procedure for less than they would be paid, they would realize a profit; if not, they would experience a loss. The result, it was hoped, would at the very least, be a slowing of the rate of increase in health costs.

As of the year 2010, we find that various versions of this system are being used in at least 36 countries around the globe, and we see this as a good illustration of how the flow of policy instruments across national borders is indicative of flattening in the sense Friedman intended. Some version of the DRG patient classification system is being used in countries as diverse as Sweden, Hungary, Singapore, Italy, and Japan. This is another indicator of the globalizing of health care—similar policy instruments are being adopted by countries in very different parts of the world with very different health systems, and are influencing management practice as a consequence. Patients seeking care across national borders, health professionals finding jobs across national borders, and similar policy instruments being used across national borders are all examples that suggest a flattening of the world of health care and health care management.

# THE DRIVERS OF CROSS-BORDER FLOW

Why have DRG-based patient classification systems spread so widely around the globe? Perhaps the most obvious reason is that this particular policy instrument is seen at the macro level as having the potential to help countries contain, if not control, the cost of health care—a problem that nearly every country has faced for decades and that only seems to be growing in significance with the passage of time. Additionally, at the micro or provider level, it encourages investment in capabilities that allow a given provider to understand its cost structure in a more detailed fashion and to make certain operational and investment decisions with a greater degree of managerial sophistication. Finally, it allows clinicians and managers to engage in dialogue around questions of resource consumption and performance in a data-driven, as opposed to a more rhetorical and intuitive, fashion.

While the cost-containing potential of DRG-based patient classification systems may help to explain their spread across national borders, other factors have played and continue to play an important role as well. If we think of the business aspects of health care, and if we consider the kinds of opportunities that lie behind the flow of policy instruments across national borders, we are led to examine how the development and spread of these systems was motivated by market forces and opportunities to benefit as perceived by a variety of interested parties—researchers, policy makers, consultants, and software developers, to name only the most obvious. Individual members in each of these groups saw opportunities for gain, and a few invested time, effort, and, in many cases, money very early in the process to explore the potential further. The research group at Yale, for example, became actively involved in helping to develop awareness of the instrument's potential by holding seminars on campus and in a number of locations around the globe, including France, England, Australia, and New Zealand. Once the system had been adopted by the federal government in the United States, policy makers were invited to speak about its structure and advantages in other countries. A number of consulting firms began offering advice on the design and implementation of patient classification systems both in the United States and in other countries. 3M began actively marketing the grouper software it had developed to providers and national systems both at home and abroad.

In 1987, as awareness of the instrument and its potential spread across national borders, a group of researchers and policy makers interested in sharing experiences and in defining "best practices" formed PCS Europe, which later, as interest in patient classification systems grew further, became PCS International. The organization they founded played an important role both as a focal point for information about patient classification systems and as a catalyst for further dissemination. It is difficult to determine exactly when what Malcolm Gladwell (2000) has called a "tipping point" was reached, but the formation and growth of PCS International is a key indicator of the extent to which the DRG-based policy instrument had achieved a level of credibility and interest that has drawn in others from various parts of the world.

## Barriers to Cross-Border Flow

Resources and ideas do not cross national borders seamlessly. A host of possible barriers exists, including regulatory, political, economic, and cultural barriers. As any company doing business in more than one county knows, differences in labor laws, product safety codes, political priorities, economic vibrancy, and underlying values and habits all influence the character and outcomes of multi-country business ventures. One size does not necessarily fit all, and it is always a challenge to balance the advantages of standardization with the need for sensitivity to local customs and preferences. Nowhere is this more true than in health care, where local practices, medical knowledge, and available resources vary widely, not only from one country to the next, but from one region to another within any particular country.

In the case of health workers, one barrier could be the exporting of Western-style medical training to many developing countries. Cuba's "training for context" serves to highlight the potential that can be realized with the removal of such a barrier. In the case of DRG-based patient classification systems, a significant potential barrier is the fact that the original system was developed in the United States. Although the United States is widely recognized as a leader in medical research and education, it is also widely criticized for its lack of universal access to care. It may also be a matter of national pride in some cases to avoid adopting a policy instrument that was developed elsewhere. Known as the **not-invented-here syndrome**, this simply refers to the well-known skepticism about the appropriateness or relevance of something not invented at home for the home. The Japanese, for example, might question the relevance for

## DEBATE TIME: Global Flows and Health

Many experts are suggesting that the health care world is flattening with migration of patients to seek the highest quality and more affordable treatments available, and with health care workers also migrating to find best positions for their careers and to meet the needs of their families. The flow of technology is also substantial, and even the flow of diseases themselves has accelerated. Although best practices regarding routine clinical care are disseminated by the international public health arm of the United Nations (UN), World Health Organization (WHO), this body is largely advisory with little financial and regulatory power over national health systems. Regulations including the approval of use of drugs or the licensure of health workers to perform various treatments are overseen largely by national and professional agencies and ministries. This leads to tremendous diversity in the availability and approach to medical problems across differing countries, even within the same overall economic environment. Consider the impact of these aspects of globalization for quality, cost, and accessibility of medical care and for global health more generally.

their country of a system developed in a country with different medical practices and different epidemiological characteristics.

In point of fact, different countries have used the system in quite different ways to meet idiosyncratic situations and particular needs (Kimberly et al., 2008). The flexibility and adaptability of the system have allowed it to be adopted for multiple uses in a variety of contexts. Thus, the potential impact of the NIH syndrome has been mitigated to a certain extent.

### The Situation Today

As of the year 2010, two conclusions can be drawn clearly from the history of cross-border flow of patient classification systems in general and the DRG-based systems in particular. First, the flow has been substantial. The number of countries using some version of the DRG-based system continues to grow and, perhaps most important, the operations management mind-set as applied to the management of hospitals and other health care facilities continues to spread and profoundly change the way policy makers and managers think about the intersection of clinical and managerial practice. In this sense, we have seen a globalizing of managerial practice in health care or, as Friedman would argue, a flattening of such practice. Second, and just as important, the search for improved instruments, tools, and practices that will help to contain costs in health care continues. The DRG-based PCS may have been the first of its kind to have had a certain degree of global uptake, but it has also spawned a host of initiatives intended to replace it. This pattern is just what we would expect in a robust, globalizing industry that is ripe for innovation. The process of globalizing opens new markets and rewards those who identify new opportunities and meet pressing needs.

# ADDITIONAL CONSIDERATIONS

So far we have made the case that flows of a variety of types across national borders are increasing in the world of health care and health care management, and that these increases indicate that the business of health care is globalizing, or that this world is becoming "flatter." To illustrate, we have presented three concrete examples of how this process is unfolding: one dealing with flows of patients across national borders, a second focusing on flows of health workers across national borders, and a third describing the spread of a policy instrument across national borders.

We turn now to three additional considerations. First, the **directionality of flows** is important. We should not assume that what the developed countries have should flow to the less developed countries, nor should we assume that increased flows are necessarily beneficial to all concerned. As we saw with patient flows, in some cases, wealthy patients from less developed countries seek care in more developed ones, the assumption being that care will be "better" in the latter. But we also see patients from developed countries seeking care in less developed countries because that care is less expensive and is of comparable quality. We also see health workers from less developed countries migrating to more developed countries, a pattern that further exacerbates shortages of qualified health workers in the countries they leave behind, and which can hardly be viewed as beneficial to those countries. Yet, if you ask any U.S. health professional who has worked in a low-income country about their experience, they will invariably refer to it as a life-changing experience and enthuse about how much they have learned. As Immelt, Govindarajan, and Trimble (2009) contend, the developed countries have a lot to learn from others if they will only be open to the possibility. They make the case for what they call **reverse innovation**, by which they mean that rather than modifying products and services developed in the West for emerging markets, innovation should be sourced in smaller, less developed markets and then introduced into larger, more developed markets. For example, the innovations in skill mix and task shifting adopted by many African countries may have lessons for the West. This argument turns the generally accepted thought process upside down and encourages us to ask what might be learned about health maintenance, health promotion, health care delivery, and health care management through careful observation and analysis of practices used in less developed settings. The point we are making is simple, but not simplistic. Flows are multidirectional, and we must be careful not to overlook how flattening may lead to unexpected value-creating possibilities.

Second, we should be mindful of how technological innovation can change the landscape of health care across national borders. A particularly vivid example is teleradiology, the ability to read and interpret images taken in one place and sent digitally to another. Effectively, this means that the reading and interpretation of radiological images is "borderless," and consequently that it depends only on the expertise of the reader, no matter where he or she may be located. The technology enables virtually instantaneous transmission of the images, making "place" irrelevant. Another example is robotic surgery, a technology that permits a surgeon located in one part of the world to operate on a patient located elsewhere. Again, this technology makes traditional borders irrelevant and hinges primarily on the availability of the technology and the surgical and support capabilities.

Finally, we must remember that not all cross-border flows in health care are positive. The enhanced frequency and volume of cross-border flows has a dark side as well. We have already discussed the problem that the movement of health workers from less developed to more developed countries poses for the countries the workers leave. There are more sinister examples as well. Global trafficking in human organs is a case in point, as are global markets for blood supplies. In both cases, cross-border flows are enabled by a combination of sophisticated communication and logistical technologies, and in both cases, we see systematic exploitation of the underprivileged for the benefit of the wealthier.

# CONCLUSION

The world of health care and health care management is flattening. Patients are seeking care outside their home countries; health workers are relocating to new countries; new policy instruments and management practices are spreading from country to country. Although health care is still primarily a "local" business—local practice patterns and health-seeking behavior vary considerably, both within and across national borders—there are signs that at least some aspects of the business are becoming more global as awareness of opportunities increases and as enabling technologies become available. The challenge is to encourage the spread of those technologies and practices that are welfare-enhancing and to discourage the spread of those that are not. History tells us that this challenge is daunting. Globalization is not, in and of itself, a force for good or a force for evil. Ultimately, the challenge is to maintain equity through a sense of global responsibility, while capitalizing on the potential benefits globalization affords to health care.

# SUMMARY AND MANAGERIAL GUIDELINES

1. The fundamental question that must be addressed in examining globalization in any domain, including health care, is how flows of various kinds—both legal and illegal—across national borders have changed.

2. Comparative advantage, when applied to health care, refers to the discovery and deployment of significant differences in a nation's cost, quality, or access such that a medical or surgical procedure, health activity, or service creates patient value. Care program for lung cancer or organ transplantation could become a "power offering" to anyone, anywhere in the world. The difference between inbound and outbound medical tourism can have a significant effect on an economy.

3. Medical tourism may be a "disruptive innovation" that deserves more clinical and managerial attention. Studies predict that in the coming years, patients traveling across country borders for the sole purpose of obtaining acute health services will grow into a multibillion-dollar global industry. The key factors for global competition will be a provider's clinical reputation, defined in terms of (1) outcomes; (2) technological backup; and (3) use of the most advanced medical procedures.

4. The number of infant deaths per 1,000 live births is highly associated with the degree of local health care infrastructure. In general, countries with high per capita GDP have low infant mortality rates. Health care managers should pay attention to these numbers.

5. Enhancing the patient experience can bring a great return to a hospital. For example, Bumrungrad Hospital in Bangkok, with five-star hotel services and accreditation from the Joint Commission for International Accreditation, receives 37 percent of its patient revenues from international patients from 154 countries. They offer deluxe rooms, VIP and royal suites, laptop computers, a swimming pool, and a fitness center. It is also within walking distance to Bangkok's most prestigious restaurants, shopping and entertainment venues. To attract loyal international patients requires substantial investments in buildings, equipment, service processes, and people who can "delight" patients. There is growing rivalry among nations to attract medical tourists with no guarantee of permanent patient loyalty.

6. The market for international patients has many risks and uncertainties—for example, of air safety, transportation costs, national rivalry for patients, the global economy, national moods, global economics, and politics. The flow of patients abroad depends on the perceived value of medical travel in relation to the perceived sacrifices.

7. Africa carries 25 percent of the world's disease burden, yet has only 1.3 percent of the world's health workers. Approximately 37 of the 47 sub-Saharan African countries (SSA) have fewer than 20 doctors per 100,000 people; the sub-Saharan average was 15.5 physicians for 100,000 people, 73.4 nurses per 100,000 people. In contrast, the average among the Organization for Economic Co-operation and Development (OECD) countries was approximately 311 physicians and 737.5 nurses per 100,000 people in 2002. On average, African countries have about 20 times fewer physicians and 10 times fewer nurses than high-income countries.

8. Countries like Angola, Congo-Brazzaville, and Sierra Leone all experienced civil war in the 1990s, and all had lost more than 40 percent of their physicians by 2000. Kenya, Tanzania, and Zimbabwe all experienced decades of economic stagnation in the late twentieth century and by its end, each had lost more than half of its physicians. Countries with greater stability and prosperity—Botswana, South Africa, and pre-collapse Côte d'Ivoire—managed to retain their doctors.

9. Migrant remittances, defined as the transfer of funds from migrants to relatives or friends in their country of origin, have become an increasingly important feature of modern economic life. Indeed, remittances are now recognized as an important source of global development finance. One report stated that international remittance flows by migrant health workers play a substantial role in alleviating poverty in recipient countries.

10. Countries need to improve their workforce planning and monitoring and to assess incentives for retaining their health workers. By developing flexible pay systems, shorter specialist training, and improving human resources and personnel administration systems, countries can change the scale of emigration. Delegation of tasks that would traditionally fall within the scope of practice of doctors or nurses to other health workers who have undergone shorter periods of training is another effective strategy to alleviate health worker shortages.

11. Non-physician clinicians (NPCs) are trained with less cost than physicians for an average period of 3–4 years post secondary school. In sub-Saharan Africa, 25 countries use NPCs, and, in nine of these countries, NPCs equaled or exceeded numbers of physicians. NPCs do basic diagnosis and medical treatment, but some are trained in specialty activities such as caesarean section, ophthalmology, and anesthesia.

12. Countries that attract health workers may do so for short time periods. Ireland had a critical shortage of nurses and began to recruit hundreds of Filipino nurses to fill gaps in the services. However, the nurses who had been in the country for 4–5 years and who therefore had gained excellent experience were now moving on to the United States or Canada in search of higher salaries and greater opportunities for skill development. Retaining health workers is as important as recruiting them.

13. DRGs were developed in the United States in the late 1960s. They were adopted in the United States in 1983. In 2010, various versions of this system are being used in at least 36 countries around the globe, and this illustrates how the flow of policy instruments across national borders is indicative of "flattening" in the sense Friedman intended. Some version of the Diagnosis Related Groups (DRG) patient classification system is being used in countries as diverse as Sweden, Hungary, Singapore, Italy, and Japan.

14. DRGs have the potential to help countries contain, if not control, the cost of health care. Additionally, DRGs encourage investment in capabilities that allow a given provider to understand its cost structure. Finally, DRGs allow clinicians and managers to engage in dialogue around questions of resource consumption and performance in a data-driven fashion rather than a more rhetorical, intuitive fashion.

15. Although health care is still primarily a "local" business—local practice patterns and health-seeking behavior vary considerably, both within and across national borders—there are signs that at least some aspects of the business are becoming more global as awareness of opportunities increases and as enabling technologies become available.

# DISCUSSION QUESTIONS

1. What explains the directionality of flows in health care? Patients, health workers, managerial practices?

2. Discuss the implications of the following statement: "We came to believe that quality of care in facilities credentialed by the Joint Commission International (JCI) in foreign countries, and in India in particular, is as good as or better than that in the United States, and offers a 70–80 percent cost differential in many cases."

3. What are the five segments of patients who are willing to travel across borders to obtain health care? Are there other patient segments beside these five?

4. What explains the global price differential among hospitals? Why would countries like the United States have 10 times the charges for procedures like hip replacements?

5. Why is there growing rivalry for inbound international patients? Under what conditions should a hospital make capital investments to attract international patients?

6. The Cleveland Clinic's goal is to bring world-class medical care to the people of the world wherever possible. Will it work? Will they attract medical tourists?

7. What is the scale of the outflow of health workers? What are the financial implications of health worker flows from low and middle income countries?

8. With respect to worker flows, what international and national responses have been effective?

9. The Ethiopian government has a novel approach to addressing the health worker shortage. Will they retain these newly trained professionals and achieve an equitable distribution of health care workers?

10. What lessons does Cuba have for training health professionals? Is training for context one way to address the migration problem?

11. Why is there an insufficient supply of health professionals to meet current service demands? Should higher income countries follow Ethiopia and adopt shorter training, more specialized training, and task shifting to allied health professionals?

12. Are some professionals overtrained for the work that they do? Can we afford to continue training health professionals for periods of 5–10 years? With increasingly sophisticated technological and medical diagnostic aids, how important is the human element in the process?

13. How many countries have adopted DRGs? Why?

14. Have DRGs actually reduced health care costs?

15. Are there policy instruments or management practices that can reduce social injustices such as the outflow of health workers or racial or ethnic disparities that lead to poor quality of care?

# CASE: Canada's High-Quality, Low-Cost Hernia Hospital*

Shouldice Hospital in Ontario, Canada, is an 89-bed hospital with five operating theaters. Founded in 1945, the hospital focuses on the surgical repair of simple inguinal hernias. They are not only efficient, but they offer high-quality care and can attract many medical tourists.

The Shouldice hernia repair almost never uses general anesthesia; in well over 95 percent of the cases, operations are performed under local infiltration and a light sedative (Glassow, 1986). The avoidance of general anesthesia significantly reduces the risk of harm to patients. Moreover, Shouldice surgeons are carefully selected and trained for over four months before they are allowed to operate. Whereas a general surgeon may perform 50 hernia repairs a year, each Shouldice surgeon performs over 600 per year. Additionally, the surgery is not done on an outpatient basis; each patient stays for a minimum of three days. What makes the clinical work challenging and rewarding for a Shouldice surgeon is repairing a hernia that another surgeon was unable to repair.

Every day at noon, the surgeons operate on patients with a hernia recurrence. These patients may have already had one or two hernia procedures, but the hernia returned because it was not properly repaired. Performing a procedure over old scar tissue is tricky work for any surgeon. Nevertheless, these are the cases that motivate Shouldice surgeons, because they provide clinical evidence of the superiority of the Shouldice technique with its specialized incision, suturing, and early ambulation. Shouldice surgeons can guarantee their patients (and themselves) that they are the best hernia surgeons in the world.

Shouldice is not just a hernia repair technique; it is a well-designed service proposition that has clinical value for specific group of patients (Urguhart and O'Dell, 2004). The care process includes a stay in a pleasant and relaxed environment, continuity of relationships, low prices, and high quality. The physician-patient interaction differs from most surgical encounters; when patients are admitted, the first person they see is their surgeon, who confirms their diagnosis and explains the procedure and what to expect.

Once selected for Shouldice, patients are educated to become partners and coproducers in every aspect of the care process, which builds both trust and self-confidence. For example, they walk into the operating room, they are awake and can talk with the surgeons during the surgery, and they are invited to get off the operating table and walk (with the help of the surgeon) to the postoperative, room because early ambulation is part of the recovery process.

Recovery is completely programmed to include wake-up, medication, breakfast, exercise classes, rest periods, lunch in the dining room, more exercise, dinner, and more activity. To encourage mobility and interaction, there are no televisions or telephones in the rooms. Meals must be eaten in a dining room, and patients must take themselves to the toilets. The facility has stairs with low risers, putting greens, exercise cycles, walking paths, and other activities aimed at a speedy recovery. Once discharged, patients are invited to annual reunions and membership in the Shouldice patient network.

Every patient, physician, nurse, and employee at Shouldice is an alumnus. Patients, providers, and staff are fully engaged, understand their roles and responsibilities, and share an attitude and a mind-set. Through mutual interaction, learning, and understanding, they are committed to the mission and goals of the clinical care process and adopt a Shouldice identity. The nurses know that their job is not to perform menial tasks, but to educate patients, help them to exercise, and relieve physicians

---

*Information for this case study is from Chilingerian and Savage (2005), based on interviews in October 1985 at Shouldice, and on October 2000 with Mr. Alan Odell.

of simple nonclinical tasks. These are powerful lessons in the repositioning of the primary clinical activities and the role of management in the formulation of care practices into a care process. Value is created for patients; value is created for clinicians; and value is created for the organization.

## Questions

1. From a medical tourist perspective, compare Shouldice with the traditional hospital in terms of the key factors of competition.

2. Why would Shouldice attract patients from outside the local province?

3. How is value created for patients, for clinical and nonclinical professionals, and for the Shouldice Hospital as an organization?

4. Which segment or type of medical travelers would Shouldice attract?

# REFERENCES

Al-Hammouri, F. (2008). Jordan as medical destination: A spotlight on Middle East. *World Medical Tourism & Global Health Congress*, San Francisco.

Alkire, S., & Chen, L. (2004). "Medical exceptionalism" in international migration: Should doctors and nurses be treated differently? JLI Working Paper 7-3, Global Health Trust; 2004 Retrieved January 26, 2007, from http://www.globalhealthtrust.org/doc/abstracts/WG7/Alkirepaper.pdf

Anderson, D. H. A., Modrow, R. E., & Tan, J. K. H. (1992). Surgical waiting lists: definition, desired characteristics, and uses. *Healthcare Management FORUM, 5*(2), 17–22.

Alsagoff, F. (2005) Singapore General Hospital: On local shores and beyond. Unpublished master's thesis, INSEAD, Fontainebleau, France.

Awases, M., Gbary, A., Nyoni, J., & Chatora, R. (2004). *Migration of health professionals in six countries: A synthesis report* (p. 38). Brazzaville, Rep. of Congo: World Health Organization Regional Office for Africa.

Bach, S. (2003) International migration of health workers: Labour and social issues. Sectoral Activities Programme, Working Paper. Geneva: International Labour Office.

Bach, S. (2004, August) Migration patterns of physicians and nurses: Still the same story? *Bulletin of the World Health Organisation, 82*(8).

Beecham, L. (2002). British patients willing to travel abroad for treatment. *British Medical Journal, 325,* 10.

Benveniste, I. (2008). High quality of care available in the Middle East: Is developing coutnries' trend for getting treatment in the USA now reversed? Medical Tourism Association Conference. Acibadem Healthcare Group, Turkey.

Buchan, J., & Perfilieva, G. (2006). Health worker migration in the European region: Country case studies and policy implications. Copenhagen: WHO Regional Office for Europe.

Chen, L., Evans, T., Anand, S., Boufford, J. I., Brown H., Chowdhury, M., et al. (2004). Human resources for health: overcoming the crisis. *Lancet, 364,* 1984–1990.

Chilingerian, J. A. (2004). Who has star quality? In R. E. Herzlinger (Ed.), *Consumer-driven health care: Implications for providers, payers, and policy-makers* (pp. 443–453). San Francisco: Jossey-Bass.

Chilingerian, J. A., & Savage, G. T. (2005). The emerging field of international health care management. In G. T. Savage, J. A. Chilingerian, & M. Powell, *Advances in health care management* (Vol. 5). Boston: Elsevier JAI.

Chilopora, G., Pereira, C., Kamwendo, F., Chimbiri, A., Malunga, E., & Bergstrom, S. (2007). Postoperative outcome of caesarean sections and other major emergency obstetric surgery by clinical officers and medical officers in Malawi. *Human Resources for Health, 5*, 17.

Clemens, M. A. & Pettersson, G. New data on African health professionals abroad. Working Paper Number 95, Centre for Global Development, February.

Cleveland Clinic Abu Dhabi to be operational in 2011.(2008). *Arab Health Online,* April 20.

Comarow, A. (2008). Saving on surgery by going abroad. *U.S. News & World Report,* May 1 (pp. 42–50). *USNews.com,* September 16. Retrieved October 10, 2009, from <http://health.usnews.com/articles/health/special-reports/2008/05/01/saving-on-surgery-by-going-abroad.html>.

Commonwealth Secretariat. (2003) Companion document to the Commonwealth Code of Practice for International Recruitment of Health Workers, London.

Cooper, R. A., Laud, P., & Dietrich, C. L. (1998) Current and projected workforce of non-physician clinicians. *Journal of the American Medical Association, 280,* 788–794.

Cortez, N. (2008). Patients without borders: the emerging global market for patients and the evolution of modern health care. *Indiana Law Journal, 83*(71), 71–132.

Cumming, I. (2009, October 30). Unpublished interview with Jon Chilingerian, Boston, MA.

Department for International Development, UK. (2006) *BME remittance survey—research report.* July 27.

Dovlo, D., & Martineau, T. (2004). A review of the migration of Africa's health professionals. A Joint Learning Initiative: Human Resources for Health and Development Working Paper.

Dovlo, D., Sagoe, K., Ntow, S., & Wellington, E. (1998). Ghana case study: staff performance management. In *Reforming health systems* (research report). Retrieved February 17, 2006, from http://www.liv.ac.uk/lstm/research/documents/ghana.pdf.

Douglas, D. E. (2007). Is medical tourism the answer? *Frontiers of Health Services Management 24*(2), 35–40.

Erhart, M. (2008, February 10). Unpublished interview with Jon Chilingerian. Abu Dhabi, UAE.

Ehrbeck, T., Guevara, C., & Mango, P. D. (2008) Mapping the market for medical travel. *McKinsey & Company Quarterly Report.* McKinsey & Company

Fares, Z. (2009, February 13). Unpublished interview with Jon Chilingerian. Abu Dhabi, UAE.

Fleni. (2008). Fundacion de lucha contra las enfermedadaes neurologicas de la infancia. World Medical Tourism & Global Health Congress. San Francisco.

Friedman, T. (2005) *The world is flat: A brief history of the twenty-first century.* New York: Farrar, Straus and Giroux.

Frank, M., & Reed, G. (2008). Doctors for the (developing) world, training physicians for global health. *MEDICC Review.* Retrieved August 5, 2010, from http://www.medicc.org/publications/medicc_review/0805/spotlight.html

Fried, B. J., & Harris, D. M. (2007). Managing healthcare services in the global marketplace. *Frontiers of Health Services Management, 24*(2), 3–17.

Garman, A. N. (2008). International travel for essential medical care: Niche specialty or disruptive innovation? Final Report to the Alfred P. Sloan Foundation. Rush University Medical Center.

Ghemawat, P. (2007). Businesses beware: the world is not flat. Interview, Harvard Business School Working Knowledge, October 15.

Gladwell, M. (2002). *The tipping point: How little things can make a big difference.* New York: Little, Brown & Company.

Grote, K. D., Newman, J. S., & Sutaria, S. S. (2008). A better hospital experience. *McKinsey & Company Quarterly Report*. McKinsey & Company.

Gruber, N. (2007). Will globalization impact the delivery of healthcare in America? *Frontiers of Health Services Management, 24*(2), 31–33.

Hediger, V., Lambert, T. M., & Mourshed, M. (2007). Private solutions for health care in the Gulf. *McKinsey & Company Quartery Report*. McKinsey & Company.

Heyman, Joe. (2008). AMA perspective on globalization. World Medical Tourism & Global Health Congress. San Francisco.

Hospital Association of South Africa. (2008). Healthcare in South Africa. World Medical Tourism & Global Health Congress. San Francisco.

Immelt, J., Govindarajan, V., & Trimble, C. (2009). How GE is disrupting itself. *Harvard Business Review*, October.

Intel Corporation. (2004). *Bumrungrad hospital transforms healthcare delivery with integrated information system on Intel architecture*. Retrieved March 24, 2005, from http://www.intel.com/business/casestudies/bumrungrad.pdf

Kapur, D., & McHale, J. (2005a). The global migration of talent: What does it mean for developing countries? Centre for Global Development Brief. Retrieved August 6, 2010, from http://www.cgdev.org

Kapur, D., & McHale, J. (2005b). Policy options. In *Give us your best and brightest: The global hunt for talent and its impact on the developing world*. Washington, DC: Center for Global Development.

Keckley, P. H. and Underwood, H. R. (2008). *Medical tourism: Consumers in search of value*. Washington, DC: Deloitte Center for Health Solutions.

Keckley, P. H. and Underwood, H. R. (2009). *Medical tourism: An update*. Washington, DC: Deloitte Center for Health Solutions.

Kimberly, J. R., Pouvourville, G., & D'Aunno, T. (2008). *The globalization of managerial innovation in health care*. London: Cambridge University Press.

Kruk, M. E., Pereira, C., Vaz, F., Bergstrom, S., & Galea, S. (2007). Economic evaluation of surgically trained assistant medical officers in performing major obstetric surgery in Mozambique. *BJOG, 114*, 1253–1260.

Labonte, R., Packer, C., & Klassen, N. (2006). Managing health professional migration from sub-Saharan Africa to Canada: a stakeholder inquiry into policy options. *Human Resources for Health, 4*, 22.

Landers, S. J. (2002). Heightened security keeping international patients away: U.S. hospitals with substantial international programs see a decline in revenue; doctors see a boost in telemedicine consults. Retrieved March 20, 2005, from http://www.ama-assn.org/amednews/2002/09/16/hlsc0916.htm

Lehman, U. (2008). Mid-level health workers: The state of the evidence on programmes, activities, costs and impact on health outcomes, a literature review. World Health Organization, Department of Human Resources for Health. Geneva, July 2008.

Lowell B. L. & Findlay, A. M. (2001). Migration of highly skilled persons from developing countries: Impact and policy responses. Synthesis report, International Labor Office, Geneva.

Marquez, M. (2009) Health-workforce development in the Cuban health system. *Lancet, 374*(9701), 1574–1575.

Martin P., Abella, M., & Kuptsch, C. (2006). *Managing labor migration in the twenty-first century*. New Haven, CT: Yale University Press.

Matejowsky, T. S. (2006) Overseas contract labor, remittances, and household consumption: A case study from San Fernando City, the Philippines. *Research in Economic Anthropology, 24*, 11–36.

McAuliffe, E., Manafa, O., Maseko, F., Bowie, C., & White, E. (2009) Understanding job satisfaction amongst mid-level cadres in Malawi: The contribution of organisational justice. *Reproductive Health Matters, 17*(33): 80–90.

McAuliffe, E., Manafa, O., Bowie, C., Makoae, L., Maseko, F., Moleli, M., & Hevey, D. (2010). Managing and motivating: Pragmatic solutions to the brain drain. In S. Kebane (Ed.), *Human resources in healthcare, health informatics and health systems*. Hershey, PA: IGI Global.

Medical Tourism Association. (2008, September 25). Quality of care project. Retrieved October 10, 2009, from http://www.medicaltourismassociation.com.

Merrit, M. G., et al. Involvement abroad of U.S. academic health centers and major teaching hospitals: The developing landscape. *Academic Medicine, 83*(6), 541–549.

Mullan, F., & Frehywot, S. (2007). Non-physician clinicians in 47 African countries. *Lancet, 370,* 2158–2163.

Odell, Alan. (2000, October). Unpublished interview with Jon Chilingerian. Harvard Business School, Cambridge, MA.

OECD. (2002). GATS: The case for open services markets. Paris.

Pang, T., Lansang, M. A., & Haines, A. (2002). Brain drain and Health professionals. *BMJ, 324,* 499–500.

Pereira, C., Cumbi, A., Malalane, R., Vaz, F., McCord, C., Bacci, A., & Bergstrom, S. (2007). Meeting the need for emergency obstetric care in Mozambique: Work performance and histories of medical doctors and assistant medical officers trained for surgery. *BJOG, 114*(12), 1530–1533.

Porter, M. (1987). Changing patterns of international competition. In D. J. Teece (Ed.), *The competitive challenge.* Cambridge: Ballinger Publishing Company.

Roy, C. W., & Hunter, J. (1996). What happens to patients awaiting arthritis surgery? *Disability and Rehabilitation, 18*(2), 101–105.

Rowley, S. D. (2008). Medical tourism in Asia. *World Medical Tourism & Global Health Congress*. San Francisco.

Rugman, A., & Oh, C. (2008) Friedman's follies: Insights on the globalization/regionalization debate. *Business and Politics, 10*(2), 1–14.

Sanders, D., & Lloyd, B. (2005). South African health review 2005. In P. Ijumba & P. Barron (Eds.), *Human resources: International context* (pp. 76–87). Durban, South Africa: Health Systems Trust.

Schiano, T. D., & Rhodes, R. (2010). The dilemma and reality of transplant tourism: An ethical perspective for liver transplant programs. *Liver Transplantation, 16,* 113–117.

Schroth, L., & Khawaja, R. (2007). Globalization of healthcare. *Frontiers of Health Services Management, 24*(2), 19–30.

Solomon, J. (2004, April 26). Traveling cure: India's new coup in outsourcing: Inpatient care; Facing expense, long waits at home, Westerners fly in; A hospital empire grows; Mr. Salo has "real doubts." *Wall Street Journal,* p. A1.

Timmons, K. (2007). The value of accreditation: why Americans needing health care abroad should choose JCI-accredited facilities. *Joint Commission International 2007.* Retrieved October 10, 2009, from http://www.jointcommissioninternational.org.

Troy, P., Wyness, L., & McAuliffe, E. (2007) Nurses' experiences of recruitment and migration from developing countries: A phenomenological approach. *Human Resources for Health, 5,* 15.

Urquhart, D. J. B., & O'Dell, A. (2004). A model of focused health care delivery. In R. E. Herzlinger (Ed.), *Consumer-driven health care: Implications for providers, payers, and policy-makers* (pp. 627–634). San Francisco: Jossey-Bass.

Vequist, D. G. (2008). The impact of medical tourism on medical equipment sales. World Medical Toursim and Global Health Congress. San Antonio, TX.

Vujicic, M., Zurn, P., Diallo, K., Adams, O., & Dal Poz, M. (2004). The role of wages in slowing the migration of health care professionals from developing countries. Department of Health Services Provision, World Health Organization, Geneva, Switzerland.

Weiners, W. W. (2007). Going global: Delivering healthcare services in a "flat" world. *Frontiers of Health Services Management, 24*(2), 41–43.

Williams, J. I., Llewellyn Thomas, H., Arshinoff, R., Young, N., & Naylor, C. D. (1997). The burden of waiting for hip and knee replacements in Ontario. *Journal of Evaluation in Clinical Practice, 3*(1), 59–68.

Woodman, H. (2008) *Patients without borders: Everybody's guide to affordable world-class medical travel.* Durham: Health Travel Media.

World Health Organization (WHO). (1996). Strengthening nursing and midwifery: Progress and future directions, 1996–2000. Geneva, WHO.

World Health Organization (WHO). (2006). Working together for health. World Health Report. Geneva, WHO.

# Acronyms

| | | | |
|---|---|---|---|
| ACF | Agency for Children and Families | CCAD | Cleveland Clinic Abu Dhabi |
| ACHE | American College of Healthcare Executives | CCC | Convenient Care Clinic |
| ACO | Accountable Care Organization | CCCA | Convenient Care Clinic Association |
| ACTION | Acclerating Change in Transforming Networks | CCR | Continuity of Care |
| | | CDC | Centers for Disease Control and Prevention |
| AFDC | Aid to Families with Dependent Children | CDHP | Consumer Directed Health Plan |
| AHA | American Hospital Association | CEO | Chief executive officer |
| AHIP | America's Health Insurance Plans | CER | Comparative clinical effectiveness research |
| AHRQ | Agency for Healthcare Research and Quality | CFO | Chief financial officer |
| AIDET | Acknowledge, Introduce, Duration, Explanation, Thank You | CHCS | Composite health care system |
| | | CHIP | Children's Health Insurance Program |
| AIDS | Acquired Immune Deficiency Syndrome | CHP | Comprehensive health program |
| AKS | Anti-Kickback Statute | CIA | Corporate integrity agreement |
| AMA | American Medical Association | CIO | Chief information officer |
| ANA | American Nursing Association | CITI | Collaborative Institutional Training Initiative |
| AoA | Administration on Aging | CMS | Centers for Medicare and Medicaid Services |
| ARRA | American Recovery and Reinvestment Act | COGME | Committee on Graduate Medical Education |
| ART | Antiretroviral therapy | CON | Certificate of need |
| ASQ | American Society for Quality | COO | Chief operating officer |
| ATSDR | Agency for Toxic Substances and Disease Registry | COSTAR | Computer stored ambulatory record |
| | | CPOE | Computerized physician order entry |
| BATNA | Best Alternative to a Negotiated Agreement | CPR | Computer-based patient records |
| BCG | Boston Consulting Group | CQI | Continuous quality improvement |
| BIDMC | Beth Israel Deaconess Medical Center | CRM | Crew resource management |
| BPR | Business process reengineering | CSHSC | Center for Studying Health System Change |
| CAHME | Commission on the Accreditation of Healthcare Management | DHCP | Decentralized hospital computer system |
| | | DMAIC | Define, Measure, Analyze, Improve, Control |
| CAM | Complementary and Alternative Medicine | DO | Doctor of Osteopathy |
| CBO | Congressional Budget Office | DOJ | Department of Justice |

| | | | |
|---|---|---|---|
| DOL | Department of Labor | HRO | High reliability organization |
| DRAM | Dynamic Random Access Memory | HRSA | Health Resources and Services |
| DRG | Diagnosis related group | | Administration |
| DTC | Direct-to-consumer advertising | HSA | Health Savings Account |
| EHR | Electronic health record | IBM | International Business Machines |
| EI | Emotional intelligence | ICU | Intensive Care Unit |
| EMR | Electronic medical record | IDN | Integrated Delivery Network |
| EMTALA | Emergency Medical Treatment and Labor Act | IDS | Integrated Delivery System |
| EPHTI | Ethiopa Public Health Training Initiative | IHS | Indian Health Service |
| ERISA | Employee Retirement Income Security Act | IOM | Institute of Medicine |
| FCA | False Claims Act | IOR | Interorganizational Relationship |
| FDA | Food and Drug Administration | IPA | Independent Practitioner Association |
| FSA | Flexible Spending Accounts | IPP | Implementation policies and practices |
| FTC | Federal Trade Commission | IRB | Institutional Review Board |
| GAO | Government Accountability Office (formerly General Accounting Office) | IRS | Internal Revenue Service |
| | | IS | Information Systems |
| GATS | General Agreement on Trade in Services | ISM | Integrated Salary Model |
| GAVI | Global Alliance for Vaccines and Immunization | IT | Information Technology |
| | | JAMA | Journal of the American Medical Association |
| GDP | Gross domestic product | JCI | Joint Commission International |
| GE | General Electric | JLI | Joint Learning Initiative |
| GHWA | Global Health Workforce Alliance | LMX theory | Leader member exchange theory |
| GPO | Group Purchasing Organization | M&A | Merger and Acquisition |
| HCA | Hospital Corporation of America | M&M Rounds | Morbidity and Mortality |
| HCO | Health care organization | MBO | Management by objectives |
| HCQIA | Health Care Quality Improvement Act | MCO | Managed-care organization |
| HDHP | High-deductible health plan | MDGs | Millenium Development Goals |
| HELP | Health, Education, Labor, and Pensions Committee (U.S. Senate) | MedPAC | Medicare Payment Advisory Commission |
| | | MELD | Model for end-stage liver disease |
| HELP | Health Evaluation through Logical Processing | MHA | Master's in Health Administration |
| HEWs | Health extension workers | MRI | Magnetic resonance imaging |
| HHS | Department of Health and Human Services | MSA | Medical savings account |
| HIE | Health Information Exchange | MSO | Management Services Organization |
| HIMSS | Health Information and Management Systems Society | NCHL | National Center for Healthcare Leadership |
| | | NCI | National Cancer Institute |
| HIPAA | Health Insurance Portability and Accountability Act | NCQA | National Committee for Quality Assurance |
| | | NCSL | National Conference of State Legislatures |
| HIT | Health information technology | NEJM | New England Journal of Medicine |
| HIV | Human Immunodeficiency Virus | NHCL | National Center for Healthcare Leadership |
| HLA | Health Leadership Alliance | NHE | National Health Expenditures |
| HMO | Health Maintenance Organization | NHS | National Health Service |
| HPR | Hospital-physician relationships | NIH | National Institutes of Health |
| HPWP | High-performance work practices | NIHS | Not-invented-here Syndrome |
| HR | Human resources | NPCs | Non-physician clinicians |
| HRA | Health Reimbursement Accounts | NPDB | National Practitioner Data Bank |

| | | | |
|---|---|---|---|
| NQF | National Quality Forum | SSA | Sub-Saharan Africa |
| NRH | Norman Regional Hospital | SSI | Supplemental Security Income |
| OHRP | Office for Human Research Protections | SWOT | Strengths, Weaknesses, Opportunities, Threats |
| OIG | Office of the Inspector General | | |
| P4P | Pay-for-Performance | TQM | Total quality management |
| PA | Physician's Assistant | TVA | Tennessee Valley Authority |
| PBRN | Provider base research network | UBIT | Unrelated business income tax |
| PCS | Patient Classification System | UNCTAD | United Nations Conference on Trade and Development |
| PDA | Personal Digital Assistant | | |
| PHI | Protected health information | UNOS | Network of Organ Sharing |
| PHO | Physician Hospital Organization | USD | United States dollars |
| PHQID | Premier Hospital Quality Incentive Demonstration | VA | Veterans Administration (Department of Veterans Affairs) |
| PHR | Personal health record | VBP | Value-based purchasing |
| PPO | Preferred Provider Organization | VHA | Veterans Health Administration |
| PPP | Public-private partnership | VIP Model | Virtual integrated practice model |
| PPS | Prospective Payment System | VISN | Veterans Integrated Service Network |
| ProPAC | Prospective Payment Assessment Commission | VP | Vice president |
| | | WHO | World Health Organization |
| PSQIA | Patient Safety and Privacy Act | | |
| PVC | Preventative Services Chart | | |
| QI | Quality improvement | | |
| QIO | Quality Improvement Organization | | |
| QM | Quality management | | |
| QUERI | Quality Enhancement Research Initiative | | |
| R&D | Research and development | | |
| RAC | Recovery audit contractor | | |
| RBRVS | Resource Based Relative Value System | | |
| RD Teams | Research and development teams | | |
| RFID | Radio Frequency Identification | | |
| RFP | Request for Proposal | | |
| RHIOs | Regional Health Information Organizations | | |
| ROI | return on investment | | |
| SADC | Southern African Development Cooperation | | |
| SAMHSA | Substance Abuse and Mental Health Services Administration | | |
| SBU | Strategic Business Unit | | |
| SDLC | Systems Development Life Cycle | | |
| SEPT | South Essex Partnership University NHS Foundation Trust | | |
| SMART | Specific, Measurable, Achievable, Realistic and Time Bound | | |
| SNA | Social network analysis | | |
| SNS | Social network sites | | |
| SOP | Standard operating procedure | | |

# Glossary

**Accountability in Teams:** The entities to which teams are formally accountable, which may be internal to the team as well as external to the team and organization.

**Accreditation:** An entity receives accreditation when it meets the quality standards defined by the accrediting organization.

**Adaptive Learning:** A form of learning in which problem solvers adjust their behavior and work processes in response to changing events or trends. Adaptive learning is similar to single-loop learning.

**Administrative Leadership:** The instrumental and interpersonal support provided by those who hold senior positions in the organization such as chief executive officer, chief operating officer, and vice president for performance improvement.

**Alliance Objectives:** The goals pursued by the parties in a strategic alliance and thus serve as the stated purpose of the alliance.

**Alliance Problems versus Symptoms:** This distinction highlights that there is often disagreement as to why alliances fail, and that this disagreement is often rooted in mistaking a root cause for a mere symptom.

**Alliance Process:** The flow of activities in the life cycle of a strategic alliance.

**Alliance Risk:** The risk that a strategic alliance will fail. This risk must be balanced against the expected rewards.

**Alliances:** Informal, voluntary agreements among individuals or groups of similar or complementary interests for purposes of achieving objectives.

**Ambassador Activities:** Activities carried out by team members involving communication with those above them in the organizational hierarchy, often carried out to protect the team from outside pressures, to persuade others to support the team, and to lobby for resources.

**Ambidexterity:** An important attribute of high-performing organizations, which is based on the ability to conduct two seemingly opposed sets of activities.

**Anchoring Bias:** A psychological effect whereby an initial offer in negotiation tends to influence subsequent thinking.

**Anti-Kickback Statute (AKS):** Prohibits the knowing and willful solicitation or receipt of renumeration by any person in connection with items or services for which payment could be made by Medicare or Medicaid.

**Antiretroviral Therapy (ART):** A set of medications for the treatment of infection by retroviruses, primarily HIV.

**Antitrust Law:** The body of law intended to promote competition.

**Autonomy:** Relates to the freedom to follow or act according to one's own will.

**Balancing Feedback Loops:** Feedback loops that counteract or oppose whatever is happening in a system.

**Barriers to Communication:** The psychological factors that distort the substance of a message, such as credibility, relationships, beliefs, interests, and communication styles.

**Barriers to Entry:** The existence of obstacles that prevent competitors from attempting to enter an industry or market.

**BATNA:** This stands for "Best Alternative to a Negotiated Agreement" and represents the best option left with if the current negotiations fail and an agreement cannot be reached.

**Behavioral Norms:** Rules that standardize how people act at work on a day-to-day basis, while performance norms are rules that standardize employee output.

**Behavioral Theories:** Leadership theories that examine how those in leadership roles act toward those they are influencing.

**Belmont Report:** A result of work by the National Commission for the Protection of Human Subjects of Biomedical and Behavioral Research in the 1970s with revisions by the Department of Health and Human Services (HHS) in the late 1970s and early 1980s for the protection of human subjects.

**Benchmarking:** A key feature of many QI approaches, benchmarking is the process of comparing an organization's performance metrics (e.g., quality, cost, operational efficiency) to those of other "best practice" or peer organizations.

**Bending the Cost Curve:** This refers to reducing health spending relative to projected trends in spending.

**Beneficence:** The obligation to do good, prevent or remove harm, and to act in a kind or benevolent manner.

**Bioethics:** The discipline concerned with ethical questions and actions in medicine and biology.

**Boundary-Spanning Roles:** Individuals who help enhance communication and coordination with other organizations or teams.

**Bounded Rationality:** This refers to the limits on the correctness of managerial decisions due to limits on managers' cognition of all variables and forces in the environment.

**Brain Drain:** An imbalance in the distribution of health workers, due to increasing demand for health workers and the ability of high-income countries to offer more attractive remuneration packages.

**Bureaucracy:** Literally, this means government by bureaus or offices. More generally, it refers to an organization structured on bureaucratic principles with clear roles, lines of authority and accountability, procedures, and rules.

**Business Models:** The core elements of a firm and how it is organized to deliver value to its customers and generates revenues.

**Buyer Power:** The ability of buyers and/or customers to exert pressure on lower price and higher quality.

**Centers for Medicare and Medicaid Services (CMS):** One of the largest programs in HHS which manages the Medicare and Medicaid programs.

**Centralization:** The concentration of responsibilities and authority vertically at higher levels or horizontally within one or only a few people or organizational units.

**Certificate of Need:** A form of approval that is sometimes legally required for the creation of a health care organization, purchase of equipment, or provision of a service. State agencies grant this approval based on their determination of community need.

**Classical School of Administration:** The management school that emphasized general principles and the best way to structure organizations.

**Clayton Act:** Prohibits mergers, acquisitions, and joint ventures that threaten to substantially lessen competition or are likely to create a monopoly.

**Clinical Leadership:** Instrumental and interpersonal support provided by those who hold clinical positions, such as physicians and nurses

**Clinical Practice Guidelines:** Typically developed by expert panels, clinical practice guidelines synthesize evidence from the literature and make recommendations regarding treatment for specific clinical conditions. The National Guideline Clearinghouse (http://www.guideline.gov) is a publicly available resource for evidence-based guidelines covering a full range of clinical conditions.

**Coalition:** A limited-term alliance among individuals or groups that is formed in order to increase power and further the respective interests.

**Coercion:** The use of subtle influence dynamics to achieve desired goals.

**Cognitively Active:** Constantly and intentionally focusing on all parties instead of only focusing on oneself.

**Collaborating:** A negotiation strategy where parties try to help each other get what they want and in the process maximize the value created in the negotiation.

**Combinatorial complexity:** Also known as "detail" complexity, this arises from the number of constituent elements of a system or the number of interrelationships that might exist among them.

**Communication:** The exchange of information among individuals. Especially important, in the context of achieving coordination in an organization, are the frequency, timeliness, accuracy, and focus on problem solving in information exchange.

**Communication Networks and Structure:** The manner and patterns through which communication is disseminated in an organization; these include both formal and informal modes of communication.

**Communication Technology:** The variety of methods used for communication within an organization or team.

**Community Benefit Standard:** To maintain tax-exempt status as charitable organizations under section 501(c)(3) of the federal Internal Revenue Code, nonprofit health care providers must meet a community benefit standard. Examples of relevant factors under this standard include the presence of a community board, the operation of an emergency room open to all, and the provision of charity care.

**Comparative Advantage:** The discovery and deployment of significant differences in a nation's cost, quality, or access such that a medical or surgical procedure, health activity, or service creates patient value.

**Comparative Clinical Effectiveness:** A type of research that involves a systematic comparison of the impact of drugs, devices, procedures, or services on patient health outcomes.

**Competencies:** The knowledge, skills, and abilities needed to be an effective leader of an organization.

**Competing:** A negotiation strategy where one party tries to get as much value for themselves as possible, with little, if any, concern for the other party.

**Competitive Advantage:** The long-term market position and uniqueness that is not easily duplicable by rivals that enables a firm to outperform its rivals. It could also be called "key success factors."

**Complex Adaptive System:** A system that is comprised of people and activities that mutually influence each other in complex ways with often unpredictable outcomes. Elements of the system co-evolve as people and activities move forward together and interact over time.

**Compliance:** An organization's compliance program consists of the steps it takes to ensure that it follows applicable statutes, regulations, and rules.

**Compromising:** A negotiation strategy where the parties in the negotiation divide value and find a solution that partially satisfies everyone.

**Confidential:** An expectation of a certain privacy and nondisclosure regarding information relayed to another person.

**Confidentiality:** The nature of a confidence or confiding of secrets or private information from one to another.

**Confirming Evidence Bias:** The tendency for people to seek out and pay attention only to information that confirms prior beliefs.

**Conflict Management:** The study of how parties approach, deal with, and resolve conflict and those personal, social, and environmental factors that affect that process.

**Consumer Driven Health Care:** A strategy that encourages and enables people to take charge of their personal health through: (1) knowledge of their current status and needs; (2) informed decision making; (3) wise use of health care dollars; and (4) confident and active participant in their own health care decisions and treatment choices.

**Consumer Driven Health Plan (CDHP):** A health plan designed to allow the employee greater choice in their health care, thus enabling them to be wise consumers.

**Consumer:** A person who uses up a commodity. Also known as a purchaser of goods or services, or a customer.

**Consumerism:** A social and economic order that is based on the systematic creation and fostering of a desire to purchase goods or services in ever greater amounts.

**Contingency Theory:** This theory posits that the selection of the most appropriate form of organization is dependent upon the particular circumstances of the environment in which the organization operates. Contingency theory does not advocate an either/or approach but rather views the process as a continuum from mechanistic/bureaucratic to organic forms.

**Continuous Quality Improvement (CQI):** A participative, systematic approach to planning and implementing a continuous organizational improvement process.

**Control:** Control indicates influence, and an influence can come from many sources, of which ownership is only one.

**Convenient Care Association (CCA):** An organization of health care systems and companies that offer accessible, cost-effective, quality health services located in retail-based environments.

**Convenient Care Clinic (CCC):** Walk-in services for a limited scope of medical conditions, usually staffed by advanced practice health professionals such as nurse practitioners (NPs) or physician assistants (PAs).

**Convenient Care Clinic Association:** An organization of health care systems and companies that offer accessible, cost-effective, quality health services located in retail-based environments.

**Coordination:** Achievement of synchronized action among individuals and work units so that their work is mutually reinforcing and contributing to organizational goals.

**Corporate Integrity Agreement:** An agreement imposed by the HHS Office of the Inspector General on a health care provider in the aftermath of a health care fraud investigation. It is intended to promote adherence to health care laws and regulations by imposing specific compliance obligations on a health care provider.

**Cost Reduction versus Revenue Enhancement:** This distinction highlights that the strategic intent behind alliances may differ on fundamental dimensions, such as cost versus value, and that such differences imply different bases for evaluating the success of an alliance.

**Culturally Derived Power:** Power that derives from the informal aspects of organization, such as norms, values, beliefs, and assumptions.

**Curse of Knowledge:** The problem of imagining another person's state of mind when you have a piece of knowledge that they lack.

**Decentralization:** The delegation of responsibilities and authority vertically to lower levels or horizontally among many people or organizational units. (*See also* centralization.)

**Decisional Authority:** The continuum of roles that teams may play in decision making from no decision authority to being able to make all decisions.

**Decision-Making School:** The management school that emphasized how decisions are made and how goals are set within the firm, with a view towards controlling managerial behavior.

**Deeming Authority:** Authority granted to an accreditation organization such that a provider meeting accreditation requirements is deemed to also meet certain Medicare requirements.

**Delphi Technique:** An approach to decision making in which a panel of experts is asked for their views on an issue followed up by controlled feedback and repeated until consensus is reached. This technique encourages member participation.

**Department of Health and Human Services (HHS):** The principle federal government agency for health care under which the Public Health Service and 11 other public health agencies are governed.

**Department of Justice (DOJ):** The DOJ, along with the Federal Trade Commission (FTC) is responsible for federal enforcement of the antitrust laws. These federal agencies coordinate their efforts in investigating and prosecuting antitrust cases.

**Detail Complexity:** Another name for combinatorial complexity.

**Diagnosis-Related Groups (DRGs):** The patient classification system adopted by Congress and developed by a team of researchers at Yale University in the late 1970s.

**Differentiation:** The segmentation of an organization into units together with the structuring of those units and development of organizational practices and systems and employees' cognitive and emotional orientations that are suited to each unit's unique tasks and sub-environment.

**Direct Contact:** A structural alternative for coordination in which individuals in different functional departments coordinate efforts through direct interaction with each other. Direct contact is a weak structural alternative to coordination.

**Discovery:** A form of learning in which innovators learn about possible action alternatives, outcome preferences, and contextual factors. Discovery is similar to double-loop or generative learning in that it opens up and investigates possibilities.

**Distortion:** Factors that affect how a listener understands a message. These factors include the content of the message, the medium of the message (face-to-face, written, or electronic communication), and the listeners themselves.

**Diversity in Teams:** Multiple dimensions upon which team members vary, including age, professional background, and tenure in the organization.

**Double-Loop Learning:** A form of learning in which problem solvers attempt to close the gap between desired and actual states of affairs by questioning and modifying those organization's policies, plans, values, and rules that frame organizational problems and guide organizational action. Double-loop learning is similar to generative learning.

**Dynamic complexity:** A form of complexity that arises from the operation of feedback loops.

**Economies of Scale:** When the average cost per unit decreases from increased volumes.

**Electronic Health Record (EHR):** An electronic record of health-related information on an individual that conforms to nationally recognized interoperability standards and that can be created, managed, and consulted by authorized clinicians and staff across more than one health care organization.

**Electronic Medical Record (EMR):** An electronic record of health-related information on an individual that can be created, gathered, managed, and consulted by authorized clinicians and staff in one health care organization.

**Emergence:** New ideas, products, practices, and relationships that arise spontaneously and are neither predicted nor anticipated by participants or observers.

**Emotional Contagion:** When emotions are transmitted from one party to another.

**Empowerment:** A strategy in which employees are given information, knowledge and power to make decisions when the traditional hierarchical management structure and the command-and-control management techniques are no longer viable. Teams, when used as an extension of the general employee empowerment strategy, occur along four dimensions: potency, meaningfulness, autonomy, and consequences.

**EMTALA (Emergency Medical Treatment and Labor Act):** Established in 1986, the EMTALA is designed to prevent institutions from denying care to anyone seeking emergency medical treatment, regardless of citizenship, insurance status, or ability to pay.

**Environmental Context:** The mix of external factors that significantly affect or may affect the team or organization.

**Equity:** Fairness in the relationships among individuals and groups. In equity theory, employees compare their perceived inputs and outcomes with their perceptions of others' inputs and outcomes.

**Equity versus Non-Equity Alliances:** This distinction highlights that alliances may differ in terms of whether the alliance partners invest equity capital in the alliance's formation and thus have ownership stakes tied to such investments.

**ERISA (Employee Retirement Income Security Act):** A statute which imposes minimum requirements on retirement and health benefit plans.

**Ethos, Pathos, Logos:** Aristotle's terms for "character," "emotion," and "logic," the three modes of communicating one's message.

**Evidence-Based Medicine:** The systematic identification and application of available scientific information for clinical decision making by health care professionals. Scientific information includes findings related to process and outcome-based measures of quality, as well as findings related to cost and cost-effectiveness.

**Expectancy:** The perceived link between effort and performance (e.g., the relationship between how hard an employee tries and how well he or she does in terms of job performance).

**External Environment:** The conditions, entities, and factors surrounding an organization that influences its activities and choices.

**FCA (False Claims Act):** A law that prohibits knowingly submitting or causing to be submitted a false claim to the government, such as a Medicare claim for a service different from the one that was actually provided.

**Feedback:** Feedback approaches to coordination entail the exchange of information among staff usually while work is being carried out. Feedback approaches permit staff to change or modify work activities in response to unexpected requirements. Feedback also refers to the part of the communication process through which the sender and receiver engage in a two-way process of communication. It reverses the sender and receiver roles so that information can be shared, recycled, and fine-tuned to achieve unambiguous and mutual understanding in the communication process.

**Feedback Approaches to Coordination:** One of two major categories of approaches to coordination at the micro or process level. Feedback approaches, which include supervision, mutual adjustment and group coordination, rely upon personal interaction among the people involved. Feedback approaches are sometimes also called "personal approaches."

**Fidelity:** The obligation to honor commitments.

**First Mover Advantage:** The advantage an organization attains by being the first competitor to pursue a particular source of competitive advantage.

**Flexible Spending Account (FSA):** A blanket term for financial accounts where pretax monies are held to be used for reimbursement for noncovered medical expenses.

**Followership:** Those who share a common purpose with the leader, believes in what the organization is trying to accomplish, and wants both the leader and the organization to succeed.

**Formal Groups:** An organizationally based social system that is formally recognized, has defined boundaries, and maintains differentiated yet interdependent member roles.

**Formal Leadership:** Leadership based on formal authority conferred by the organization to an individual.

**Fractioning:** A negotiation tactic that involves separating out the various components of a specific issue.

**Free Rider:** A team member who obtains the benefits of group membership but does not accept a proportional share of the costs of membership (synonymous with Social Loafing).

**Frontline Managers:** Those who provide supervision directly to care providers.

**Functional Fixedness:** When a negotiator bases his or her strategy on familiar, rather than the most effective, methods.

**Functional Organization Structure:** The organizational form that is based on segmentation, at the highest level of an organization structure, of responsibilities and authority for achievement of an organization's primary task, into units that represent different functions. In industrial firms, these functions are typically research, engineering, manufacturing, marketing, and sales. In health care organizations, the functions are typically professions and disciplines directly involved in delivery of services to patients, such as medical specialties and subspecialties, nursing, social work, therapies, and transportation.

**General Agreement on Trade in Services (GATS):** A 1995 treaty of the World Trade Organization (WTO) created to extend the multilateral trading system to the service sector, in the same way that the General Agreement on Tariffs and Trade (GATT) provides such a system for merchandise trade.

**Generative Learning:** a form of learning in which problem solvers attempt to eliminate problems by changing the underlying structure of the system. This underlying structure includes the "operating policies" of the decision makers and actors in the system (e.g., their values and assumptions). Generative learning is similar to double-loop learning.

**Generic Strategies:** The label Michael Porter gave to two prominent position strategies—low cost and high differentiation. He argued that most firms naturally gravitate to one or the other, and thus he called these "generic" positions.

**Gini Index:** A measurement tool used to estimate income disparities between rich and poor countries on a scale of 0 to 1.

**Global Health Workforce Alliance (GHWA):** An international partnership established in 2006 to identify and implement solutions to the global health workforce crisis.

**Globalization:** A process by which regional economies, societies, and cultures have become integrated through a global network of communication, transportation, and trade.

**Goals:** The larger aspirations of the organization.

**Goal Setting:** A motivational technique based on the concept that the practice of setting specific goals enhances performance, and that setting difficult goals results in higher performance than setting easier goals.

**Governance:** The activities and decisions that focus on the determination of mission, strategy and goals of an organization, as well as its broad policies. In addition, it is the governance structure that holds the organization's leadership accountable for their actions and performance. Typically, the board of trustees performs the governance functions in a health care organization, and a collective body representing the medical staff performs its governance activities, such as determining its policies and regulations.

**Group Coordination:** The exchange of information among more than two people, such as through meetings, rounds, and conferences, for the purpose of coordinating their interdependent activities. It is one of three types of feedback approaches to coordination.

**Groupthink:** A team decision-making phenomenon in which a desire for consensus overrides the full exploration of alternative courses of action.

**HCQIA (Health Care Quality Improvement Act):** At the time of its enactment in 1986, HCQIA reflected two primary concerns, one relating to weaknesses in existing peer review processes, and the other to the ease with which incompetent physicians were able to move between states without a record of their malpractice experience or professional disciplinary action.

HCQIA is designed to address these issues by encouraging physicians to identify and discipline fellow physicians who are incompetent or who engage in unprofessional behavior, so as to improve the quality of care.

**Health Information Exchange (HIE):** Refers to the technology, standards, and governance that enables the exchange of data between the information systems of various health care stakeholders.

**Health Information Technology:** A general term used to describe a broad range of technologies for transmitting and managing health information for use by consumers, providers, payers, insurers, and others interested in health care.

**Health Insurance Portability and Accountability Act (HIPAA):** Federal legislation that specifies regulations for the privacy of personal health information, portability of health insurance, and the organization of the interchange of electronic data for certain financial and administrative operations.

**Health Reimbursement Account (HRA):** A financial arrangement that is used for reimbursement of substantiated medical expenses.

**Health Savings Account (HSA):** A tax-exempt financial account used to reimburse medical expenses not covered under existing health plans.

**Health Systems:** Arrangements among hospitals, physicians, and other provider organizations that involve direct ownership of assets on the part of the parent system.

**Hierarchy of Authority:** The arrangement of responsibilities and authority for actions and decisions such that successively higher levels in the organization have authority over units below them. The hierarchy of authority is used specifically in this book as a macro-level approach to coordination.

**Hierarchy of Needs:** Five psychological need levels that must be satisfied sequentially in order to motivate an employee. In terms of rank from lower to higher, these include psychological needs, security needs, belongingness needs, esteem needs, and self-actualization needs.

**High Deductible Health Plan (HDHP):** A type of consumer-driven health plan that offers a broad provider network, limited involvement with medical management, higher deductibles, and lower premiums.

**High-Performance Work Practices (HPWPs):** Workforce or human resource practices that have been shown to improve an organization's capacity to effectively attract, select, hire, develop, and retain high-performing employees.

**HITECH Act:** The Health Information Technology for Economic and Clinical Health (HITECH) Act is a section of the American Recovery and Reinvestment Act of 2009 that establishes a formal plan for advancing the use of health information technology to improve care and enable the electronic exchange and use of health information systems.

**Hospital-Physician Relationships:** The array of economic, noneconomic, and clinical integration mechanisms designed to link hospitals more closely with their medical staffs and community-based physicians.

**Human Relations School:** The management school that focuses on the individual and the group, and the importance of their participation in organizational decision making.

**Human Subjects:** In the context of research, human subjects are living individual(s) who provides data or other material with which researchers conduct studies.

**Hybrid Organization:** An organization that maintains its traditional functional structure and creates program structures for just one or two programs.

**Hygiene Factors:** Factors related to the work environment (such as extrinsic factors) whose presence prevents dissatisfaction but does not lead to satisfaction or motivation.

**Implementation:** The processes involved and occurring between the decision to adopt the QI innovation and the routine use of the QI innovation, or the integration of a new idea or practice into the operating system of the organization.

**Inert Knowledge Problem:** The inability for negotiators to draw on information they have to solve novel situations.

**Infant Mortality Rates:** An often-used health statistic measured in the number of infant deaths per 1,000 live births; shown to be highly associated with the degree of local health care infrastructure.

**Informal Groups:** Groups that are not formally established or sanctioned by the organization, but are formed naturally by individuals in the organization to fill a personal or social interest need.

**Informal Leadership:** Leadership that is not formally established or sanctioned by the organization, but develops as a result of other sources of power and authority.

**Innovation:** An idea, practice, or object that is perceived as new by an individual or other unit adopting it. Innovation also refers to the act (or process) of introducing something new into an environment or setting.

**Institutional Review Boards:** Administrative entities established by institutions to protect the ethical rights of human subjects who participate in research conducted under their supervision.

**Institutional Theory:** The management school that emphasizes that organizations face environments characterized by external norms, rules, and requirements to which they must conform in order to receive support and legitimacy.

**Integrated Delivery System:** An organization consisting of subunits that provide different types of care across the continuum. Integrated delivery systems typically include hospitals, long-term care facilities, rehabilitation facilities, ambulatory care facilities, and home health agencies, and structurally they vertically integrate these different suborganizations. They may provide services in one or several geographic regions.

**Integration:** Coordination of activities among organizational units, including the management of conflict among the units, to achieve synchronized actions and decisions.

**Integrators:** Individuals whose primary responsibility is coordination. Care managers are a prime example of integrators in health care. (*See also* Lateral Relations.)

**Interconnectedness of Work:** The property of work itself that inherently requires differ parts or elements to fit together to be performed well. For example, the decisions and actions performed in the care of an individual patient are interconnected elements of work.

**Interdependence:** The nature and degree to which the performance of work (taking actions and making decisions) by an individual or organization unit is dependent upon or is (potentially) affected by the performance of work by other individuals or organization units.

**Intergroup Relationships and Conflict:** Patterns and types of interactions and interdependence among groups in an organization, including conflicts among groups.

**Internal Environment:** The conditions and elements within an organization, including employees, management, and culture, that affect the firm's choices and activities.

**Iron Triangle:** Refers to the difficulty of seeking to improve quality of care, improve access to care, and reduce the cost of care simultaneously.

**Job Redesign:** Altering certain aspects of the job to better satisfy an employee's psychological needs. Examples include task identity, skill variety, task significance, knowledge of results, and feedback.

**Joint Commission International (JCI):** A private sector, U.S.-based, not-for-profit organization focused on improving the safety of patient care through the provision of accreditation and certification services.

**Joint Venture:** A legal entity formed between two or more parties to undertake an economic activity together.

**Justice:** The quality of being (morally) just or righteous, including just conduct, integrity, and conformity to a moral right or reason.

**Knowledge-Based Sources of Power:** Power that derives from a group's control over the expertise needed to make key decisions and organize production.

**Kohl and Dekker Cases:** Two cases by the European Court of Justice in 1998, which established that health care resources should be treated as any other part of the European Union economy with regard to the free movement of goods and services.

**Lateral Relations:** A set of mechanisms to achieve coordination across specialized departments. Lateral relations are invoked in organizations when information processing requirements exceed the capacity of vertical coordinating mechanisms (use of the organization's hierarchy).

**Leadership:** The process in which one engages others to set and achieve a common goal, often an organizationally defined goal.

**Lean:** A management and operations improvement approach, often described as a "transformation" that focuses on eliminating waste across "value streams" that flow horizontally across technologies, assets, and departments (as opposed to improving within each). The intent of a Lean approach is cost-effectiveness, error reduction, and improved service to customers. The term "Lean" was originally coined by Jim Womack, to describe innovations in Toyota's manufacturing processes (http://www.lean.org).

**Learning:** The acquisition of knowledge or skills through study, instruction, or experience. Learning is essentially a feedback process.

**Learning Organization:** An organization skilled at creating, acquiring, and transferring knowledge, and at modifying its behavior to reflect new knowledge and insights.

**Liaison Roles:** A boundary-spanning role within a unit or department whose responsibilities are to serve as a point of contact and coordinator with other units or departments.

**Licensure:** State agency-granted authority to practice a profession or operate a facility.

**Logrolling:** A negotiation tactic that involves trading off on issues of different value to each party.

**Macro Perspective:** The unit of analysis in organizational theory and research that focuses on the organization as a social system in the context of other organizations.

**Managed Migration:** The linkage of international migration to the health policy goals of individual states; the regulation of the flows of health workers in a way that benefits both source and destination countries.

**Management:** The process of accomplishing predetermined objectives through the effective use of human, financial, and technical resources.

**Management Teams:** Teams that coordinate and provide direction to the subunits under their jurisdiction; such subunits may exist at multiple organizational levels.

**Market Niche Strategy:** A strategy in which a competitive seeks advantage by focusing on a single or small number of product lines or population segments.

**Market Structure:** The organizational features of a market (e.g., seller concentration, entry barriers, degree of product differentiation) that condition or influence the conduct and strategies of competitors.

**Matrix Organization:** The organization form in which responsibilities and authority are allocated between two equally powerful hierarchies, one representing functions and the other representing programs, overlaid on each other. The "matrixed" individuals have two supervisors—a functional supervisor, and a program supervisor.

**Medical Innovation:** A new development that improves patient care (e.g., new medications), helps doctors care for patients (e.g., electronic medical records), or lowers the cost of delivery.

**Medical Savings Account:** A type of tax-exempt financial account created to offset non-covered medical expenses for self-employed individuals or employees of small businesses (fewer than 50 workers).

**Medical Tourism:** The practice of travelling across international borders to obtain health care.

**Medicare Payment Advisory Commission (MedPAC):** An independent congressional agency, MedPAC has played a significant role in shaping a variety of Medicare reform initiatives. MedPAC advises Congress on a broad range of issues and is also tasked with analyzing access to care, quality of care, and other issues affecting Medicare.

**Membership Fluidity and Boundary Permeability:** The extent to which, and the frequency with which, team membership changes; this is related in part to boundary permeability, or the extent to which a team's core membership is maintained over time and the ease with which new members can enter and current members exit the team.

**Mental Models:** The discipline of constantly surfacing, testing, and improving our assumptions about how the world works.

**Message:** Communication that is delivered using one or more of the three persuasive means of conveying a message—ethos (character), pathos (emotion), and logos (logic).

**Micro Perspective:** The unit of analysis in organizational theory and research that focuses on the individual, group, and departments within the organization.

**Middle Managers:** Those who have responsibility for entire units within a health care organization.

**Migrant Remittances:** The transfer of funds from migrants to relatives or friends in their country of origin. Migrant remittances have become an increasingly important feature of modern economic life.

**Millennium Development Goals (MDGs):** Eight time-bound goals, agreed upon by world leaders in 2000, that provide a framework for the entire international community to work together towards a common end of global development.

**Mission:** The foundation for strategic direction. A mission provides the reason for the company's existence and forms the basis for strategy. It should guide the firm to focus its energies and frame its choices of strategy and commitments of resources.

**Model for End Stage Liver Disease (MELD):** A scoring system for assessing the severity of chronic liver disease that later was adopted for determining prognosis and prioritizing for receipt of a liver transplant.

**Monopolistic Competition:** A market structure that is characterized by a large number of small firms that have similar, but not identical products. There is relative free entry and exit and knowledge of prices and technology is common. Competition is relatively vigorous, but each firm, depending on the degree of their differentiation, has some control over their prices.

**Monopoly:** A market when there is only one provider of a supply or service.

**Motivation:** A state of feeling or thinking in which one is engaged or aroused to perform a task or engage in a particular behavior.

**Motivators:** Factors related to the work content (i.e., intrinsic factors) whose presence increases job satisfaction and motivation but whose absence does not lead to job dissatisfaction. Motivators include achievements, recognition, work, responsibility, and advancement.

**Mutual Adjustment:** The direct communication between two individuals who are not in a hierarchical relationship for the purpose of coordinating their interdependent activities. It is one of three types of feedback approaches to coordination.

**National Practitioner Data Bank:** A federal repository of data on medical malpractice payments made on behalf of and adverse actions taken against health care practitioners (such as license terminations or hospital privileges revocations). A federal statute specifies what information state licensing boards, hospitals, insurers, and others are required to report and how often they are expected to report.

**Network Centrality:** A situation within an organization where one work group or unit lays at the intersection of other work groups or units, as a result becoming a repository of knowledge about how the entire organization works.

**Network of Organ Sharing (UNOS):** A nonprofit, scientific, and educational organization whose mission is to advance organ availability and transplantation.

**Nominal Group Technique:** A model of team decision making in which members pool their individual judgments in a guided systematic manner. This technique encourages member participation.

**Nonmaleficence:** The obligation to do no harm upheld by physicians by virtue of their Hippocratic Oath.

**Nonspecific Compensation:** A negotiation tactic that involves adding issues that are not tied to money or compensation.

**Non-Physician Clinician (NPC):** Health care professionals trained with less cost than physicians for an average period of 3–4 years post secondary school.

**Notice of Proposed Rulemaking:** A precursor to the creation of a new federal regulation. Agencies' notices of proposed rulemaking describe the rules they intend to enact and then solicit public comments; the agencies may subsequently revise initially proposed rules in light of comments received.

**Not-Invented-Here Syndrome (NIHS):** The well-known skepticism about the appropriateness or relevance of something not invented in one's homeland.

**Objectives:** Subordinate goals that must be achieved to accomplish the overall organizational goal.

**Office for Human Research Protections:** A branch of the U.S. Department of Health and Human Services that provides leadership regarding protection of human subjects involved in research activities.

**Office of the Inspector General:** With the cooperation of the Department of Justice, the Office of the Inspector General dedicates considerable resources to enforcing federal fraud and abuse laws.

**Oligopoly:** A market in which there are a small number of firms, and the competitors believe that their rivals have sufficient market power to influence their long-term survival. They therefore consciously adapt their strategies in response to their assessments of rival competitive advantages and expected strategic maneuvers.

**Open Systems Theory:** The management school that emphasizes that organizations are part of the external environment and, as such, must continually change and adapt to meet the challenges posed by the environment. The need for openness, adaptability, and innovation are consistent with the open system view.

**Organization Design:** The arrangement of authority, responsibilities, and flow of information by segmentation into organizational subunits, designation of scopes of authority and responsibility vertically and horizontally, and creation of structures to facilitate coordination among those subunits. A broader view of organization design also includes development of policies and design of control, reward, evaluation, and information systems.

**Organization Structure:** The graphical representation of segmentation of authority and responsibility into organization units and their interrelationships, resulting from organization design. Also called "table of organization."

**Organizational Culture:** The deepest level of beliefs, values, and norms that are shared by members of the organization. These beliefs, values, and norms represent the unique character of the organization and provide the context for action and behavior.

**Organizational Learning:** An organization-wide process that involves the systematic integration and collective interpretation of new knowledge.

**Organizational Politics:** The ongoing interplay of interests and power among people and groups in an organization. Different coalitions of interest or influence vie for the opportunity to achieve their desired goals.

**Outcome Measures of Quality:** Metrics based on the results of work performed. Examples include health status, patient satisfaction, and mortality.

**Ownership and Control:** Ownership stakes in an alliance do not necessarily result in greater control of an alliance. Control indicates influence, and an influence can come from many sources, of which ownership is only one.

**Parallel Organization:** An organization structure that operates "parallel" to the primary structure. Parallel organizations are often used for large-scale change programs. Parallel structures also refer to

integrating mechanisms that are used for managing programs that cross a functional structure.

**Parallel Teams:** Teams typically composed of people from different work units or jobs who carry out functions not regularly performed in the organization.

**Partner Orientation:** A summary characterization of the degree to which an alliance partner is interested in working cooperatively with his or her partner.

**Patient Classification System:** A policy instrument that allows for output comparisons to be made across hospitals and provides a basis on which hospitals can be paid in a standardized, consistent fashion for the products they produce.

**Patient-Centered Communication:** A model of communication designed to maximize the effectiveness of communication between health care providers and patients.

**Pay-for-Performance (P4P):** Reimbursement for health care services that is designed to link payment incentives to quality and performance outcomes. Demonstration programs to test various approaches have been under way through the Centers for Medicare and Medicaid Services.

**Perfect Competition:** The most fragmented of markets, which is characterized by many buyers and sellers, and many products that are similar and undifferentiated. Markets in perfect competition have few barriers to entry, and prices are generally the means of competition.

**Performance Norms:** Formal or informal rules that standardize employee output in a team.

**Performance Outcomes:** A management tool used to clarify goals and document progress toward achieving those goals.

**Personal health record (PHR):** An electronic record of health-related information on an individual that conforms to nationally recognized interoperability standards and that can be drawn from multiple sources while being managed, shared, and controlled by the individual.

**Personal Mastery:** The discipline of individual learning, without which organizational learning cannot occur. Personal mastery involves continuously clarifying our individual sense of purpose and vision, and continuously learning how to see the world as it is without distortion.

**Planning and Goal Setting:** Global-level approaches to coordination that are used in addition to hierarchy of authority when an organization faces relatively low levels of uncertainty.

**Policy Resistance:** The tendency for interventions to be delayed, diluted, or defeated by the response of the system to the intervention itself.

**Pooled Interdependence:** A type of interdependence among team members in which each member makes a contribution to group output without the need for interaction among members. (*See also*

Reciprocal Interdependence, Sequential Interdependence, Simulutaneous Interdependence.)

**Pooling Alliances:** Pooling alliances reflect two or more organizations contributing similar resources for mutual gain.

**Population Ecology:** The management school that emphasizes the environment's "selecting out" of certain organizations for survival. Organizational success is more dependent upon environmental selection than managerial decision making and implementation.

**Porter's Five Forces Framework:** A framework developed by Michael Porter of Harvard University to analyze the five main forces that affect competition in a market.

**Portfolio Analysis:** A method that compares the value of the strategic business units (SBUs) of firms. Components of companies are categorized by their competitive market position and the environmental attractiveness.

**Power:** The ability to exert influence or control over others.

**Power Abuse:** Situations where one or more organizational stakeholders use power in ways that are generally not acceptable, often involve self-interest, and can inflict negative outcomes on the organization.

**Power Stratification:** When different stakeholders have unique opportunities to access power based upon their particular characteristics or circumstances.

**Preemption:** The displacement of one law by another, rendering the displaced law ineffective. When federal and state statutes conflict, the federal statute preempts the state statute.

**Privacy:** The right or choice to be alone, undisturbed, or free from public attention or intrusion.

**Process Measures of Quality:** Refer to indicators of the activities involved in carrying out work in an organization. Activities such as reviewing medical records to ensure completion of patient education, monitoring physician and nurse compliance with organizational standards for cleanliness, or evaluating the use of central lines are examples of process metrics.

**Product Life Cycle:** A phase or life cycle that relates to its level of costs and sales, which have strategic implications. Life cycles occur because of the inherent limited life of any products, as a result of technological advances and adapting consumer preferences.

**Program Organization Structure:** The organization structure resulting from segmentation of authority and responsibilities corresponding to different programs. Individuals from different professions and disciplines providing services for a given program (e.g., providing mental health care) are aggregated into an organizational unit and have a reporting relationship to the head of that program. (For contrast, *see* Functional Organization Structure.)

**Programmable Work:** Work, or components of work, that is relatively certain, predictable or well understood. Programmable work can largely be coordinated by programming or standardized approaches to coordination.

**Programming Approaches to Coordination:** One of two major categories of approaches to coordination at the micro or process level. Programming approaches, which include standardization of work, skills, and output, function best when work is relatively certain. Programming approaches are sometimes also called "standardized approaches." (*See also* Feedback Approaches to Coordination.)

**Project Management:** A collection of techniques for planning, organizing, and managing resources to bring about the successful completion of a one-time endeavor (project) that includes multiple tasks, including the management of project scope, time, cost, and human resources.

**Project Teams:** Teams that are typically time limited, producing one-time outputs such as a new product, service, or support function (e.g., a new information system) in the organization.

**Prospective Payment:** A financial incentive created as a result of DRGs that financial encourages more cost-efficient management of medical care.

**Psychological Safety:** An individual's perceptions about the consequences of taking interpersonal risks in the work environment. It is a largely taken-for-granted belief about how others will respond when one puts oneself on the line, such as by asking a question, seeking feedback, reporting a mistake, or proposing a new idea.

**Quality Improvement (QI):** An organized approach to planning and implementing continuous improvement in performance. QI emphasizes continuous examination and improvement of work processes by teams of organizational members trained in basic statistical techniques and problem-solving tools, and empowered to make decisions based on their analysis of the data.

**Quality Improvement (QI) Interventions:** Interventions designed to decrease medical errors and enhance patient safety.

**Quality Measures:** Structural, process, and outcome measures, including both organizational and clinical metrics.

**Receiver:** The person for whom a message is intended in the communication process.

**Reciprocal Interdependence:** A type of interdependence among team members in which the outputs of each member become inputs for the others. (*See also* Pooled Interdependence, Sequential Interdependence, and Simultaneous Interdependence).

**Reciprocity:** The tendency for others to exchange equal levels of goods and services.

**Recovery Audit Contractor:** Entity under contract with Medicare to review claims for the purpose of identifying payment errors and fraud.

**Regional Health Information Organization (RHIO):** An organization that provides an health information exchange to health care stakeholders in a specific region, such as a city or multicounty area.

**Regulation:** Governmental oversight of the private marketplace.

**Reinforcing Feedback Loops:** Feedback loops that amplify or intensify whatever is happening in a system.

**Relational Coordination:** A relational process involving a network of communication and relationship ties among people whose tasks are interdependent to achieve coordination.

**Relationship Conflict:** Conflict regarding some inherent characteristic of the other party.

**Relationships:** One of the two interacting components of relational coordination, relationships can be seen as consisting of shared goals, shared knowledge, and mutual respect.

**Research:** A systematic investigation, including research development, testing and evaluation, designed to develop or contribute to generalizable knowledge.

**Resource Dependence Theory:** The management school that emphasizes the importance of the organization's abilities to secure needed resources from its environment in order to survive.

**Retail Medicine:** Health care services that are provided in "retail settings" or nonhospital, nontraditional medical environments.

**Retrospective Reimbursement:** A payment method in which rates are set on the basis of costs already incurred.

**Reverse Innovation:** An innovation either seen first or used first, in small or less developed markets before spreading to the larger, more developed markets.

**Rivalry:** Competition levels that influence the strategies of firms and determine the overall profitability of the industry. Many factors affect the rivalry in a market. The number and type of firms are significant factors. In an industry where new rivals can enter relatively easily, increasing the number of firms, or firms can grow in size via merger and acquisition, the industry tends to be more competitive, and firms are less likely to enjoy high average profitability. Rivalry is likely to occur in markets where competitors differ substantially from one to another.

**Rules and Procedures:** Approaches to coordination specifying how work is to be done and providing guidance to behavior. Rules and procedures augment use of an organization's hierarchy in coordinating work that is programmable.

**Safety Zones:** In antitrust guidelines, safety zones are outlines of the factual elements of business arrangements viewed as acceptable by the Department of Justice and the Federal Trade Commission. Such arrangements will generally not be prosecuted for antitrust violations, barring extraordinary circumstances.

**Scientific Management School:** The management school that emphasizes the application of scientific methods (e.g., time-motion studies) to maximize worker productivity and conformance to the one best way of production.

**Scout Activities:** Activities carried out by team members involving general scanning for ideas and information about the external environment.

**Self-Actualization:** Realizing one's potential for continued growth and individual development. The top level of the hierarchy of needs.

**Self-Care:** The process of managing oneself.

**Self-Fulfilling Prophecy:** The process by which one party's beliefs cause another party to behave in such a way which supports that belief.

**Sender:** The person who is delivering a message in the communication process.

**Senior Management:** A team member who holds a leadership role in a health care organization, such as the CEO. According to the IOM, all individuals in leadership roles must develop, implement, and sustain systems that improve the safety, timeliness, efficiency, cost-effectiveness, equity, and patient-centeredness of care delivered in their organizations.

**Sequential Interdependence:** A type of interdependence in which one group member must act or produce an output before another one can begin or complete a task. (*See also* Pooled Interdependence, Reciprocal Interdependence, Simulutaneous Interdependence.)

**Service Line:** An organizational arrangement designed to coordinate the work of people from multiple professions and disciplines for a specific service in a health care organization. A service line is a health care variant of the general program organization. There are several variations of service line structures, characterized by the degree to which they facilitate integration. Service lines in health care can focus on diseases, patient populations, or technologies.

**Shared Vision:** The discipline of generating a common answer to the question, "What do we want to create?"

**Sherman Act:** Section 1 of this antitrust law prohibits contracts and other agreements that unreasonably restrain trade. This provision applies to situations where individuals or organizations that are in a competitive situation with one another also collaborate to achieve common business objectives. Section 2 prohibits activities that are undertaken to obtain or achieve a monopoly. This section is aimed at the conduct of a single entity that undertakes anticompetitive activities to strengthen its competitive position.

**Single-Loop Learning:** A relatively simple error-and-correction process whereby problem solvers look for solutions within an organization's policies, plans, values, and rules. Single-loop learning is similar to adaptive learning.

**Six Aims:** The goals for improvement in a high-performing health care system; care should be safe, effective, patient-centered, timely, efficient, and equitable.

**Six Sigma:** A data-driven methodology for eliminating defects in any process by applying a consistent framework of DMAIC (define, measure, analyze, improve, control) to minimize variation and improve processes. Six Sigma was started at Motorola and has been widely adopted at other companies, including GE. (http://www.isixsigma.com)

**Skill-Based Pay:** A type of reward system in which employees are rewarded for acquiring new value-added skills, knowledge, or competencies.

**SMART:** An acronym that means specific, measurable, achievable, realistic, and time bound. It is commonly used to describe the types of objectives that are most effective in strategic problem solving.

**Social Capital:** In health and human service systems, the web of co-operative relationships between providers that involve interpersonal trust, norms of reciprocity, and mutual aid.

**Social Loafing:** In teams, behaviors associated with obtaining the benefits of group membership without accepting a proportional share of the costs of membership (synonymous with Free Rider).

**Social Media:** Web 2.0 interactive communication technology.

**Social Network Approach:** The management school that emphasizes the role of social relationships among individuals and groups in explaining organizational behavior.

**Social Networks:** The connections among a group of people and the broader environment in which they live and work.

**Speaker-Listener Model:** A model of communication in which the speaker sends a message directly to the listener.

**Specialization:** The process of focusing on a narrow field of work to develop a depth of expertise. In organization design, developing different work units so that each unit can perform work that differs from that in other units in terms of its character, content and information requirements (e.g., medical specialties). Specialization is one component of differentiation.

**Stages of Team Development:** A relatively predictable series of developmental stages experienced by teams. A team's stage of development may be related to team functioning and effectiveness.

**Stakeholder:** A person or group of people who are affected by an idea or message.

**Stakeholder Analysis:** The mapping of stakeholders according to power and interests.

**Standardization of Output:** The specification of goals or of characteristics of a product or service for the purpose of coordinating the interdependent activities of two or more people or organizational units. It is one of three types of programming approaches to coordination.

**Standardization of Skills:** The specification of specific training or skills required for people in different jobs, for the purpose of coordinating the interdependent activities of people in those jobs or the organizational units in which those jobs reside. Often this is achieved through specification of minimum levels and types of education, certification as evidence of meeting minimum qualifications, or on-the-job training. It is one of three types of programming approaches to coordination.

**Standardization of Work:** The use of rules, regulations, schedules, plans, procedures, policies, and protocols to specify activities to be performed. It is one of three types of programming approaches to coordination.

**Stark Physician Self-Referral Law (Stark):** A federal fraud and abuse law that prohibits physicians from referring patients to certain health services providers with which the physicians have a financial relationship.

**Status Differences:** A characteristic of a team defined by the extent of variation in the status of each team member.

**Strategic Alliance:** Any formal agreement between two or more organizations for purposes of ongoing cooperation and mutual gain.

**Strategic Group:** A concept to identify organizations within an industry that have similar business models or strategic orientations so that they directly compete with each other.

**Strategic Management:** The creation, implementation, and overall direction for a firm. As such, it requires both internal and external management functions to facilitate the development, implementation, and monitoring of strategy within an organization.

**Strategic Management Approach:** A set of management schools that emphasize how firms achieve competitive advantage in the context of competitive forces and market structure.

**Strategic Management Perspective:** The strategic management perspective emphasizes the importance of positioning the organization relative to its environment and competitors in order to achieve its objectives and assure its survival.

**Strategic Problem Solving:** An eight-step approach to integrating the strategic function of leadership involving goal and objective setting, with the subsequent organizational action required to achieve the set objectives.

**Strategy:** The development of a broad formula prescribing a way in which a business competes and collaborates, sets goals, and establishes policies to carry out those goals in order to achieve the organizational mission.

**Structural Measures of Quality:** Measures based on aspects of an organization or an individual's actions that could impact overall quality or organizational performance. Examples include indicators such as the number and type of beds in a given organization, the presence of shared governance structures, and the existence of a computerized provider order entry (CPOE) system with decision support features.

**Structurally Derived Power:** Power that is derived from the formal or bureaucratic aspects of an organization.

**Supervision:** The exchange of information among two or more people, one of whom is responsible for the work of the others. It reflects the use of an organization's hierarchy for the purpose of coordinating interdependent activities of people or organizational units. It is one of three types of feedback approaches to coordination.

**Supplier Power:** The ability of suppliers to influence price and quality.

**Support Teams:** Teams that enable others in the organization to do their work, serving such functions as quality improvement, strategic planning, and search committees.

**Switching Cost:** The cost incurred when a customer changes from one supplier or product to another.

**SWOT Analysis:** A simple analytical framework that includes assessments of strategically important factors both internal (strengths and weaknesses) and external (opportunities and threats) to organizations.

**Symbiotic versus Competitive Interdependence:** This distinction highlights that alliances often have mixed motives, whereby parties can create joint value, but often will compete in the claiming of that value.

**System Perspectives:** A set of new perspectives on individual and organizational behavior, emphasizing the wider social and societal systems that condition this behavior.

**Systems Development Life Cycle (SDLC):** A general methodology for selecting, acquiring, implementing, and maintaining an information system. The SDLC has various stages including definition (planning), construction (analysis, design and testing), implementation, and maintenance.

**Systems Thinking:** The discipline of seeing wholes, perceiving the structures that underlie dynamically complex systems, and identifying high-leverage change opportunities.

**Task Conflict:** Conflict regarding differences amongst the parties in understanding and carrying out tasks.

**Task Coordinator Activities:** Activities carried out by team members involving communication and coordination with other groups and persons at lateral levels in the organization. These activities include discussing problems with others, obtaining feedback, and coordinating and negotiating with outsiders.

**Task Force:** A temporary, interdisciplinary group formed to coordinate work of different departments, usually for a specific objective, such as planning a new service. Task forces are one of several types of lateral relations, or structural mechanisms to achieve coordination across specialized departments. (*See also* Integrators, Team.)

**Task Interdependence:** The level and manner in which information or resources are exchanged in carrying out team tasks; this often refers to the degree in which sub-tasks in a team are related to each other in carrying out the work of a team.

**Task Uncertainty:** A characteristic of work reflecting lack of knowledge of cause-and-effect relationships and/or predictability of events affecting task performance. Task uncertainty is a central factor in design of organizational units (*see also* differentiation) and in interdependence, which directly affects the need for coordination.

**Tax Exemption:** Freedom from an obligation to pay taxes, such as income or property taxes. Nonprofit health care providers seeking to maintain tax exempt status are subject to a number of legal obligations not shared by for-profit entities.

**Team:** In the context of coordination, an enduring interdisciplinary group of people working together to achieve one or more common goals. Teams are one of several types of *lateral relations*, or structural mechanisms to facilitate coordination across specialized departments. (*See also* Integrators, Task Force.)

**Team-Based Rewards:** Financial or nonfinancial rewards given to team members for the accomplishment of team goals. This sometimes refers to rewarding team members for their contributions to the work of the team.

**Team Cohesiveness:** The extent to which members are committed to each other, often related to trust, emotional support, and ability to mutually adjust to changes in the behavior of others.

**Team Composition:** Membership on a team, which may be defined in aggregate numbers or according to another characteristic, such as professional status or gender.

**Team Goals:** The formal purposes of a team, which may vary by goal clarity, complexity of goals, and diversity of goals. This should be distinguished from informal team goals, which may or may not be related to the formal purposes of a team.

**Team Interdependence:** A situation in which team members diagnose, solve problems, and collaborate as a group while performing work or work-related activities. Team interdependence requires a workflow that is simultaneous and multidirectional.

**Team Leadership:** Team members who are formally assigned leadership roles, or who informally assume such roles.

**Team Learning:** Activities carried out by team members through which a team obtains and processes data that allows it to adapt and improve.

**Team Norms:** Standards that are shared by team members and regulates member behavior.

**Team Performance:** Formal measures of the effectiveness of a team in achieving its goals.

**Team Processes:** Methods of interacting and performing work by team members alone and in interaction with each other.

**Team Size:** A measure of team membership, often related to a variety of measures of team performance, member satisfaction, and other team processes.

**Temporal Nature of Teams:** A measure of the permanence of a team over time.

**Tenure Diversity:** The length of time during which members have been on a team.

**Testing:** A form of learning in which innovators learn about action-outcome relationships. In particular, they learn through successive experimentation which actions reliably produce desired outcomes. Testing is similar to single-loop or adaptive learning.

**Threat of Substitution:** Threats from firms that produce products and services that differ from, but perform the same function as those of extant competitors in the market. The threats depend on the market structure, environmental changes, and the relative competitive advantages of rivals and of those firms that produce substitute products and services.

**Threat Rigidity Effect:** When individuals feel threatened, their thinking becomes rigid or inflexible.

**Top Managers:** Those who are responsible for managing the entire organization and hence have responsibility for all of the units within the organization.

**Trading Alliances:** Trading alliances are based on the notion of combining dissimilar—but complementary—resources for mutual gain.

**Trait Theories:** Theories of leadership that examine personality traits associated with leadership success.

**Transactional Leadership:** A leadership theory composed of these four behavioral elements: (1) making rewards contingent on performance, (2) correcting problems actively when performance goes wrong, (3) refraining from interruptions of performance if it meets standards (i.e., passive management of exceptions), and (4) a laissez-faire approach to organizational change.

**Transformational Leadership:** An influential model of leadership style in contemporary theories that includes four key behaviors: (1) influence through a vision, (2) motivating through inspiration, (3) stimulating the intellect of subordinates, and (4) individualized consideration.

**Transparency:** Proponents of transparency in the health care setting advocate wide dissemination of information about health care providers and their services, including information about service quality and prices.

**Triple Aim:** The attempt to improve the experience of care, improve the health of populations, and reducing per capita costs of health care.

**Turbulent Environment:** This refers to the situation whereby an organization is facing rapidly changing external circumstances and greater interconnectedness and interdependence between itself and other organizations.

**Uncertainty Reduction:** An important benefit of strategic alliances, when compared with alternative approaches to growth, given the exit options typically found in alliance agreements.

**Unobtrusive Controls:** Controls over managerial decisions, behaviors, and the flows of information needed to make them.

**Value:** In economics, value is the quotient of quality divided by cost, the combined benefits among all the parties in the negotiated agreement.

**Value Chain:** This refers to the interlinked activities among a set of organizations whereby suppliers provide raw material inputs to manufacturers who process them and produce outputs for downstream markets.

**Values:** The expression of the ethics that guide employees' actions. They should constrain how the mission and vision is accomplished.

**Vertical Information Systems:** Approaches to coordination based on increasing the information-processing capacity of the hierarchy by facilitating information flow up and down the hierarchy and by increasing the capabilities of various managers to handle more information.

**Vision:** A statement about what the organization wants to become. It focuses on the future.

**Winner's Curse:** The feeling of unhappiness after a reached settlement where one side feels that they should have asked for more.

**Work Teams:** Groups of people responsible for producing goods or providing services.

# Author Index

# Subject Index